AF327969

Monographs on Pathology of Laboratory Animals

Sponsored by the
International Life Sciences Institute

The following volumes have appeared so far

Endocrine System
1983. 346 figures. XV, 366 pages. ISBN 3-540-11677-X

Respiratory System
1985. 279 figures. XV, 240 pages. ISBN 3-540-13521-9

Digestive System
1985. 352 figures. XVIII, 386 pages. ISBN 3-540-15815-4

Urinary System
1986. 362 figures. XVIII, 405 pages. ISBN 3-540-16591-6

Genital System
1987. 340 figures. XVII, 304 pages. ISBN 3-540-17604-7

Nervous System
1988. 242 figures. XVI, 233 pages. ISBN 3-540-19416-9

Integument and Mammary Glands
1989. 468 figures. XI, 347 pages. ISBN 3-540-51025-7

The following volumes are in preparation

Musculoskeletal System
Cardiovascular System
Special Sense

T. C. Jones J. M. Ward U. Mohr
R. D. Hunt (Eds.)

Hemopoietic System

With 351 Figures and 47 Tables

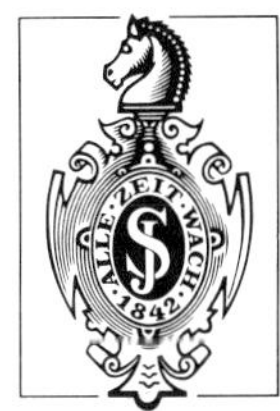

Springer-Verlag Berlin Heidelberg New York
London Paris Tokyo Hong Kong Barcelona

Thomas Carlyle Jones, D. V. M., D. Sc.
Professor of Comparative Pathology, Emeritus
Harvard Medical School
New England Regional Primate Research Center
One Pine Hill Drive, Southborough, MA 01772, USA

Jerrold Michael Ward, D. V. M., Ph. D.
Chief, Tumor Pathology and Pathogenesis Section
Laboratory of Comparative Carcinogenesis
Division of Cancer Etiology
National Cancer Institute, National Institutes of Health
Frederick, MD 21701, USA

Ulrich Mohr, M. D.
Professor of Experimental Pathology
Medizinische Hochschule Hannover
Institut für Experimentelle Pathologie
Konstanty-Gutschow-Strasse 8
3000 Hannover 61, Federal Republic of Germany

Ronald Duncan Hunt, D. V. M.
Professor of Comparative Pathology
Harvard Medical School
New England Regional Primate Research Center
One Pine Hill Drive, Southborough, MA 01772, USA

ISBN 3-540-52212-3 Springer-Verlag Berlin Heidelberg New York
ISBN 0-387-52212-3 Springer-Verlag New York Berlin Heidelberg

Library of Congress Cataloging-in-Publication Data
Hemopoietic system/T. C. Jones . . . [et al.], eds.
p. cm. – (Monographs on pathology of laboratory animals)
ISBN 0-387-52212-3 (U.S.)
1. Hematopoietic system – Pathophysiology. 2. Hematopoietic system – Diseases.
3. Laboratory animals – Diseases. I. Jones, Thomas Carlyle. II. Series.
RB145.H42974   1990   616.4'1-dc20   90-9584

Typesetting, Printing, and Binding: Appl, Wemding
2123/3140-543210 – Printed on acid-free paper

Foreword

The International Life Sciences Institute (ILSI) was established in 1978 to stimulate and support scientific research and educational programs related to nutrition, toxicology, and food safety, and to encourage cooperation in these programs among scientists in universities, industry, and government agencies to assist in the resolution of health and safety issues.

To supplement and enhance these efforts, ILSI has made a major commitment to supporting programs to harmonize toxicologic testing, to advance a more uniform interpretation of bioassay results worldwide, to promote a common understanding of lesion classifications, and to encourage wide discussion of these topics among scientists. The *Monographs on the Pathology of Laboratory Animals* are designed to facilitate communication among those involved in the safety testing of foods, drugs, and chemicals. The complete set will cover all organ systems and is intended for use by pathologists, toxicologists, and others concerned with evaluating toxicity and carcinogenicity studies. The international nature of the project – as reflected in the composition of the editorial board and the diversity of the authors and editors – strengthens our expectations that understanding and cooperation will be improved worldwide through the series.

Alex Malaspina
President
International Life Sciences Institute

Preface

This book, on the hemopoietic system, is the eighth volume of a set prepared under the sponsorship of the International Life Sciences Institute (ILSI). One aim of this set on the pathology of laboratory animals is to provide information which will be useful to pathologists, especially those involved in studies on the safety of foods, drugs, chemicals, and other substances in the environment. It is expected that this and future volumes will contribute to better communication, on an international basis, among people in government, industry, and academia who are involved in protection of the public health.

The arrangement of this volume is based, in part, upon the philosophy that the first step toward understanding a pathologic lesion is its precise and unambiguous identification. Therefore, the microscopic and ultrastructural features of a lesion that are particularly useful to the pathologist for definitive diagnosis are considered foremost. Diagnostic terms preferred by the author and editors are used as the subject heading for each pathologic lesion. Synonyms are listed although most are not preferred and some may have been used erroneously in prior publications. The problems arising in differential diagnosis of similar lesions are considered in detail. The biologic significance of each pathologic lesion is considered under such headings as etiology, natural history, pathogenesis, and frequency of occurrence under natural or experimental conditions.

Comparison of information available on similar lesions in man and other species is valuable as a means to gain broader understanding of the processes involved. Knowledge of this nature is needed to form a scientific basis for safety evaluations and experimental pathology. References to pertinent literature are provided in close juxtaposition to the text in order to support conclusions in the text and lead toward additional information. Illustrations are an especially important means of nonverbal communication, especially among pathologists, and therefore constitute important features of each volume.

The subject under each heading is covered in concise terms and is expected to stand alone but, in some instances, it is important to refer to other parts of the volume. A comprehensive index is provided to enhance the use of each volume as a reference.

Some omissions are inevitable and we solicit comments from our colleagues to identify parts which need strengthening or correcting. We have endeavored to include important lesions which a pathologist might encounter in studies involving the rat, mouse, or hamster. Newly recognized lesions or better understanding of old ones may make revised editions necessary in the future.

The editors wish to express their deep gratitude to all of the individuals who have helped with this enterprise. We are indebted to each author and member of the Editorial Board whose name appears elsewhere in the volume. We are especially grateful to the Officers and Board of Trustees of the International Life Sciences Institute for their support and understanding. Several people have worked directly on important details in this venture. These include Mrs. Nina Murray,

Executive Secretary; Mrs. Ann Balliett, Editorial Assistant; Mrs. June Armstrong, Medical Illustrator; Mrs. Sydney Fingold, Librarian; Mrs. Lori MacInnes, Secretary. Ms. Sharon K. Coleman, ILSI Coordinator for External Affairs, Mrs. Karen A. Taylor, ILSI Manager of Publications, and Ms. Sharon Senzik, Associate Director, ILSI Research Foundation, were helpful on many occasions.

We are particularly grateful to Dr. Dietrich Götze and his staff at Springer-Verlag for the quality of the published product.

The death of Mr. Roger D. Middlekauff, Secretary-Treasurer of ILSI, occurred unexpectedly at his home in Washington, D.C. while this volume was in production. Mr. Middlekauff took an active part in developing the plans for these volumes and worked to support their completion.

March 1990

THE EDITORS

T.C. Jones
J.M. Ward
U. Mohr
R. D. Hunt

Contents

Contributors

Victor O. Anosa, D. V. M., M. V. M., Ph. D., M. R. C. Path.
Professor and Head
Department of Veterinary Pathology, University of Ibadan
Ibadan, Nigeria

Yves Bailly, V. M.
Senior Toxicologist, Laboratoires Merck Sharp & Dohme-Chibret
Riom, Cedex, France

Henry J. Baker, D. V. M.
Professor, Department of Comparative Medicine
Bowman Gray School of Medicine, Wake Forest University
Winston-Salem, North Carolina, USA

Nabila Barsoum, M. D., FRCP (C)
Director of Pathology, Parke Davis Research Institute
Ontario, Canada

Dr. Rudolf B. Beems
Head of Pathology, TNO-CIVO Toxicology and Nutrition Institute
Zeist, The Netherlands

John Bienenstock, M. D.
Professor, Medicine and Pathology, McMaster University
Ontario, Canada

Donald V. Cramer, D. V. M., Ph. D.
Associate Professor of Pathology
University of Pittsburgh School of Medicine
Pittsburgh, Pennsylvania, USA

David N. Crichton, B. Sc.
Senior Research Officer
MRC Clinical and Population Cytogenetics Unit
Western General Hospital, Edinburgh, United Kingdom

Orsolya Csuka, Ph. D.
Research Institute of Oncopathology
National Oncological Institute
Budapest, Hungary

L. H. J. C. Danse, MSc., Ph. D.
Head, Department of Toxicological Pathology
National Institute of Public Health and Environmental Protection
Bilthoven, The Netherlands

Deborah E. Devor, B. S.
Biologist, Supervisor-Technical Operations, TPPS
National Cancer Institute
Frederick Cancer Research Facility, Maryland, USA

Christine D. Dijkstra, M. D., Ph. D.
Associate Professor
Department of Cell Biology, Vrije Universiteit
Amsterdam, The Netherlands

Pierre Duprat, D. V. M., Ph. D.
Director of Pathology, Laboratoires Merck Sharp & Dohme-Chibret
Riom, Cedex, France

Kara Eberly, Ph. D.
Assistant Professor
Department of Biology, St. Mary's College
Notre Dame, Indiana, USA

Peter B. Ernst, D. V. M., Ph. D.
Assistant Professor of Pathology, McMaster University
Hamilton, Ontario, Canada

Torgny N. Fredrickson, D. V. M., Ph. D.
Professor, Department of Pathobiology
University of Connecticut
Storrs, Connecticut, USA

Arnold S. Freedman, M. D.
Assistant Professor of Medicine
Harvard Medical School, Dana-Farber Cancer Institute
Boston, Massachusetts, USA

Charles H. Frith, D. V. M., Ph. D.
Consultant in Pathology and Toxicology
Toxicology Pathology Associates
Little Rock, Arkansas, USA

Ferenc Gal
Senior Scientist, Research Institute of Oncopathology
National Oncological Institute
Budapest, Hungary

M. Gonda, Ph. D.
Laboratory of Cell and Molecular Structure Prog. Resources Inc.
Frederick Cancer Research Facility-National Cancer Institute
Frederick, Maryland, USA

Angela C. Hanglow, Ph. D.
Senior Scientist, Department of Pharmacology and Chemotherapy
Hoffmann-La Roche
Nutley, New Jersey, USA

Johannes H. Harlemann, D. V. S., Ph. D.
Head of Experimental Pathology, ASTA Pharma AG
Bielefeld, FRG

Victor M. H. Hollanders, Ph. D.
Research Scientist, TNO-CIVO Toxicology and Nutrition Institute
Zeist, The Netherlands

Kiyoshi Imai, D. V. M., Ph. D.
Head of Pathology Laboratory
Hatano Research Center-Food and Drug Safety Center
Kanagawa, Japan

Tohru Inoue, M. D., D. M. Sc.
Associate Professor
School of Medicine, Yokohama City University
Yokohama, Japan

Wolfgang Jahn, Dr. med. vet.
Head of Institute of Toxicology, ASTA Pharma AG
Bielefeld, FRG

S. H. M. Jeurissen, Ph. D.
Faculteit der Geneeskunde, Vrije Universiteit
Amsterdam, The Netherlands

E. W. A. Kamperdijk, Ph. D.
Faculteit der Geneeskunde, Vrije Universiteit
Amsterdam, The Netherlands

Jiro J. Kaneko, D. V. M., Ph. D., D. V. Sc. (h. c.)
Professor of Clinical Pathology
School of Veterinary Medicine, University of California
Davis, California, USA

David G. Keyes, B. S., M. T. (ASCP)
Project Leader, Mammalian & Environmental Toxicology Research
Laboratory, The Dow Chemical Company
Midland, Michigan, USA

Gary J. Kociba, D. V. M., Ph. D.
Professor, Department of Veterinary Pathobiology
Ohio State University
Columbus, Ohio, USA

Richard J. Kociba, D. V. M., Ph. D.
Research Scientist in Pathology, The Dow Chemical Company
Midland, Michigan, USA

Robert M. Kovatch, D. V. M.
Veterinary Pathologist, Pathology Associates Inc.
Frederick, Maryland, USA

Magda A. M. Krajnc-Franken, Ph. D.
Senior Pathologist
National Institute of Public Health & Environmental Protection
BA Bilthoven, The Netherlands

Gerhard R. F. Krueger, M. D.
Professor of Pathology and Immunopathology
Institute of Pathology/University of Cologne
Cologne, FRG

C. Frieke Kuper, Ph. D.
Staff Member, TNO-CIVO Toxicology and Nutrition Institute
Zeist, The Netherlands

Patricia S. Latham, M. D.
Assistant Professor of Medicine and Pathology
University of Maryland School of Medicine
Baltimore, Maryland, USA
and Laboratory of Molecular Immunoregulation
National Cancer Institute
Frederick, Maryland, USA

Norman L. Letvin, M. D.
Associate Professor of Medicine, Harvard Medical School
New England Regional Primate Research Center
Southborough, Massachusetts, USA

Robert M. Lewis, D. V. M.
Professor of Pathology
New York State College of Veterinary Medicine
Cornell University
Ithaca, New York, USA

Larry G. Lomax, D. V. M., Ph. D.
Research Leader, Pathologist
Mammalian and Environmental Toxicology Research Laboratory
The Dow Chemical Company
Midland, Michigan, USA

Mutsushi Matsuyama, M. D.
Professor, Second Department of Pathology
Nagoya University School of Medicine
Nagoya, Japan

Toshiaki Ogiu, M. D.
Section Head, Division of Physiology and Pathology
National Institute of Radiological Sciences
Anagawa, Chiba, Japan

Paul K. Pattengale, M. D.
Head, Hematopathology Section
Children's Hospital of Los Angeles
Los Angeles, California, USA

Catherine A. Picut, V. M. D.
Senior Scientist, Veritas Laboratories, Inc.
Burlington, North Carolina, USA

Morris Pollard, D. V. M., Ph. D.
Coleman Professor of Biological Sciences
University of Notre Dame
Notre Dame, Indiana, USA

James A. Popp, D. V. M., Ph. D.
Chemical Industry Institute of Toxicology
Research Triangle Park, North Carolina, USA

David J. Prieur, D. V. M., Ph. D.
Professor, Department of Veterinary Microbiology and Pathology
Washington State University
Pullman, Washington, USA

Barbara Reed, R. T.
Hematology Manager, Environmental Contaminants Section
Environmental and Occupational Toxicology Division
Health and Welfare Canada
Ottawa, Ontario, Canada

Sabine Rehm, Dr. med. vet.
Visiting Scientist, National Cancer Institute
Frederick, Maryland, USA

Craig W. Reynolds, Ph. D.
Program Director and Corporate Liaison
Biological Resources Branch/National Cancer Institute
Frederick Cancer Research Facility
Frederick, Maryland, USA

Bernard Sass, D. V. M.
Senior Scientist
Registry of Experimental Cancers/National Institutes of Health
Bethesda, Maryland, USA

Thomas J. Sayers, Ph. D.
Section Head, Biological Carcinogenesis Development Program
National Cancer Institute/Frederick Cancer Research Facility
Frederick, Maryland, USA

Masatoshi Seki, M. D.
Scientific Advisor, Koenji-Kita, Suginami-ku
Tokyo, Japan

Taede Sminia, M. D.
Professor, Chairman
Department Cell Biology/Histology, Vrije Universiteit
Amsterdam, The Netherlands

Graham Smith, B. V. M. S., M. R. C. V. S., M. Sc.
Section Director of Clinical Laboratories
Parke Davis Research Institute
Mississauga, Ontario, Canada

Robert A. Squire, D. V. M., Ph. D.
Professor, Division of Comparative Medicine
The Johns Hopkins University School of Medicine
Baltimore, Maryland, USA

Paul C. Stromberg, D. V. M., Ph. D.
Associate Professor
Department of Veterinary Pathobiology, Ohio State University
Columbus, Ohio, USA

Janos Sugar, M. D., D. MSc.
Director, Research Institute of Oncopathology
National Oncological Institute
Rath Gyorgy utca 7–9, Budapest 1122, Hungary

Victor E. Valli, D. V. M., M. Sc., Ph. D.
Professor of Pathology
Ontario Veterinary College
Guelph, Ontario, Canada

Gerda van der Brugge-Gamelkoorn, Ph. D.
Faculteit der Geneeskunde, Vrije Universiteit
Amsterdam, The Netherlands

Marja B. van der Ende
Technician, Vahgroep Celbiologie, Vrije Universiteit
Amsterdam, The Netherlands

Luigi Varesio, Ph. D.
Section Chief, Laboratory of Molecular Immunoregulation
National Cancer Institute
Frederick, Maryland, USA

A. J. P. Veerman, M. D., Ph. D.
Professor, Faculteit der Geneeskunde, Vrije Universiteit
Amsterdam, The Netherlands

David C. Villeneuve, Ph. D.
Head, Environmental Contaminants Section
Environmental and Occupational Toxicology Division
Health and Welfare Canada
Ottawa, Ontario, Canada

J. G. Vos, D. V. M., Ph. D.
Director of Immunology
National Institute of Public Health & Environmental Protection
BA Bilthoven, The Netherlands

Jerrold M. Ward, D. V. M., Ph. D.
Chief, Tumor Pathology and Pathogenesis Section
Lab. of Comparative Carcinogenesis/National Cancer Institute
Frederick, Maryland, USA

Bone Marrow
and Peripheral Blood

Regulation of Hemopoiesis

Donald V. Cramer

Introduction

The bone marrow is responsible for the generation of cells of the blood and many of the principal components of the immune system. Early in embryonic life a small population of multipotent stem cells, capable of extensive self-renewal, are formed. Some of these stem cells undergo differentiation to produce progenitor cells for each of the different erythroid, myeloid, and lymphoid lineages. Continued division and maturation of individual progenitors result in mature cells for each of several lines, including granulocytes (neutrophils), eosinophils, mast cells, macrophages, erythrocytes, megakaryocytes, and lymphocytes.

The control of this complex process of renewal and differentiation is largely mediated by specific glycoprotein growth factors. Recent advances in the ability to culture bone marrow progenitor cells in vitro and discovery of the molecular characteristics of the growth factors has greatly increased our understanding of how these factors regulate hemopoiesis. It is becoming increasingly clear that hemopoietic growth factors mediate overlapping interactions with each other, including the proliferation and differentiation of individual cell lineages and important cell-to-cell communications between subsets of lymphocytes of the immune system. The interaction of the myeloid system, including granulocytes, erythrocytes, megakaryocytes, and the lymphoid system is teleologically consistent with the importance of these systems for host defense. The focus of this review will be on the current models of the structure of the hemopoietic system, the control of the development of individual cell lineages by hemopoietic growth factors and the areas of interaction between the myeloid and lymphoid systems.

Structure of the Hemopoietic System

The generally accepted models of the structure of the hemopoietic system consist of the existence of a pluripotent stem cell that gives rise to all of the cells produced in the bone marrow (Fig. 1). This cell divides to produce other pluripotent stem cells and a series of more differentiated progenitor cells for each individual cell line. The functional existence of pluripotent stem cells in vivo has been inferred from experiments that demonstrate that irradiated mice can regenerate a complete hemopoietic system following transplantation of bone marrow (Dexter and Moore 1986). The assay for these pluripotent stem cells has been the measurement of colony formation (colony-forming units-spleen or CFU-s) in the spleens of irradiated mice following the injection of bone marrow. The injection of bone marrow is followed by the localization of the stem cells in the spleen, differentiation into progenitor cells, and growth of colonies that produce macroscopically visible foci containing myeloid, erythroid, and additional pluripotent CFU-s cells (Schrader 1983). CFU-s are known to be a heterogeneous group of cells with differing potentials for self-renewal (Magli et al. 1982; Metcalf 1984). Although the CFU-s assay is generally thought to represent pluripotent cell activity, it is possible that more primitive stem cells exist that are not detected with this assay.

Recent advances in in vitro culture have led to the long-term culture of bone marrow, including pluripotent stem cells, myeloid cells, and lymphocytes (Dexter et al. 1977). The more differentiated progenitors can also be cultured in vitro, and these techniques have provided the opportunity to study the development of progenitor colony-forming cells (CFC) for several cell lineages. Under the appropriate conditions, the existence of cells committed to the formation of a specific cell line can be demonstrated. It is possible, for example, to assay for the presence of

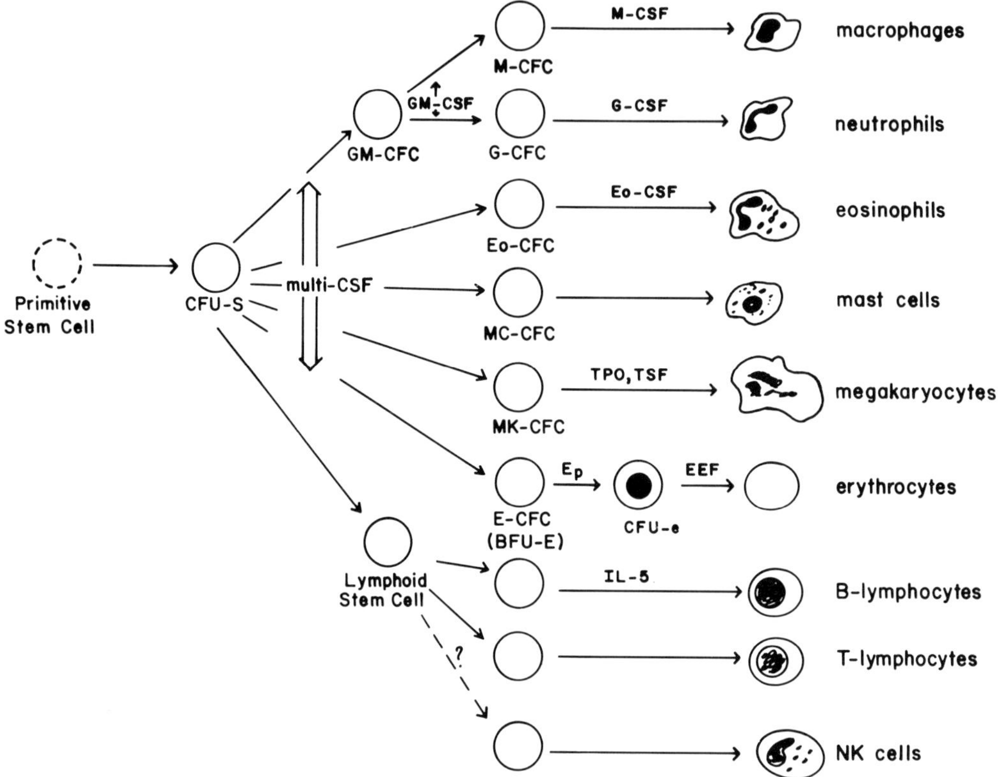

Fig. 1. Structure of the hemopoietic system. See text and Table 1 for abbreviations of cell progenitors and growth factors

progenitor cells for macrophages (M-CFC), granulocytes (G-CFC), megakaryocytes (MK-CFC), eosinophils (Eo-CFC), and mast cells (MC-CFC). Erythroid progenitors are assayed either as early progenitors (E-CFC) or burst-forming units-erythroid (BFU-E). In some cases, progenitors with the capacity to produce more than one cell line, such as the GM-CFC (macrophages and granulocytes), can be cultured in vitro. While lymphocytes and natural killer (NK) cells) are derived from the bone marrow, the progenitors for these cells have not been identified in vitro.

The commitment of a progenitor cell to a specific cell line leads to the proliferation of cells with greater levels of differentiation. The mature myeloid and erythroid cells produced by the bone marrow do not have the potential to regenerate to more primitive progenitor cells and are terminally committed. The exception to this developmental scheme is the lymphocyte populations, which retain the potential for additional development at distant sites. Bone marrow-derived (B) and thymic-derived (T) lymphocytes, NK cells, and cells of the mononuclear-phagocytic system are all derived from bone marrow precursors and retain the potential for additional development in peripheral tissues.

Cytokine Regulation of Hemopoiesis

All of the in vitro assay systems for bone marrow stem and progenitor cells depend upon the presence of soluble growth factors. The hemopoietic progenitor cells are not capable of division without the presence of growth factors. They have traditionally been referred to as colony-stimulating factors (CSF). Early colony assays utilized poorly characterized supernatants from cell cultures that empirically contained soluble factors necessary for the growth of various progenitor cells. As with inflammatory mediators and lymphokines, the use of different cell lines and culture conditions led to the creation of a large and complex group of "factors" that could influence hemopoiesis. It became clear, however, that stimulated lymphocyte cultures provided a particularly rich source of bone marrow growth factors. The isolation, characterization, and production via recombinant DNA technology of these "lymphokines" has demonstrated that many of the growth factors originally thought to be specific for hemopoiesis are identical to those factors that mediate the interactions of lymphocyte subpopulations.

Stem Cells

The development of pluripotent stem cells can be influenced by at least two growth factors, multi-CSF (IL-3) and H-1 (IL-1). The first of these, murine multipotential colony-stimulating factor (multi-CSF) is produced by stimulated T lymphocytes, leukemia cell line WEHI-3B, and T-lymphocyte hybridomas (Metcalf 1986; Sachs 1987). As with other CSFs, multi-CSF can be produced by a wide variety of normal cells. Genomic and complementary (cDNA) clones have been isolated for multi-CSF, and the locus responsible for production of the factor in mice is present as a single copy gene on chromosome 11. Although generally small amounts of CSF can be isolated from many tissues, the isolation and purification of individual CSFs typically require cell lines or cultures with a cell density sufficient to produce factors in the quantities necessary for isolation. Recombinant multi-CSF has been produced, and both the native and recombinant molecules exhibit a wide capacity for stimulating hemopoietic and lymphoid cells. Multi-CSF stimulates pluripotent stem cells, CFU-s, and progenitor cells for granulocytes, macrophages, eosinophils, erythroid cells, mast cells, and megakaryocytes.

The human pluripotent growth factor, H-1, has been isolated from supernatants of a human bladder tumor cell line and has been reported to have the ability to stimulate a variety of hemopoietic stem cells (Welte et al. 1985; Bartelmetz and Stanley 1985). H-1 apparently acts by enhancing the expression of receptors for CSF-1 on primitive hemopoietic cells (Stanley et al. 1986) and IL-2 on bone marrow NK cell precursors (Migliorati et al. 1987). Treatment of early mouse hemopoietic cells with H-1 enhances the generation of NK cells in the presence of IL-2. Similar results are not seen when IL-3 (multi-CSF) is included.

Progenitor Cells

The stimulus for division, differentiation, and functional development of hemopoietic lineages are individual CSFs that have been defined by in vitro culture systems. For each cell line, individual CSFs are thought to be responsible for stimulating the division of the progenitor cells, for their commitment to a particular lineage, and for the establishment of the functional activity of the mature end stage cells. CSFs have been operationally defined for stimulation of the development of hemopoietic progenitor cells, including those for erytrocytes, macrophages, granulocytes (neutrophils) eosinophils, mast cells, basophils, and megakaryocytes (Metcalf 1984; Zoumbos et al. 1986). The definition of a factor(s) by its ability to stimulate the differentiation of a recognizable hemopoietic colony, however, should not be interpreted to mean that individual factors for the development of each cell line exist. The high specific activity and difficulties of purification have limited the characterization of these factors, but the overlap in the function of many CSFs suggests that operational definition of CSFs for different cell lines may include factors that stimulate many different progenitor cells, such as multi-CSF, or the stimulation of one progenitor (i. e., M-CFU) with multiple different factors.

While many of these growth factors are incompletely characterized, those that stimulate the development of granulocyte/macrophage colonies have been studied in detail and can function as a model for describing this general class of factors. In the mouse there are at least three well-characterized factors that function primarily to mediate the development of granulocytes (neutrophils) and macrophages (Table 1). They include GM-CSF, G-CSF, and M-CSF. In the mouse, GM-CSF is a glycosylated polypeptide (124 amino acids) coded for by a single locus on chromosome 11. The factor is produced by a variety of tissues and has the property of stimulating both granulocyte and macrophage colony formation at very low concentrations (10^{-12} mol/l). As is characteristic for many CSFs, GM-CSF has the ability at high concentrations to enhance the development of other types of hemopoietic colonies, including eosinophils, megakaryocytes, and erythrocytes (Metcalf 1986).

Two other factors, G-CSF and M-CSF, are polypeptides that are structurally distinct from GM-CSF and function to stimulate the development of granulocyte and macrophage colonies, respectively. In mice M-CSF (originally CSF-1) is a 70 000 dalton glycoprotein that consists of two 35 000 dalton subunits. A similar dimeric glycoprotein has been described in humans (Das and Stanley 1982). M-CSF acts principally to stimulate the development of macrophages and has little effect on other hemopoietic cells. Stimulation of two or three cell divisions of macrophage progenitor cells by M-CSF induces a permanent commitment to macrophage development, even though other CSFs may still be able to stimulate continued proliferation of the cell

Table 1. Hemopoietic growth factors

Name	Synonyms	Activity
multi-CSF	IL-3 HCGF BPA MK-CSF HCGF PSF H-2 E-CSF	Growth and development of pluripotent stem cells and hemopoietic progenitors; negative NK regulation
H-1 (hemopoietin-1)		Pluripotent stem cell and T-lymphocyte activation
IL-1	H-1 (?)	Activation of T lymphocytes and macrophage/granulocyte progenitors
GM-CSF		Stimulation of macrophage and neutrophil colonies
M-CSF	CSF-1	Stimulation of macrophage colonies
G-CSF		Stimulation of neutrophil colonies
Eo-CSF		Stimulation of eosinophil colonies
IL-2	TCGF	Activation of T lymphocytes, NK cells, and B-lymphocyte growth and differentiation
IL-4	BCGF-1 BSF-1	Stimulates activation of resting lymphocytes and development of hemopoietic progenitor cells
IL-5	BCGF-2 BCDF	Growth and differentiation of B lymphocytes
γ-Interferon	MAF	Macrophage activation Inhibits in vitro myelopoiesis and stem cell production
Erythropoietin	Ep	Erythropoiesis
Thrombopoietin	TPO	Stimulates megakaryocyte differentiation and platelet production
TSF (thrombopoiesis-stimulating factor)		Stimulates megakaryocyte differentiation and platelet production

line (Metcalf and Burgess 1982). In general, granulocyte and macrophage progenitors have a heterogeneous response to stimulation with CSFs, many responding to higher levels of factors whose primary activity is directed at other cell lines. G-CSF is a glycoprotein monomer of approximately 25000 daltons that, at low to moderate concentrations, exclusively stimulates the formation of granulocyte (neutrophil) colonies. It is capable of stimulating the proliferation of other GM progenitors but only for limited periods of time (Metcalf 1986).

The proliferation and differentiation of erythroid progenitor cells into mature erythrocytes depends upon the burst-promoting activity (BPA) of growth factors that stimulate the growth of early erythrocyte precursors (E-CFC or BFU-E; Aye 1977; Johnson and Metcalf 1977). The BPA growth factors are found in the supernatants of leukocyte cultures and have been shown to copurify with IL-3 (multi-CSF) (Iscove et al. 1982). It seems probable that the same pluripotent growth factors that stimulate the development of myeloid cells also act to stimulate the development and commitment of early erythroid precursors.

The continued development of erythrocytes is regulated by erythropoietin (Kurtz 1987). Erythropoietin (Ep) is a glycoprotein with a molecular weight of 34000 daltons and is produced by the liver and kidneys of adults. Ep circulates in the peripheral blood and regulates erythropoiesis by stimulating the proliferation of primitive erythroid precursors (E-CFC or BFU-E) and more differentiated progenitor cells (CFU-e). Ep acts in vivo to stimulate erythropoiesis, primarily in response to conditions, including anemia and hypoxia, that result in insufficient oxygen supply to the tissues. In the absence of sufficient oxygen, the levels of Ep become elevated, followed in approximately 24 h by increased levels of erythropoiesis. The gene that codes for erythropoietin has been recently cloned from both the kidney (Lee-Huang 1984) and the liver (Jacobs et al. 1985).

Megakaryocyte colony formation is thought to be the result of factors that initially promote the proliferation of the primitive mononuclear precursor cell, combined with a second group of factors that stimulate megakaryocyte differentiation (Williams et al. 1982, 1984). One of the primary promoters of megakaryocyte proliferation is a factor (MK-CSF) present in the supernatant of the WEHI-3 cell line. MK-CSF has been shown to copurify with IL-3 (multi-CSF), and comparison of the biological properties of the two suggests that they are identical molecules

(Ihle et al. 1982; Sparrow and Williams 1986). A number of factors act then on the proliferating cells to promote cytoplasmic and nuclear maturation of the megakaryocytes (see Evatt et al. 1986). These include two factors, thrombopoietin (TPO) and thrombopoiesis-stimulating factor (TSF), that appear to be specific for megakaryocytes. Both have similar in vivo and in vitro effects and stimulate megakaryocyte differentiation and platelet production.

Role of Lymphokines in Hemopoiesis

Recent advances in our ability to characterize biochemically molecules that control cell growth (cytokines) have demonstrated that many growth factors have broader biological functions than originally anticipated. The designation of soluble factors produced by lymphocytes as lymphokines does not necessarily imply that their primary function is in the regulation of lymphocyte interactions. The lymphokine IL-3, for example, was originally defined as a unique factor thought to be responsible for the stimulation of differentiation of T lymphocytes (Ihle et al. 1981). Subsequent characterization of the molecule, however, has shown that it is identical to growth factors capable of stimulating the development of all hemopoietic cell lineages and has received no less than 15 different names or acronyms including multi-CSF, MK-CSF, BPA, PSF, HCGF, hemopoietin-2 (H-2), and E-CSF. Ironically, the original association of IL-3 with the induction of T-lymphocyte differentiation has proven to be incorrect; its primary function is that of a factor with a broad range of hemopoietic activity on cell lines other than lymphocytes (Schrader 1986). The lymphokines that have been associated with the regulation of different aspects of hemopoiesis include interleukin 1 (IL-1), interleukin 2 (IL-2), interleukin 3 (IL-3), interleukin 4 (IL-4 or B cell growth factor 1), interleukin 5 (IL-5 or B cell growth factor 2), α-interferon, and γ-interferon (see Table 1). Each of these cytokines is involved in hemopoiesis, either due to regulation of hemopoietic cell or lymphocyte development. Although primarily characterized as soluble growth factors produced by lymphocytes, many are produced by other cells and, alternatively, some hemopoietic factors, such as IL-4, IL-5, Eo-CSF, and GM-CSF, are secreted by activated T lymphocytes.
A brief summary of the major regulatory effects of the hemopoietic growth factors is presented in

Table 1. Interleukin 1 has been included as both a well-characterized lymphokine and as a potential pluripotent stem cell regulator. Clearly, IL-1 fulfills an important role as a stimulant for T-lymphocyte development, but there are also suggestions that it may have a more general role in regulating the production of GM-CSF and G-CSF (Broudy et al. 1987) and the expression of IL-2 and M-CSF receptors on progenitor cells (Migliorati et al. 1987) and may share functional and biochemical characteristics with the stem cell hemopoietin H-1. IL-4 is produced by T lymphocytes and stimulates the activation of resting T and B lymphocytes, particularly for the regulation of immunoglobulin synthesis. It has been shown to regulate the activity of a wide variety of hemopoietic precursor cells including the early precursors of the erythroid and myeloid lineages, megakaryocytes, mast cells, and macrophages (Paul 1987). The activities regulated by IL-4 are not the same for each cell line, suggesting that the effect may be due to local cell-to-cell interactions or to the binding of the cytokine with cell surface molecules, such as class II histocompatibility antigens, that may be expressed at different times on individual cell lines.

Synthesis

Hemopoietic growth factors represent a structurally diverse group of cytokines with similar and overlapping functional activities. The close similarity of functional activities assures close coordination and control of the development of individual cell lineages, including the lymphoid system. CFSs apparently are capable of functioning at two levels, local and systemic, to provide for the regulation of cell growth and the interaction of different cell lines. The broad range of target cell activity exhibited by many CSFs suggests that CSFs may be produced and act locally on cells in response to the need for hemopoietic cell production. Since the proliferation of bone marrow cells in vitro depends upon the presence of CSFs, the differentiation and production of normal levels of hemopoietic cells probably reflects close cell-to-cell interaction of CSFs at low levels. The CSFs can also, however, increase the functional activity of granulocytes and macrophages in the periphery, providing an opportunity for more effective inflammatory responses (Metcalf 1984). CSFs are known to be stimulated by bacterial breakdown products, especially endotoxin, leading to the potential for local stimulation of the activity of mature inflammatory cells and the recruitment of new cells from the bone marrow.

Bone marrow cells in mice are known to express specific, high affinity receptors for individual CSFs (Nicola 1987). The type of receptor and its distribution parallels the stimulatory activity of the multiplural CSFs and CSFs with more restricted activity on specific progenitor cells. The receptors for multi-CSF and GM-CSF are small (50000–75000 daltons), are widely distributed on different cell lineages, and decrease in number with the maturity of the cells. In contrast, M-CSF and G-CSF are larger glycoproteins with a restricted distribution and higher concentrations on the surface of more mature cells. M-CSF shares structural features with other growth factor receptors, including immunochemical cross-reactivity with the proto-oncogene *c-fms* (Rettenmeir et al. 1986). Under normal conditions CSFs such as G-CSF have the ability to bind to their receptors and stimulate the production of daughter cells, some of which remain as progenitor cells and others that are irreversibly committed to terminal differentiation.

The relationship between the mechanism(s) responsible for CSF stimulation of proliferation and differentiation is not known. These processes are of considerable interest, however, because of the potential relationship between oncogenes, growth factors, and/or growth factor receptors. The neoplastic transformation of cells may be mediated by cellular oncogenes that have mutated or become subject to abnormal regulation and subsequently stimulate increased synthesis of either growth factors or their receptors. The leukemic cells from patients with myeloid leukemia require the presence of CSF to grow in vitro. Some CSFs such as G-CSF have the ability to stimulate at low concentrations the proliferation of the myelomonocytic leukemia line WEHI-3B and at slightly higher levels the terminal differentiation of these neoplastic cells (Metcalf 1982). Similar results have been obtained in mice as administration of CSF preparations have been shown to suppress the growth of experimental leukemias in vivo (Lotem and Sachs 1981).

The clarification of the role that growth factors play in regulating the proliferation, differentiation, and function of hemopoietic cells has led to the recognition of the important potential clinical applications of purified CSFs. At present recombinant lymphokines, such as IL-2, are being employed in the immunotherapy of cancer, and there is increasing interest in other modulators of lymphocyte development and function as therapy for immune diseases including immunodeficiencies, autoimmune diseases, and neoplastic diseases. It is clear that multiplural CSFs could be important agents for stimulating recovery from primary or secondary bone marrow failure, including the large group of patients who experiences bone marrow toxicity following high-dose chemotherapy for metastatic neoplastic diseases. As described above, for certain forms of neoplasms, especially those of bone marrow origin, there is the additional potential of using selected CSF reagents to modify directly their neoplastic behavior.

References

Aye MT (1977) Erythroid colony formation in cultures of human marrow: effect of leukocyte conditioned medium. J Cell Physiol 91: 69–77

Bartelmez SH, Stanley ER (1985) Synergism between hemopoietic growth factors (HGFs) detected by their effects on cells bearing receptors for a lineage specific HGF: assay of hemopoietin-1. J Cell Physiol 122: 370–378

Broudy VC, Kaushansky K, Harlan JM, Adamson JW (1987) Interleukin 1 stimulates human endothelial cells to produce granulocyte-macrophage colony-stimulating factor and granulocyte colony-stimulating factor. J Immunol 139: 464–468

Das SK, Stanley ER (1982) Structure-function studies of a colony-stimulating factor (CSF-1). J Biol Chem 257: 13679–13684

Dexter TM, Moore M (1986) Growth and development in the haemopoietic system: the role of lymphokines and their possible therapeutic potential in disease and malignancy. Carcinogenesis 7: 509–516

Dexter TM, Allen TD, Lajtha LG (1977) Conditions controlling the proliferation of haemopoietic stem cells in vitro. J Cell Physiol 91: 335–343

Evatt BL, Kellar KL, Ramsey RB (1986) Thrombopoietin: past, present and future. In: Levine RF et al. (eds) Megakaryocyte development and function. Liss, New York, pp 143–155

Ihle JN, Pepersack L, Rebar L (1981) Regulation of T cell differentiation: in vitro induction of 20-alpha-hydroxysteroid dehydrogenase in splenic lymphocytes from athymic mice by a unique lymphokine. J Immunol 126: 2184–2189

Ihle JN, Keller J, Greenberger JS, Henderson L, Yetter RA, Morse HC III (1982) Phenotypic characteristics of cell lines requiring interleukin 3 for growth. J Immunol 129: 1377–1383

Iscove NN, Roitsch CA, Williams N, Guilbert LJ (1982) Molecules stimulating early red cell, granulocyte, macrophage and megakaryocyte precursors in culture: similarity in size hydrophobicity and charge. J Cell Physiol (Suppl) 1: 65–78

Jacobs K, Shoemaker C, Rudersdorf R, Neill SD, Kaufman RJ, Mufson A, Seehra J, Jones SS, Hewick R,

Fritsch EF, Kawakita M, Shimizu T, Miyake T (1985) Isolation and characterization of genomic and cDNA clones of human erythropoietin. Nature 313: 806–810

Johnson GR, Metcalf D (1977) Pure and mixed erythroid colony formation in vitro stimulated by spleen conditioned medium with no detectable erythropoietin. Proc Natl Acad Sci USA 74: 3879–3882

Kurtz A (1987) Erythropoietin: structure, function, origin. Adv Nephrol 16: 371–378

Lee-Huang S (1984) Cloning and expression of human erythropoietin c-DNA in *Escherichia coli*. Proc Natl Acad Sci USA 81: 2708

Lotem J, Sachs L (1981) In vivo inhibition of the development of myeloid leukemia by injection of macrophage- and granulocyte-inducing protein. Int J Cancer 28: 375–386

Magli MC, Iscove NN, Odartchenko N (1982) Transient nature of early haematopoietic spleen colonies. Nature 295: 527–529

Metcalf D (1982) Regulator-induced suppression of myelo-monocytic leukemia cells: clonal analysis of early cellular events. Int J Cancer 30: 203–210

Metcalf D (1984) The hematopoietic colony stimulating factors. Elsevier, Amsterdam

Metcalf D (1986) The molecular biology and functions of the granulocyte-macrophage colony-stimulating factors. Blood 67: 257–267

Metcalf D, Burgess AW (1982) Clonal analysis of progenitor cell commitment to granulocyte or macrophage production. J Cell Physiol 111: 275–283

Migliorati G, Cannarile L, Herberman RB, Bartocci A, Stanley ER, Riccardi C (1987) Role of interleukin 2 (IL2) and hemopoietin-1 (H-1) in the generation of mouse natural killer (NK) cells from primitive bone marrow precursors. J Immunol 138: 3618–3625

Nicola NA (1987) Why do hemopoietic growth factor receptors interact with each other? Immunol Today 8: 134–140

Paul WE (1987) Interleukin 4/B cell stimulatory factor 1: one lymphokine, many functions. FASEB J 1: 456–461

Rettenmeir CW, Sacca R, Furman WL, Roussel MF, Holt JT, Nienhuis AW, Stanley ER, Sherr CJ (1986) Expression of the human c-*fms* proto-oncogene product (colony-stimulating factor-1 receptor) on peripheral blood mononuclear cells and choriocarcinoma cell lines. J Clin Invest 77: 1740–1746

Sachs L (1987) The molecular control of blood cell development. Science 238: 1374–1379

Schrader JW (1983) Bone marrow differentiation in vitro. CRC Crit Rev Immunol 4: 197–277

Schrader JW (1986) The panspecific hemopoietin of activated T lymphocytes (Interleukin 3). Annul Rev Immunol 4: 205–230

Sparrow RL, Williams N (1986) Megakaryocyte colony stimulating factor: its identity to interleukin-3. In: Levine RF (ed) Megakaryocyte development and function. Alan R Liss, New York, pp 123–128

Stanley ER, Bartocci A, Patinkin D, Rosendaal M, Bradley TR (1986) Regulation of very primitive, multipotent, hemopoietic cells by hemopoietin-1. Cell 45: 667–674

Welte K, Platzer E, Lu L, Gabrilove JL, Levi E, Mertelsmann R, Moore MAS (1985) Purification and biochemical characterization of human pluripotent hematopoietic colony-stimulating factor. Proc Natl Acad Sci USA 82: 1526–1530

Williams N, Eger RR, Jackson HM, Nelson DJ (1982) Two-factor requirement for murine megakaryocyte colony formation. J Cell Physiol 110: 101–104

Williams N, Jackson H, Iscove NN, Dukes PP (1984) The role of erythropoietin, thrombopoietic stimulating factor, and myeloid colony-stimulating factors on murine megakaryocyte colony formation. Exp Hematol 12: 734–740

Zoumbos N, Raefsky E, Young N (1986) Lymphokines and hematopoiesis. Prog Hematol 14: 201–227

Evaluation of Blood and Bone Marrow, Rat

Victor E. Valli, David C. Villeneuve, Barbara Reed, Nabila Barsoum, and Graham Smith

Introduction

The examination of blood and bone marrow is a relatively universal feature of dose-response studies which utilize the laboratory rat. Changes in the hemopoietic system may arise as primary effects on the blood cells themselves or secondarily due to irritation in the tissues exposed by the route of administration of the test substance. Thus, myeloid hyperplasia may result without an apparent target in response to lithium or with a direct target in response to injury in the gut, lung, or skin. Similarly, erythropoiesis may be directly depressed by toxic exposure or increased due to hypoxia, hemolysis, or blood loss. While the changes in the blood may be readily apparent, the mechanisms by which these alterations occurred may be less clear. In general, the marrow and blood need to be considered together in a precursor-product relationship and changes interpreted with knowledge of the type and extent of lesions occurring elsewhere in the body.

Much has been learned from basic studies of rat marrow in terms of stem cell physiology (Gong 1978; Maniatis et al. 1971; Schuit and Krebs 1982; Tavassoli et al. 1971), iron kinetics (Murray et al. 1970; Hershko et al. 1973), and functional anatomy (DeBruyn 1981; Lichtman 1981; Weiss 1965). Recent texts have provided essential information on age-related changes in the hemopoietic system of the rat (Burek 1978) and on mechanisms of hemopoietic injury (Irons 1985) and tumors (Greaves and Faccini 1984). More general texts provide information on collection techniques and normal value (Benirschke et al. 1978; Archer and Jeffcott 1977; Jain 1986). The purpose of this report is to provide tabular data on rat blood and marrow and to illustrate dose-related nonneoplastic responses.

Collection Techniques

Serial blood samples from rats may be collected from the orbital sinus, tail vein, or cardiac puncture. Considerable skill is required to obtain samples suitable for automated analysis without loss of the animals. Large volume collections are most effectively carried out at termination under anesthesia by syringe and 22 ga. needle from the abdominal aorta. The blood should be transferred immediately to anticoagulant-containing tubes preferably with a larger bore needle to minimize turbulent cell injury. Vials should be placed on an agitator or inverted 25 times to ensure adequate anticoagulation and avoid platelet clumping or clotting. Blood films are best made at the time of collection and may utilize blood from the tip of the collection needle. Films should be rapidly waved or fan dried. Fixation may be delayed unless ambient humidity is high. The level of blood constituents may be affected by the site chosen for blood collection (Quimby et al. 1948; Beckhardt et al. 1983).

In general, stress-related collections from the tail or orbital sinus of unanesthetized rats are characterized by higher leukocyte and erythrocyte counts although the magnitude in the change in the red cells is proportionately far less than for the leukocytes. Anesthesia preceding blood collection can be expected to cause some excitement, but the overall results following the anesthesia tend to be less variable regardless of the site of collection (heart, artery, or vein). Since the cellular content of blood is raised by physical activity, the choice site of collection is the one which can be employed with the minimum of struggling by the rat. Factors which increase the variability of results independent of the site of collection include: too large a collection vial causing a dilution by anticoagulant, free alcohol

on the skin leading to hemolysis, prolonged venous stasis (>1 min) causing an increase in hematocrit, and excessive tissue injury leading to platelet aggregation and spuriously lower counts.

Marrow collection for cytologic examination must be made before blood clotting occurs and within 2–3 min of death. Marrow aspiration from an isolated bone is most easily obtained where there is red marrow free of cancellous spicules. The midfemoral cavity is a reliable site for evaluation of hemopoiesis throughout life and free of cancellous bone. Collection is most efficiently accomplished by exposure of the metaphyseal cavity by the prosector with collection carried out by aspiration of marrow into a 5 µl pipette containing EDTA anticoagulated sera from a control rat. Marrow films are prepared as for blood and are best made by the person who will be carrying out the microscopic examination. Optimal results can only be obtained if there is skilled teamwork (Table 2).

Marrow for histological examination can be obtained from the femoral medulla, and this site will yield superior cytologic detail since the marrow can be obtained free of bone, thus obviating

Table 2. Critical steps in conducting bone marrow differential counts

Procedure	Technical requirements
Marrow collection	Must be performed to avoid blood coagulation leading to cell injury.
Slide preparation	Essential to use the "granule trail" rather than the crush method to minimize dilution by sinusoidal blood. If the aspirate is dilute, a concentration technique is required to increase the density of marrow granules placed on the slide.
Staining	Examine test slides prior to mounting cover slips to ensure adequacy of stain with good differentiation of cytoplasmic granules. Restain if necessary.
Slide examination	Identify granules which have a dense trail of well-stained marrow cells. Move the stage only within the trail of cells to reduce bias of selection and dilution of marrow cell counts by peripheral blood cells. Count at least 200 cells for determining M/E ratios and 500 cells for complete differentials. Avoid over-classification of injured or unidentifiable cells.

the need for decalcification. In contrast, the sternum has the advantage of providing sections in which the marrow architecture is undisturbed in its relation to endosteal bone. Spontaneous trabecular thickening and cartilage necrosis may frequently be found in the sternebra of rats 130–180 days of age (Jasty et al. 1986), but these changes appear to have little effect on hemopoiesis.

Processing Techniques

Blood and marrow films are routinely fixed in methanol and stained with a standard Romanovsky procedure. With most staining protocols, the greater cellularity of marrow films requires a doubling of the staining time. For optimal cytologic detail in tissue section, the bone marrow should be fixed in situ after removal of the femoral metaphyses. A core of the fixed marrow can then be processed and sectioned without decalcification. If the architecture is of equal importance, the sternum should be removed for fixation, then decalcified, and processed for sectioning. Gentle agitation for 24 h in fixative is essential for proper penetration of formalin into marrow fixed in situ. If immunohistochemical procedures are anticipated, the target tissues should be fixed separately in a B5 type solution and preferably embedded in methacrylate (Beckstead 1985; Dacie and Lewis 1985).

Normal Values

Data presented in Tables 3–5 are derived from control groups of male and female Sprague-Dawley rats. Blood analysis was carried out on a Baker 7000 cell counter using a 100 μm aperture with 0.50 mA of current and 0.95 V for leukocytes and 0.40 V for erythrocytes. Red cells were diluted in Baker Haemaline for counting and leukocytes were counted after the red cells were destroyed using Baker Haemolyse. Platelets were counted on a Baker 810 platelet analyser. In order to facilitate the comparison of dose-related changes with control levels of peripheral blood cells, all values are given in absolute numbers rather than percentages.

Variations in Blood and Bone Marrow

Most hemologic changes observed in toxicologic testing appear to be physiologic responses of the bone marrow to peripheral lesions in the body such as pneumonia or hemorrhage from skin

Table 3. Complete blood counts of peripheral blood cells from normal Sprague-Dawley rats at various ages

	Age of animals						Pregnant	
	2 months		4 months		1 year			
	M	F	M	F	M	F		
WBC	8.1 +1.70	6.4 ±1.76	7.7 ⊥2.50	4.5 ±1.80	6.9 ±1.25	3.3 ±1.0	6.1 ±1.70	
RBC	6.80 ±0.38	6.91 ±0.39	7.86 ±0.44	7.20 ±0.29	7.60 ±0.36	6.90 ±0.32	5.82 ±0.50	
HGB	138.2 ±5.20	135.0 ±5.73	143.2 ±7.60	133.1 ±5.30	145.8 ±5.0	139.2 ±4.60	120.0 ±10.0	
HCT	0.395±0.02	0.400±0.02	0.415±0.03	0.388±0.01	0.422±0.01	0.403±0.01	0.332±2.50	
MCV	58.5 ±1.94	58.6 ±2.52	52.7 ±3.70	53.7 ±1.30	55.3 ±2.0	58.6 ±1.40	57.1 ±1.40	
MCH	20.5 ±0.72	20.4 ±0.84	18.2 ±0.70	18.5 ±0.50	19.1 ±0.74	20.3 ±0.62	20.5 ±0.30	
MCHC	349.4 ±6.2	348.8 ±6.1	345.6 ±8.1	342.6 ±4.6	345.2 ±4.6	345.5 ±8.1	360.0 ±6.0	
Plts	1191 ±132	1095 ±161	1074 ±123	1029 ±158	882 ±103	792 ±112	1196 ±190	
Retics	128 ±55	90 ±52	118 ±47	65 ±36	206 ±69	189 ±26	184 ±75	
Neuts	0.95 ±0.67	0.57 ±0.22	0.80 ±0.35	0.45 ±0.17	1.34 ±0.53	0.73 ±0.24	2.04 ±0.44	
Bands	0.0	0.0	0.0	0.005	0.0	0.0	0.0	
Lymphs	6.58 ±0.70	5.34 ±0.33	6.31 ±0.40	3.88 ±0.23	4.95 ±0.99	2.18 ±0.92	3.81 ±0.49	
Monos	0.52 ±0.26	0.41 ±0.15	0.41 ±0.28	0.14 ±0.08	0.62 ±0.26	0.22 ±0.07	0.24 ±0.15	
Eosinos	0.08 ±0.09	0.06 ±0.07	0.10 ±0.10	0.04 ±0.03	0.06 ±0.07	0.05 ±0.04	0.02 ±0.04	
Rubris	0	0	0	0	0	0	0	
n	40	49	10	10	19	18	11	

Values are means and standard deviations of counts on 100 cells on each animal. Leukocytes, reticulocytes, and platelets are expressed as $\times 10^9/l$ and erythrocytes as $\times 10^{12}/l$. Hemoglobin and indices are expressed in SI units. The number of animals in each group is indicated by *n*. Blood was collected under ether anesthesia from the abdominal aorta into EDTA anticoagulant.
WBC, white blood cells (leukocytes); RBC, red blood cells; HGB, hemoglobin; HCT, hematocrit; MCV, mean corpuscular volume; MCH, mean corpuscular hemoglobin; MCHC, mean corpuscular hemoglobin concentration; Plts, platelets; Retics, reticulocytes; Neuts, mature neutrophils; Bands, immature (unsegmented) neutrophils; Lymphs, lymphocytes; Monos, monocytes; Eosino, eosinophils; Rubris, rubriblasts.

Table 4. Mean proportions of bone marrow cells from normal Sprague-Dawley rats at various ages

Age	Sex	Myeloid cells	Erythroid cells	M/E ratio	Eosinophil total	Lymphos/ Monos	Plasma cells	Injured/ unidentified
2 months	m $n=$ 9	166 ± 24	141 ± 22	$1.2\ \pm0.27$	8 ± 5	186 ± 32	4 ± 3	3 ± 3
	f $n=10$	196 ± 22	156 ± 25	$1.3\ \pm0.4$	19 ± 5	144 ± 17	3 ± 2	1 ± 1
4 months	m $n=81$	203 ± 25	190 ± 29	$1.1\ \pm0.18$	13 ± 5	90 ± 41	2 ± 2	15 ± 8
	f $n=63$	208 ± 25	182 ± 25	1.17 ± 0.27	21 ± 8	88 ± 22	1 ± 1	21 ± 8
1 year	m $n=20$	224 ± 19	186 ± 18	1.22 ± 0.2	12 ± 4	63 ± 14	–[a]	26 ± 11
	f $n=18$	196 ± 19	189 ± 20	1.06 ± 0.21	14 ± 5	84 ± 26	–[a]	31 ± 18
Pregnant 21 days	$n=68$	224 ± 31	181 ± 26	1.28 ± 0.3	18 ± 7	79 ± 42	3 ± 3	15 ± 13

[a] Plasma cells included with lymphocytes. Eosinophils are included in total myeloid cells and the myeloid/erythroid (M/E) ratio. "Total eosinophils" are the proportion of 500 marrow cells which are of this cell lineage. The number of animals in each group is indicated by n; means $\pm$ SD given.

Table 5. Marrow differential counts and maturation indices from normal Sprague-Dawley rats

Cell type	Age and Sex									
	4 months				1 year				Pregnant	
	m	total	f	total	m	total	f	total	f	total
Erythroblast	$0.2\ \pm0.5$		$0.7\ \pm0.4$		$0.3\ \pm0.3$		$0.5\ \pm0.4$		$0.4\ \pm0.3$	
Prorubricyte	$1.3\ \pm1.0$		$1.6\ \pm0.8$		$1.7\ \pm0.8$		$2.1\ \pm1.3$		$1.9\ \pm0.9$	
Basorubricyte	$5.6\ \pm1.7$	7.1 p	$6.3\ \pm1.5$	8.6 p	$6.3\ \pm1.6$	8.3 p	$3.7\ \pm1.2$	6.3 p	$6.3\ \pm1.1$	8.6 p
Polyrubricyte	$6.9\ \pm4.0$		$7.9\ \pm1.7$		$7.4\ \pm1.9$		$7.7\ \pm1.7$		$10.8\ \pm2.1$	
Normorubricyte	$8.3\ \pm2.3$		$9.1\ \pm2.2$		$6.9\ \pm1.7$		$7.5\ \pm1.2$		$9.9\ \pm2.8$	
Metarubricyte	$15.4\ \pm4.3$	30.6 m	$14.5\ \pm2.9$	31.5 m	$13.2\ \pm2.0$	28.2 m	$14.8\ \pm2.5$	30.0 m	$9.2\ \pm3.3$	29.9 m
Maturation index (p/m)[a]	0.24 ± 0.13		0.28 ± 0.08		0.30 ± 0.08		0.22 ± 0.10		0.30 ± 0.08	
Myeloblast	$0.6\ \pm0.6$		$0.2\ \pm0.1$		$1.0\ \pm0.9$		$0.9\ \pm0.5$		$0.3\ \pm0.2$	
Promyelocyte	$3.4\ \pm1.0$		$1.5\ \pm0.9$		$2.0\ \pm0.9$		$1.9\ \pm0.6$		$2.0\ \pm0.6$	
Myelocyte	$4.5\ \pm1.4$	8.5 p	$3.8\ \pm1.6$	5.5 p	$4.4\ \pm0.9$	7.4 p	$6.0\ \pm2.0$	8.8 p	$7.0\ \pm1.1$	9.3 p
Metamyelocyte	$9.5\ \pm2.5$		$7.7\ \pm2.2$		$6.8\ \pm1.4$		$8.5\ \pm1.5$		$9.9\ \pm0.8$	
Band cell	$17.6\ \pm2.9$		$17.1\ \pm3.3$		$14.8\ \pm2.7$		$10.9\ \pm3.1$		$14.4\ \pm3.1$	
Segmented	$5.3\ \pm2.2$	32.4 m	$4.6\ \pm2.4$	29.4 m	$11.9\ \pm3.3$	33.4 m	$9.9\ \pm1.9$	29.3 m	$9.0\ \pm1.6$	33.3 m
Maturation index (p/m)[a]	0.27 ± 0.09		0.21 ± 0.12		0.21 ± 0.05		0.28 ± 0.11		0.26 ± 0.06	
Lymph + Mono	$14.8\ \pm3.5$		$14.2\ \pm3.4$		$18.7\ \pm3.6$		$20.4\ \pm5.2$		$15.1\ \pm4.4$	
Eosinophil	$3.4\ \pm2.3$		$5.4\ \pm1.4$		$2.7\ \pm0.9$		$3.2\ \pm1.0$		$2.5\ \pm1.3$	
Plasma cell	$0.3\ \pm0.3$		$0.5\ \pm0.6$		$0.4\ \pm0.5$		$0.5\ \pm0.7$		$0.9\ \pm0.5$	
Unidentified	$3.0\ \pm2.6$		$4.8\ \pm3.1$		$0.4\ \pm0.3$		$0.5\ \pm0.5$		$0.3\ \pm0.2$	
n	12		13		10		10		10	

Values are means and standard deviations of counts of 500 cells on each animal. The number of animals in each group is indicated by n.
[a] Maturation index (p/m) = total of proliferative phase cells (p) divided by the total of the maturation phase cells (m).

trauma or a necrotic tumor. In 2-year studies hyperplastic responses are often lymphoproliferative and do not present a problem in diagnosis although the pathogenesis may be less clear.

In short-term studies the hemologic system is infrequently affected in a primary manner, and the changes observed are generally of mild degree and part of a general pattern of injury to a number of organ systems. Thus, careful examination of tissues and data is essential to detect primary effects on the marrow and its products. Agents which affect early marrow precursors may be expected to cause an increase or decrease in marrow cellularity without alteration in the sequence of maturation or cell morphology (Cronkite et al. 1985). If there is injury to the marrow stroma such as myelofibrosis with an intact stem cell system, extramedullary hemopoiesis (see p. 232, this volume) will most likely result as the precursors seek fertile ground in other tissues such as the liver and spleen. If, however, there is primary injury to the stem cells, the marrow will become hypoplastic or aplastic and extramedullary proliferation will not be found (Figs. 2–4). In general, most of the toxic effects observed on rat marrow are benign variations in cellularity or

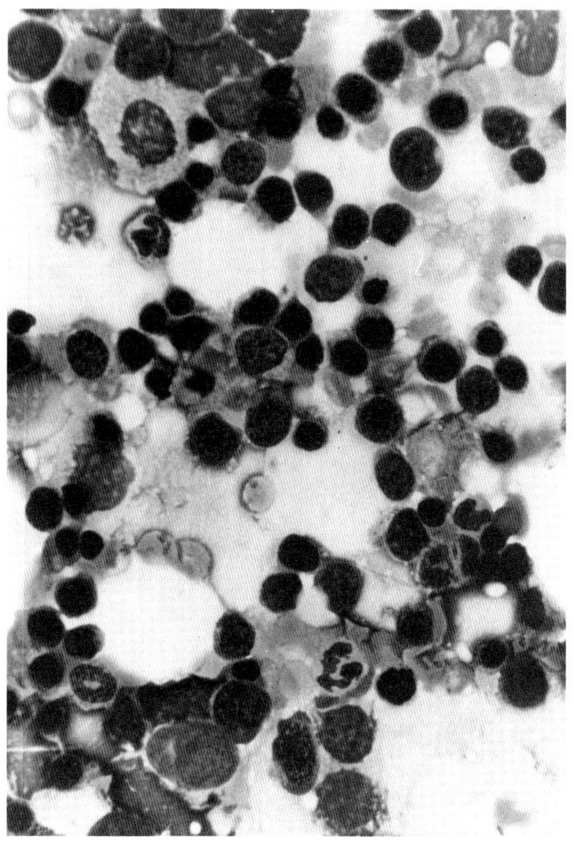

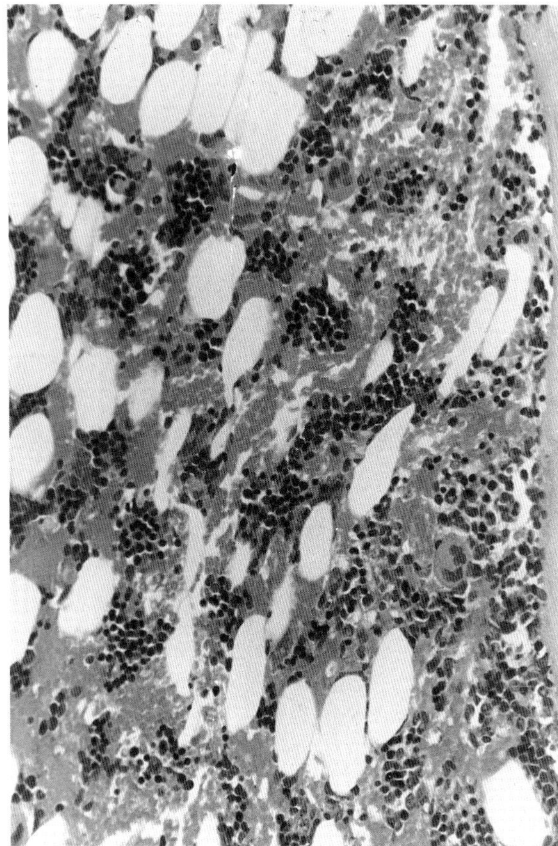

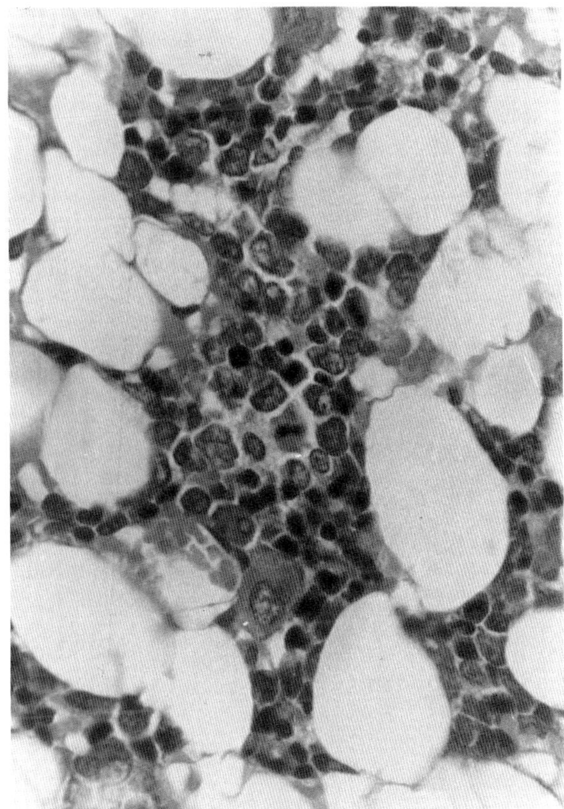

Fig. 2 *(upper left)*. Myeloid hypoplasia. Bone marrow from a 4-month-old male Wistar rat given a prazosin analogue for 13 weeks. Marrow cytology: remaining cells are largely erythroid. Wright's, ×670

Fig. 3 *(upper right)*. Myeloid hypoplasia, same rat as in Fig. 2. Marrow histology: normal proportion of fat cells with reduced density of hemopoietic cells and greatly expanded sinusoidal volume filled with red cells. H and E, ×270

Fig. 4 *(lower right)*. Higher magnification of Fig. 3. Note paucity of mature granulocytes. H and E, ×670

Table 6. Summary of adverse marrow changes[a]

Conditions	Morphology of change		Kinetics of change	
	Marrow	Blood	Marrow	Blood
Myeloid hyperplasia	Synchronous myelopoiesis; increased M/E	Normal or increased WBC, often with left shift	Increased stem cell input and granulocyte output	Lesion-related increase in granulocyte consumption
Myeloid metaplasia	Late asynchrony; increased M/E	Normal or increased WBC, often with left shift	Increased stem cell input and granulocyte output	No apparent target tissue or lesion
Myeloid hypoplasia	Late asynchrony; decreased M/E	Leukopenia; neutropenia; minimal left shift	Decreased stem cell input and granulocyte output	Shortened granulocyte $t_{1/2}$ due to tissue deficit
Dysmyelopoiesis	Early asynchrony; M/E variable	Normal or reduced WBC; minimal left shift	Adequate stem cell input with impaired maturation	Tissue deficit due to leukopenia and or impaired migration
Megakaryocytic hyperplasia	Synchronous thrombopoiesis; hyperdiploidy	Usually thrombocytopenia with platelet immaturity	Increased stem cell input and platelet output	Shortened $t_{1/2}$ due to increased consumption
Megakaryocytic hypoplasia	Early asynchrony; hypodiploidy	Thrombocytopenia; small pale platelets without immaturity	Decreased stem cell input and platelet output	Normal or shortened platelet $t_{1/2}$ with reduced turnover
Dysthrombopoiesis	Normal or increased ploidy with reduced cytoplasmic volume and maturation	Variable level of small, pale, and poorly granulated platelets	Adequate stem cell input with impaired maturation	Usually reduced platelet $t_{1/2}$ and turnover
Erythroid hyperplasia	Synchronous erythropoiesis; decreased M/E	Increased or decreased red cells with immaturity; anisocytosis	Increased stem cell input and red cell output	Normal red cell $t_{1/2}$, (hypoxic) or reduced (hemolysis); increased turnover
Erythroid hypoplasia	Late asynchrony; increased M/E	Normochromic normocytic anemia without immaturity	Decreased stem cell input and red cell output	Normal red cell $t_{1/2}$; reduced turnover
Dyserythropoiesis	Early asynchrony with binucleation, micronuclei, and late stage mitoses	Normochromic normocytic anemia without immaturity	Adequate stem cell input with impaired maturation	Normal red cell $t_{1/2}$; reduced turnover

M/E, myeloid/erythroid ratio.
[a] The changes listed here may be caused by toxic, immune, or idiopathic mechanisms.

frank tumors with the spontaneous myelodysplastic syndromes as seen in humans, cats, and dogs occurring rarely (Table 6).

Hyperplastic Changes

Figures 5–15 form relatively straightforward interpretations with subjective evaluations made on marrow histology easily verified by differential counts on marrow cytologic spreads. If an apparently increased marrow production appears in the blood as increased cell counts or increases in immature cells (bands, reticulocytes, shift platelets), then a diagnosis of hyperplasia is ap-

Fig. 5 *(upper left).* Myeloid hyperplasia. Bone marrow ▶ from a 4-month-old male Sprague-Dawley rat dosed dermally with a coal liquefaction product at 400 mg/kg body weight daily for 13 weeks. Marrow cytology: increased proportion of myeloid cells many of which are mature neutrophils. Wright's, × 670

Fig. 6 *(lower left).* Myeloid hyperplasia, same rat as in Fig. 5. Marrow histology: hypercellularity. H and E, × 1070

Fig. 7 *(upper right).* Myeloid hyperplasia, detail of Fig. 6 showing increased mature granulocyte reserves. H and E, × 1070

Fig. 8 *(lower right).* Myeloid hyperplasia. Unusual hyperplasia in an untreated 2-year-old male Wistar rat. Marrow cytology: myeloid foci. Wright's, × 670

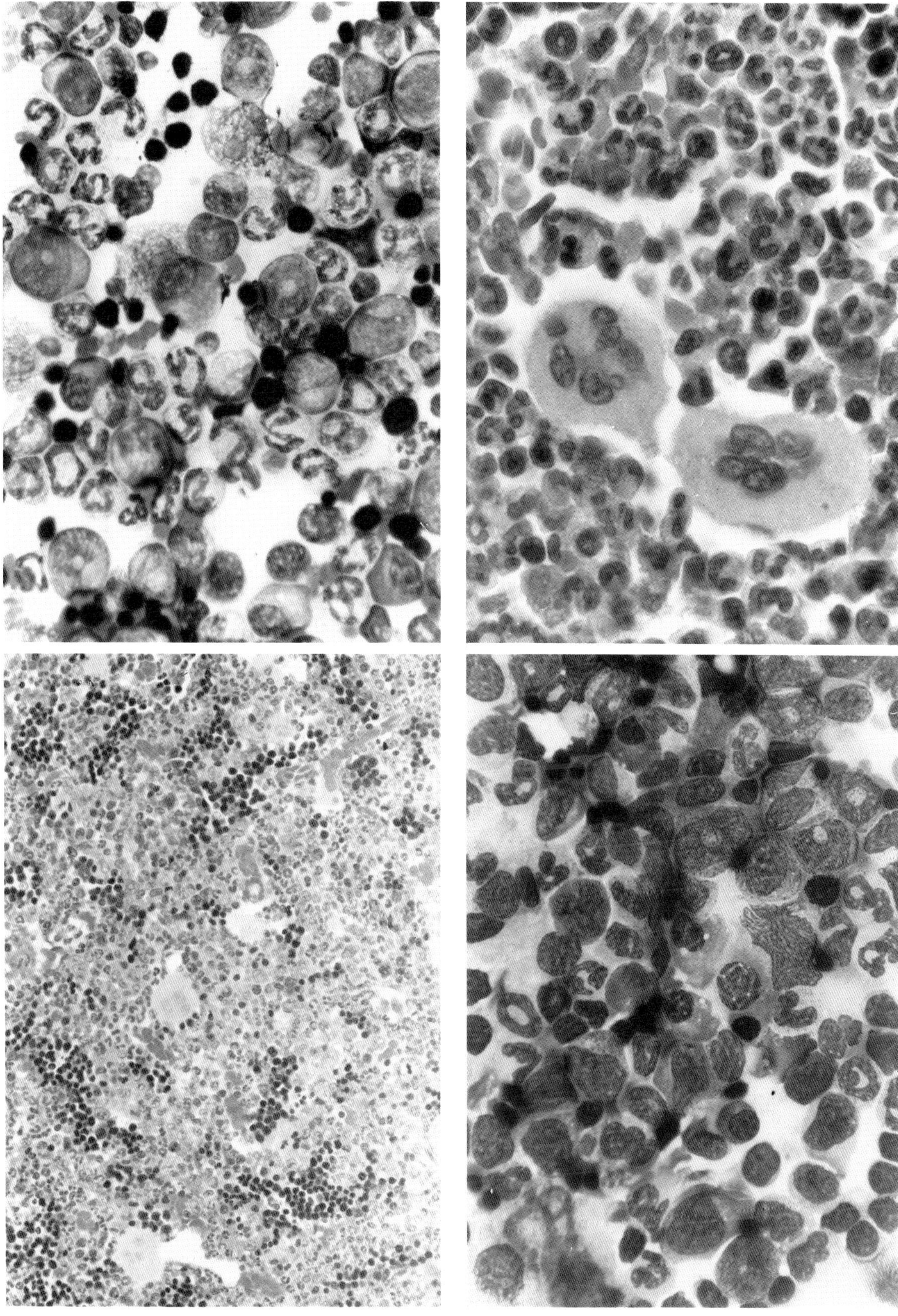

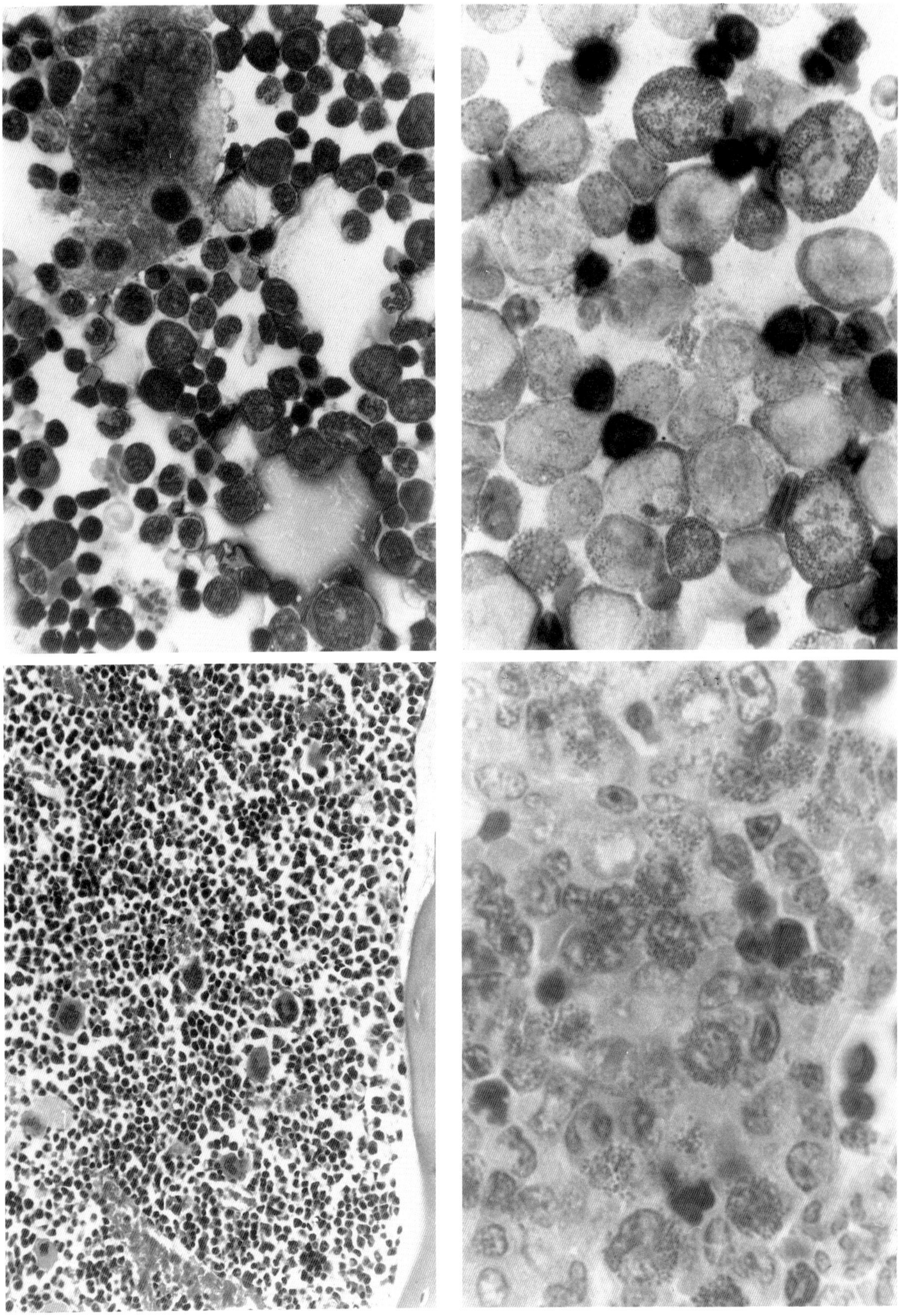

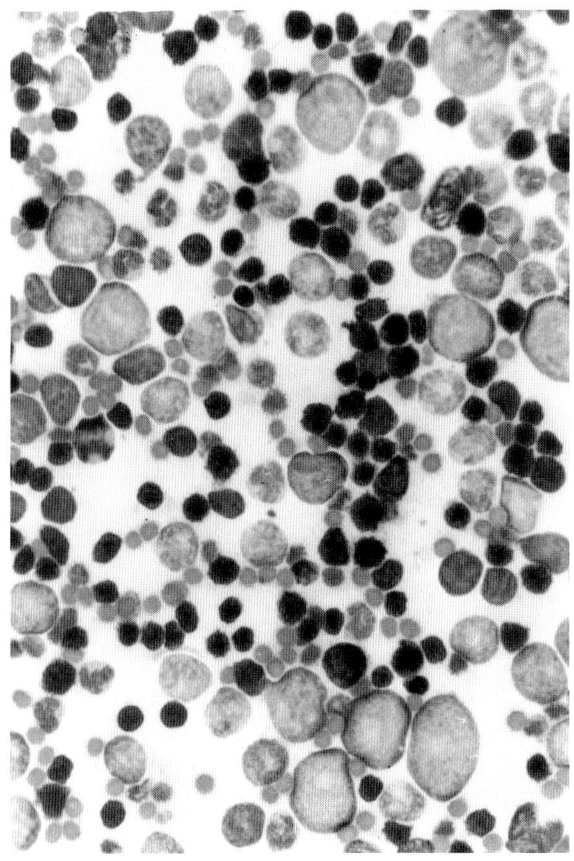

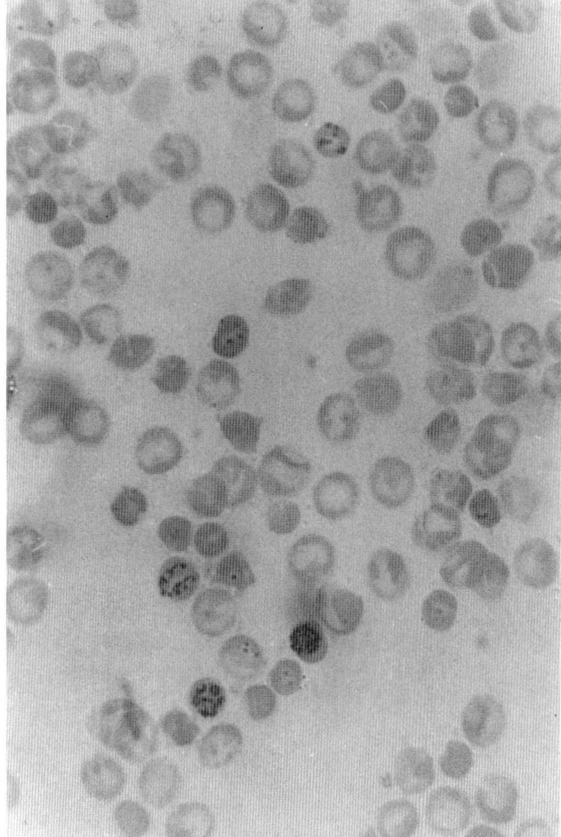

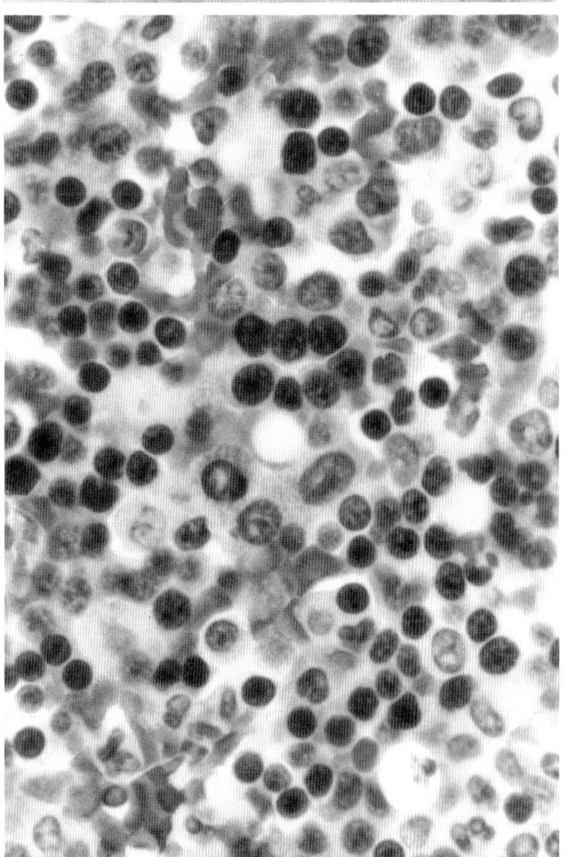

◄ **Fig. 9** *(upper left)*. Myeloid hyperplasia, same animal as in Fig. 8. Erythroid foci. Wright's, × 670

Fig. 10 *(lower left)*. Myeloid hyperplasia, same animal as in Fig. 8. Marrow histology: hypercellularity. H and E, × 270

Fig. 11 *(upper right)*. Myeloid hyperplasia. Eosinophil hyperplasia in a 3-month-old Sprague-Dawley rat dosed dermally with a coal processing product at 800 mg/kg bw daily for 6 weeks. Marrow cytology: area of dense eosinopoiesis. Wright's, × 1070

Fig. 12 *(lower right)*. Myeloid hyperplasia, same animal as in Fig. 11. Histology. H and E, × 1700

Fig. 13 *(upper left)*. Erythroid hyperplasia. Bone marrow ► from a male Sprague-Dawley rat in the same group as that of Fig. 16. Marrow cytology: an erythroid area with numerous rubricytes most of which are in maturation phase. Wright's, × 670

Fig. 14 *(upper right)*. Erythroid hyperplasia. Blood, increased level of young red cells and a polychromatic rubricyte. Reticulocyte stain, × 1070

Fig. 15 *(lower right)*. Erythroid hyperplasia. Marrow histology: increased proportion of erythroid cells with normal maturation sequence. H and E, × 1070 propriate. If, on the contrary, marrow hyperplasia is not accompanied by evidence of increased cell release to the blood, then a dysplastic (Figs. 16–19) or metaplastic condition may be present. Myeloid hyperplasia with synchronous maturation and no apparent target in the peripheral system suggests myeloid metaplasia, especially if the leukocyte count is near normal levels. Comparable changes in the erythroid system are rare or do not occur. Hyperplasia with an increased proportion of proliferative phase cells and accompanied by morphologic abnormalities and with or without peripheral blood cytopenia suggests dyshemopoiesis that may be primarily myeloid (Figs. 16–19) or erythroid (Figs. 20, 21), or affect both systems.

These conditions occur as dose-related effects in the rat. Their recognition, however, is not easy, and actual determination of the proportions of proliferating to maturing cells is the most convincing evidence that an asynchronous pattern of maturation exists. In human medicine a paradoxical condition of hyperplastic marrow with cytopenia(s) was referred to as "myelokathexis" (Zeulzer 1964) and the "preleukemic syndrome" (Linman and Saarni 1974). The recognition that a number of syndromes with a varying tendency to evolve into frank malignancy were included in these definitions led to the current terminology of myelodysplastic syndromes (Coiffier et al. 1987). These diseases have been described in domestic animals (Baker and Valli 1986), but the autonomous diseases as described in humans have not been recognized in the rat.

The elucidation of separate systems controlling proliferation and maturation in the erythroid (Shibuya et al. 1982), myeloid (Sachs 1987), and megakaryocytic (Mazur 1987) series puts understanding of the asynchronous maturation of the dysmyelopoietic syndromes on a much more logical basis. Further, these insights into the normal control mechanisms of the hemopoietic system provide a conceptual basis of the treatment of leukemia based on induced differentiation rather than on largely nonspecific cell killing. (Klein 1987; Jiminez and Yunis 1987).

Hypoplastic Changes

These are relatively uncommon responses which present little problem in interpretation since the reduced marrow activity is accurately refleced in reduced cell numbers in the peripheral blood (Figs. 2–4, 22–24). In terms of cell lineage the erythroid system is much more volatile than the myeloid, and "pure" erythroid hypoplasia and aplasia are much more common than hypoplasia involving only the myeloid system. Myeloid aplasia that persists is not compatible with life, and the relatively more resilient myeloid system may have evolved as a change benefitting survival. Rarely, the rat megakaryocytic system suffers both hypoplasia and aplasia with predictable results. An animal such as a parturient female which has gone through a phase of hyperplasia may subsequently develop a relatively hypoplastic-appearing marrow without peripheral cytopenia because of the expanded volume of red marrow.

The proportions of red to yellow marrow may vary quite widely without being abnormal. In general, most young rats have a very cellular marrow with the hemopoietic area occupying 70%–90% of the marrow volume. Older animals have a marrow with a relatively decreased cellularity. We have, however, observed older rats with a very high cellularity in both test and control groups without apparent cause. The marrow tends to have a higher level of hompoiesis near the endosteal bone and near the metaphyses. It is therefore highly desirable to have a consistent pattern of sampling to avoid errors based on normal variation in marrow anatomy.

True *hypoplasia* (Figs. 2–4) will be evident by reduced cellular packing as well as a reduced hemopoietic area. Sections of marrow with normally dense packing of hemopoietic cells but a low proportion of red to yellow marrow is most likely

Fig. 16 *(upper left).* Dysmyelopoiesis. Bone marrow from a 4-month-old male Sprague-Dawley rat dosed with an inorganic lead compound by gavage at 300 mg/kg bw daily for 13 weeks. Marrow areas of myelopoiesis with increased proportion of proliferative phase cells. Cytology, Wright's, × 1070

Fig. 17 *(lower left).* Dysmyelopoiesis, same rat as in Fig. 16. Histology, H and E, × 1370

Fig. 18 *(upper right).* Dysmyelopoiesis. Bone marrow from a male Sprague-Dawley rat given a dermal application of a coal processing product for 6 weeks (same group as in Fig. 11 and 12). Marrow areas of myelopoiesis with an increased proportion of "donut" metamyelocytes and some "giant" forms of these cells. Number of mature granulocytes is increased in proportion to the proliferative phase cells, and they often appear hypersegmented. Cytology, Wright's, × 1070

Fig. 19 *(lower right).* Dysmyelopoiesis, same rat as in Fig. 18. Histology, H and E, × 1370

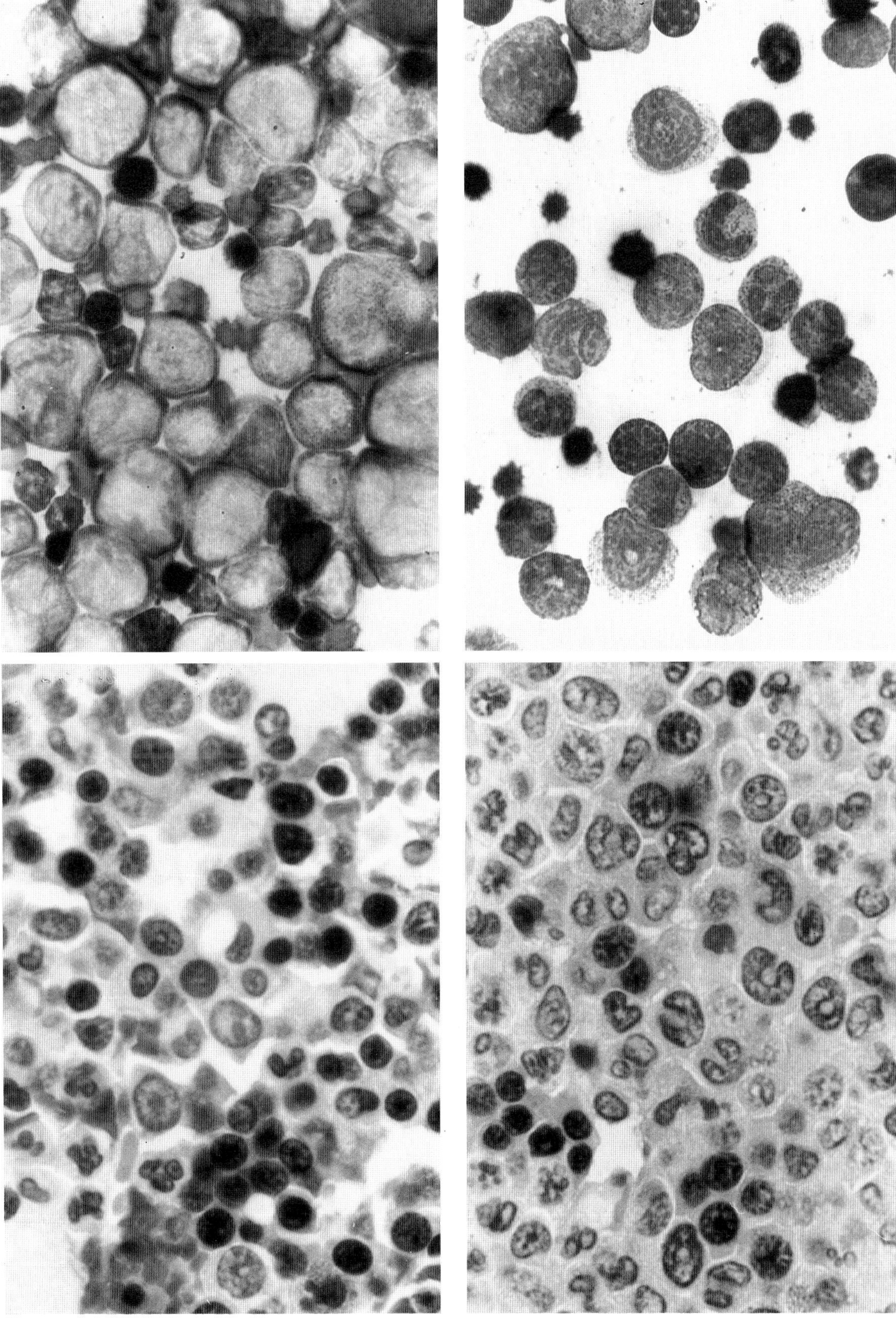

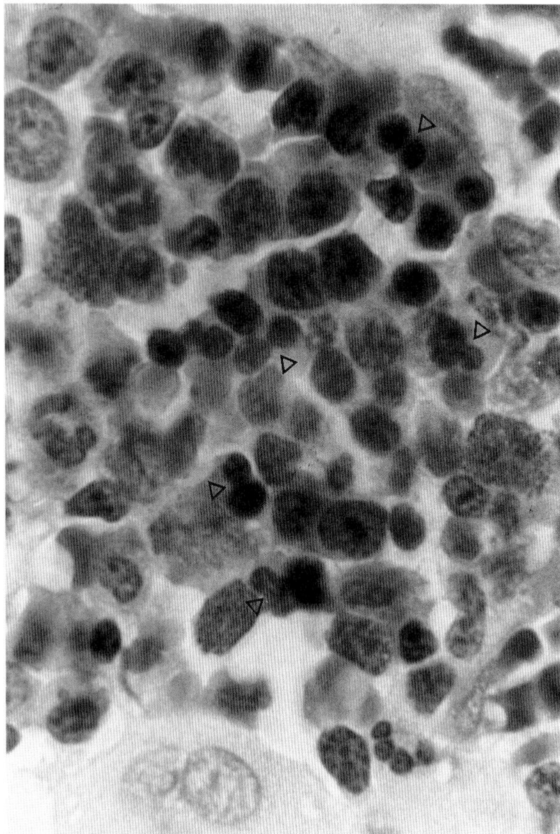

◀ **Fig. 20** *(above)*. Dyserythropoiesis. Bone marrow from a male Sprague-Dawley rat in the same group as that of Figs. 16 and 13 given inorganic lead for 90 days. Changes in the proportion of erythroid cells are accompanied by morphologic abnormalities. Note: asymmetrical binucleation or budding of rubricyte nuclei *(arrowhead)*. H and E, × 1700

Fig. 21 *(below)*. Dyserythropoiesis. Bone marrow, same rat as in Figs. 16 and 13. Increased frequency of erythroid mitoses. *Arrowheads* indicate a prophase *(1)*, metaphase *(2)*, anaphase *(3)*, and telophase *(4)*. H and E, × 1700

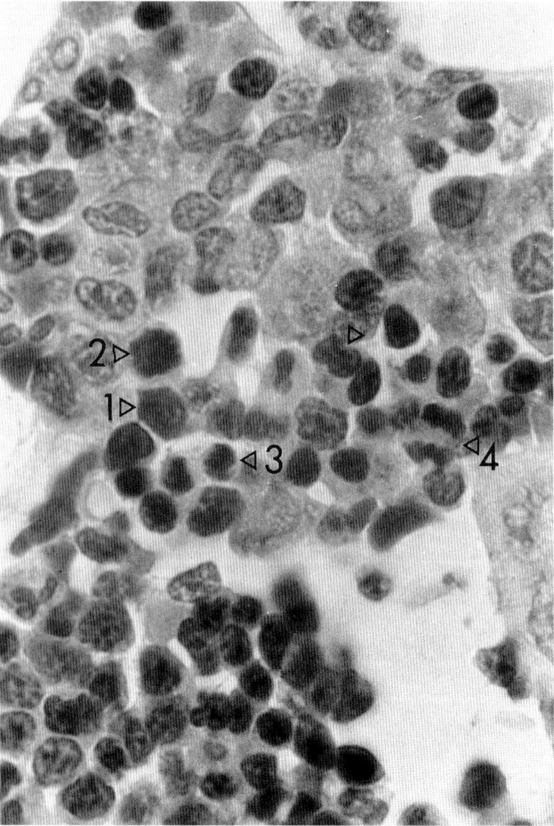

normal and from an area with normally low cellularity. Thus, it is essential to evaluate both cellularity (hemopoietic to fatty area) and cell density or cellular packing.

Maturation Index

In normal mammals the proportion of proliferating to maturing marrow cells tends to remain close to a 1:4 ratio. The kinetic basis for this relationship has been described for humans (Killman et al. 1963), dogs (Raab et al. 1964), rats (Lapin et al. 1969), and the calf (Valli et al. 1971). These studies are compatible with the concept that the proliferative phase cells of the myeloid and erythroid systems divide to produce two heteromorphogenic (differently appearing) progeny. Thus, the output of a single unipotential stem cell produces: one myeloblast, two promyelocytes, four myelocytes, and eight metamyelocytes. Some homomorphogenic (similarly appearing) metamyelocyte and probable myelocyte and basophylic rubricyte divisions occur to produce about ten maturing cells. These seven proliferative phase cells (1 + 2 + 4) and thirty (10 + 10 + 10) maturation phase cells constitute the typical 1:4 relationship characteristic of normal marrow.

The *maturation index* is the ratio between the number of proliferative phase cells to the number of maturation phase cells counted in the bone marrow. For convenience this ratio has been expressed as a fraction (8/30 = 0.23) in this report. The consistency of the maturation indices in normal rats is remarkable, as can be seen in Table 5 where the overall mean of the ten ratios is 0.253. The utility of this concept was investigated in dogs (Hoff et al. 1985) with the conclusion that these ratios were not frequently altered in spontaneous diseases of that species. We conclude that these measures of synchronous maturation

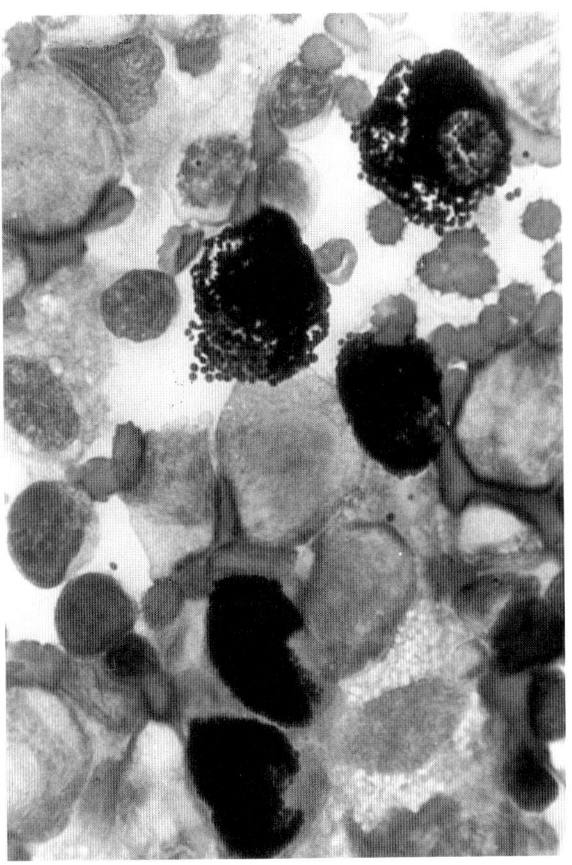

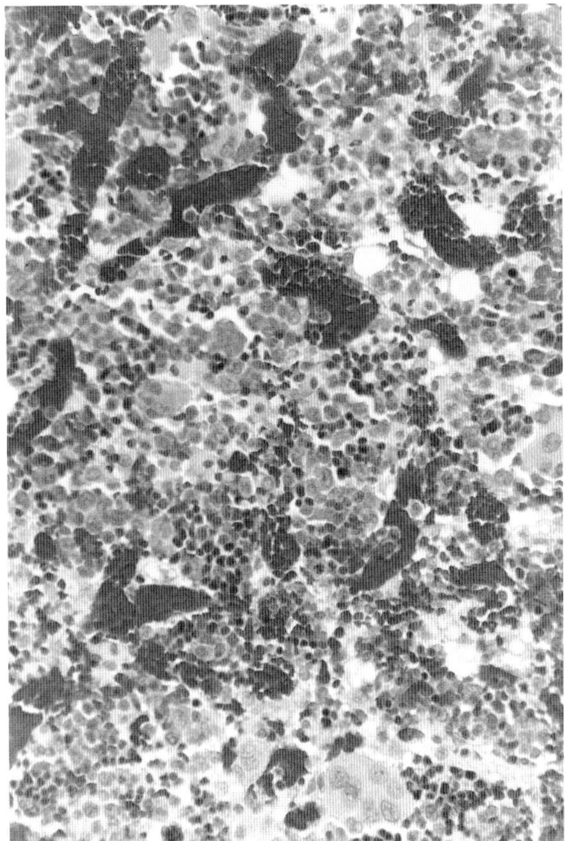

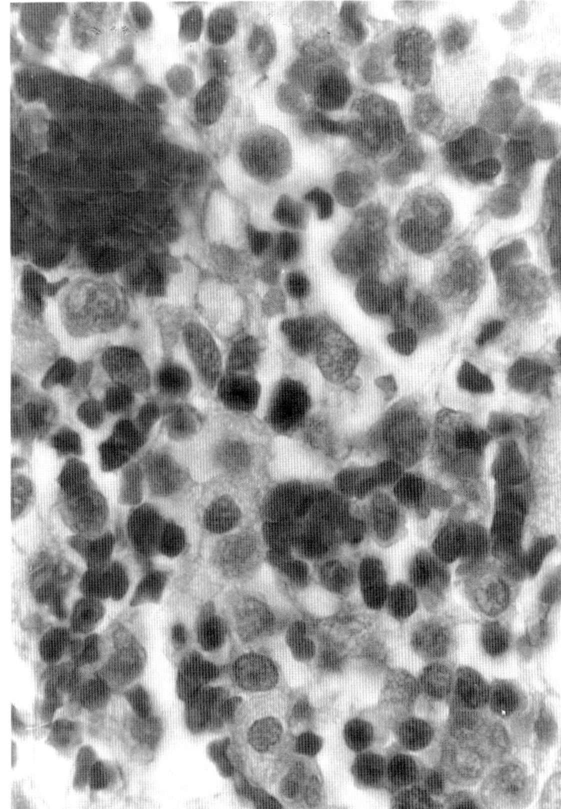

Fig. 22 *(upper left).* Erythroid hypoplasia. Bone marrow from a male Sprague-Dawley rat given a coprocessing product intratracheally at 75 mg/kg bw daily, 5 days/week for 2 weeks. Marrow cytology: erythroid atrophy and mast cell hyperplasia. Mature granulocytes are reduced in number. Wright's, × 1070

Fig. 23 *(upper right).* Eythroid hypoplasia. Marrow histology: a hypercellular marrow with few fat cells and an early loss of cell density evident by prominent sinusoidal dilatation and reduced cellular packing. H and E, × 270

Fig. 24 *(lower right).* Erythroid hypoplasia. Higher magnification of Fig. 23 with erythroid atrophy, early myeloid asynchrony, and dilated, congested vessels. H and E, × 1070 are useful to verify subjective interpretations of ineffective hemopoiesis. Good marrow spreads are essential for an accurate assessment of marrow function and especially for determining proliferative indices since marrow diluted with peripheral blood may have an excess of maturing myeloid cells.

Dose-Related Changes in Blood and Bone Marrow

Myeloid Hyperplasia

This is a condition characterized by an increased proportion of myeloid cells as indicated by an increase in the myeloid/erythroid ratio with a normal synchrony of cellular maturation or in other words a normal ratio of proliferating to maturing myeloid cells. In the case illustrated in Figs. 5–7 the mean total leukocyte count for the treated group increased from 7.7 to $11.7 \times 10^9/l$, and the total neutrophils increased from 0.80 to $3.1 \times 10^9/l$. The myeloid/erythroid ratio for this specific animal increased to 1.45 compared with 1.10 for controls (Table 4) while the Maturation Index for myeloid cells (0.22) remained in the normal range. The Maturation Index for erythroid cells was increased out of the normal range to 0.39. This change indicates a competent myeloid marrow response to increased peripheral demands induced by dermal injury and/or systemic toxicity. The increased erythroid Maturation Index is indicative of stress on this system. This animal was mildly anemic with the lowest hemoglobin level in this group (118 g/l) and had increased reticulocytes ($176 \times 10^9/l$) as compared with means of 143.2 g/l of hemoglobin and reticulocytes of $118 \times 10^9/l$ for the control group.

Myeloid Hypoplasia

This is a relative and absolute reduction in marrow granulocytes without a major change in the other cell lines. In the case illustrated in Figs. 2–4 the total leukocyte count was reduced to one-half that of the control group and total neutrophils to one-third that of the controls. The mean myeloid/erythroid ratio of the controls was 1.0 and 0.4 in the group from which this animal was derived. Maturation indices were not determined. The red cell and platelet systems were relatively unaffected.

Dysmyelopoiesis

Dysmyelopoiesis, or less appropriately, *myelodysplasia*, is a condition characterized by asynchronous maturation of the granulocytic cells. The animal given inorganic lead illustrated in Figs. 16, 17 had an increase in the Maturation Index of both myeloid cells (0.39; control level of 0.21; Table 5) and erythroid cells (0.31) while the myeloid/erythroid ratio (1.17) was near normal. The mean total leukocyte count of the treated group was reduced, but total granulocytes were at normal levels without immaturity. The normal level of marrow myeloid cells and blood neutrophils with an increased proportion of proliferative phase cells indicates ineffective myelopoiesis with early asynchrony. The animal was not anemic, but the reticulocyte count was increased to $333 \times 10^9/l$. The animal given the dermal coal processing product (Figs. 18, 19) had neutrophilia with a mean leukocyte count in the treated group of $13.65 \times 10^9/l$ (controls, 7.82) and an myeloid/erythroid ratio increased to 1.88 (controls, 1.10). The Maturation Index was reduced for both myeloid (0.15) and erythroid (0.17) systems, with increased proportions of mature cells. There was mild anemia in the treated group. These changes indicate ineffective hemopoiesis of both systems with late asynchrony that may be associated with impaired release of mature cells (Dormer et al. 1987).

Megakaryocytic Hyperplasia

In Figs. 25, 26 it can be seen that like myeloid hyperplasia, megakaryocytic hyperplasia is characterized by increased numbers of cells of the lineage with a normal sequence of maturation. The platelet counts are decreased in the treated group to a mean of $692 \times 10^9/l$ from a control mean of $1035 \times 10^9/l$, and the animal depicted had a count of $751 \times 10^9/l$. The hemoglobin level of the treated animals was slightly decreased to 143 g/l from 149 g/l in the controls, and the mean leukocyte count was increased to $13.3 \times 10^9/l$ from $7.8 \times 10^9/l$ in the controls. The blood platelets had increased basophilia and granulation with some large oval forms. These changes suggest increased marrow output of platelets with this level of hyperplasia inadequate to compensate completely for increased peripheral consumption.

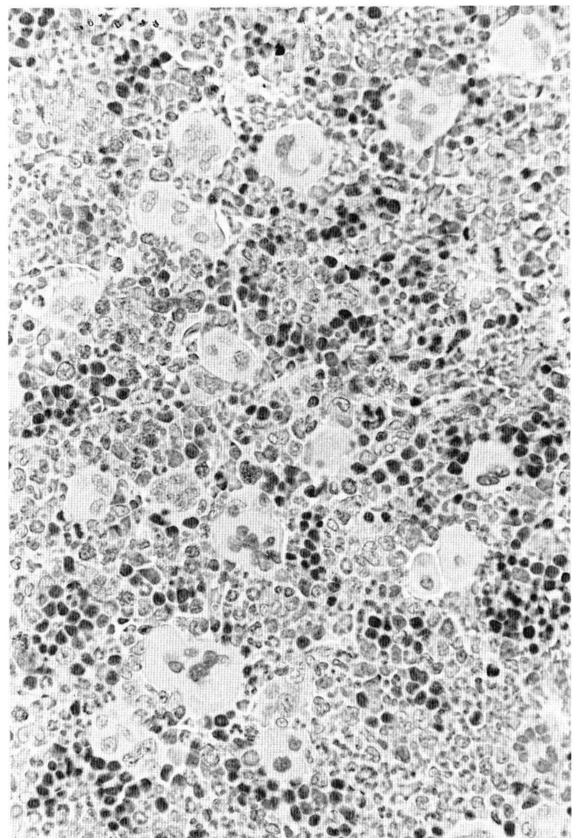

◄ **Fig. 25** *(above)*. Megakaryocytic hyperplasia. Bone marrow from a 3-month-old male Sprague-Dawley rat administered a coprocessing product by dermal application at 1000 mg/kg bw daily, 5 days a week for 2 weeks. High cellularity with increased density of normal appearing megakaryocytes. Histology, H and E, × 430

Fig. 26 *(below)*. Megakaryocytic hyperplasia, same rat as Fig. 25. H and E, × 1070

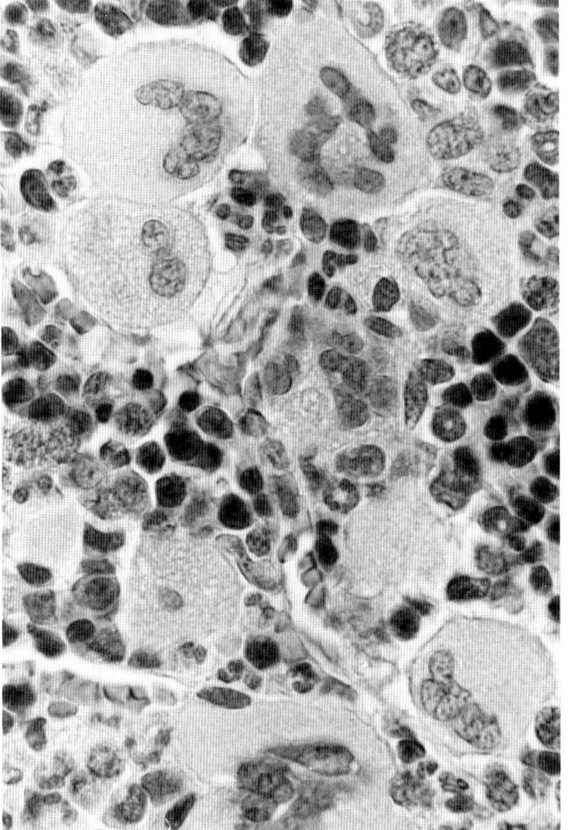

Dysthrombopoiesis

This is a condition of abnormal maturation of the megakaryocytes. The animal illustrated in Figs. 27–29 had a normal platelet count with small, poorly granulated cells. The reduced megakaryocyte cytoplasmic volume relative to nuclear volume with increased numbers of precursors without increased output suggests ineffective thrombopoiesis. In Fig. 30 the female rat given the coal processing product had increased numbers of megakaryocytes and a platelet count nearly double that of the controls. The platelets were small and poorly granulated and may have had decreased functional capacity. This case demonstrates mild impairment of a hyperplastic response. The anmial given inorganic lead (Fig. 31) had one-third the level of platelets of the controls despite increased numbers of megakaryocytes. In this case the impairment of maturation was more severe, with well-developed, ineffective thrombopoiesis.

Erythroid Hyperplasia

This is characterized by an increase in erythroid precursors which results in an increase in reticulocytes in the peripheral blood. In Figs. 13–15 the animal illustrated had only a slight reduction in its myeloid/erythroid ratio (1.06) with an increase in the Maturation Index of erythroid cells to 0.38 and myeloid cells to 0.52 (controls, erythroid 0.24 and myeloid 0.27; Table 5). The reticulocyte count was increased from a mean of $97 \times 10^9/l$ in the controls to $175 \times 10^9/l$ in this animal. The mean erythrocyte count for the treated group increased while the mean red cell indices and hemoglobin level decreased. This demonstrates a functional response of the erythroid system in terms of stem cell generation and cell output but the lack of macrocytosis and poor cell saturation are indications of toxic impairment of hemoglobin synthesis.

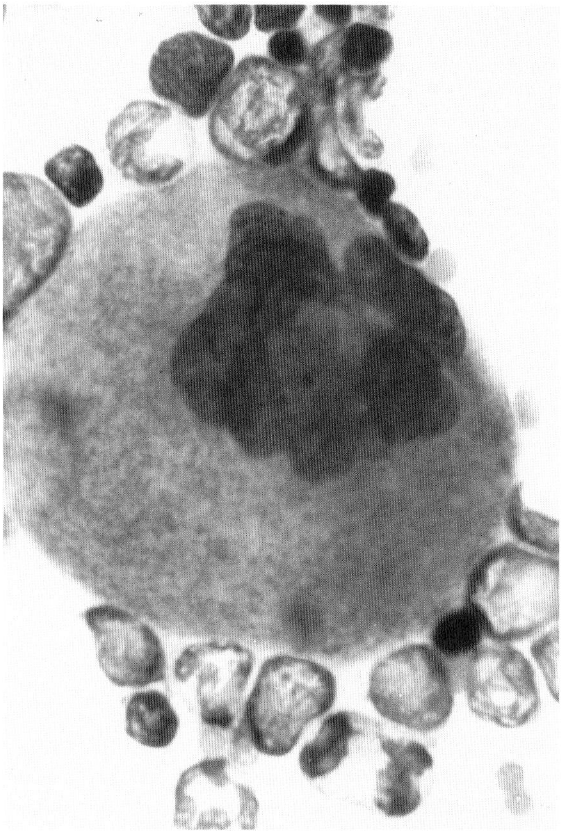

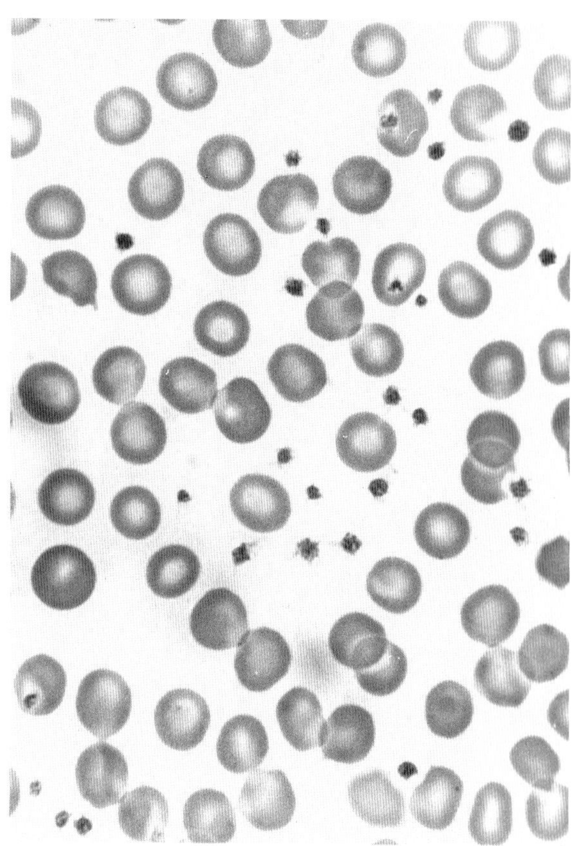

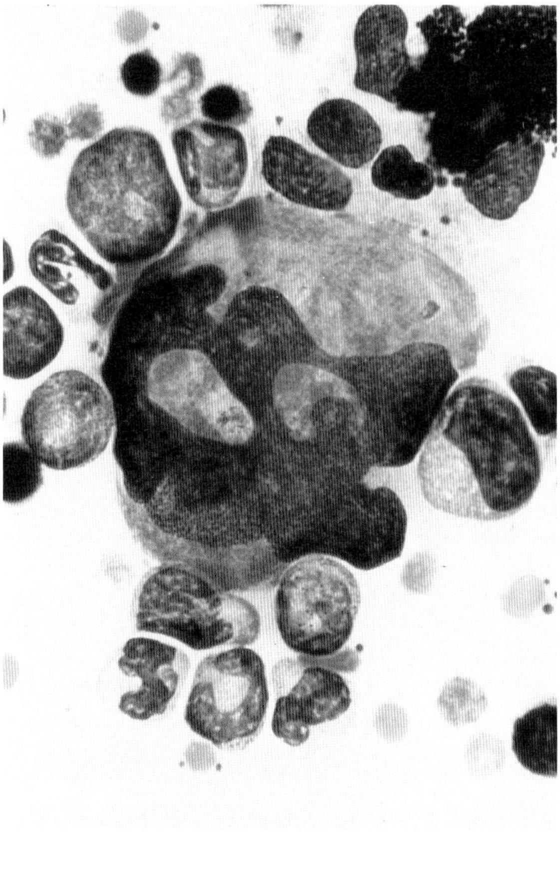

Fig. 27 *(upper left).* Dysthrombopoiesis. Bone marrow from a 3-month-old male Sprague-Dawley rat dosed orally with a coal processing product at 100 mg/kg bw daily for 28 days. Marrow cytology: normal-appearing megakaryocyte with abundant, well-granulated cytoplasm and vesicular nucleus in early regression. Wright's, × 1070

Fig. 28 *(lower left).* Dysthrombopoiesis, same rat as Fig. 27. Megakaryocyte with low volume of poorly granulated cytoplasm, large hyperchromatic nucleus with atypical fusion of nuclear lobes. Wright's, × 1070

Fig. 29 *(upper right).* Dysthrombopoiesis. Blood, platelets are all small and highly basophilic. Wright's, × 1070

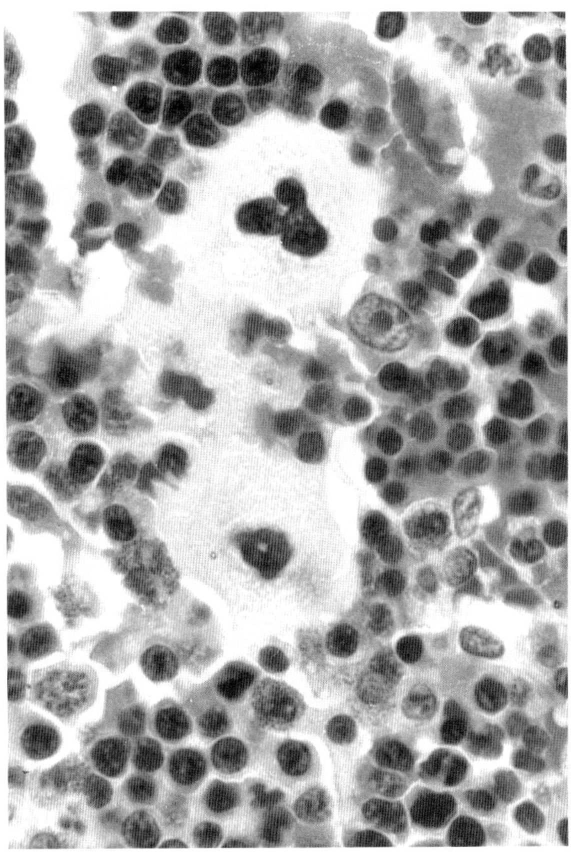

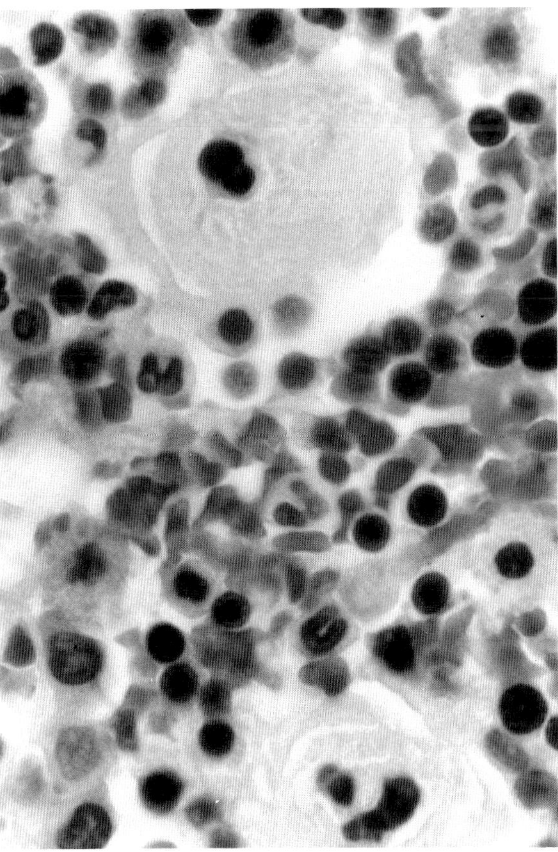

◀**Fig. 30** *(above)*. Dysthrombopoiesis. Bone marrow from a pregnant Sprague-Dawley rat dosed dermally with a coal liquefaction product at 500 mg/kg bw daily on days 6–15 of gestation. Histology: megakaryocytes have a slightly reduced volume of poorly granulated cytoplasm with asynchronous early pyknosis. H and E, × 1070

Fig. 31 *(below)*. Dysthrombopoiesis. Bone marrow from a male Sprague-Dawley rat given inorganic lead orally for 90 days. Histology: megakaryocytes have reduced cytoplasmic granulation with artefactual fracturing and early pyknosis. H and E, × 1070

Erythroid Hypoplasia

This is characterized by a reduction in erythroid precursors and peripheral blood reticulocytes with minimal alteration in the other cell lines. The animal illustrated in Figs. 22–24 had lost weight at termination, and anemia was most likely masked by blood volume contraction and dehydration. Red cell indices were not altered, but the mean reticulocyte count was $196 \times 10^9/l$ in the control group and $134 \times 10^9/l$ in the treated group and $87 \times 10^9/l$ or less than half of normal in this animal. The animal had mild leukopenia with an increased proportion of neutrophils. The myeloid Maturation Index was near normal at 0.30. The myeloid/erythroid ratio was 1.32 (control level 1.06; Table 4), and the erythroid Maturation Index was reduced to 0.16 (control level 0.23; Table 5). This demonstrates a reduced stem cell input into the erythroid series, mild late asynchrony, and depressed reticulocyte response.

Dyserythropoiesis

This ist characterized by morphologic abnormalities of the rubricytes consisting of nuclear duplication, satellitism, and "budding". The animal illustrated in Figs. 20, 21 had a near normal red cell count with reticulocytes increased slightly from a mean of $97 \times 10^9/l$ in the controls to $120 \times 10^9/l$. The myeloid/erythroid ratio was near normal at 1.0; the Maturation Index for erythroid cells was increased from a control level of 0.24 (Table 5) to 0.44, and the myeloid Maturation Index (0.34) was high normal. This demonstrates a normal level of stem cell input with early asynchrony and largely effective production despite morphologic changes of heavy metal toxicity.

References

Archer RK, Jeffcott LB (1977) Comparative clinical haematology. Blackwell Scientific, Oxford

Baker RJ, Valli VEO (1986) Dysmyelopoiesis in the cat: a hematological disorder resembling refractory anemia with excess blasts in man. Can J Vet Res 50: 3–6

Beckstead JH (1985) Optimal antigen localization in human tissues using aldehyde-fixed plastic-embedded sections. J Histochem Cytochem 33: 954–958

Benirschke K, Garner FM, Jones TC (1978) Pathology of laboratory animals, vol 1. Springer, Berlin Heidelberg New York

Beckhardt K, Büttner D, Müschen U, Plonait H (1983) Influence of bleeding procedure and some environmental conditions on stress-dependent blood constituents of the laboratory rat. Lab Anim 17: 161–165

Burek JD (1978) Pathology of aging rats. CRC Press, Boca Raton

Coiffier B, Adeleine P, Gentilhomme O, Felman P, Treille-Ritouet DC, Bryon PA (1987) Myelodysplastic syndromes: a multiparametric study of prognostic factors in 336 patients. Cancer 60: 3029–3032

Cronkite EP, Burlington H, Chanana AD, Joel DD (1985) Regulation of Granulopoiesis. Prog Clin Biol Res 184: 129–144

Dacie JV, Lewis SM (1975) Practical haematology, 5th edn. Churchill Livingstone, Edinburgh

De Bruyn PPH (1981) Structural substrates of marrow function. Semin Hematol 18: 179–193

Dormer P, Hershko C, Wilmanns W (1987) Mechanisms and prognostic value of cell kinetics in the myelodysplastic syndromes. Br J Haematol 67: 147–152

Gong JK (1978) Endosteal marrow: a rich source of hematopoietic stem cells. Science 199: 1443–1445

Greaves P, Faccini JM (1984) Rat histopathology. A glossary for use in toxicity and carcinogenicity studies. Elsevier, Amsterdam

Hershko C, Cook JD, Finch CA (1973) Storage iron kinetics. III. Study of desferrioxamine action by selective radioiron labels of RE and parenchymal cells. J Lab Clin Med 81: 876–886

Hoff B, Lumsden JH, Valli VEO (1985) An appraisal of bone marrow biopsy in assessment of sick dogs. Can J Comp Med 49: 34–42

Irons RD (ed) (1985) Toxicology of the blood and bone marrow. Target organ toxicology series. Raven, New York

Jain NC (1986) Schalm's veterinary hematology, 4th edn. Lea and Febiger, Philadelphia

Jasty V, Bare JJ, Jamison JR, Porter MC, Kowalski RL, Clemens GR, Jackson GE, Hartnagel RE Jr (1986) Spontaneous lesions in the sternums of growing rats. Lab Anim Sci 36: 48–51

Jiminez JJ, Yunis AA (1987) Tumor cell rejection through terminal cell differentiation. Science 238: 1278–1280

Killmann S-A, Cronkite EP, Fleidner TM, Bond VP, Brecher G (1963) Mitotic indices of human bone marrow cells. II. Use of mitotic indices for estimation of time parameters of proliferation in serially connected multiplicative cellular compartments. Blood 21: 141–163

Klein G (1987) The approaching era of the tumor suppressor genes. Science 238: 1539–1544

Lapin DM, LoBue J, Gordi AS, Zanjani ED, Schultz EF (1969) Mechanisms of leukocyte production and release. IX. Kinetics of leukocyte release in leukocytapheresed rats. Proc Soc Exp Biol Med 131: 756–759

Lichtman MA (1981) The ultrastructure of the hemopoietic environment of the marrow: a review. Exp Hematol 9: 391–410

Linman JW, Saarni MI (1974) The preleukemic syndrome. Semin Hematol 11: 93–98

Maniatis A, Tavasolli M, Crosby WH (1971) Factors affecting the conversion of yellow to red marrow. Blood 37: 581–586

Mazur EM (1987) Megakaryocytopoiesis and platelet production: a review. Exp Hematol 15: 340–350

Murray MJ, Stein N, Bjerke R (1970) Do iron stores affect absorption and distribution of iron in pregnancy? J Lab Clin Med 75: 747–753

Quimby FH, Saxon PA, Goff LG (1948) Total white cell counts of peripheral and heart blood of the rat. Science 107: 477

Raab SO, Athens JW, Haab OP, Boggs DR, Ashenbrucker H, Cartwright GE, Wintrobe MM (1964) Granulokinetics in normal dogs. Am J Physiol 206: 83–88

Sachs L (1987) The molecular control of blood cell development. Science 238: 1374–1379

Shibuya T, Niho Y, Mak TW (1982) Erythroleukemia induction by friend leukemia virus. J Exp Med 156: 398–414

Schuit KE, Krebs RE (1982) Depressed blood neutrophil response to lithium stimulation in newborn rats. J Reticuloendothel Soc 31: 523–527

Tavassoli M, Maniatis A, Binder RA, Crosby WH (1971) Studies on marrow histogenesis. II. Growth characteristics of medullary marrow autotransplants. Proc Soc Exp Biol Med 138: 868–870

Valli VEO, Hulland TJ, Mcsherry BJ, Robinson GA, Gilman JPW (1971) The kinetics of hematopoiesis in the calf. I. An autoradiographical study of myelopoiesis in normal, anaemic and endotoxin treated calves. Res Vet Sci 12: 535–550

Weiss L (1965) The structure of bone marrow. Functional interrelationships of vascular and hematopoietic compartments in experimental anemia: an electron microscopic study. J Morphol 117: 467–538

World Health Organization (1977) The SI for the Health professions. WHO, Geneva

Zeulzer WW (1964) 'Myelokathexis' a new form of chronic granulocytopenia report of a case. N Engl J Med 270: 699–704

Normal Blood Cell Values, Rat

Yves Bailly and Pierre Duprat

Introduction

The blood (and bone marrow) constitutes a highly dispersed organ system which includes a widely heterogeneous population of cells, each having a specialized function in the total body system. Hematology is a science laid down on validated methodologic approaches, and it has seen many advances in the past 2 decades as a result of the growth of knowledge of blood cell functions and interactions. Hematology provides insights into the understanding of pathologic processes involved in toxicity or safety profile of drugs and chemical compounds and complements information obtained from clinical signs, biochemical and urine analysis, and gross and microscopic examinations. Baseline control data are established and available for comparison during critical analysis of the hematologic profile for possible disease or compound-induced or spontaneous changes in parameters. Variations are known to occur as a result of different analytical procedures (Nachtman et al. 1985), sampling sites (Duprat et al. 1975; Upton and Morgan 1975; Archer and Riley 1981; Suber and Kodell 1985; Smith et al. 1986; Duprat 1987), handling at the time of sampling (anesthetized versus nonanesthetized), type of anesthetic used, frequency of sampling (Nachtman et al. 1985), nutrition, and environment (Yamanuchi et al. 1981). However, these key points can usually be identified and controlled. There appears to be few fundamental differences in hematologic parameters between different rat strains (Creskoff et al. 1949; Didisheim et al. 1959; Youatt et al. 1961; Burns and DeLannoy 1966; Schermer 1967; Vondruska and Greco 1973; Ringler and Dabich 1979; Lewi and Marsboom 1981; Yamanuchi et al. 1981; Archer et al. 1982; Weil 1982; Jain 1986; Leonard and Ruben 1986). This section will focus on a brief summary of the light and ultrastructural morphology of peripheral blood cells, blood cell counts, and their variations as a function of age in Sprague-Dawley rats of Crl:CD (SD) BR stock from Charles River (France), maintained under standardized conditions between 1982 and 1987.

Biologic Features (Light and Electron Microscopy)

Erythrocytes

Erythrocytes are 6–7 µm in diameter, flat, biconcave discs. They form the greatest population of blood cells with minimal variation in size (almost no anisocytosis) and hemoglobin content (neither polychromasia nor polychromatophilia) in healthy adult rats (Ringler and Dabich 1979). Polychromasia and macrocytosis are common in very young rats and anisocytosis and anisochromasia in "aged" rats above 22 months of age in this stock.

Scanning electron microscopy (SEM) reveals the biconcave disc shape of erythrocytes (Fig. 32). Transmission electron microscopy (TEM) confirms that fact and also the total absence of intracytoplasmic organelles.

Erythrocytes carry hemoglobin and transport oxygen to body systems but normally do not leave the cardiovascular system. Hemoglobin structure as studied by Shaw and MacLean (1971) and Garrick et al. (1974) is thought to be composed of five globin chains: two alpha and three beta; since then it has received little attention, especially in this strain of rats. Their second function, deformability, allows them to pass through capillaries and this deformability depends on the flexibility of the lipid membrane (Gerrard 1985).

Platelets (Thrombocytes)

In fixed and stained blood smears, platelets are small (2–4 µm), anucleate, membrane-bound fragments of cytoplasm, with a denser central cytoplasm compared with the clearer periphery.

Almost biconvex under scanning illumination, thrombocytes fixed for TEM appear homogeneous as opposed to after fixation in blood smears. They have a fuzzy membrane surface (with numerous penetrating invaginations) and contain cytoplasmic organelles: small mitochondria; several types of vacuoles containing glycogen, fibrinogen, factor VIII, and several other substances involved in blood clotting; microfila-

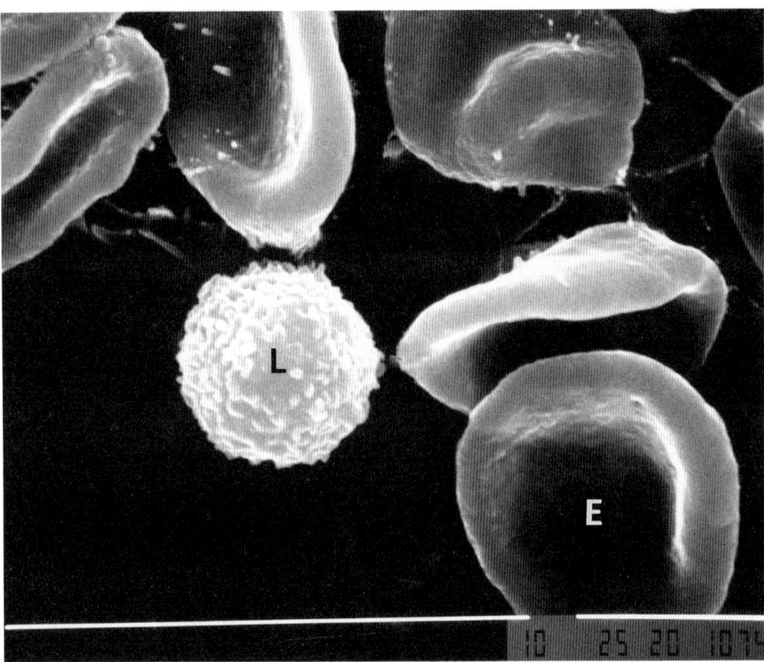

Fig. 32. Erythrocyte *(E);* lymphocyte *(L),* rat. SEM, *bar*= 10 µm

ments and microtubules and membranes of smooth endoplasmic reticulum (Gerrard 1985) forming a system of smooth interconnected tubules (Rhodin 1974), also called the surface-connected canalicular system (Gerrard 1985), which is an important site for calcium storage.

They circulate for a few days in the blood before removal by the spleen and lungs. They play an important role in the response of the blood to vessel wall injury, i. e., the formation of a hemostatic platelet-fibrin plug.

Leukocytes

Lymphocytes. In blood smears, rat lymphocytes vary in size. Small lymphocytes (6–8 µm) represent the vast majority of this type of cell. They are characterized by a nucleus with densely packed chromatin and a scanty rim of cytoplasm. Large lymphocytes (12–15 µm) represent the minority of the lymphocyte population. They have a clearer nucleus which is often eccentrically located and has clumped heterochromatin. An abundant pale cytoplasm often contains azurophilic granules.

When examined by TEM, lymphocyte nuclei are usually round (but sometimes indented) and contain heterochromatin (peripheral clumps) and euchromatin (central core) with occasionally a nucleolus. Sparse cytoplasm occupies a rim around the nucleus and contains small mito-

chondria, numerous free monoribosomes, and profiles of granular endoplasmic reticulum. Short microvilli are present on the cell membrane surface; this has been confirmed by SEM (Fig. 32) and TEM (Fig. 33).

Lymphocytes were viewed as a homogeneous population over the past decades, but they must now be considered as made up of functionally distinct subsets of cells which interact. They contribute to cell-mediated (sensitization to T-cell-dependent antigens; skin hypersensitivity; mitogen reponses) and humoral (antibody formation) immunities, host-resistance, and NK cell functions which are analyzed in immunotoxicity tests.

Polymorphonuclear Leukocytes (Granulocytes; Polymorphs). Circulating polymorphonuclear leukocytes are approximately 12 µm in diameter. In rat blood smears their nuclei are coiled or twisted (Ringler and Dabich 1979), but the nuclear lobulation of these neutrophils is not as pronounced as in humans. Band cells have a ring-shaped nuclear pattern. The cytoplasm of granulocytes contains granules with characteristic staining affinity. Neutrophilic granules are less stainable than in human granulocytes. Eosinophilic granules are prominent and brilliant (birefringent) and tend to mask the nucleus which usually is annular and often twisted. Basophilic granulocytes are very rare in rat blood smears.

TEM reveals granulocytes to have lobulated nuclei and contain clumps of chromatin. Cross sec-

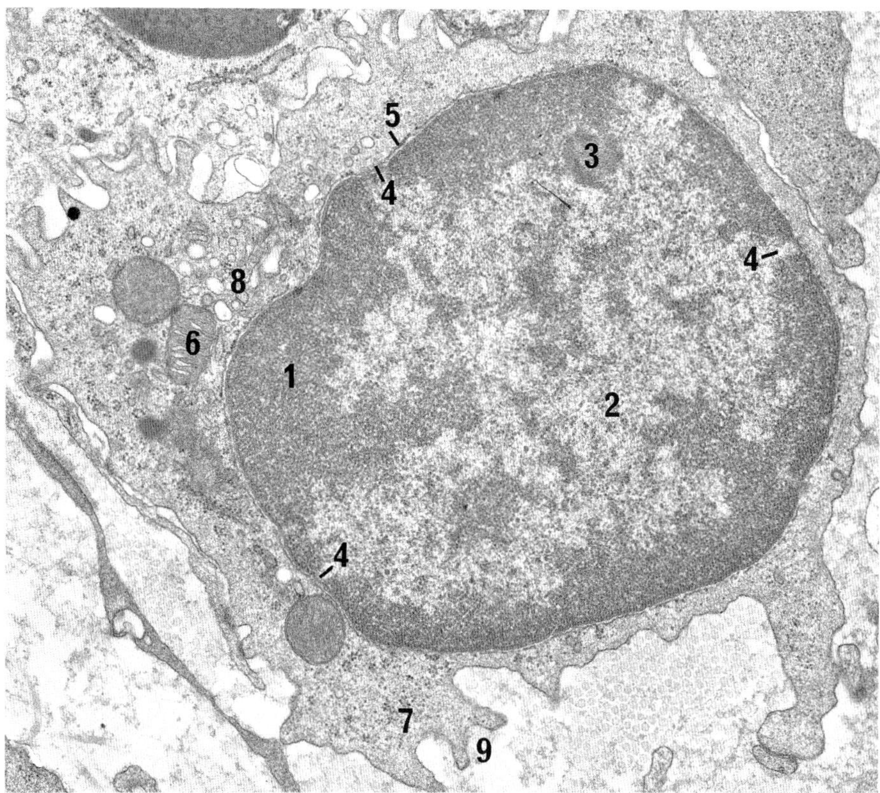

Fig. 33. Lymphocyte, rat. *1,* heterochromatin; *2,* euchromatin; *3,* nucleolus; *4,* nuclear pore areas; *5,* nuclear membrane; *6,* mitochondria; *7,* free monoribosomes; *8,* Golgi system; *9,* microvilli. TEM, × 15 000

tions often indicate separate nuclear profiles, especially in neutrophils and basophils. In eosinophils, chromatin has the same pattern, but the nuclei are less indented. The cytoplasm of granulocytes contains a centrosome, Golgi apparatus, and usually limited endoplasmic reticulum (more abundant and persisting longer in eosinophils than in neutrophils; Gerrard 1985), mitochondria (larger in eosinophils), and cell-specific granules.

The granules are small, heterogeneous, and limited in number in neutrophilic granulocytes. These consist of peripheral primary granules, which correspond to azurophilic granules in smears (specialized lysosomes), and specific (secondary) granules (Fig. 34). These secondary granules are larger and ovoid with more or less electron-dense crystalloids in eosinophilic granulocytes (Fig. 35), as in humans (Gerrard 1985). They are also larger, round, membrane-bound, and filled with electron-dense material in basophilic granulocytes. Microvilli or pseudopodia (Fig. 34) are seen at the periphery of granulocytes (except eosinophils), and, in addition, the cytoplasm of neutrophils contains vacuoles near the cell surface.

Polymorphonuclear cells are motile and exhibit chemotaxis; the prime function of neutrophils is phagocytosis and inactivation of phagocytized materials. As an example, bacteria are killed, neutrophils become degranulated and often die; the accumulation of dead polymorphs form S pus. Eosinophils also phagocytize material with a preference for antigen-antibody complexes, and lytic lysosomal enzymes digest engulfed material. An eosinophilic response is seen when a parasitic infestation or hyper-sensitivity reaction occurs, but, in general, little is known about any other functions or mechanism of action. Rats are known to have, under normal conditions, numerous eosinophilic polymorphs in the lamina propria of the gastrointestinal tract, especially in the submucosa of the stomach at the limiting ridge of both gastric mucosae and, to a lesser extent, in some other organs (uterus, urinary bladder). Basophils react to very small stimuli, but their prime function is synthesis and storage in granules of heparin and histamine. They are discharged (cell degranulation) by exocytosis under numerous conditions, and large amounts of these substances may be detrimental to the host (allergy and anaphylactic reactions).

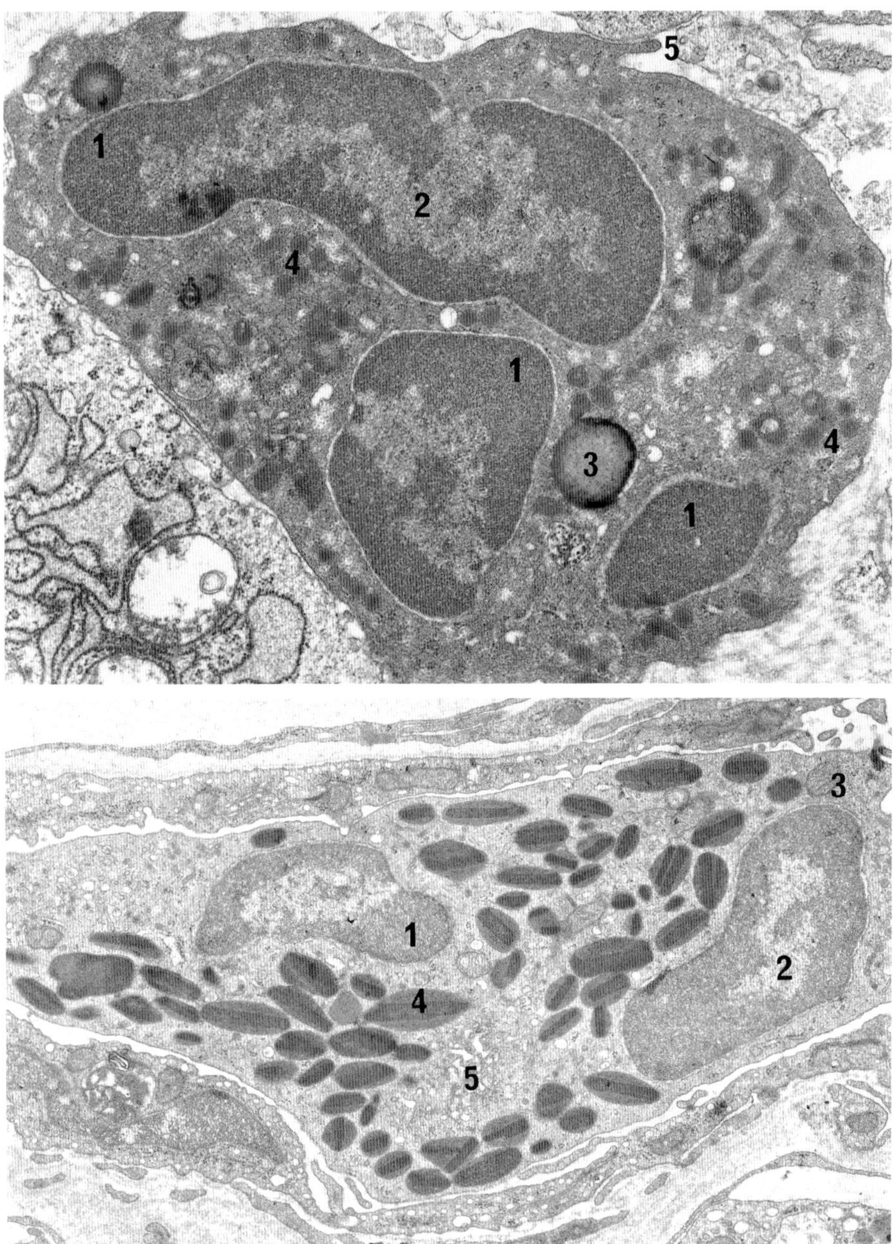

Fig. 34 *(above)*. Neutrophil polymorphonuclear leukocyte, rat. *1*, heterochromatin of multilobulated nucleus; *2*, euchromatin; *3*, azurophilic (primary) granule; *4*, specific (secondary) granule; *5*, microvilli. TEM, × 15000

Fig. 35 *(below)*. Eosinophil polymorphonuclear leukocyte, rat. *1*, heterochromatin of bilobed nucleus; *2*, euchromatin; *3*, mitochondria; *4*, specific granules; *5*, Golgi system. TEM. × 10000

Neutrophilic granulocytes contain, in lysosomes, phosphatase (Hardy 1967) and peroxidase (Schermer 1967), enzyme activities which are known to vary in quantity with age and give an indication of granulocyte turnover and which thus can be used as markers (Duprat and Gradiski 1978). Presence of these enzyme activities can also be used as diagnostic markers in hemopoietic tumors.

Monocytes. Monocytes are the largest circulating leukocytes and have typical features in blood smears: large, lobulated, sometimes kidney-shaped nuclei and abundant cytoplasm with more or less numerous azurophilic granules. They vary in size from 14 to 20 µm, and the smaller ones with granules may resemble large lymphocytes.

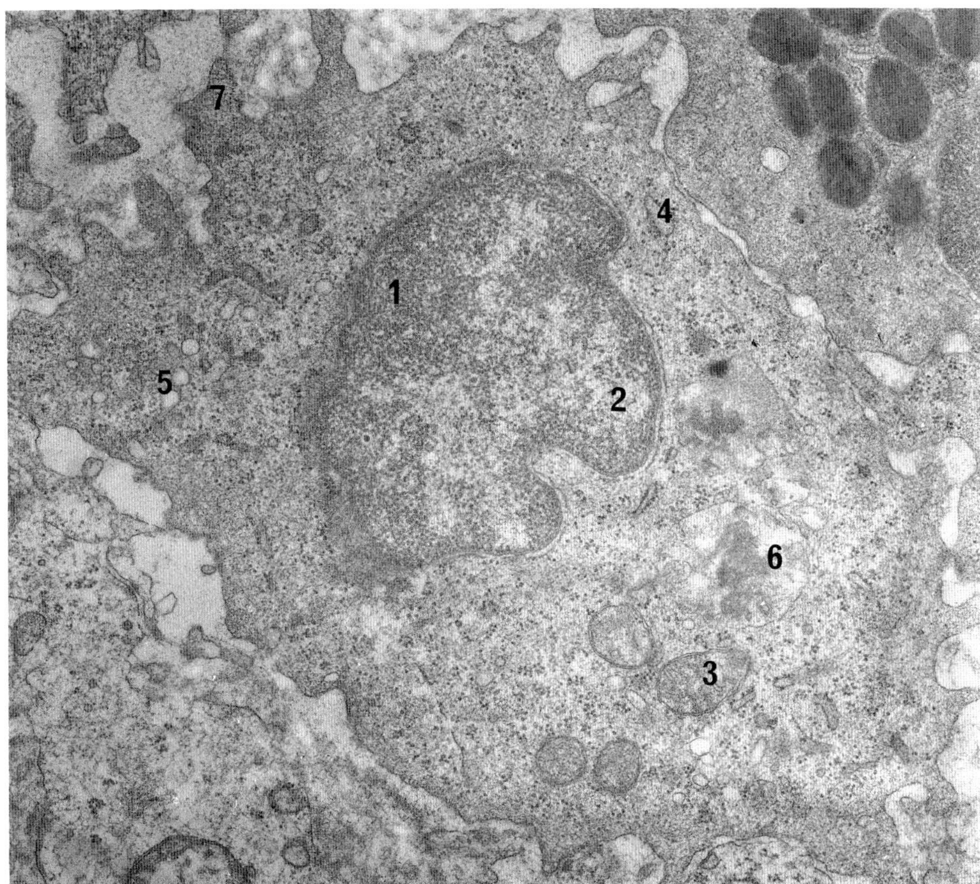

Fig. 36. Monocyte, rat. *1*, heterochromatin; *2*, euchromatin; *3*, mitochondria; *4*, short profile of granular endoplasmic reticulum; *5*, vesicles; *6*, lysosome; *7*, pseudopod. TEM, × 19000

Monocytes are the most pleomorphic leukocytes; SEM reveals an irregular surface and large pseudopodia. Under TEM (Fig. 36) microvilli are present at the membrane surface and vacuoles (pinocytic vesicles) are seen nearby. Nuclei have abundant peripheral clumps of heterochromatin and one or two nucleoli. The cytoplasm is more abundant than in lymphocytes and contains a well-developed and active Golgi apparatus with centrosome (often opposite indentation of the nucleus), glycogen granules, primary lysosomes (small dense and homogeneous granules with a peripheral membrane and containing acid phosphatase activity), some round mitochondria, microtubules, and filaments (Fig. 36).

Monocytes contain a nonspecific esterase used as a marker of the monocyte/macrophage lineage. Monocytes can be shown to have mobility (less than granulocytes), chemotaxis, and active phagocytic and killing activities. Many antigens require initial processing by monocytes/macrophages before lymphocyte presentation or recognition. Monocytes stay a few days in the circulat-

ing blood and then cross capillary walls and become wandering macrophages (see p. 114, this volume).

Blood Cell Counts and Age-Related Changes

Red (RBC) and white (WBC) blood cells counts, platelet count (PLT), hemoglobin concentration (HGB), and mean cell volume (MCV) were measured electronically on a Coulter S Plus instrument (Coulter Electronics, Lyon, France). Mean cell hemoglobin (MCH), mean corpuscular hemoglobin concentration (MCHC), and hematocrit (HCT) were calculated from previous measurements. The leukocyte differential counts were made on smears obtained by centrifugation with a Uni Smear Spinner (Perkin Elmer Coleman Instrument Division, Paris, France) and automatically stained by the modified Wright's procedure with a Hematek Staining System (Ames, Miles Products, Tour Bayer, Puteaux, France). Blood cell counts and erythrocyte inde-

Table 7. Hematology reference range data for female rats, all ages

Age	7–10 weeks ($n = 784$)			30–34 weeks ($n = 89$)			56–60 weeks ($n = 105$)			100–104 weeks ($n = 24$)			115–140 weeks ($n = 29$)		
	Median value	95% Spread		Median value	95% Spread		Median value	95% Spread		Median value	95% Spread		Median value	95% Spread	
		2.5%	97.5%		2.5%	97.5%		2.5%	97.5%		2.5%	97.5%		2.5%	97.5%
RBC ($10^6/mm^3$)	7.77	6.67	8.80	7.95	6.84	8.76	8.01	7.19	8.92	7.00	4.27[a]	8.14[a]	6.58	3.61[a]	8.41[a]
HCT(%)	46.0	41.0	50.0	44.0	38.4	48.4	45.0	40.8	49.6	40.5	27.0[a]	47.0[a]	40.0	24.2[a]	49.0[a]
HGB (g/dl)	16.6	15.0	18.0	16.5	14.4	17.8	16.4	14.7	17.9	15.5	10.2[a]	18.2[a]	14.9	9.5[a]	17.8[a]
PLT ($10^3/mm^3$)	1281	971	1656	1189	880	1515	1109	821	1431	1048	755[a]	1378[a]	973	605[a]	1419[a]
WBC ($10^3/mm^3$)	8.8	4.8	16.6	7.4	4.0	14.3	6.2	3.8	9.0	7.3	4.3[a]	14.1[a]	8.1	4.9[a]	22.7[a]
Differential count (%)															
Neutrophils	8.0	3.0	21.8	11.0	4.5	34.5	17.0	8.0	33.2	27.5	8.0[a]	68.0[a]	30.0	14.0[a]	69.5[a]
Lymphocytes	90.0	77.0	96.0	84.5	62.5	93.5	79.0	65.0	87.9	66.5	29.0[a]	85.0[a]	63.5	25.5[a]	85.0[a]
Eosinophils	0.0	0.0	2.0	1.0	0.0	4.0	1.0	0.0[a]	3.5[a]	1.0	0.0[a]	4.0[a]	1.0	0.0[a]	9.0[a]
Monocytes	1.0	0.0	4.0	2.0	0.0	7.0	2.0	0.0	5.0	4.0	0.0[a]	7.0[a]	4.0	0.5[a]	8.0[a]
Basophils	0.0	0.0	0.0	0.0	0.0	0.0	0.0	0.0	0.0	0.0	0.0[a]	0.0[a]	0.0	0.0[a]	0.0[a]
Erythrocytes indices															
MCV (μ^3)	59.0	55.0	64.0	55.6	52.2	59.0	56.0	53.0	59.1	58.5	50.0[a]	80.0[a]	60.4	54.9[a]	68.8[a]
MCH (μg)	21.4	19.4	24.2	20.6	18.7	23.0	20.3	19.0	22.6	22.3	18.9[a]	31.5[a]	22.6	20.6[a]	26.3[a]
MCHC (g/ml)	36.2	34.3	39.0	37.1	34.8	40.5	36.4	34.8	39.4	38.4	35.7	40.0	38.0	35.4	39.7

n, number of blood samples.

[a] Range of actual values instead of 95% spread values (not sufficient number of blood samples).

Table 8. Hematology reference range data for male rats, all ages

Age	7-10 weeks ($n = 784$)			30-34 weeks ($n = 89$)			56-60 weeks ($n = 105$)			100-104 weeks ($n = 24$)			115-140 weeks ($n = 29$)		
	Median value	95% Spread		Median value	95% Spread		Median value	95% Spread		Median value	95% Spread		Median value	95% Spread	
		2.5%	97.5%		2.5%	97.5%		2.5%	97.5%		2.5%	97.5%		2.5%	97.5%
RBC (10^6/mm^3)	7.69	6.53	8.76	9.08	7.60	10.25	9.28	7.80	10.29	8.53	4.77	9.60	7.54	3.53	8.99
HCT (%)	45.1	40.7	50.0	46.0	42.0	50.0	47.5	41.2	50.9	45.0	26.2	49.0	41.2	20.2	48.8
HGB (g/dl)	16.6	15.0	18.2	17.0	15.1	18.1	16.6	14.7	18.3	17.1	10.6	18.6	15.4	7.8	17.7
PLT (10^3/mm^3)	1291	995	1713	1146	834	1670	1102	869	1510	1144	769	1875	1236	771	2122
WBC (10^3/mm^3)	11.6	6.6	20.5	11.8	7.9	17.2	9.9	6.0	16.1	10.6	7.4	21.8	11.7	5.4	28.6
Differential count (%)															
Neutrophils	9.0	3.0	24.7	13.0	5.5	34.8	15.0	8.0[a]	35.5[a]	24.5	6.1	60.7	28.5	13.0[a]	58.0[a]
Lymphocytes	89.0	73.5	96.0	84.0	58.8	94.0	81.0	58.5[a]	90.0[a]	69.5	30.4	85.0	65.5	21.0[a]	80.0[a]
Eosinophils	0.0	0.0	2.0	1.0	0.0	4.0	1.0	0.0[a]	3.5[a]	1.0	0.0	4.0	1.0	0.0[a]	9.0[a]
Monocytes	1.0	0.0	4.0	2.0	0.0	6.1	2.0	0.0[a]	4.0[a]	3.0	0.0	11.0	4.0	0.0[a]	23.0[a]
Basophils	0.0	0.0	0.0	0.0	0.0	0.0	0.0	0.0[a]	0.0[a]	0.0	0.0	0.0	0.0	0.0[a]	0.0[a]
Erythrocyte indices															
MCV (μ^3)	59.0	55.0	64.6	50.7	47.4	54.0	51.0	47.0	54.9	53.0	49	61.9	54.0	48.5	65.6
MCH (μg)	21.6	19.8	24.6	18.8	16.1	20.7	18.0	15.9	20.0	20.0	17.8	23.6	20.4	17.8	24.8
MCHC (g/ml)	36.7	34.9	39.2	36.9	34.0	39.2	34.8	33.4	38.2	37.6	35.5	40.2	38.0	34.0	39.7

n, number of blood samples.
[a] Range of actual values instead of 95% spread values (not sufficient number of blood samples).

xes for Sprague-Dawley Crl:CD (SD) BR rats, measured in blood obtained by retro-orbital puncture, are expressed for each sex as means with 95% confidence limits in Tables 7 (females) and 8 (males) for five time points: 7–10 weeks, 30–34 weeks, 56–60 weeks, 100–104 weeks, and 115–140 weeks. These time points corresponded approximately to those for toxicity studies with duration of 1 month, 3 months, 6 months, 1 year, 2 years, and over 2 years. The number of values per hematologic determination ranged from 40 to 792 for males and from 24 to 784 for females. However, it is felt that diagrammed displays are more indicative of the trend of age-related changes (Figs. 37–43).

Red blood cell counts in males (approximately $8 \times 10^6/\text{mm}^3$ at 2 months of age) undergo an initial increase (approximately $+15\%$ up to $9.4 \times 10^6/\text{mm}^3$ at 8 months of age) (Fig. 37). These values in both sexes reach a plateau then decrease after 16 months of age and have a greater dispersion (boxes are wider in Figs. 37–43). Hemoglobin values are not as variable, and values in both sexes appear almost parallel through 20 months of age. At this age the hemoglobin levels fall, sharply in females, reaching mean levels below 14 g/100 ml of blood (Fig. 38). Platelet values have the most pronounced sex-related difference: values in female rats tend to decrease slightly over a 32-month period while those of male rats increase over a similar period (30

months) with a final drop at 32 months of age to values almost equal to those of females (Fig. 39)).

All cell counts (RBC, PLT, and WBC) are generally higher in males than in females, and age-related changes are also somewhat different. In addition, greater individual variations are commonly seen in almost all blood cell counts of young rats (4 months of age and sometimes up to 6 months) and in "aged" rats (usually at 22/24 months of age and above). This is clearly evident in Figs. 37, 39–41, in which the boxes are wider.

Total WBC counts in females are always lower than those of males: the lowest mean in females is around $7 \times 10^3/\text{mm}^3$ and in males about $10 \times 10^3/\text{mm}^3$. Total WBC counts vary in young rats of both sexes (2 and 4 months of age). Mean WBC counts in both sexes decrease slightly with time up to 16–18 months and then either stabilize (males) or tend to increase (females) with a wider spread of values in the oldest animals (Fig. 40).

In addition to these variations in total count there is a shift of the leukocyte population with a marked decline in numbers of lymphocytes, both in percentage and absolute numbers (not shown). This decrease is accompanied by an increase of granulocytes, mainly neutrophils, both in percentage and absolute counts. This blood picture correlates with the age-associated lymphoid depletion commonly seen in Sprague-Dawley rats

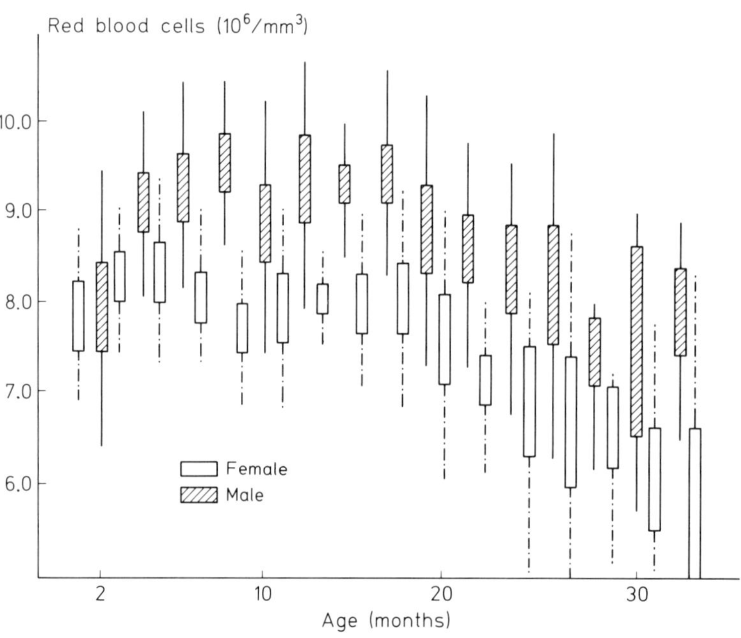

Figs. 37–43. For each schematic plot, the bottom of each box is at the 25th percentile, the top at the 75th percentile. *Vertical bars* delineate confidence limits (bottom: 5% and top: 95%). Fig. 38–43 see pp. 35–37

and the multiple pathologic lesions seen in old rats which Zurcher and Hollander (1982) consider the "hallmark of aging".

Most of these variations are in agreement with the hematologic findings in healthy Sprague-Dawley rats (Hardy 1967; Schermer 1967; Ringler and Dabich 1979; Weil 1982; Jain 1986; Wolford et al. 1986, 1987). In our stock, as in other Sprague-Dawley rats, eosinophil counts tend to increase slightly with age. This is in contrast to the findings of Everitt and Webb (1958) who re-ported decreased eosinophil counts in older animals. The baseline hematology values for this strain of rats (Charles River: Crl: CD (SD) BR as functions of sex and age (as reported by the Charles River Breeding Laboratories Technical Bulletin, 1982) have trends similar to those seen in our data. However, the experimental conditions of blood sampling were different: they used unfasted animals, cardiac puncture, and carbon dioxide anesthesia which resulted in decreased RBC counts (approximately -32%). These results

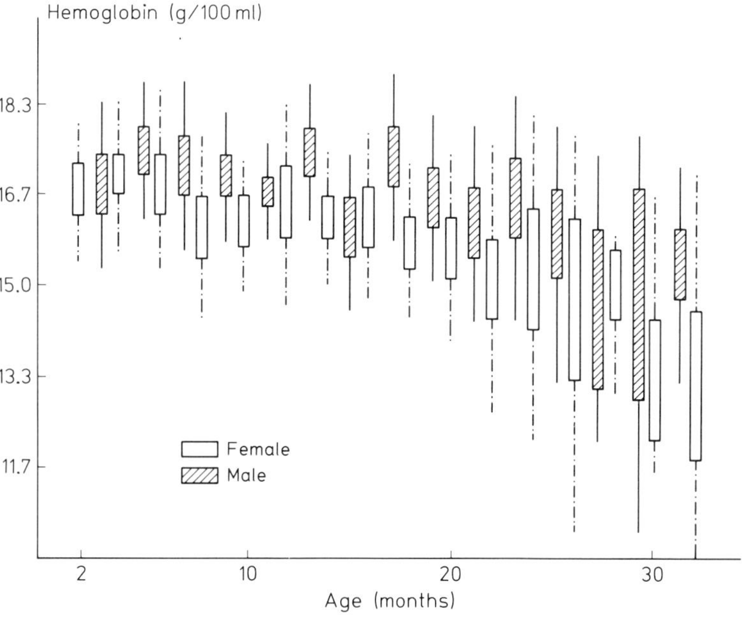

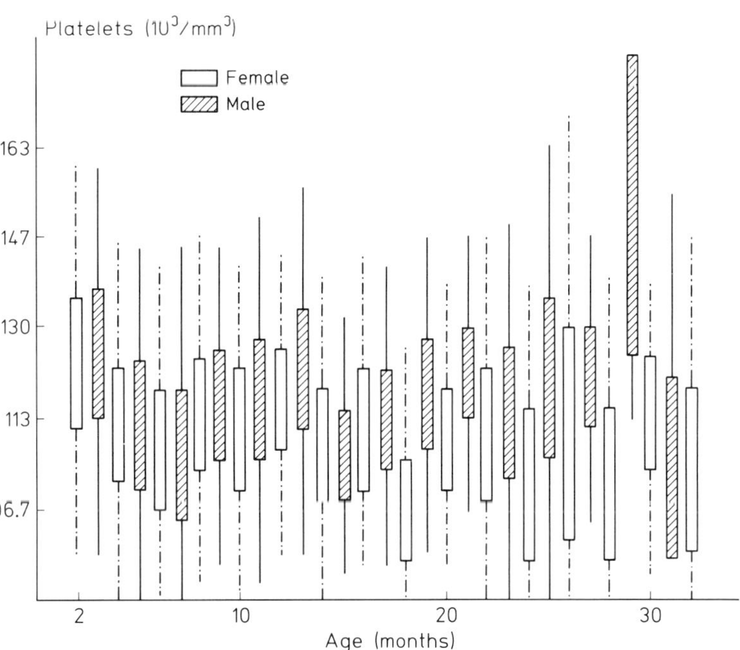

Fig. 38 *(above),* **39** *(below).* Legend see p. 34

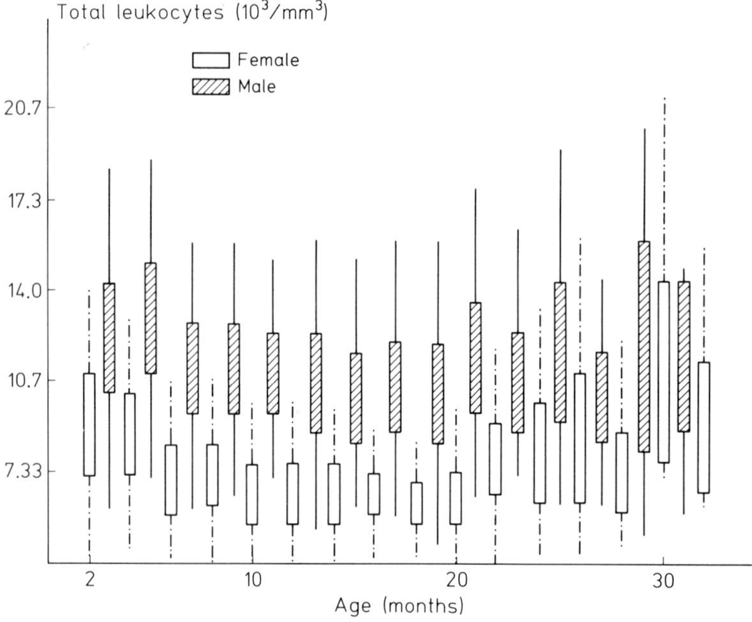

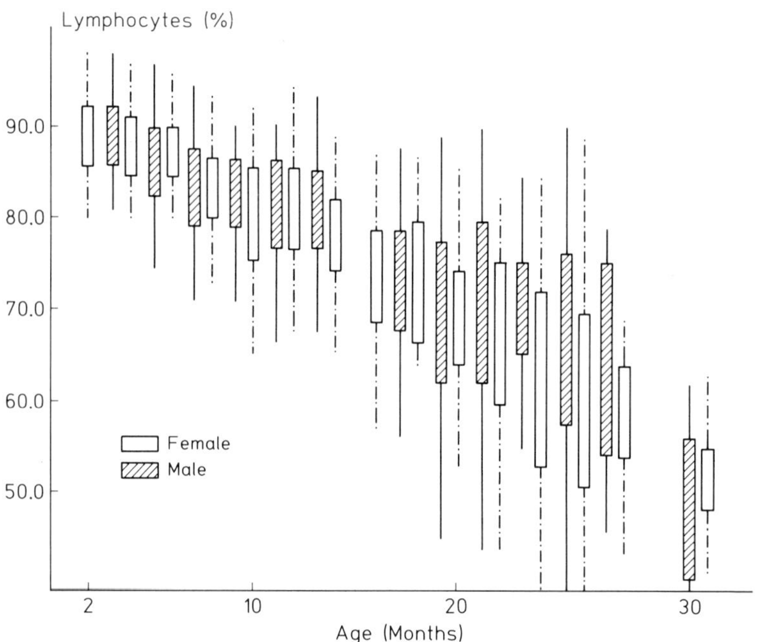

Fig. 40 *(above)*, **41** *(below)*. Legend see p. 34

are not unexpected for this site of blood sampling as mentioned by Smith et al. (1986) for Fischer 344 rats. In our stock, percentages of monocytes increase with time as reported in the Wistar rat (Lewi and Marsboom 1981; Sanderson and Phillips 1982) and Long Evans and Sprague-Dawley rats (Jain 1986).

Comparison with Other Species

All rat blood cells (RBC, WBC, PLT) as well as those of other small laboratory animals, are smaller than those of humans but are similar structurally and functionally. Morphologically, rat leukocytes are less lobulate than those of humans.

The hematologic profile of the rat typically contains more RBC (approximately 1.5 times) than humans and dogs, with hemoglobin and hematocrit values similar to those of these two species.

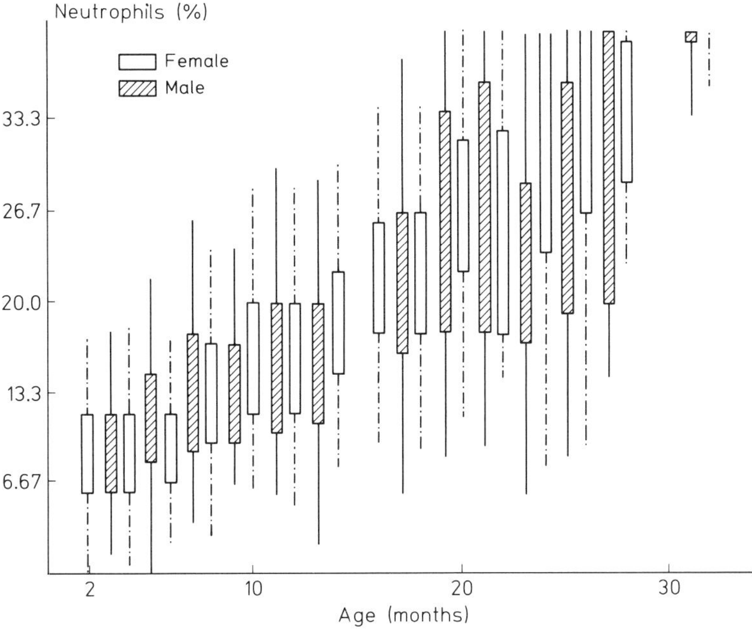

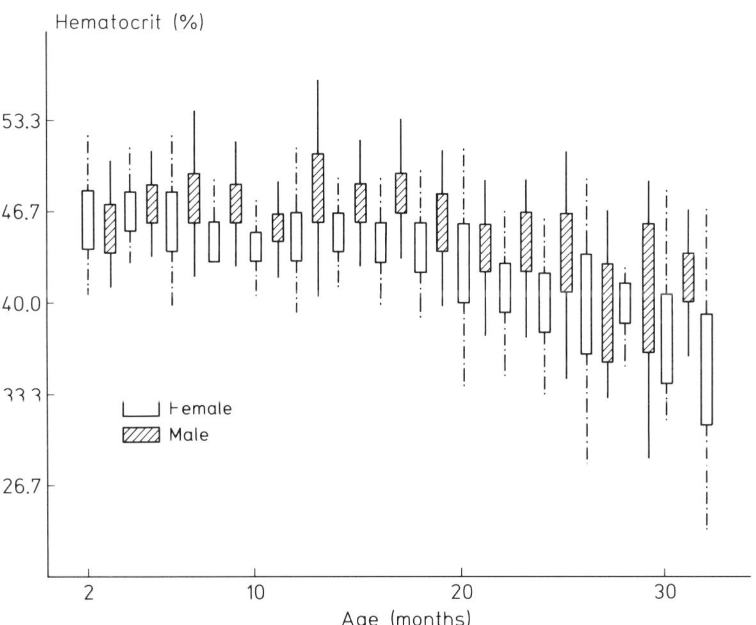

Fig. 42 *(above),* **43** *(below).* Legend
see p. 34

Rats also have much more numerous reticulocytes (not reported here) in circulating blood than humans (up to 10 times) or dogs (up to approximately 4 times) (Ringler and Dabich 1979). The platelet counts are also much higher in rats than in humans (approximately 5–8 times) and even greater then in dogs ($\times 1.5$–2.0 approximately). The range of white blood cell counts is broader in rats than in humans but similar to that in dogs, although the values are slightly higher (Sobotta and Hammersen 1985).

The striking features of the rat hemogram are the percentages of neutrophilic granulocytes (less than 10%) and lymphocytes (80%–85%). These values contrast with percentages in the blood of humans (neutrophils: 50%–70%; lymphocytes: 20%–40%) and dogs (neutrophils: 60%; lymphocytes: 30%). In addition, monocytes are found in smaller numbers in the blood of rats and dogs (less than 5% in both species) than in humans (less than 10%).

References

Archer RK, Riley J (1981) Standardized method for bleeding rats. Lab Anim 16: 25–28

Archer RK, Festing MFW, Riley J (1982) Haematology of conventionally-maintained lac: P outled Wistar rats during 1st year of life. Lab Anim 16: 198–200

Burns KF, DeLannoy CW Jr (1966) Compendium of normal blood values of laboratory animals with indication of variations. I. Randomsexed populations of small animals. Toxicol Appl Pharmacol 8: 429–437

Creskoff AJ, Fitz-Hugh T, Farris EJ (1949) Hematology of the rat. In: Farris EJ, Griffiths JQ (eds) The rat in laboratory investigation, 2nd edn. Lippincott, Philadelphia, pp 406–420

Didisheim P, Hattori K, Lewis JH (1959) Hematologic and coagulation studies in various animal species. J Lab Clin Med 53: 866–875

Duprat P (1987) Prélèvements et injections. In: Swynghedauw B (ed) Expérimentation animale en cardiologie. INSERM, Flammarion, Paris, pp 16–20

Duprat P, Gradiski D (1978) Intoxication benzenique chez le rat. Etude numérique et cytochimique du sang periphérique. Analyse du renouvellement des cellules médullaires. Arch Mal Prof 39: 445–457

Duprat P, Gradiski D, Delsaut L (1975) Etude de quelques paramètres sanguins chez le rat. Influence du lieu de prélèvement. Rev Méd Vét 126: 1159–1179

Everitt AV, Webb C (1958) The blood picture of the aging male rat. J Gerontol 13: 255–260

Garrick LM, Sharma VS, Ranney HM (1974) Structural studies of rat hemoglobins. Ann NY Acad Sci 241: 434–435

Gerrard JM (1985) Prostaglandins and leukotrienes. Blood and vascular cell function. In: Brinkhous KM (ed) Hematology, vol 1. Dekker, New York

Hardy J (1967) Hematology of rats and mice. In: Cotchin E, Roe FJC (eds) Pathology of laboratory rats and mice. Blackwell, Oxford, pp 501–536

Jain NC (1986) Schalm's veterinary hematology, 4th edn. Lea and Febiger, Philadelphia, pp 288–298

Leonard R, Ruben Z (1986) Hematology reference values for peripheral blood of laboratory rats. Lab Anim Sci 36: 277–281

Lewi PJ, Marsboom RP (1981) Toxicology reference data. Elsevier/North Holland, Amsterdam

Nachtman RG, Dunn CDR, Driscoll TB, Leach CS (1985) Methods for repetitive measurements of multiple hematological parameters in individual rats. Lab Anim Sci 35: 505–508

Rhodin JAG (1974) Histology. A text and atlas. Oxford University Press, London p 96

Ringler DH, Dabich L (1979) Hematology and clinical biochemistry. In: Backer HJ, Lindsey JR, Weisbroth SH (eds) The Laboratory Rat. Academic, New York, pp 105–121

Sanderson JH, Phillips CE (1982) An atlas of laboratory animal haematology. Oxford University Press, Oxford, pp 38–87

Schermer S (1967) The blood morphology of laboratory animals, 3rd edn. Davis, Philadelphia

Shaw ARE, MacLean N (1971) A reevaluation of the haemoglobin electrophoretogram of the Wistar rat. Comp Biochem Physiol [B] 40: 155–163

Smith CN, Neptun DA, Irons RD (1986) Effect of sampling site and collection method on variations in baseline clinical pathology parameters in Fisher-344 rats. II. Clinical hematology. Fundam Appl Toxicol 7: 658–663

Sobotta J, Hammersen F (1985) Histology – Color atlas of microscopic anatomy. Urban and Schwarzenberg, Baltimore, p 115

Suber RL, Kodell RL (1985) The effect of the phlebotomy techniques on hematological and clinical chemical evaluation in Sprague-Dawley rats. Vet Clin Pathol 14: 23–30

Technical bulletin (1982) Baseline hematology and clinical chemistry values for Charles River Cr:CD (SD) BR rats as a function of sex and age. Charles River Breeding Laboratories, Inc., Wilmington

Upton PK, Morgan DJ (1975) The effect of sampling technique on some blood parameters in the rat. Lab Anim 9: 85–91

Vondruska JF, Greco RA (1973) Certain hematologic and blood chemical values in Charles River CD albino rats. Clin Pathol 2: 3–17

Weil CS (1982) Statistical analysis and normality of selected hematological and clinical chemistry measurements used in toxicologic studies. Arch Toxicol 5: 237–253

Wolford ST, Schroer RA, Gohs FX, Gallo PP, Brodeck, Falk HB, Ruhren R (1986) Reference range data base for serum chemistry and hematology values in laboratory animals. J Toxicol Environ Health 18: 161–188

Wolford Sk, Schroer RA, Gallo PP, Gohs FX, Brodeck M, Falk HB, Ruhren R (1987) Age-related changes in serum chemistry and hematology values in normal Sprague-Dawley rats. Fundam Appl Toxicol 8: 80–88

Yamanuchi C, Fujita S, Obara T, Veda T (1981) Effects of room temperature on reproduction body and organ weights, food and water intake, and hematology in rats. Lab Anim Sci 31: 251–258

Youatt WG, Fay LD, Howe DL, Harte HD (1961) Hematologic data on some small animals. Blood 18: 758–763

Zurcher C, Hollander CF (1982) Multiple pathological changes in aging rat and man. Exp Biol Med 7: 56–62

Granulocytic Leukemia, Rat

Ferenc Gal, Janos Sugar, and Orsolya Csuka

Synonyms. Myeloid leukemia; myelogenous leukemia; chloroleukemia.

Gross Appearance

Splenomegaly and occasionally hepatomegaly are so severe that these organs become palpable in the living animal. The spleen is enlarged and may weigh 3–16 g (10 times the normal value; Swaen and Van Heerde 1973; Gal et al. 1973). Both spleen and liver are fragile with smooth and even capsular surfaces. In some cases the cut surface of the spleen exhibits tiny grayish areas. The liver edges are rounded. Lymph nodes are slightly or only moderately enlarged and of grayish-white cast; in the case of chloroleukemia (eosinophilic leukemia), they are greenish. Infiltrations are frequently found in other organs such as the lungs, kidneys, testicles, and ovaries.

Microscopic Features

The white blood cell (WBC) count may reach a very high value, 120000–680000/mm^3 (Moloney 1974) in the final stage of the disease. At the same time, however, there is a fall in the number of red blood cells (RBC), lymphocytes, and platelets in the peripheral blood (Gal et al. 1973). In blood smears stained by May-Grünwald-Giemsa, myeloid elements representing all degrees of maturation can be identified (Fig. 44). Quite often nucleated red blood cells are also found in the peripheral blood; Pelger-Huët anomaly is, however, seldom detectable (Moloney 1974) (Table 9). In all the peripheral blood smears, bone marrow sediment, and imprint smears of liver and spleen, the ratio of peroxidase and Sudan Black B-positive cells is elevated to some 70%–80% (Moloney 1974) (Fig. 45). The number of alkaline phosphatase and nonspecific esterase active cells is de-

Table 9. Blood picture of rats with advanced granulocytic leukemia induced by 7,12-dimethylbenz [α] anthracene

Peripheral blood	%	$\pm$ SD ($n=15$)
Blasts – promyelocytes	30.4	5.6
Myelocytes – metamyelocytes	24.0	3.5
Bands	22.1	3.2
Lymphocytes	20.0	2.4
Undefinable	3.5	2.5
Nucleated red blood cells	sporadically 1–10/100 WBC	

From Gal et al. 1973.

creased (Gal et al. 1973). In some cases, however, Moloney et al. (1962) and Ioachim et al. (1971) observed rising values, even in the immature forms (see Table 9). Lysozyme activity is enhanced both in the serum and urine (Osserman and Lawlor 1966).

Histologic studies reveal that cells which are found in the blood also infiltrate the bone marrow, spleen, liver, kidneys, testicles, and ovaries. These mature and immature myeloid elements are polygonal with clear, eosinophilic cytoplasm, quite often dotted with minute granules. The nuclei of these cells are kidney- or ring-shaped, lobular, and contain one or more nucleoli. Abnormal myeloblasts are also present: they have large, slightly lobular nuclei and pale, mildly reticular chromatin substance. The bone marrow is highly cellular, fat tissue is completely displaced, and normal myelopoiesis or erythropoiesis cannot be observed. Only the occasional presence of megakaryocytes indicates the remains of the original cellular content of the bone marrow (Figs. 46–49) (Ioachim et al. 1972; Moruichi et al. 1983).

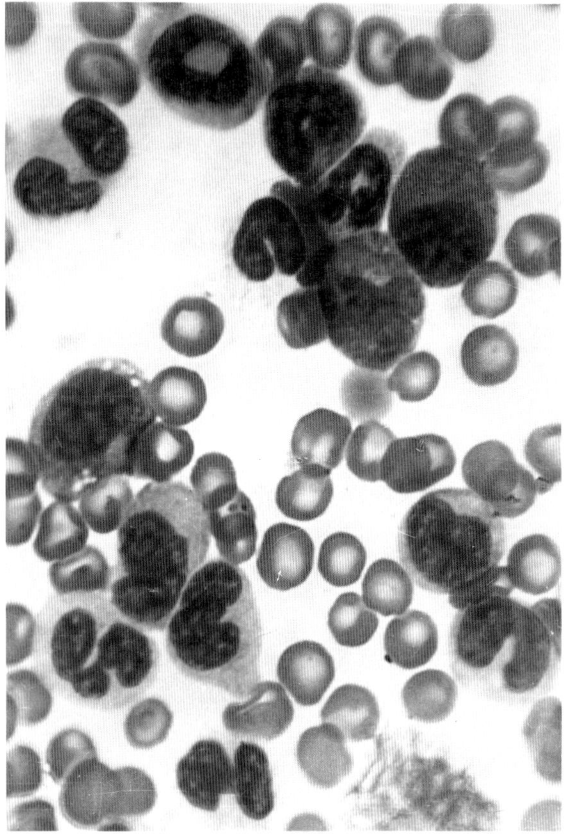

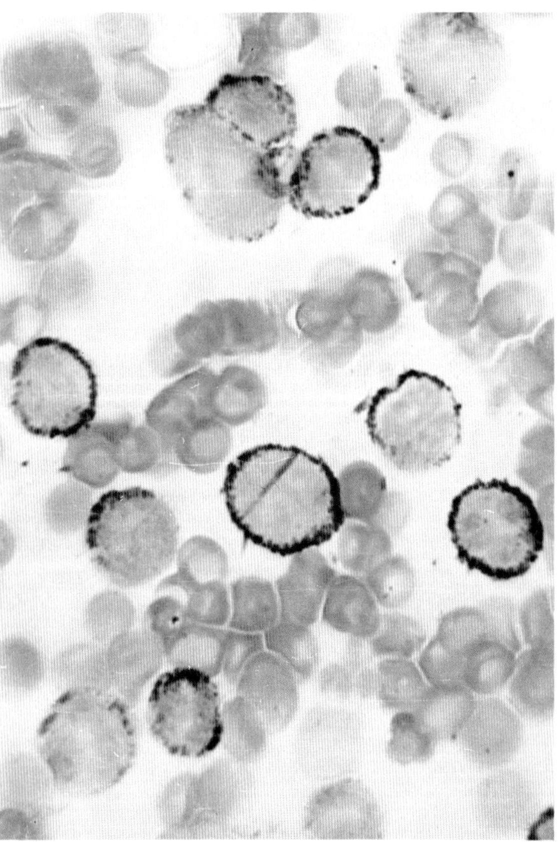

◄ **Fig. 44** *(above).* Peripheral blood of rat with advanced granulocytic leukemia induced by 7,12-dimethylbenz[a]-anthracene. WBC 120000/mm³. Note the presence of leukocytes in all stages of maturity. May-Grünwald-Giemsa, ×420

Fig. 45 *(below).* Same rat as in Fig. 44. Peroxidase reaction, ×420

Fig. 46 *(upper left).* Rat, bone marrow, most frequent his- ► tological alterations caused by 7,12-dimethylbenz[a]anthracene induced granulocytic leukemia. Normal myelopoiesis or erythropoiesis in the bone marrow displaced by leukemic cells. H and E, ×920

Fig. 47 *(lower left).* Rat, spleen, granulocytic leukemia induced by 7,12-dimethylbenz[a]anthracene; spleen pulp is infiltrated by leukemic cells, but the follicles are preserved. H and E, ×255

Fig. 48 *(upper right).* Rat, granulocytic leukemia induced by 7,12-dimethylbenz[a]anthracene. Liver is infiltrated around the central veins and in the portal areas. H and E, ×255

Fig. 49 *(lower right).* Rat, granulocytic leukemia induced by 7,12-dimethylbenz[a]anthracene, lymph node. The structure is distended by the infiltration of leukemic cells. The capsule is also infiltrated (not shown). H and E, ×350

Ultrastructure

So-called endogenous myeloperoxidase activity in the neutrophils of rat chloroma cells has been demonstrated (Ioachim et al. 1972). Endogenous peroxidase activity even in the endoplasmic reticulum of the myeloblasts lends further support to the myeloid origin of induced leukemia (Fig. 50). The degree of cellular differentiation ranges from myeloblast to mature granulocyte in the bone marrow (Fig. 51).

In this type of leukemia the presence of viral particles could not be observed by electron microscopy. The occurrence of C type viruses, however, has been detected in rat chloroleukemia (Chen et al. 1972); moreover, the presence of intracisternal A particles in rat immunocytoma has also been reported (Burtonboy et al. 1978). The lack of mature virus particles in our rats with this leukemia suggests that the viruses have become integrated into the DNA of the host cells.

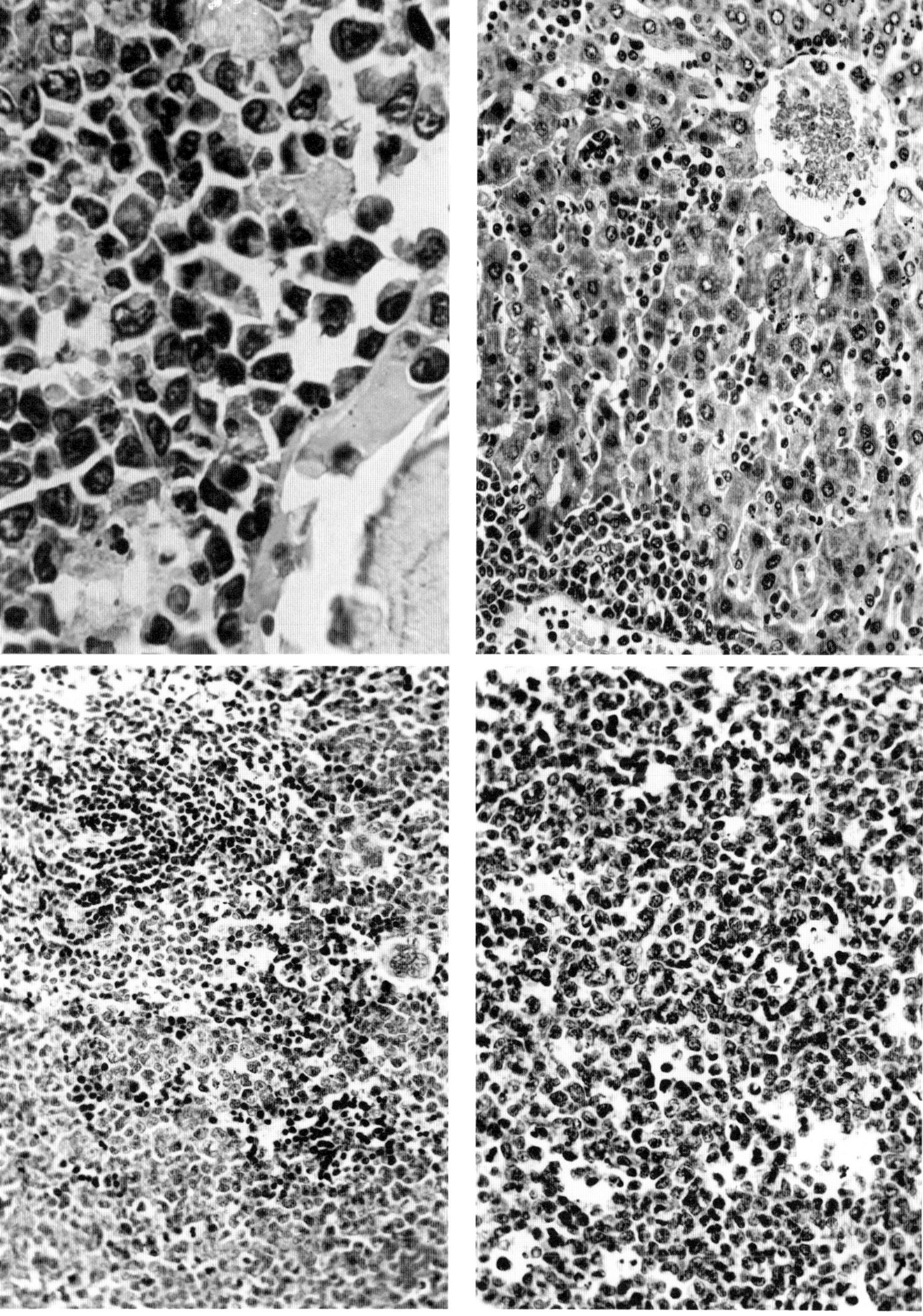

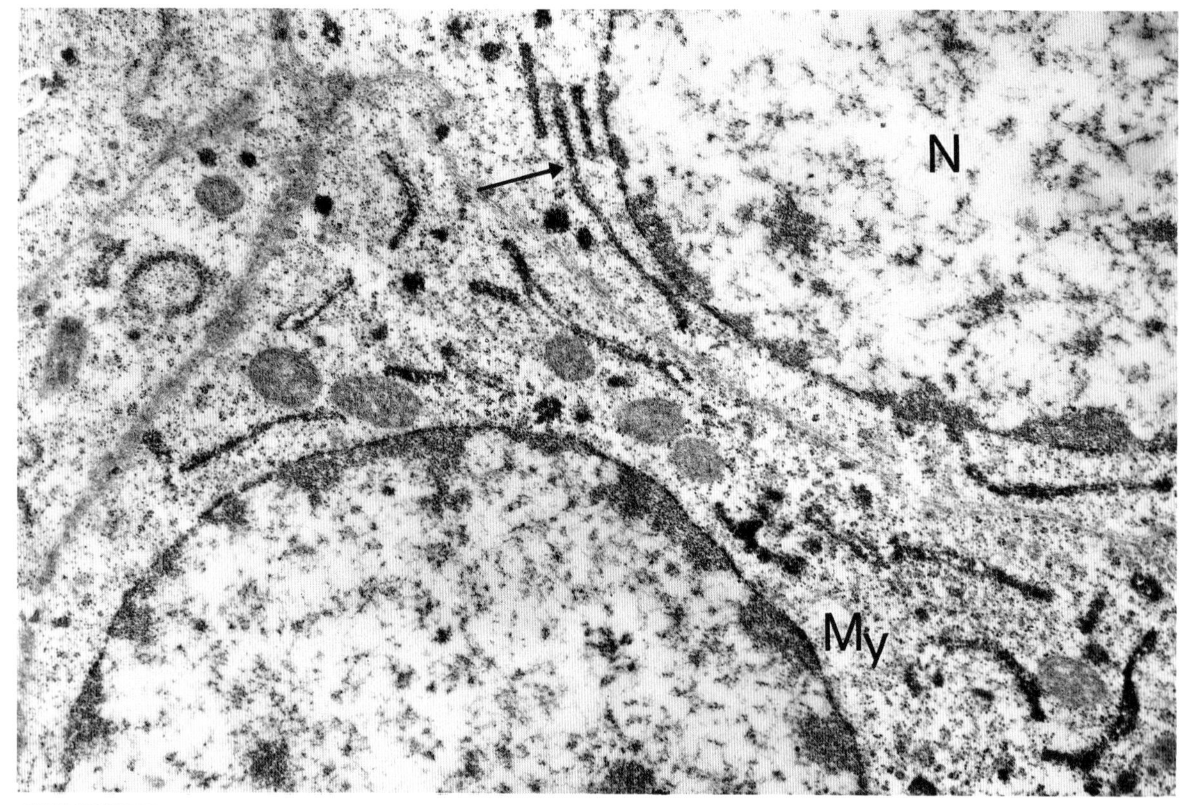

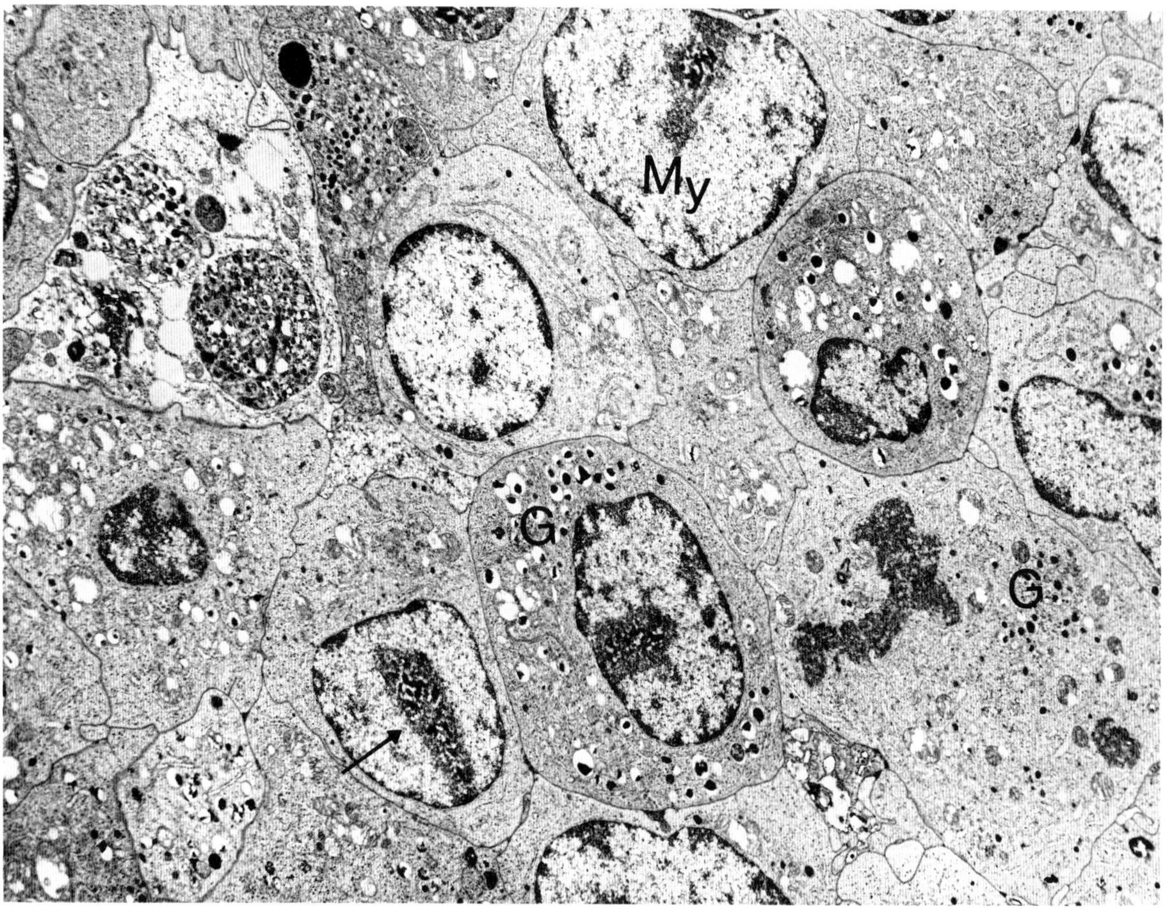

◄ **Fig. 50** *(above).* Rat, induced granulocytic leukemia. Endogenous peroxidase activity detected in the endoplasmic reticulum *(arrow)* of the myeloblast *(My)* by DAB method. *N,* nucleus. TEM, ×9920

Fig. 51 *(below).* Bone marrow, rat, with induced granulocytic leukemia. Note several myeloblasts *(My)* with prominent nucleolus *(arrow).* Immature granulocytes *(G)* were also observed. TEM, ×2800

Differential Diagnosis

Differentiation of granulocytic from lymphoid leukemia is generally easy on the basis of blood smears since the granulocytic form contains high numbers of myeloid elements with different degress of maturation. Diagnosis is facilitated by the use of various cytochemical procedures and staining techniques, such as peroxidase, Sudan Black B, lysozyme, alkaline phosphatase and esterase. Histologic examinations naturally also confirm the diagnosis. Leukemoid reaction that may occur under septic conditions and malignant tumors giving a sometimes misleading high leukocyte count must be excluded. In such cases alkaline phosphatase is elevated above normal values.

Biologic Features

Granulocytic leukemia, either spontaneous or induced by carcinogens, can be recognized in quantitative and differential blood counts. As a rule, the spontaneous form occurs in aging animals. Experimental leukemia develops within 5–8 months after application of the carcinogen. In both cases the WBC is only slightly increased at the beginning, but immature myeloid elements are already present in the peripheral blood in the early stage of the disease. The number of peroxidase-positive cells also increases as does the lysozyme activity of blood serum and urine.

Progression of the disease is accompanied either by a gradual or abrupt rise (blastic crisis) of the WBC. When studying rat granulocytic leukemias it is usual to distinguish acute, subacute, and chronic forms. Distinction is based on the maturation degree of cells causing the lesion rather than on the clinical course of the disease (Swaen and Van Heerde 1973; Moloney 1974). In the acute and subacute forms the leukocyte counts are lower (25000–190000/mm^3) than in the chronic form, and there is a predominance of immature myeloid elements. In chronic granulocyt-

ic leukemia myeloblasts and promyelocytes are less numerous in the peripheral blood. The WBC, however, becomes extremely elevated, reaching 600000/mm^3 or even higher (Swaen and Van Heerde 1973; Zeller et al. 1981). Basophilic leukemia is even less frequent than granulocytic leukemia (Eccleston et al. 1973).

Etiology and Frequency

Granulocytic leukemia does not occur frequently as a spontaneous disease in rats. Its incidence can be enhanced by chemical carcinogens, magnesium deficiency (Battifora et al. 1968), and ionizing irradiation (Table 10). Different rat strains have varying sensitivity to carcinogens. Table 10 includes some examples of known carcinogens and rat strains used in leukemogenesis studies. Attempts have usually failed to transmit either spontaneous or induced granulocytic leukemia by cell-free filtrate even when C type viruses were present in the material (Svec and Michalides 1977). In those rare cases, however, when cell-free transmission was successfully accomplished, the presence of a retrovirus not identical with RaLV, the endogenous C type helper virus, was demonstrated (Keszeghová et al. 1985).

In our studies, granulocytic leukemia was induced in Wistar rats by intravenous administration of 7,12-dimethylbenz [α] anthracene (DMBA). The leukemia could be successfully transplanted in 98% of the cases by intravenous or intraperitoneal injection of spleen or liver cells. Survival time was 18 ± 3.4 days (n − 300) (Gal et al. 1973).

Comparison with Other Species

Human and rat granulocytic leukemias are morphologically similar: leukemic cells infiltrate the same solid organs and the peripheral blood in similar numbers and stages of maturity. In acute human myeloid leukemia, Auer bodies can be found in the cytoplasm of myeloblasts. In rats, however, these bodies are absent. Another notable difference is that chloroleukemia is more frequent in rats than in humans. Acute granulocytic leukemia in humans results in only slight splenomegaly, but in the rat the spleen is greatly enlarged. Survival rates also differ. In rats most types of leukemia have a rapid course, lasting for a few weeks at most. In humans, however, chronic granulocytic leukemia may persist for years. In

Table 10. Some chemical carcinogens and rat strains used for the induction of myeloid leukemia

Carcinogens	Rat strains	References
20-methylcholanthrene	Wistar noninbred	Shay et al. 1951
	Wistar noninbred, W/Fu and Fischer inbred	Moloney 1974
		Moloney et al. 1969, 1971
7,12-dimethylbenz [α] anthracene	W/Fu, Sprague-Dawley, Long Evans noninbred	Ioachim et al. 1971, 1972
		Pollard and Kajima 1967
	Wistar, Sprague-Dawley, Fischer noninbred	Huggins et al. 1982
		Huggins and Sugiyama 1965
	Long Evans noninbred	Kurita et al. 1968
	Long Evans noninbred	Gál et al. 1973
	Wistar noninbred, WOP inbred	
9,10-dimethyl-1,2-benzanthracene	BN inbred	Hagenbeeck and Van Bekkum 1977
Ethylnitrosourea	BDIX inbred	Ivankovic and Zeller 1974
1-butyl-1-nitrosourea	Sprague-Dawley, Donryu noninbred	Odashima et al. 1975
1-propyl-1-nitrosourea	Sprague-Dawley, Donryu noninbred	Ogiu et al. 1975
	Sprague-Dawley, Donryu noninbred	Odashima et al. 1975
1-alkyl-1-nitrosoureas	Donryu noninbred	Ogiu 1978
2-naphthylamine	Wistar noninbred	Heath 1981
N,N'-fluorenylene-bisacetamide	Wistar noninbred	Takayama and Fujiwara 1976
		Fujiwara and Takayama 1976
2,6-dimethyl-m-dioxane-4-ol acetate	Wistar noninbred	Hoch-Ligeti et al. 1974
		Zeller and Schmähl 1979

rats leukemias develop in old age, while in humans acute leukemia is a frequent childhood disease.

In domestic mammals myeloid leukemias (myeloid leukosis) are very rare; they occur mainly in dogs and cats and are extremely rare in pigs. Myeloid leukemia can appear as a raspberry-red or grayish-red or grayish-white tumor tissue. It is characterized by cell proliferation in the bone marrow. In fact, tumor tissue is present both in the bone marrow and spongious interspace. As a rule, the spleen becomes considerably enlarged. On its cut surface the follicular structure can barely be discerned or is not evident at all. The diffuse infiltration initially involves the entire red pulp. The liver is also enlarged by diffuse infiltration of myeloid cells. Infiltrations are dominated by immature forms. Lymph nodes are only moderately enlarged (Lombard 1968).

Myeloid leukemia may be of leukemic or aleukemic (myeloma) character. In pigs chloroleukemia or chloroma may also appear, although very rarely. Granulocytic leukemia in the mouse is found with marked splenomegaly, hepatomegaly, and enlargement of lymph nodes. The thymus is normal or atrophic. The first histological alterations found in granulocytic leukemia can be detected in the red pulp of the spleen. First, myeloblastic foci appear which later spread throughout the entire spleen. Even in the most advanced stages, however, the lymphatic follicles may be preserved (Della Porta et al. 1979).

Myeloblastosis of chickens may be caused by several strains of avian retroviruses. The bone marrow and the peripheral blood are dominated by myeloblasts, and their chromatic content is finely and evenly distributed through the nuclei. These blast cells are prone to smudge in the smears. Spleen and liver are enlarged, and the liver surface is mottled (Squire 1964; Squire et al. 1978).

References

Battifora HA, McGeary PA, Hahneman BM, Laing GH, Hass GM (1968) Chronic magnesium deficiency in the rat. Arch Pathol Lab Med 86: 610–620

Burtonboy G, Beckers A, Rodhain J, Bazin H, Lamy ME (1978) Rat ileocecal immunocytoma. An ultrastructural study with special attention to the presence of viral particles. JNCI 61: 477–484

Chen LT, Handler EE, Handler ES, Weiss L (1972) An electron microscopic study of the bone marrow of the rat in experimental myelogenous leukemia. Blood 39: 99–112

Della Porta G, Chieco-Bianchi L, Pennelli N (1979) Tumours of the haematopoietic system. In: Turusov VS (ed) Pathology of tumours in laboratory animals. II. Tumours of the mouse. IARC Sci Publ 23: 527–576

Eccleston G, Leonard BJ, Lowe JS, Welford HJ (1973) Basophilic leukemia in the albino rat and a demonstration of the basopoietin. Nature 244: 73–76

Fujiwara M, Takayama S (1976) Influence of blood collection on incidence of 2,7-FAA-induced rat leukemia. Acta Pathol Jpn 26: 139–145

Gál F, Somfai S, Szentirmay Z (1973) Transplantable myeloid rat leukaemia induced by 7,12-dimethylbenz(α)anthracene. Acta Haematol 49: 281–290

Hagenbeek A, Van Bekkum DW (eds) (1977) Workshop on comparative evaluation of the L5222 and BNML rat leukaemia models and their relevance for human acute leukaemia. Leuk Res 1: 75–255

Heath JE (1981) Granulocytic leukemia in rats: a report of two cases. Lab Anim Sci 31: 504–506

Hoch-Ligeti C, Argus MF, Arcos JC (1974) Oncogenic activity of an m-dioxane derivative: 2,6-dimethyl-m-dioxane-4-ol acetate (Dimethoxane). JNCI 53: 791–794

Huggins CB, Sugiyama T (1966) Induction of leukemia in rat by pulse doses of 7,12-dimethylbenz(α)anthracene. Proc Natl Acad Sci USA 55: 74–81

Huggins CB, Grand L, Ueda N (1982) Specific induction of erythroleukemia and myelogenous leukemia in Sprague-Dawley rats. Proc Natl Acad Sci USA 79: 5411–5414

Ioachim HL, Keller S, Sabbath M, Andersson B, Dorsett B, Essner E (1972) Myeloperoxidase and crystalline bodies in the granules of DMBA-induced rat chloroma cells. Am J Pathol 66: 147–162

Ioachim HL, Sabbath M, Andersson B, Keller S (1971) Viral and chemical leukemia in the rat: comparative study. JNCI 47: 161–177

Ivankovic S, Zeller WJ (1974) Leukämie L5222 des Rattenstammes BDIX. Eine durch Athylnitrosoharnstoff induzierte monozytärmyeloische, transplantierbare Form für zytochemische und chemotherapeutische Studien. Blut 28: 288–292

Keszeghová V, Veselovská Z, Hlavayová E, Svec J (1985) Expression of retrovirus related functions in the methylcholanthrene-induced rat myelogenous leukemia. Neoplasma 32: 581–591

Kurita Y, Sugiyama T, Nishizuka Y (1968) Cytogenetic studies on rat leukemia induced by pulse dose of 7,12-dimethylbenz(α)anthracene. Cancer Res 28: 1738–1752

Lombard CH (1968) Les leucoses animales. Institut National de la Recherche Agronomique, Paris

Moloney WC (1974) Primary granulocytic leukemia in the rat. Cancer Res 34: 3049–3057

Moloney WC, Boschetti AE, King V (1969) Observations on leukemia in Wistar Furth rats. Cancer Res 29: 938–946

Moloney WC, Batata M, King V (1971) Leukemogenesis in the rat: further observations. JNCI 46: 1139–1144

Moloney WC, Dorr AD, Dowd G, Boschetti AE (1962) Myelogenous leukemia in the rat. Blood 19: 45–59

Moruichi T, Oikawa T, Kodama T, Yamaguchi H, Kobayashi H (1983) Establishment and characterization of a transplantable rat myelomonocytic leukemia. Cancer Res 43: 5478–5483

Odashima S, Ogiu T, Maekawa A (1975) Leukemias induced by 1-butyl- and propyl-1-nitrosoureas in the rat. Bibl Haematol 40: 107–115

Ogiu T (1978) Hematological and histopathological characteristics of leukemias induced by 1-alkyl-1-nitrosoureas in Donryu rats. Gann 69: 781–791

Ogiu T, Nakadate M, Odashima S (1975) Induction of leukemias and digestive tract tumors in Donryu rats by 1-propyl-1-nitrosourea. JNCI 54: 887–893

Osserman EF, Lawlor DP (1966) Serum and urinary lysozime (muramidase) in monocytic and monomyelocytic leukemia. J Exp Med 124: 921–951

Pollard M, Kajima M (1967) Leukemia induced by 7,12-dimethylbenz(α)anthracene in germfree rats. JNCI 39: 135–141

Shay H, Gruenstein M, Marx HE, Glazer L (1951) The development of lymphatic and myelogenous leukemia in Wistar rats following gastric instillation of methylcholanthrene. Cancer Res 11: 29–34

Squire RA (1964) Hematopoietic tumors of domestic animals. Cornell Vet 54: 97–150

Squire RA, Goodman DG, Valerio MG, Frederickson TN et al. (1978) Hemopoietic system. In: Bernischke K, Garner FM, Jones TC (eds) Pathology of laboratory animals, vol II. Springer, Berlin Heidelberg New York, pp 1091–1124

Svec J, Michalides R (1977) Biochemical properties of endogenous rat C-type viruses. Neoplasma 24: 601–614

Swaen GJV, Van Heerde P (1973) Tumours of the haematopoietic system. In: Turusov VS (ed) Pathology of tumours in laboratory animals. I. Tumours of the rat, part 1. IARC Sci Publ 5: 185–201

Takayama S, Fujiwara M (1976) Effect of a repeated bloodletting on the incidence of 2,7-FAA-induced rat leukemia. Acta Pathol Jpn 26: 435–439

Zeller WJ, Schmähl D (1979) Leukemias induced by ethylnitrosourea in Wistar rats: incidence and chemotherapy. Leuk Res 3: 239–348

Zeller WJ, Reusch K, Schmähl D (1981) Chemotherapy of autochtonous myeloid leukemias (chloroleukemias) in Wistar rats. J Cancer Res Clin Oncol 101: 243–248

Granulocytic Leukemia, Mouse

Masatoshi Seki and Tohru Inoue

Synonyms. Myelocytic leukemia; myeloblastic leukemia; chloroleukemia; myeloid leukemia (sometimes, this term includes monocytic leukemia); myelogeneous leukemia (sometimes, this term includes monocytic, erythro- and mega-karyoblastic leukemias).

Gross Appearance

The spleen is greatly swollen; its capsule is tightly stretched, and its surface is smooth. Its weight is increased several times (Table 11). The cut surface of the spleen may be dark red, yellow-white, or mottled by both colors. Rarely, it has a gray-green tone (chloroleukemia). The bone marrow is pale yellow and translucent. The liver is usually pale yellow and enlarged. Numerous small white branched patterns corresponding to Glisson's capsule can be observed on its surface. The lymph nodes are white and moderately swollen (greenish in cases of chloroleukemia). Hemorrhages in the lung or other tissues are sometimes encountered.

Microscopic Features

Granulocytic leukemia may be classified into two types based upon the morphology of cells in the blood smear: juvenile type (Fig. 52) or mature type (Fig. 53) (Table 11).
The bone marrow is usually nearly replaced by leukemic cells. A few megakaryocytes may remain. Massive necrosis due to loss of circulation is often encountered, especially in the long

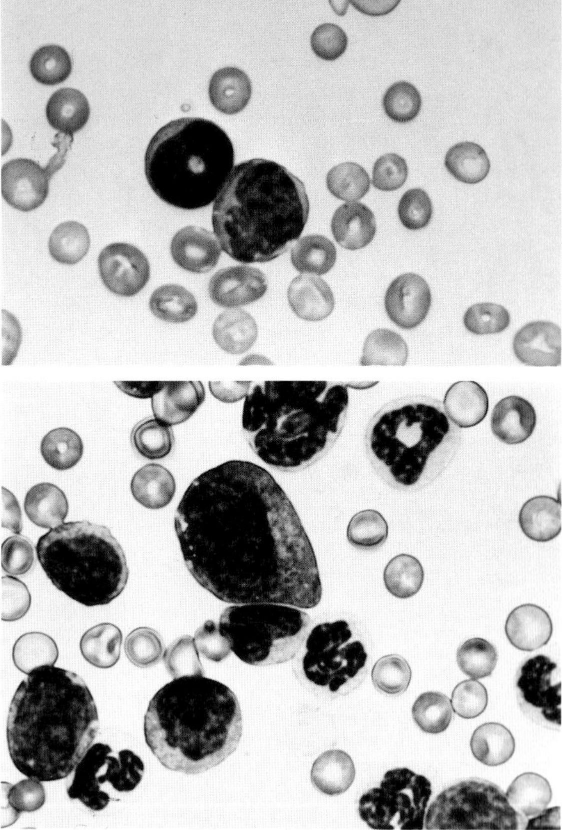

Fig. 52 *(above).* Granulocytic leukemia, juvenile type, mouse. Differentiation of leukemic cells is restricted to promyelocyte stage. May-Giemsa, × 750

Fig. 53 *(below).* Granulocytic leukemia, mature type, mouse. Leukemic cells differentiate to neutrophil stage. May-Giemsa, × 750

Table 11. Comparison of juvenile and mature type granulocytic leukemia. Figures are mean and range in parentheses

	Peripheral nucleated cell count	Hematocrit	Liver weight (mg)	Spleen weight (mg)
Juvenile Granulocytic Leukemia	27000 (3200–64000)	15.2 (8–39)	2983 (1543–4967)	1310 (324–2717)
Mature Granulocytic Leukemia	160000 (96000–218000)	9.9 (6.5–14)	2700 (811–4198)	1053 (308–1933)

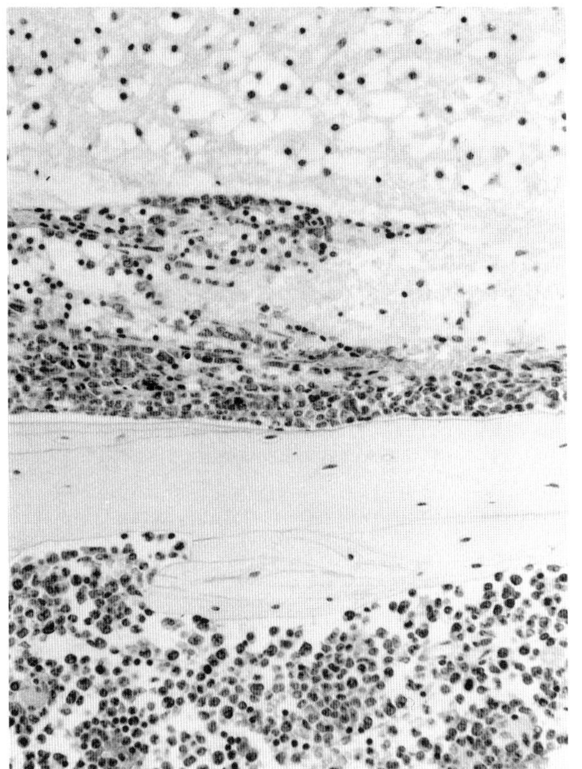

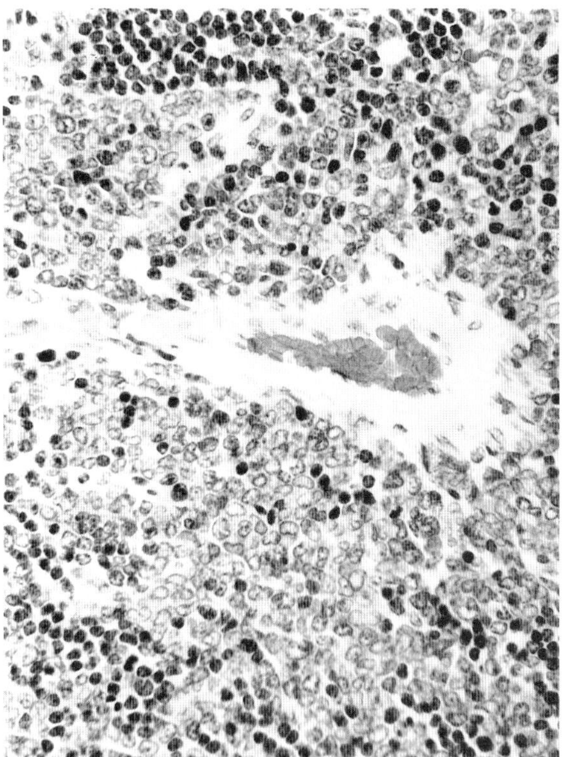

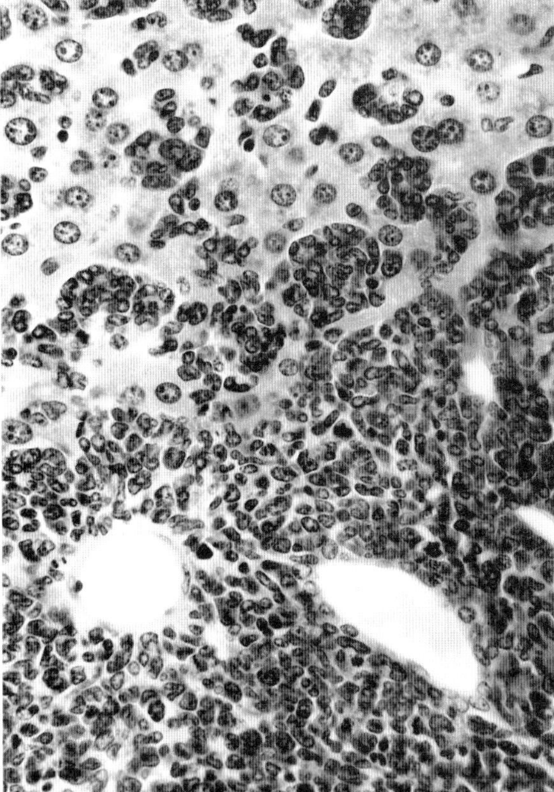

Fig. 54 *(upper left).* Skull and cerebrum, mouse. Leukemic cells have proliferated in the bone marrow of the skull and infiltrated the meninges. H and E, ×175

Fig. 55 *(upper right).* Spleen, mouse. Leukemic cells have proliferated in the white pulp, displacing lymphocytes. H and E, ×300

Fig. 56 *(lower right).* Liver, mouse. Leukemic cells have proliferated in Glisson's capsule as well as in an acinus. H and E, ×300 bones. Subperiosteal infiltration of leukemic cells may be observed. On the other hand, the meninges contiguous to the bone marrow of the skull are frequently invaded by leukemic cells (Fig. 54).

Leukemic cells proliferate not only in the red pulp of the spleen but also in the white pulp, especially surrounding the central artery where lymphocytes are replaced (Fig. 55). In the liver, leukemic cells proliferate in Glisson's capsule as well as in hepatic acini (Fig. 56).

Leukemic infiltration occurs in the kidney, adrenal glands, lymph nodes, and thymus. Generally speaking, loose connective tissue, such as in the adventitia of blood vessels, is a target of leukemic infiltration. Hemorrhage and thrombosis are often encountered in the lung.

Ultrastructure

The shape of nuclei in granulocytic leukemia cells is not uniform but varies with lobulation and segmentation (Fig. 57). An indented nucleus often surrounds the Golgi apparatus and free ribosomes. Small numbers of specific granules can be observed in part of the cytoplasm. The nucleolus is large and irregular in shape (Fig. 58).

The cytoplasm contains abundant free ribosomes and a large amount of rough endoplasmic reticulum. The mitochondria are round and have sparse irregular cristae. The outline of the leukemic cell is quite tortuous. No special attachment structures are seen between neighboring cells.

Differential Diagnosis

Extramedullary hemopoiesis in the spleen is evident by the presence of all types of developing cells of the bone marrow, including myeloid, erythroid, and megakaryocytic cells. The spleen is enlarged but of a uniform reddish color. In granulocytic leukemia the splenic parenchyma is replaced by immature cells and mature cells of the myeloid series only. Cells of the developing erythroid series are not present, nor are megakaryocytes evident in large numbers.

In blood smears from mice with granulocytic leukemia, immature and mature granulocytes are usually present in great numbers. These cells are not present in the peripheral blood of mice with extramedullary hemopoiesis (see p. 232, this volume; Barnes and Sisman 1939; Long et al. 1986). Differentiation of granulocytic leukemia from other types of murine leukemia is usually based on the histology and morphology of the neoplastic cells. Immunohistochemical identification of the cells is also definitive (see p. 126, this volume). Histologic differences between granulocytic leukemia and other myelogenous leukemias are indicated in Table 12. In erythro- and megakaryoblastic leukemia, the spleen never appears white or green. In lymphatic leukemia and lymphoma, the lymph nodes are much more enlarged than in granulocytic leukemia. Lymphoma cells proliferate in Glisson's capsule but not in acini.

Reticulum cell neoplasm type A also causes remarkable splenomegaly, but the splenic surface is rough rather than smooth. Sometimes it is accompanied by huge mesenteric lymph nodes. Histologically, characteristic granulomatous nodules are scattered in acini of the liver. No leukemic infiltration is observed in Glisson's capsule (see histiocytic sarcoma, p. 54, this volume).

Biologic Features

Progressive anemia, palpable splenomegaly, and rough respiratory movement are the triad of signs of granulocytic leukemia.

More than 95% of this type of leukemia have characteristic chromosome aberrations, i. e., partial deletion of no. 2 chromosome (Hayata et al. 1983). Most cases of granulocytic leukemia are

Table 12. Differences of leukemic infiltration among four types of leukemia

	Spleen	Liver	Thymus	Lymph node	Kidney	Adrenal gland
Granulocytic and monocytic leukemia	Red and white pulp (95.9%)	Acinus and Glisson (95.0%)	Yes (61.9%)	Often (95.4%)	Often (92.6%)	Often (80.5%)
Erythro- and megakaryoblastic leukemia	Red pulp only (100%)	Acinus only (82.4%)	No	Sometimes (28.6%)	Sometimes (45.0%)	Rare (6.7%)

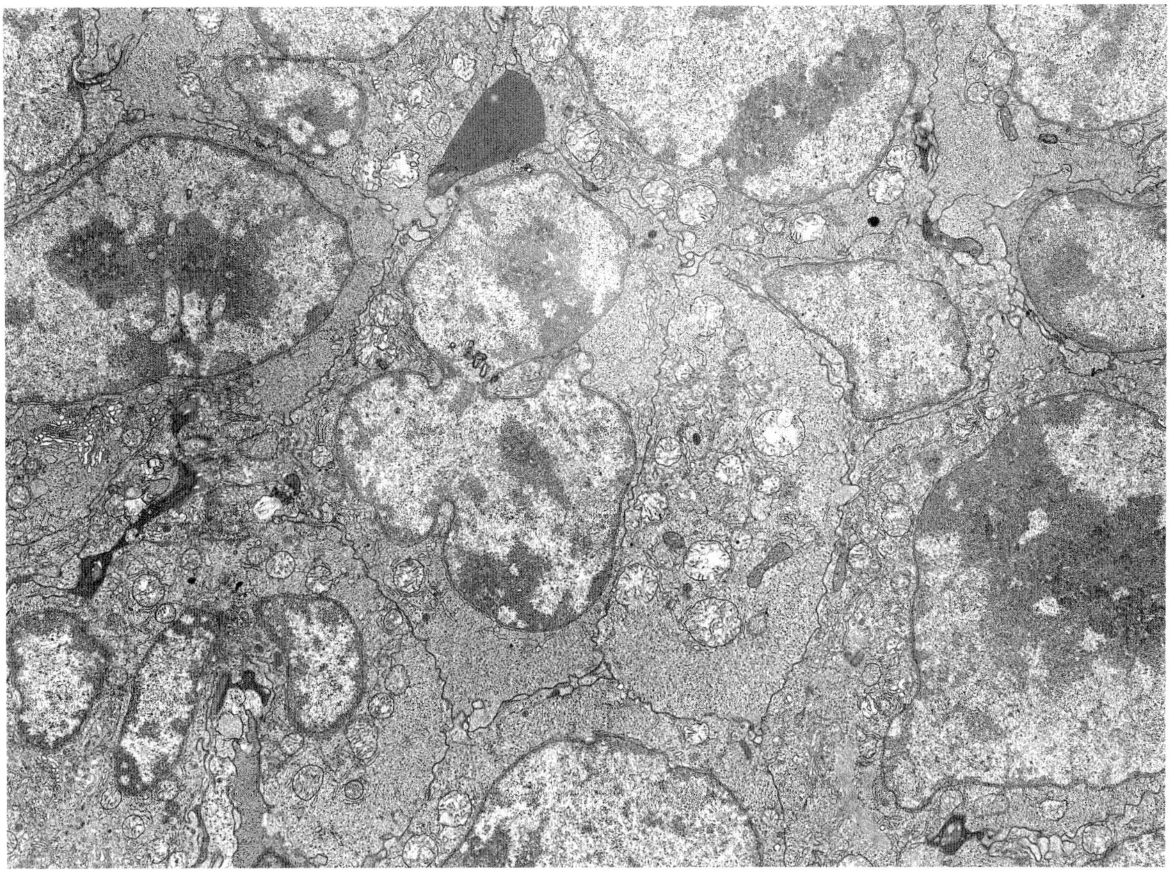

Fig. 57 *(above)*. Spleen, mouse. Splenic involvement of granulocytic leukemia. Cells with multilobulated and segmented nuclei containing prominent nucleoli are present. *Note* exaggeration of distinct myelocytic nuclear indentation and increased number of cytoplasmic organelles. TEM, × 3000

Fig. 58 *(below)*. Cell of granulocytic leukemia, mouse. *Note* rounded mitochondria, the Golgi complex, and numerous distended cristae of endoplasmic reticulum. Dense granules are few in number and vary in size, including an immature and small one with a double membrane. TEM, × 10000

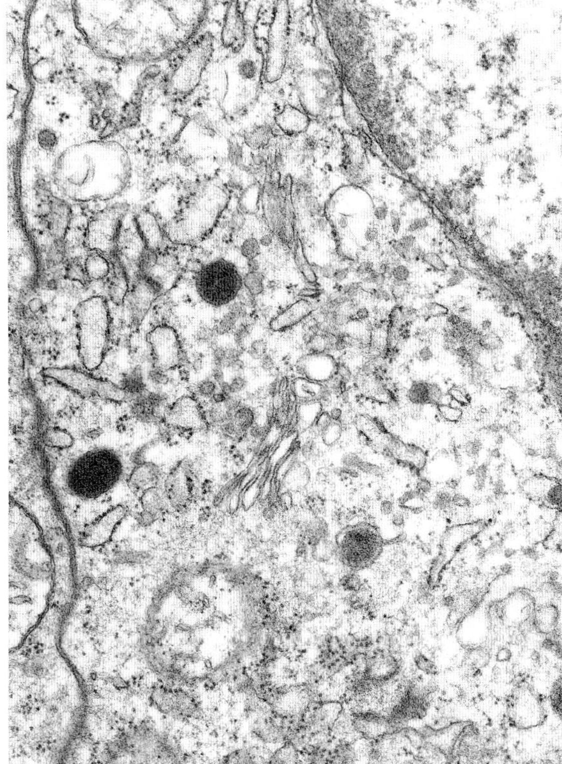

transplantable into syngeneic mice, using a suspension of spleen cells. Frequency of "takes" is about 95%. Characteristic marker chromosomes are evident even after serial transplantation.

The responsiveness of leukemic stem cells to CSFs or other hemopoietic stimulating factors varies: (a) growth independent of any factors; (b) partially dependent growth; (c) completely dependent growth; (d) unresponsive to the known factors (Yoshida et al. 1986). The last case might imply some unknown stimulating factors or cell-to-cell interaction.

Etiology and Frequency

Granulocytic leukemia is a rare disease under physiologic conditions. Only a few strains, i. e., RF (Upton et al. 1958), CBA/H (Major and Mole 1978), SJL/J (Resnitzky et al. 1987), and C3H/He (Hayata et al. 1983), are known to develop myelogenous leukemia after a single dose of whole body radiation. Natural incidence of the disease is 2%–3% in RF, 0% in CBA/H and SJL/J, 1% or less in C3H/He, respectively. The most effective radiation dose is 300 rad, which results in up to 25% incidence. Generally speaking, the frequency of radiation-induced leukemia in males is higher than that in females. In germ-free mice, the frequency is lower than in syngeneic conventional mice (Walburg et al. 1968). Administration of synthesized glucocorticoids just after irradiation increases the frequency of granulocytic leukemia significantly, from 18% to 59% in SJL/J and from 24% to 38% in C3H/He mice, respectively. The role of murine leukemia viruses in the development of granulocytic leukemia was demonstrated in the RF strain of mice (Upton et al. 1966); however, this was not proved in the C3H/He mouse strain.

Comparison with Other Species

In granulocytic leukemia, the juvenile (undifferentiated, acute) type might be comparable to human acute myelogenous leukemia (AML) and the mature (well-differentiated) type to chronic myelogenous leukemia (CML), although the time course of the disease in mice is unknown. The nucleus of the human leukemic cell does not have the doughnut shape that is characteristic in murine leukemia. Histologically, the pattern of leukemic infiltration in humans is not much different from that of the mouse; however, in most human patients the pathologic features are modified by therapeutic measures.

Induction of myelogenous leukemia by chemical carcinogens, i. e., DMBA (Huggins and Sugiyama 1966), urethane (Vesselinovitch 1968), nitrosourea (Odashima 1970; Ogiu et al. 1975), has usually been studied with rats. Pathologic features of rat granulocytic leukemia are similar to those of the mouse (see p. 39, this volume).

Acknowledgment. We thank Mr. Masachi Ikeda for his excellent technical assistance.

References

Barnes WA, Sisman IE (1939) Myeloid leukemia and non-malignant extramedullary myelopoiesis in mice. Am J Cancer 37: 1–3

Hayata I, Seki M, Yoshida K, Hirashima K, Sado T, Yamagiwa J, Ishihara T (1983) Chromosomal aberrations observed in 52 mouse myeloid leukemias. Cancer Res 43: 367–373

Huggins CB, Sugiyama T (1966) Induction of leukemia in rat by pulse doses of 7,12-dimethylbenz(a)anthracene. Proc Natl Acad Sci USA 55: 74–81

Long RE, Knutsen G, Robinson M (1986) Myeloid hyperplasia in the SENCAR mouse: differentiation from granulocyte leukemia. Environ Health Perspect 68: 117–123

Major IR, Mole RH (1978) Myeloid leukaemia in X-ray irradiated CBA mice. Nature 272: 455–456

Odashima S (1970) Leukemogenesis of N-nitrosobutylurea in the rat. I. Effect of various concentrations in the drinking water to female Donryu rats. Gann 61: 245–253

Ogiu T, Nakadate M, Odashima S (1975) Induction of leukemias and digestive tract tumors in Donryu rats by 1-propyl-1-nitrosourea. JNCI 54: 887–893

Resnitzky P, Estrov Z, Haran-Ghera N (1987) High incidence of acute myeloid leukemia in SJL/J mice after X-irradiation and corticosteroids. Leuk Res 9: 1519–1528

Upton AC, Wolff FF, Furth J, Kimball AW (1958) A comparison of the induction of myeloid and lymphoid leukemias in X-radiated RF mice. Cancer Res 18: 842–848

Upton AC, Jenkins VK, Walburg HE Jr, Tyndall RL, Conklin JW, Wald N (1966) Observations on viral, chemical and radiation-induced myeloid and lymphoid leukemias in RF mice. JNCI Monogr 22: 329–347

Vesselinovitch SD (1968) The strain difference in the induction of leukemia by urethan. Cancer Res 28: 1674–1676

Walburg HE Jr, Cosgrove GE, Upton AC (1968) Influence of microbial environment on development of myeloid leukemia in x-irradiated RFM mice. Int J Cancer 3: 150–154

Yoshida K, Nemoto K, Nishimura M, Hayata I, Inoue T, Seki M (1986) Nature of leukemic stem cells in murine myelogenous leukemia. Int J Cell Cloning 4: 91–102

Megakaryocytic Leukemia, Mouse

Torgny N. Fredrickson

Synonyms. Megakaryoblastic leukemia; megakaryocytic myelosis.

Gross Appearance

As with granulocytic and erythrocytic leukemias, the most noticeable lesion in megakaryocytic leukemia is splenic enlargement, often accompanied by marked hepatomegaly. The spleen, which can weigh over 2 g, is brownish-red without blood lakes, consolidated blood clots, or tumor nodules. The color of the liver is similar to that of the spleen, and the degree of hepatic enlargement can be severe in protracted cases. The disease is not associated with grossly discernable hemorrhage or other evidence of clotting disorders.

Microscopic Features

There is a striking increase in cells of the metakaryocytic series throughout the splenic red pulp, intermixed with myeloid and erythroid precursors (Figs. 59–61). In some preparations it is clear

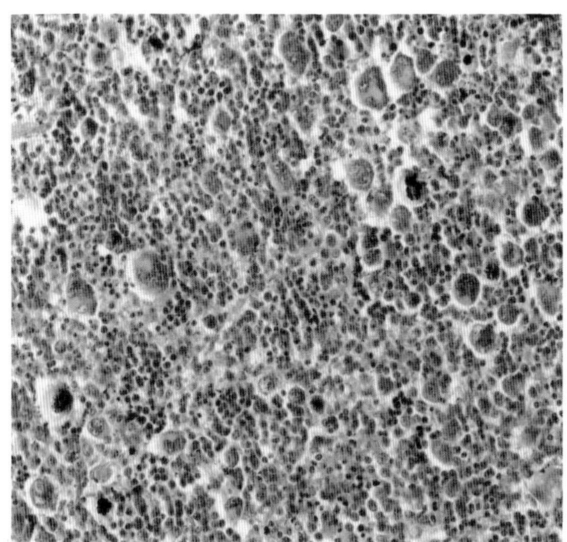

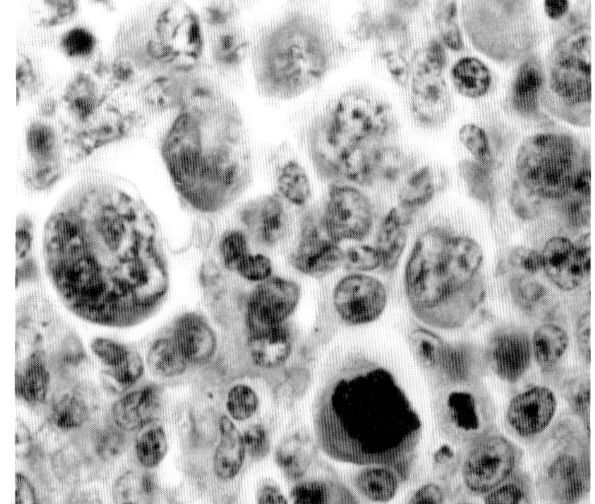

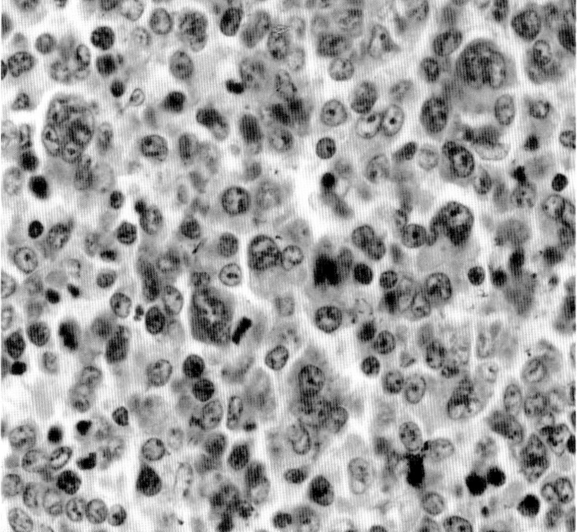

Fig. 59 *(upper left).* Spleen of an NFS/N mouse given an Mo/Fv MuLV construct. The red pulp is filled with megakaryocytes and clusters of darkly stained erythroid precursors. The degree of megakaryocytosis is attested to by the three mitotic figures *(lower left* and *upper right).* H and E, × 200

Fig. 60 *(upper right).* Spleen of mouse shown in Fig. 59 with megakaryocytic stages from megakaryoblast *(upper right)* to megakaryocyte *(left)* and mitotic figures *(lower center).* H and E, × 1000

Fig. 61 *(lower right).* Spleen of an NFS/N mouse given an Mo MuLV variant. The red pulp contains megakaryocytes and megakaryoblasts. Note numerous mitotic figures. H and E, × 600

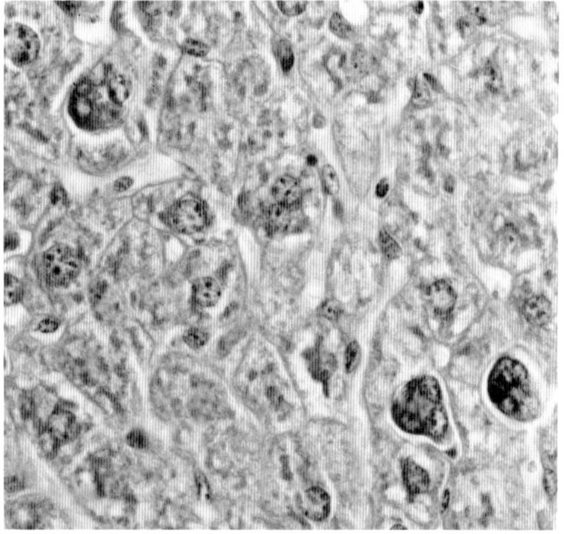

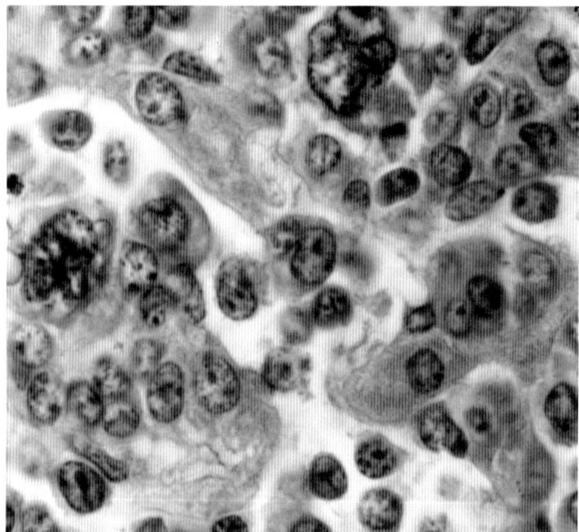

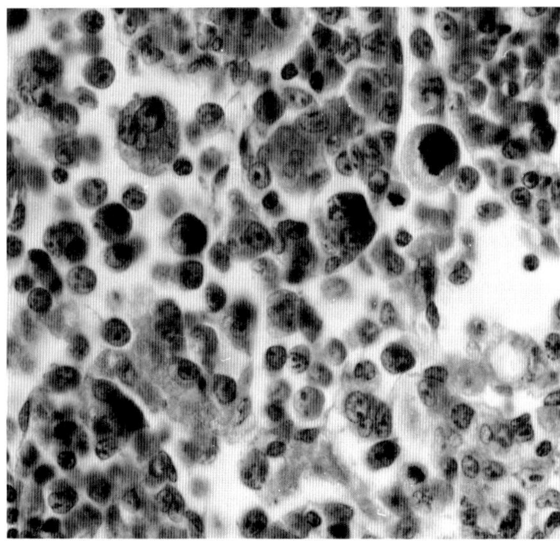

◀ **Fig. 62** *(above).* Liver of an NFS/N mouse given an Mo/Fv MuLV construct. Note three megakaryocytes in hepatic sinusoids. H and E, ×600

Fig. 63 *(middle).* Liver from the same mouse as in Fig. 61 with megakaryocytes and megakaryoblasts within hepatic sinusoids reflecting a more advanced state than in Fig. 62. H and E, ×1000

Fig. 64 *(below).* Advanced megakaryocytic leukemia in a lymph node of an NFS/Fv MuLV construct. The medullary sinuses contain numerous megakaryoblasts and megakaryocytes with mitotic figures. All nodes were equally involved. H and E, ×600

that they are mainly found within sinusoids. The white pulp is not as compressed as in erythroleukemia or myelogenous leukemia. Mitotic figures are common among megakaryoblasts and multinucleated megakaryocytes. Variable numbers of megakaryocytes, and occasionally megakaryoblasts, can also be seen within hepatic sinusoids (Figs. 62, 63) in a diffuse pattern throughout the liver. In some cases large numbers of megakaryocytes are present in the lymph nodes (Fig. 64). The cases of megakaryocytic leukemia described here were induced with retroviruses.

Ultrastructure

An outstanding ultrastructural feature of productive retroviral infection in mice is the tremendous number of viral particles that can be seen budding from the cytoplasmic demarcation membranes of megakaryocytes (LoBue et al. 1974). Despite this degree of viral replication, the megakaryocyte does not show obvious evidence of lysis, although thrombocytopenia has been noted as a component of Friend murine leukemia virus (MuLV) induced disease (Dennis and Brodsky 1965).

Differential Diagnosis

Grossly, leukemias associated with the splenic red pulp, including those of the erythroid, myeloid, megakaryocytic, and even the rare mast cell lineages all look alike with splenic and hepatic enlargement. Microscopically, the differences are quite apparent because the number of megakaryocytes and their precursors within the splenic red pulp clearly differentiated megakaryocytic leukemia. Also, megakaryocytic leukemia does not feature the splenic destructive changes common in acute erythroleukemia. In cases of chronic myelogenous leukemia there may be considerable numbers of megakaryocytes within the splenic red pulp, but they are greatly outnumbered by granulocytic precursors. Grossly, lymph nodes may be grossly enlarged in chronic myelogenous leukemia due to accumulation of myeloid cells in the medullary region. This may help in differentiating it from megakaryocytic leukemia which usually does not cause prominent nodal enlargement. Within hepatic sinusoids megakaryocytes are evenly distributed as opposed to concentrations of granulocytic cells around triad areas in chronic myelogenous leukemia and, to a lesser extent, erythroleukemia. Megakaryocytic leukemia, chronic erythroleukemia, and chronic myelogenous leukemia all have a protracted latent period of several months, and certain retroviruses can induce any of the three diseases, sometimes along with lymphomas. Therefore, histologic evaluation is required in order to make a differential diagnosis. Acetylcholinesterase is present in the cells of the megakaryocytic series in the mouse.

It is also necessary to distinguish benign megakaryocytosis since reactive conditions, such as prolonged inflammation, can lead to extensive extramedullary hemopoiesis (see p. 232, this volume) with enlargement of both the red and white pulp of the spleen, causing severe splenomegaly. Such conditions are usually associated with large numbers of megakaryocytes within the red pulp. These are, however, almost entirely mature, and their numbers are proportionately matched with increases in both myeloid and erythroid cells. Under these conditions megakaryocytes also may occasionally be seen in hepatic sinusoids, but their numbers in the liver, particularly the more immature forms, do not compare with those seen in cases of megakaryocytic leukemia. There is a single case of megakaryocytosis pictured in a recently published atlas of mouse hematopathology (Frith et al. 1985). This case appears to have splenic histologic features similar to some cases which we have diagnosed as leukemia.

Biologic Features

Effects of Friend-Moloney MuLV constructs show that megakaryocytic leukemia is induced with low frequency in groups of mice, which mainly developed either erythroleukemia or myelogenous leukemia (Li et al. 1987). This indicates that megakaryoblasts are relatively refractory to MuLV-induced transformation, a suggestion strengthened by the absence of reports on mouse megakaryocytic leukemia in the literature. Cases could have been overlooked because of their gross resemblance to other mouse leukemias, but it seems that they truly are rare. There is no wild type MuLV associated exclusively with the induction of predominantly megakaryocytic leukemia. As noted, reactive megakaryocytosis is fairly frequently seen in mice. However, there does not seem to be much doubt that the cases diagnosed as megakaryocytic leukemias and forming the basis of this report are neoplasms: firstly, splenomegaly and hepatomegaly can be very severe; secondly, one case has been analyzed at the molecular level and shown to be of clonal origin on the basis of MuLV insertion sites (Fredrickson, personal observation); thirdly, mitotic figures among megakaryoblasts and megakaryocytes are frequently seen; and fourthly, the disease is associated with MuLV known to induce leukemias.

Etiology and Frequency

Spontaneous megakaryocytic leukemia appears to be extremely rare in mice; we have observed one such case. The only other cases observed have been induced by MuLVs, including those of wild mouse origin (Fredrickson et al. 1984), Rauscher MuLV, and most frequently in mice given genetically engineered constructs, composed of different genomic fractions of Friend and Moloney MuLVs (Li et al. 1987). The number of cases encountered has been very few, and their sporadic nature and similar appearance to chronic erythroleukemia and CML has prevented any investigation of other parameters than histology because diagnosis was made only on microscopic review. Thus, the blood picture, bone marrow histology, and cytology of neoplastic megakaryocytes remain to be studied.

Comparison with Other Species

Megakaryocytic leukemia is a rare hemopoietic neoplasm in all species. Hardy (1981) mentions a single case in his survey of hemopoietic tumors of cats, however, other authors may have included this disease within the myelodystrophic syndrome. In humans the disease has been well characterized by a number of morphologic and cytochemical criteria (Bennett et al. 1985). It is well recognized that similarly stringent criteria have not been applied to the cases described here, but as noted above, there appears to be sufficient reason to accept them as true megakaryocytic leukemias.

Acknowledgment. I would like to acknowledge the help of Dr. J. W. Hartley.

References

Bennett JM, Catovsky M, Daniel MT, Flandrin G, Galton DAG, Gralnick HR, Sultan C (1985) Criteria for the diagnosis of acute leukemia of megakaryocytic lineage (M 7). A report of the French-American-British Cooperative Group. Ann Intern Med 103: 460–462

Dennis LH, Brodsky I (1965) Thrombocytopenia induced by the Friend leukemia virus. JNCI 35: 993–999

Fredrickson TN, Langdon WY, Hoffman PM, Hartley JW, Morse HC III (1984) Histologic and cell surface antigen studies of hematopoietic tumors induced by Cas-Br-M murine leukemia virus. JNCI 72: 447–454

Frith CH, Pattengale PK, Ward JM (1985) A color atlas of hematopoietic pathology of mice. Toxicology Pathology Associates, Little Rock

Hardy WD (1981) Hematopoietic tumors of cats. J Am Anim Hosp Assoc 17: 921–940

Li Y, Golemis E, Hartley JW, Hopkins N (1987) Disease specificity of nondefective Friend and Moloney murine leukemia viruses is controlled by a small number of nucleotides. J Virol 61: 693–700

LoBue J, Gordon AS, Weitz-Hamburger A, Ferdinand P, Camiscoli JF, Fredrickson TN, Hardy WD Jr (1974) Erythroid differentiation in murine erythroleukemia. In: Clarkson B and Baserga R (eds) Control of proliferation of animal cells. Cold Spring Harbor Laboratory, Cold Spring Harbor, pp 863–885

Histiocytic Sarcoma, Rat

Robert A. Squire

Synonyms. Histiocytic lymphoma; reticulum cell sarcoma.

Gross Appearance

The gross appearance of histiocytic sarcoma has not been well characterized since it is usually diagnosed only upon microscopic examination. The sites most frequently affected macroscopically are the liver, lungs, subcutis, lymph nodes, and spleen. The tumors appear as irregular, pale, tan masses or organ infiltrates.

Microscopic Features

The spectrum of microscopic features of histiocytic sarcoma in rats is very characteristic (Figs. 65–70). Most of the neoplasms are sarcomatous with minimal cellular pleomorphism. Less frequently, there is a granulomatous appearance with greater cellular pleomorphism and considerable fibrosis. Even in these cases, however, inflammatory cells are very infrequent. Histologic characteristics vary from animal to animal and even among different sites in the same animal. The tissues most frequently affected are the liver, lungs, lymph nodes, spleen, adipose tissue, retroperitoneum, mesentery, skeletal muscle, pancreas, and kidney, but any site may be involved. If only one site is affected, it is usually the liver, suggesting an origin in this tissue, at least in some cases. The earliest tumors in the liver are small collections or sheets of tumor cells in hepatic sinusoids. Early lung involvement usually consists of tumor cells in perivascular or peribronchiolar locations. Growth in all sites is both infiltrative and expansive. The tumor may spread along the serous surfaces, and tumor cells are often present in blood vessels of the liver, lung, spleen, or other tissue.

The tumor cells have a typical histiocytic appearance. The cytoplasm is relatively broad and eosinophilic and may contain vacuoles or phagocytized erythrocytes. The nuclei have little chromatin and are oval to elongated and frequently indented or folded. Nuclear membranes are delicate, and nucleoli are small and usually singular. Mitotic figures are infrequent. There may be multinucleate tumor cells of the Langhans type. Areas of tumor cell necrosis surrounded by palisaded tumor cells are very common and characteristic of histiocytic sarcoma. Fibrosis varies from minimal to extensive.

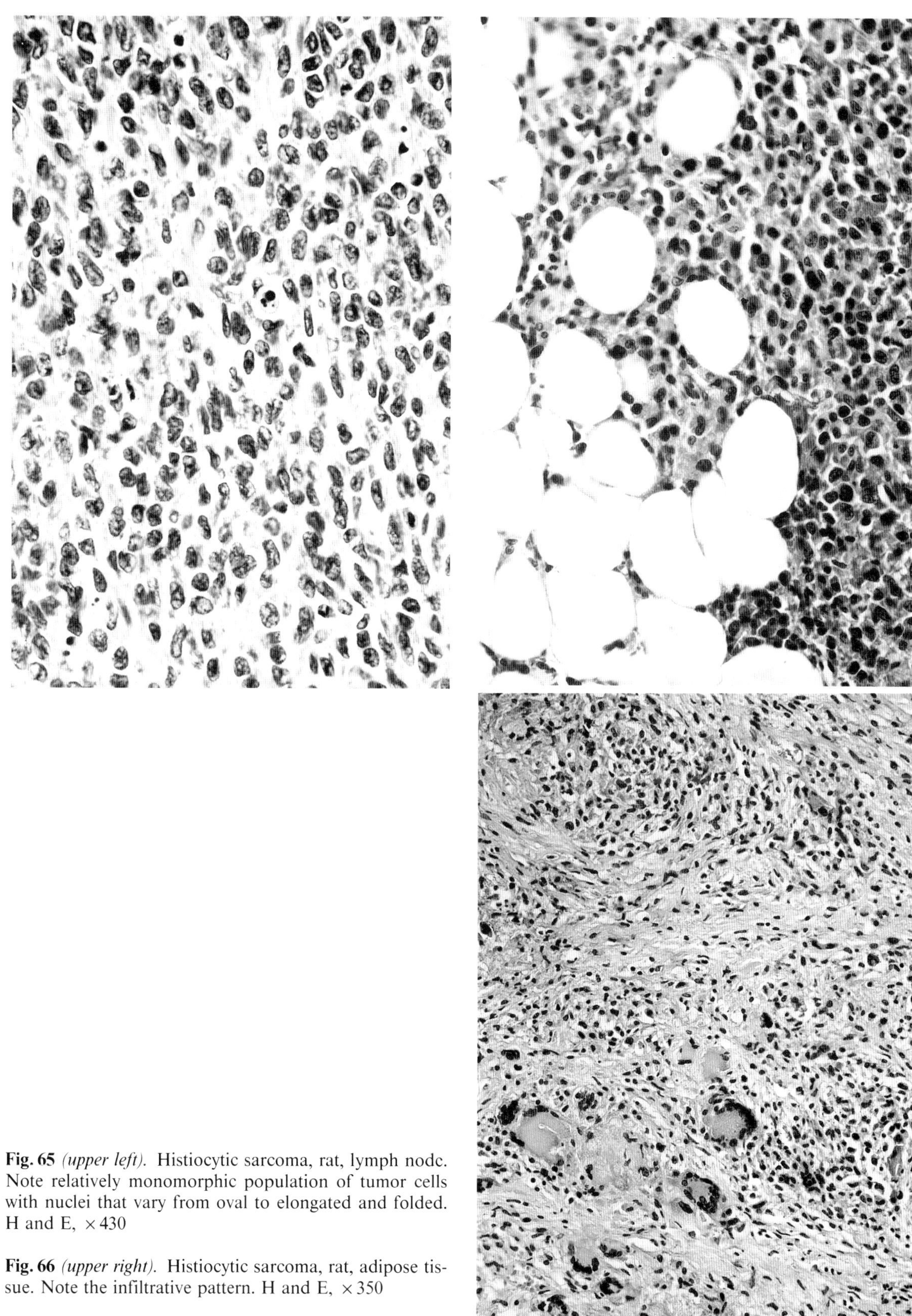

Fig. 65 *(upper left).* Histiocytic sarcoma, rat, lymph node. Note relatively monomorphic population of tumor cells with nuclei that vary from oval to elongated and folded. H and E, × 430

Fig. 66 *(upper right).* Histiocytic sarcoma, rat, adipose tissue. Note the infiltrative pattern. H and E, × 350

Fig. 67 *(lower right).* Histiocytic sarcoma, rat. Note extensive fibrosis and Langhans' giant cells. H and E, × 220

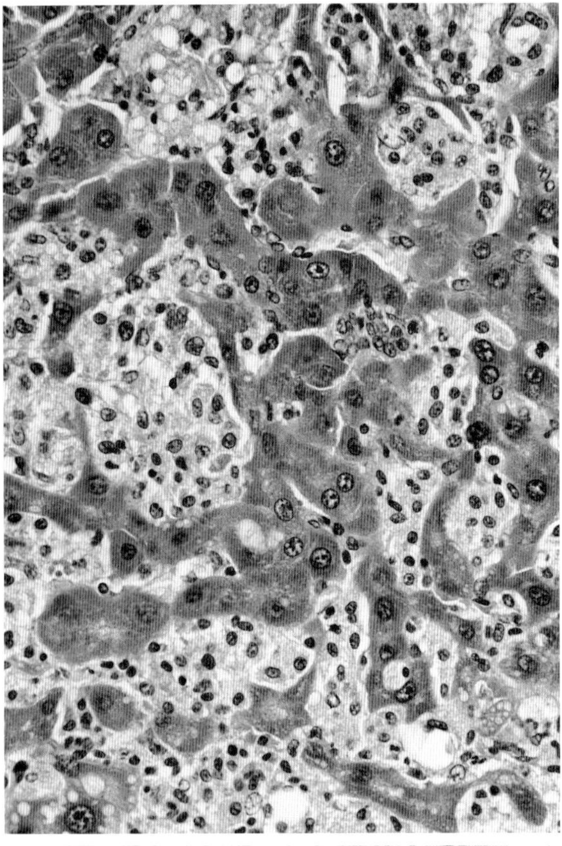

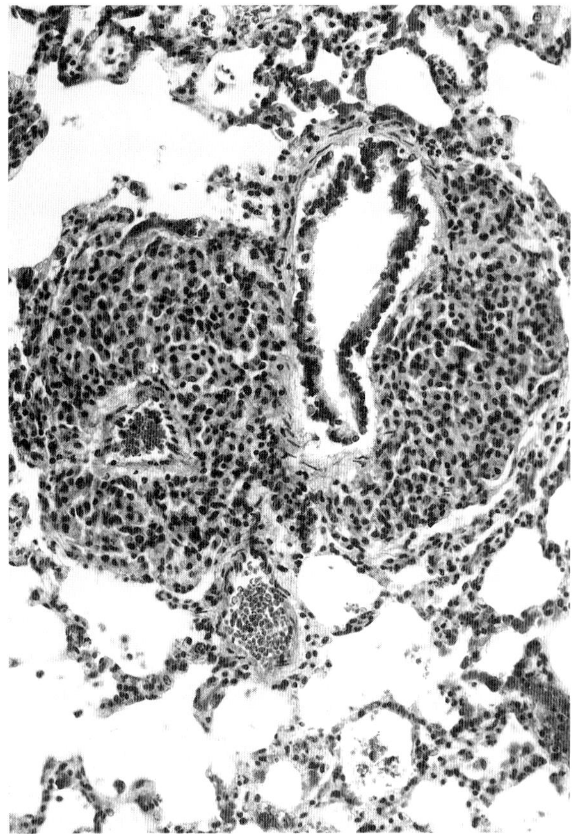

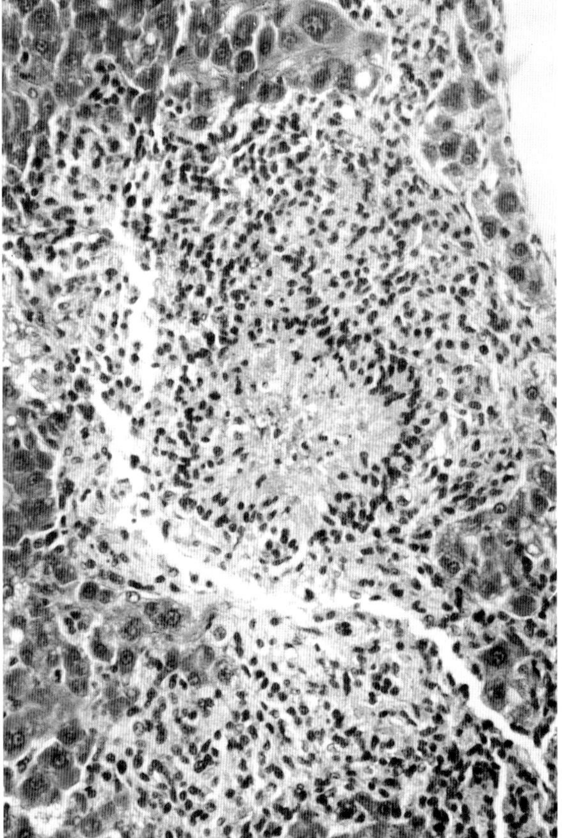

Fig. 68 *(upper left).* Histiocytic sarcoma, liver, rat. Tumor cells occupy the sinusoids and compress hepatic plates. H and E, ×350

Fig. 69 *(lower left).* Histiocytic sarcoma, liver, rat. Note tumor cell necrosis with surrounding palisaded cells. This is a frequent and characteristic histologic feature. H and E, ×190

Fig. 70 *(upper right).* Histiocytic sarcoma, lung, rat. Note typical perivascular and peribronchiolar involvement. H and E, ×220

Ultrastructure

Electron microscopic examinations have been limited (Squire et al. 1981; Ward et al. 1981; Barsoum et al. 1984). Cytoplasmic organelles are not numerous and consist of mitochondria, lipid droplets, and small amounts of rough endoplasmic reticulum. There are few or no cytoplasmic fibrils and no basement membranes. Filamentous material is occasionally present between cells without evidence of cross-banding. Immunohistochemical studies have revealed evidence of lysozyme, α_1-antitrypsin or α_1-antichymotrypsin, possible histiocytic markers (Barsoum et al. 1984).

Differential Diagnosis

Uncertainty over the classification of histiocytic sarcoma is indicated by the synonyms. This author believes that histiocytic sarcoma is a distinct disease entity that differs from so-called histiocytic lymphoma and from malignant fibrous histiocytoma, a disease originally described in humans and with which it is most frequently confused. In fact, early descriptions of histiocytic sarcoma in rats were reported as malignant fibrous histiocytoma (Squire et al. 1978; Goodman et al. 1980; Ward et al. 1981) (see p. 54, this volume).
Several histologic features serve to distinguish histiocytic sarcoma. These include: (a) tumor cell necrosis surrounded by palisaded tumor cells, (b) spread on serosal surfaces and in the vascular spaces, (c) relatively monomorphic cellularity, and (d) the presence of occasional Langhans' giant cells. Malignant fibrous histiocytoma is a more polymorphic tumor that undergoes both fibroblastic and histiocytic differentiation and does not have these characteristic features.
Histiocytic sarcoma should not be confused with granulomatous inflammation, particularly if several affected sites are examined.

Biologic Features

Histiocytic sarcoma appears to be a specific neoplasm of connective tissue histiocytes that is distinct from other soft tissue tumors (Squire et al. 1981). The morphologic features of the tumor cells and their phagocytosis of erythrocytes suggest that they are histiocytic, although this has not been completely confirmed by specific enzymatic or immunological methods (Barsoum et al. 1984). The site of origin sometimes appears to be the liver sinusoids or perhaps the Kupffer's cells. In most cases, however, the primary site cannot be determined. The tumors are malignant in that they invade locally and metastasize to distant sites. There is apparently no benign form of the disease.

Etiology and Frequency

The etiology of histiocytic sarcoma is not known. No bacteria, fungi, or viruses have been identified by special stains or limited ultrastructural studies, and no chemical has been shown to increase the incidence (Pradham et al. 1974).
Histiocytic sarcoma occurs relatively commonly as a natural event in aging rats, particularly in Sprague-Dawley derived strains. Since different diagnostic terms have been used in the past, it is difficult to determine the true historical incidences. In one large study with Sprague-Dawley rats, the overall incidence was 4.7% (Squire et al. 1981). Most tumors were observed in animals 18 months of age or older, and both sexes were affected about equally. The incidence is apparently lower in Fischer 344 and Osborne-Mendel rats, although this varies widely among different groups of animals.

Comparison with Other Species

The only similar or identical neoplasm in other species is so-called reticulum cell sarcoma type A (Dunn 1954) or histiocytic lymphoma (Frith et al. 1980) in mice. Although a different tissue distribution may occur in mice, the morphologic and biologic features of the diseases are quite similar. The term lymphoma is a misnomer in mice since the tumor cells have been shown to be histiocytes (Talmadge et al. 1981). The term histiocytic sarcoma would also be preferred for this murine disease.
As indicated, malignant fibrous histiocytoma, a tumor similar to histiocytic sarcoma, occurs in humans (Weiss and Enzinger 1978) and has been reported in dogs and cats (Gleiser et al. 1979). Greaves and Faccini (1981) described a series of "fibrous histiocytic" neoplasms in rats that appear to include both malignant fibrous histiocytoma and histiocytic sarcoma. Since there appear to be distinctive biologic and morphologic differences between these two neoplasms (see p. 58,

this volume), it is probably best not to combine them under the same term unless, in the future, a common etiology or pathogenesis is demonstrated.

References

Barsoum NJ, Hanna W, Gough AW, Smith GS, Sturgess JM, de la Iglesia FA (1984) Histiocytic sarcoma in Wistar rats; a light microscopic, immunohistochemical and ultrastructural study. Arch Pathol Lab Med 108: 802–807

Dunn TB (1974) Normal and pathologic anatomy of the reticular tissue in laboratory mice, with a classification and discussion of neoplasms. JNCI 14: 1281–1433

Frith CH, Davis TM, Zolator LA, Townsend JW (1980) Histiocytic lymphoma in the mouse. Leuk Res 4: 651–662

Gleiser CA, Raulston GL, Jardine JH, Gray KN (1979) Malignant fibrous histiocytoma in dogs and cats. Vet Pathol 16: 199–208

Goodman DG, Ward JM, Squire RA, Paxton MB, Reichardt WD, Chu KC, Linhart MS (1980) Neoplastic and nonneoplastic lesions in aging Osborne-Mendel rats. Toxicol Appl Pharmacol 55: 433–447

Greaves P, Faccini JM (1981) Spontaneous fibrous histiocytic neoplasms in rats. Br J Cancer 43: 402–411

Pradhan SN, Chung EB, Ghosh B (1974) Potential carcinogens. I. Carcinogenicity of some plant extracts and their Tannin-containing fractions in rats. JNCI 52: 1579–1582

Squire RA, Brinkhous KM, Peiper SC, Firminger HI, Mann RB, Strandberg JD (1981) Histiocytic sarcoma with a granuloma-like component occurring in a large colony of Sprague-Dawley rats. Am J Pathol 105: 21–30

Squire RA, Goodman DG, Valerio MG, Fredrickson TN, Strandberg JD, Levitt MH, Lingeman CH, Harshbarger JC, Dawe CJ (1978) Tumors. In: Benirschke K, Garner FM, Jones TC (eds) Pathology of laboratory animals, vol II. Springer, Berlin Heidelberg New York, chap 12

Talmadge JE, Kay ME, Hart IR (1981) Characterization of a murine ovarian reticulum cell sarcoma of histiocytic origin. Cancer Res 41: 1271–1280

Ward JM, Kulwich BA, Reznik G, Berman JJ (1981) Malignant fibrous histiocytoma. An unusual neoplasm of soft-tissue origin in the rat that is different from the human counterpart. Arch Pathol Lab Med 105: 313–316

Weiss SW, Enzinger FM (1978) Malignant fibrous histiocytoma: An analysis of 200 cases. Cancer 41: 2250–2266

Histiocytic Sarcoma, Mouse

Charles H. Frith

Synonyms. Reticulum cell sarcoma, type A; lymphoma, histiocytic.

Gross Appearance

The gross appearance of histiocytic sarcoma in the mouse varies depending upon the organ involved. Affected mice with the disease die quite suddenly, and the disease is usually only observed at necropsy. The liver is usually uniformly markedly enlarged (2–3 times) and is often mottled (Fig. 71). Focal nodules are seen much less frequently than diffuse involvement in the spontaneous disease. Multiple metastatic nodules in the liver are commonly seen in animals with the transplanted neoplasm (Fig. 72) (Frith et al. 1980). A small amount of serosanguinous fluid may be present in the abdominal cavity. The spleen is usually enlarged, but the enlargement is most often due to stimulated extramedullary hemopoiesis activity rather than tumor involvement (see p. 232, this volume). If the uterus is involved, a single, firm, whitish nodule is usually present in the uterine wall, often resulting in hydrometra of either one or both uterine horns.

Microscopic Features

Histiocytic sarcoma may produce clumps of neoplastic cells appearing focally in the liver, but frequently there is diffuse involvement with many neoplastic cells within the hepatic sinusoids (Fig. 73). Giant cells may or may not be a prominent feature in the liver lesions and sometimes are granulomatous (Fig. 74). The marked variation in morphology of the neoplastic histiocytic is a distinguishing feature. The basic cell has a dark basophilic nucleus and abundant, distinctly eosinophilic cytoplasm. Great variation in the size and shape of the cell and nucleus and

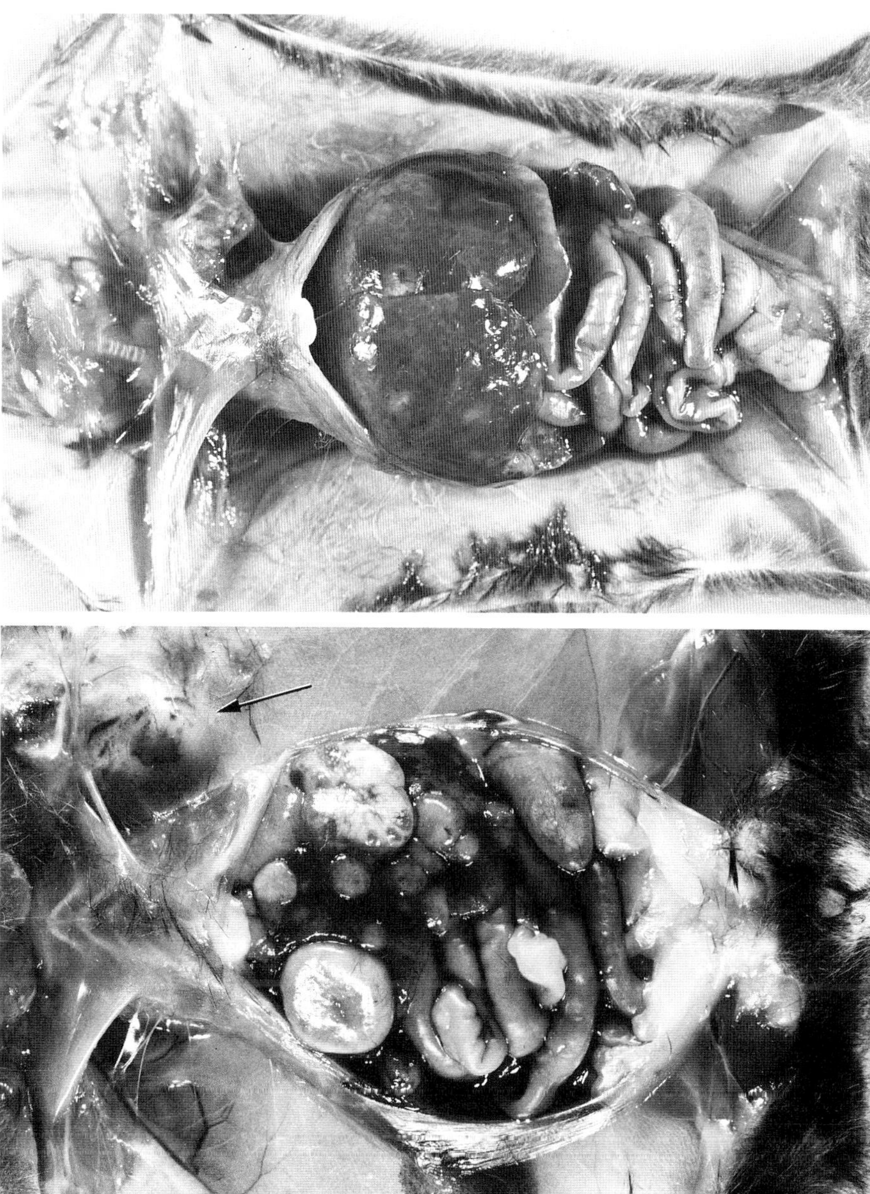

Fig. 71 *(above).* Histiocytic sarcoma, mouse, female, C 57 BL/6 strain. Enlarged liver with histiocytic sarcoma

Fig. 72 *(below).* Histiocytic sarcoma, mouse, male, C 57 BL/6 strain. Subcutaneous nodule *(arrow)* developed from transplanted cells; also note enlarged liver with numerous metastatic nodules

the nuclear-cytoplasmic ratio is common. The neoplastic cells in the uterus tend to be more spindle-shaped or fusiform and resemble fibroblasts (Fig. 75). Erythrophagocytosis may occur in both the uterus (Fig. 76) and liver, but it is more common in the liver. The ovaries may sometimes be diffusely involved by the neoplastic cells. Involvement of the lymph nodes, thymus, bone marrow (Fig. 77), and spleen is rare. If mus, bone marrow (Fig. 77), and spleen is rare. If the spleen is involved, the lesion is almost always focal in nature (Fig. 78). The gross enlargement of the spleen seen at the time of necropsy is usually due to increased extramedullary hemopoiesis rather than tumor. Neoplastic cells are prominent in the pulmonary circulation in association with liver lesions (Fig. 73). Metastases to the lungs (Fig. 79) are also quite common. Other organs including pancreas, mesentery, intestine,

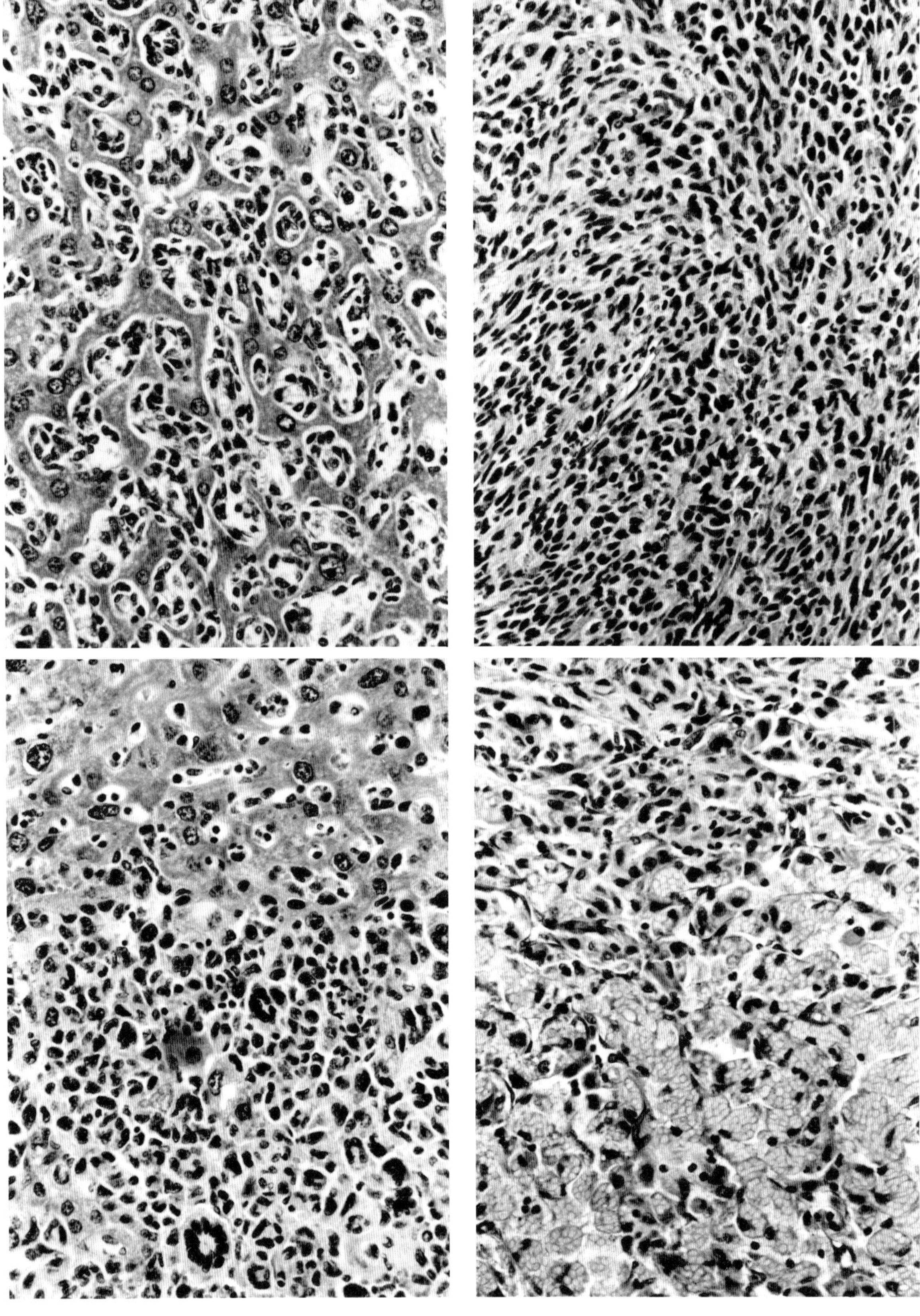

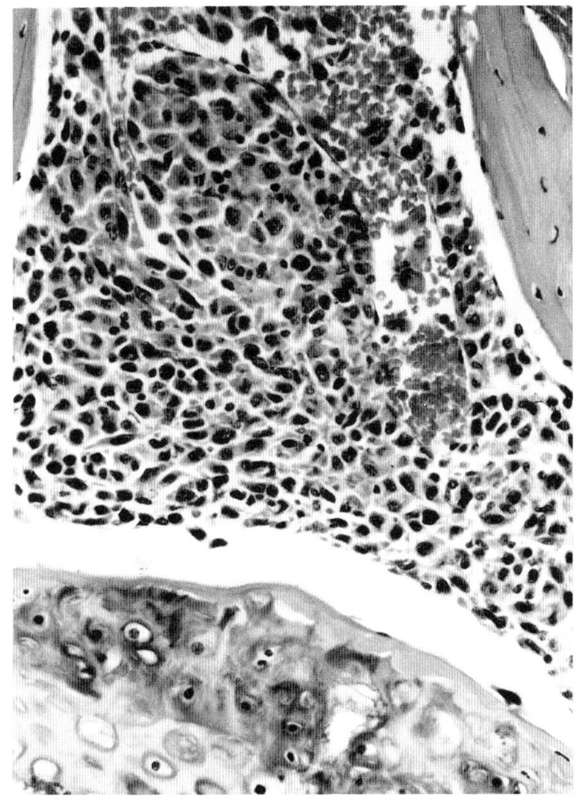

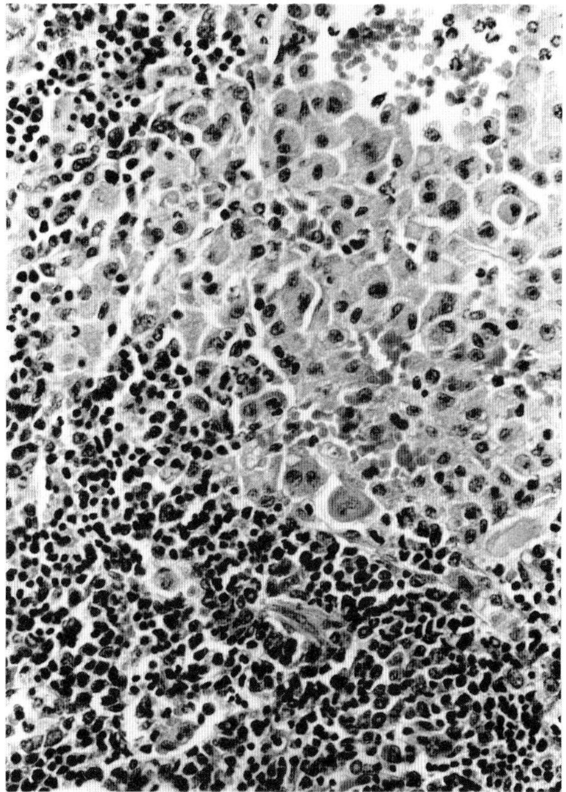

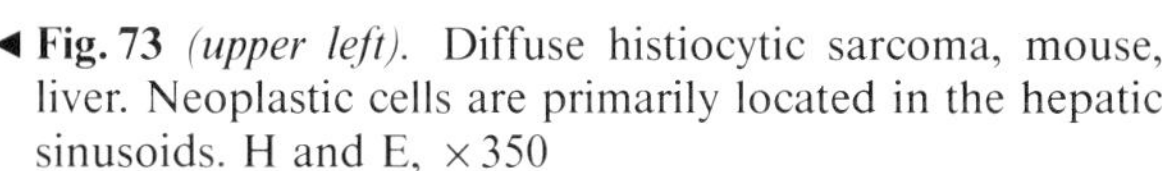

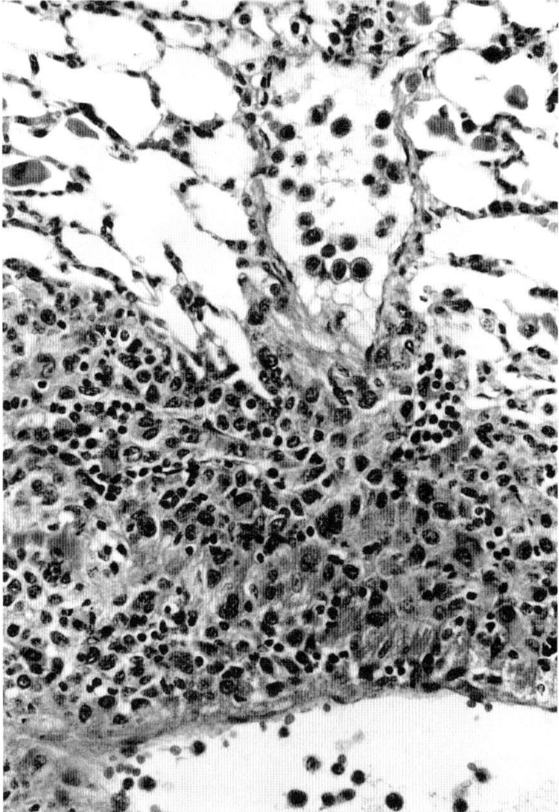

◄ **Fig. 73** *(upper left).* Diffuse histiocytic sarcoma, mouse, liver. Neoplastic cells are primarily located in the hepatic sinusoids. H and E, ×350

Fig. 74 *(lower left).* Focal histiocytic sarcoma, mouse, liver. Note numerous giant cells. H and E, ×350

Fig. 75 *(upper right).* Histiocytic sarcoma, mouse, uterus. It is made up of spindle-shaped cells. H and E, ×350

Fig. 76 *(lower right).* Histiocytic sarcoma, mouse, uterus. Erythrophagocytosis and neoplastic histiocytic cells which are filled with red blood cells. H and E, ×350

Fig. 77 *(upper left).* Histiocytic sarcoma, bone marrow, ► mouse. H and E, ×350

Fig. 78 *(upper right).* Focal histiocytic sarcoma, mouse, spleen. H and E, ×350

Fig. 79 *(lower right).* Pulmonary metastasis of histiocytic sarcoma, mouse, lung. Note large neoplastic cells in pulmonary vessel. H and E, ×350

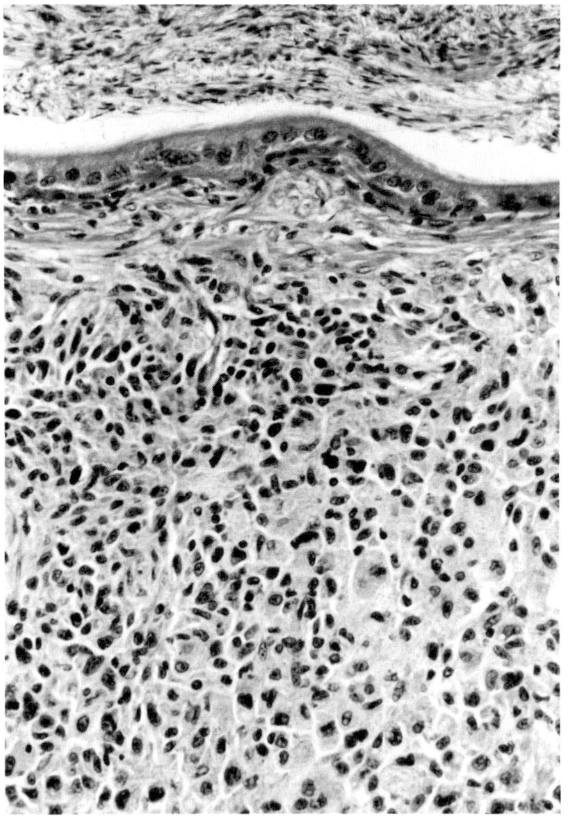

Fig. 80. Histiocytic sarcoma, mouse, epididymis. Neoplastic cells are located outside of tubule. H and E, × 350

heart, kidney, and epididymis (Fig. 80) may occasionally be involved (Frith et al. 1985; Frith and Wiley 1981). An occasional neoplastic cell can be found in a blood smear, but no cases of leukemia have been convincingly described (Della Porta et al. 1979).

Ultrastructure

Under TEM study, the neoplastic cells appear pleomorphic and variable in size and shape. The nuclei are irregular in shape, and the cytoplasm contains a moderate number of mitochondria, ribosomes, and both smooth and rough endoplasmic reticulum (Figs. 81, 82). Some of the cells may contain lysosomes, and some may have phagocytized, fragmented red blood cells. The plasma membranes of adjacent cells have prominent infolding and interdigitation, but desmosomes are not seen. A basement membrane around the tumor cells is not apparent (Fig. 82). Under SEM study, the pleomorphic cells appear

rounded, with numerous filopodia (Fig. 83). The surface of some cells contain numerous microvilli.

Differential Diagnosis

Histiocytic sarcoma in the liver does not usually present any diagnostic difficulty. If the uterus is involved, other lesions must be considered including stromal cell sarcoma, fibrosarcoma, and leiomyosarcoma. Although tumors in the liver may be present without uterine involvement, if uterine lesions are present, the liver is almost invariably involved. A general rule, that individual lesions should be diagnosed only after considering what is known to have occurred elsewhere in the animal, is particularly germane to histiocytic sarcoma in the mouse.

Biologic Features

The exact cell of origin of the histiocytic sarcoma of the mouse has not been conclusively determined. In the liver, the neoplasm may arise from Kupffer's cells. The morphologic features, erythrophagocytosis, and cytochemical characteristics certainly suggest a histiocytic origin. The lesion is definitely not of lymphoid origin and should not be referred to or grouped with lymphomas in determining the carcinogenicity of toxicants. The neoplastic cells readily transplant and produce small neoplasms at the site of inoculation (Fig. 72). However, while the transplanted neoplasm remains small, grossly and microscopically, the livers contain multiple nodules of metastatic neoplasm (Fig. 74).

Histiocytic sarcoma has been described by other investigators by a variety of other names (Chouroulinkov et al. 1969; Dawson et al. 1974; Dunn 1954; Stewart et al. 1974; and Frith et al. 1980). Dr. Thelma Dunn (1954) described the neoplasm as a reticulum cell neoplasm type A. She described the phagocytic properties of the neoplastic cells and suggested that the neoplasm arises as a primary tumor in the livers of male and female mice and in the uterus of female mice. Dawson et al. (1974) described uterine sarcomas in (C 57 BL/6 × DBA/2)F$_1$ mice, and the morphologic description suggests histiocytic sarcoma. Chouroulinkov et al. (1969) described 130 cases of endometrial sarcoma in a number of strains of mice. Their gross and microscopic findings also suggest that they were describing histio-

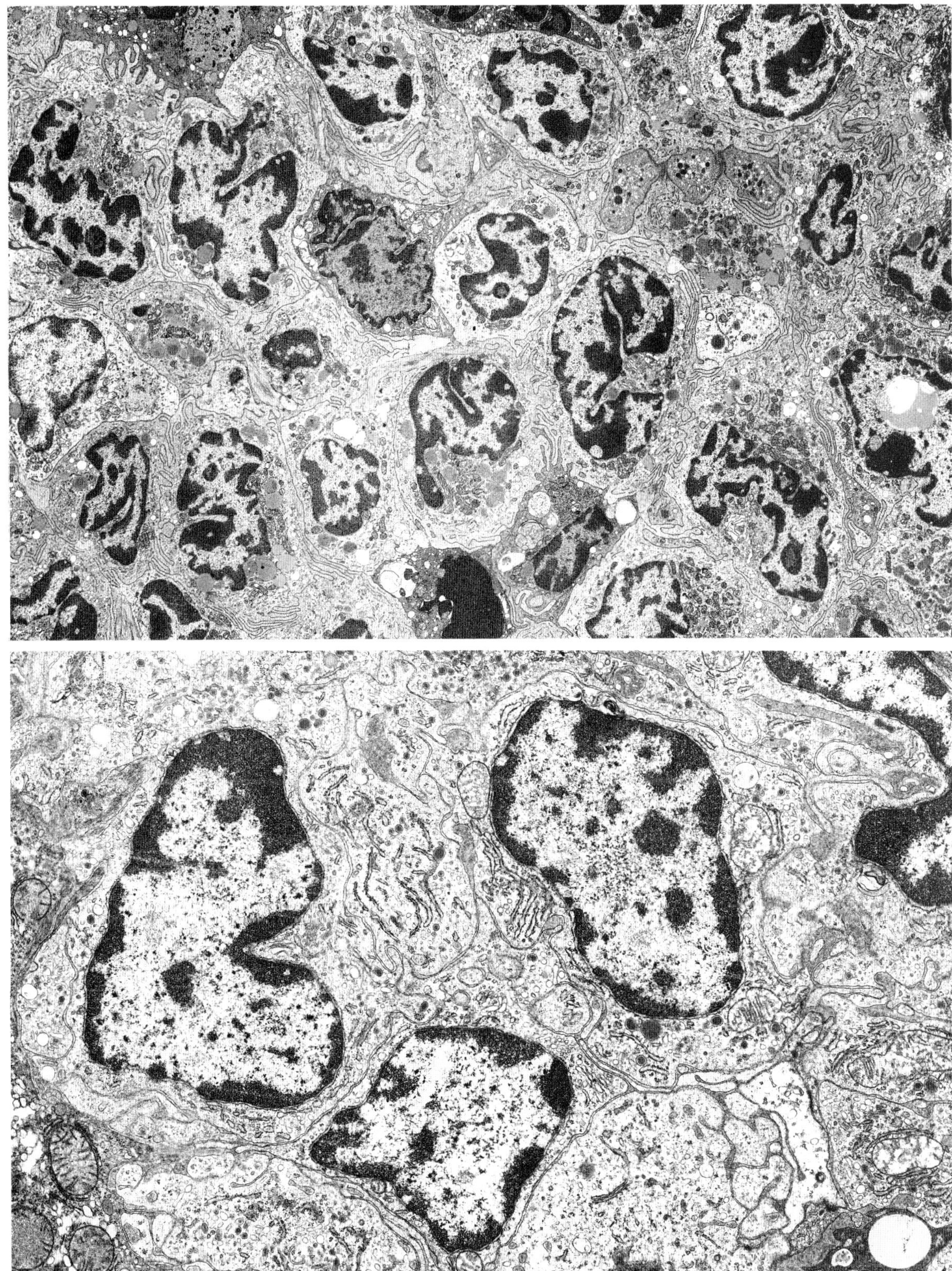

Fig. 81 *(above).* Histiocytic sarcoma, mouse, liver. Neoplastic histiocytes are quite variable in size and shape. Uranyl acetate, lead citrate, TEM, ×3540

Fig. 82 *(below).* Neoplastic histiocytes, mouse, liver. Plasma membrane has a prominent infolding, but a basement membrane is not apparent. Uranyl acetate, lead citrate, TEM, ×9090

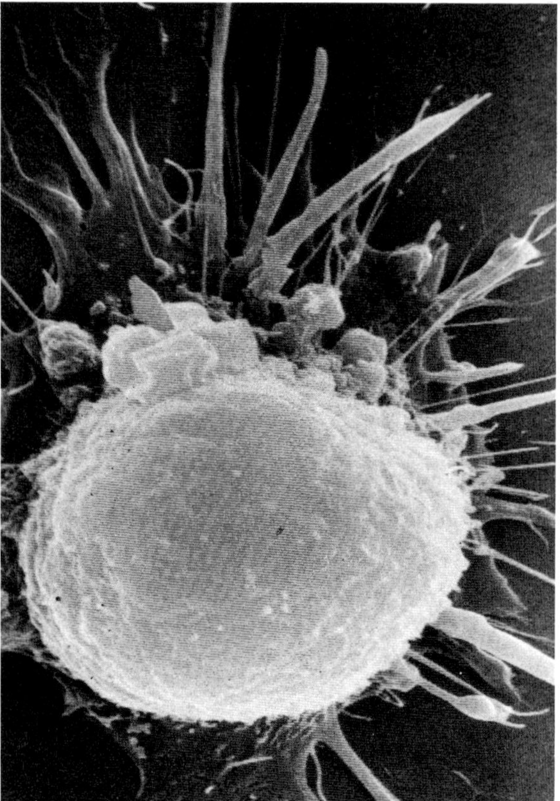

Fig. 83. Neoplastic histiocyte, mouse, liver. Rounded cell with numerous filopodia. SEM, × 3000

Table 13. Incidence (%) of histiocytic sarcoma in several strains of mice

Strain	Sex	Age (months)			
		≤6	7–12	13–18	>24
BALB/c	M	0.03	0.08	0.10	0.70
BALB/c	F	0.30	0.20	0.50	0.60
C 57 BL/6	M	0.60	0.20	0.30	22.20
C 57 BL/6	F	0.40	0.50	4.80	10.40
C 3 H-MTV−	F	0.00	0.00	0.08	0.80
C 3 H-MTV+	F	0.02	0.08	0.40	0.90

The incidence of histiocytic sarcoma varies from strain to strain as indicated in Table 13 (Frith 1987).

Comparison with Other Species

Histiocytic sarcoma is the most common non-lymphoid cell hemopoietic neoplasm in the Sprague-Dawley rat (Frith 1989). In the rat, histiocytic sarcoma also occurs in the liver, but subcutaneous neoplasms are also common. A fibrous component may be a common morphologic feature of the neoplasm in the rat, and the neoplasm has also been referred to as malignant fibrous histiocytoma (Ward et al. 1981). Although the tumor in the rat shares many morphological characteristics with the similar tumor in the mouse, they may have different causes. Histiocytic lymphoma has been diagnosed in humans, but more recent reports involving immunocytochemistry indicate that most of these neoplasms are in fact follicular center cell lymphomas (see p. 147, this volume).

cytic sarcoma. Stewart et al. (1974) described light microscopic features in 31 malignant schwannomas of the uterus, epididymis, cranial and spinal nerve roots. Their descriptions, in many ways, recall features of histiocytic sarcoma. They stated that the tumors had been misdiagnosed in the past as endometrial sarcomas and reticulum cell sarcomas. Although some of the tumors described by Stewart et al. (1974) may have been schwannomas, I do not concur in classifying all uterine or vaginal neoplasms as malignant schwannomas. Ultrastructural findings do not support the contention of Stewart (Frith et al. 1980). Basement membranes are a prominent feature of neoplastic Schwann cell tumors. Frith et al. (1980) could not confirm the presence of basement membranes ultrastructurally in histiocytic sarcoma.

Frith et al. (1980) initially referred to histiocytic sarcoma as a histiocytic lymphoma. It is clear now that this neoplasm is not derived from a lymphoid cell, and designation of lymphoma should be reserved for neoplasms derived from lymphoid cells.

References

Chouroulinkov I, Guillon JC, Guerin M (1969) Endometrial sarcomas in mice: a survey of 130 cases. JNCI 42: 593–603

Dawson PJ, Brooks RE, Fieldsteel AH (1974) Unusual occurrence of endometrial sarcomas in hybrid mice. JNCI 52: 207–214

Della Porta G, Chieco-Bianchi L, Pennelli N (1979) Tumors of the hematopoietic system. In: Turusov VS (ed) Pathology of tumours in laboratory animals, vol II. Tumours of the mouse. IARC Sci Publ 3: 527–576

Dunn TB (1954) Normal and pathologic anatomy of the reticular tissue in laboratory mice with a classification and discussion of neoplasms. JNCI 14: 1281–1433

Frith CH (1987) Incidence of neoplastic and nonneoplastic lesions in several strains of mice. Toxicology Pathology Associates, Little Rock, p 46

Frith CH (1989) Incidence of hematopoietic neoplasms in the Sprague-Dawley rat. Toxicol Pathol 16: 451–457

Frith CH, Wiley LD (1981) Morphologic classification and correlation of incidence of hyperplastic and neoplastic hematopoietic lesions in mice with age. J Gerontol 36: 534–545

Frith CH, Davis TM, Zolotor LA, Townsend JW (1980) Histiocytic lymphoma in the mouse. Leuk Res 4: 651–662

Frith CH, Pattengale PK, Ward JM (1985) A color atlas of hematopoietic pathology of mice. Toxicology Pathology Associates, Little Rock, pp 12–13

Stewart HL, Deringer MK, Dunn TB, Snell KC (1974) Malignant schwannomas of nerve roots, uterus and epididymis in mice. JNCI 53: 1749–1758

Ward JM, Kulwich BA, Reznik G, Berman JJ (1981) Malignant fibrous histiocytoma. Arch Pathol Lab Med 105: 313–316

Myelofibrosis, Mouse

Bernard Sass

Synonyms. Fibro-osseous lesion; metaphyseal osteosclerosis; myelosclerosis; endocrine osteo-myelofibrosis.

Gross Appearance

In advanced cases, the marrow cavity of affected long bones is irregularly narrowed, yellow, and rubbery.

Microscopic Features

As seen with the light microscope, areas of the marrow cavities of myelofibrotic sternebrae are replaced by acidophilic material (Fig. 84) in which there are scattered fibroblastic cells and osteoclasts (Figs. 85, 86). There is also remodeling of the cortical bone (Fig. 87).

In long bones there is remodeling of the cortices and focal areas of hyperostotic enostoses containing small foci of normal and fibrotic marrow (Figs. 84, 87). The cortex of these bones is remodeled as evidenced by osteoclastic activity and the presence of osteoid seams.

Sections colored with connective tissue stains demonstrate increased collagen in the affected areas. In a few cases the altered marrow of sternebrae contains dense bony trabeculae (Fig. 88), imparting a sclerotic appearance. The lesion of osteosclerosis is included with myelofibrosis because it is believed to represent the end stage of myelofibrosis; osteosclerosis may be found in individual bones of animals with myelofibrosis.

Differential Diagnosis

Myelofibrosis of mice needs to be differentiated from fibrous osteodystrophy which is related to the occurrence of primary or secondary parathy-roid hyperplasia or neoplasia. Fibrous osteodystrophy is characterized by the presence of periosteal new bone deposition and distortion of the bones of the skull. No description of fibrous osteodystrophy in mice has been found in the literature (Woodward and Montgomery 1978).

Osteomas induced by DNA viruses, most notably polyomavirus, C type RNA viruses, and various chemicals (Stanton 1979; Stanton et al. 1959) are difficult to differentiate histologically from myelofibrosis. Differentiation of neoplasms from osteosclerosis is easily achieved since bone marrow destruction results when the tumors have become invasive.

"Osteomas" or "hyperostoses" of the skull occur in thymectomized mice injected with gold thioglucose alone or in combination with estrogens (Rudali 1968; Rudali and Juliard 1962). However, the authors make no mention of lesions in the long bones or sternebrae. Other authors (Urist et al. 1950; Gaunt and Pierce 1985) classified estrogen-induced lesions with endosteal fibrosis and bone formation in the long bones as myelofibrosis or osteosclerosis. Spontaneously occurring changes of the marrow cavities of both the

Fig. 84 *(upper left).* Myelofibrosis, mouse. Sternebrae ▶ *(left);* fibrous replacement at ends. Tibia *(right)* with endostoses and narrowed marrow cavity *(upper right).* H and E, × 22

Fig. 85 *(lower left).* Higher magnification of one sternebra from same animal as in Fig. 84 *(center left).* H and E, × 130

Fig. 86 *(upper right).* Myelofibrosis, mouse, marrow cavity of sternebra from another animal. Fibrous tissue replaces marrow *(upper);* nuclei of giant cells are deeply stained. Normal marrow is at *bottom.* H and E, × 320

Fig. 87 *(lower right).* Myelofibrosis, mouse, tibia. Higher magnification of portion of tibia with endostotic enostosis containing small islands of marrow; normal marrow is at *left.* H and E, × 220

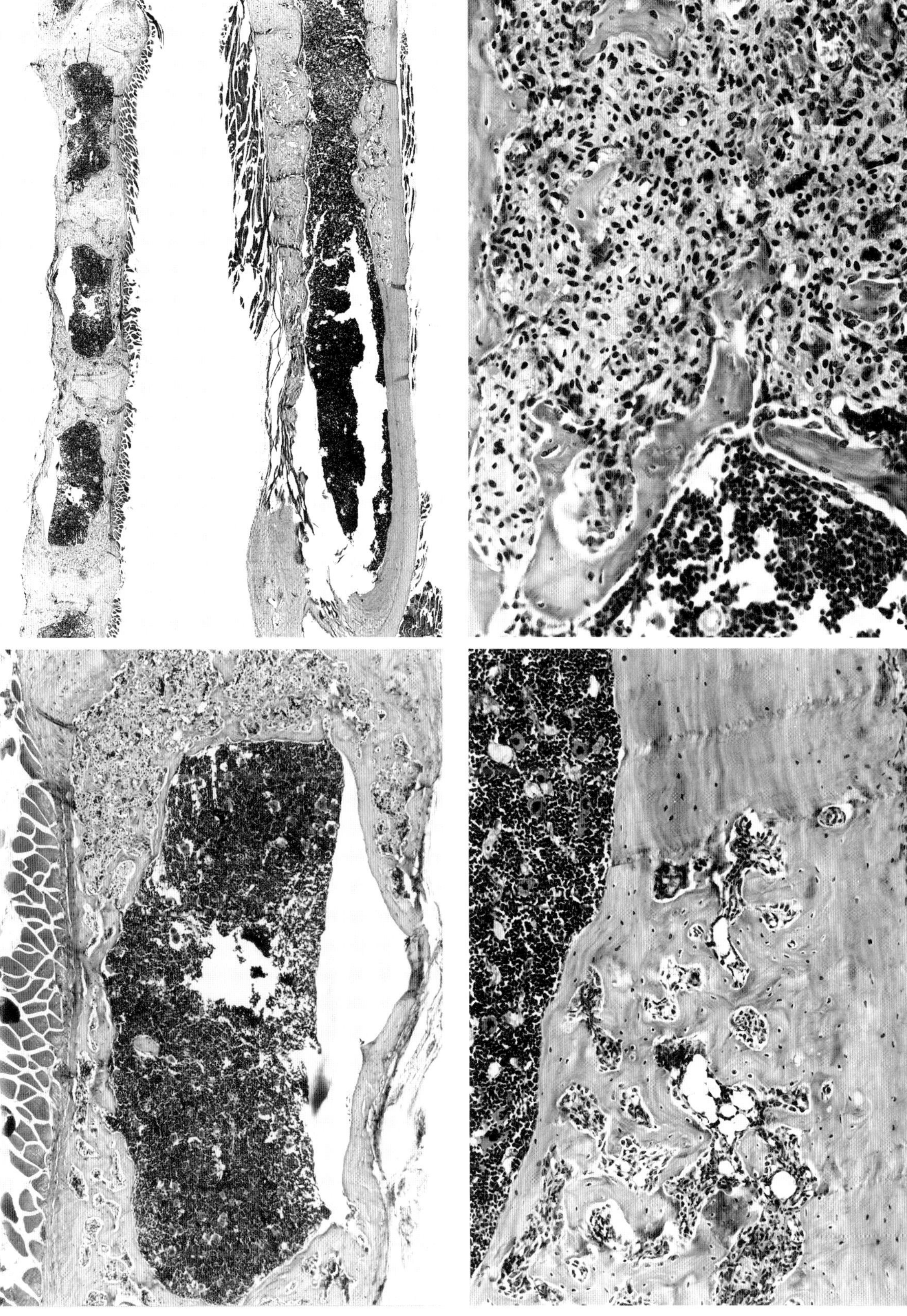

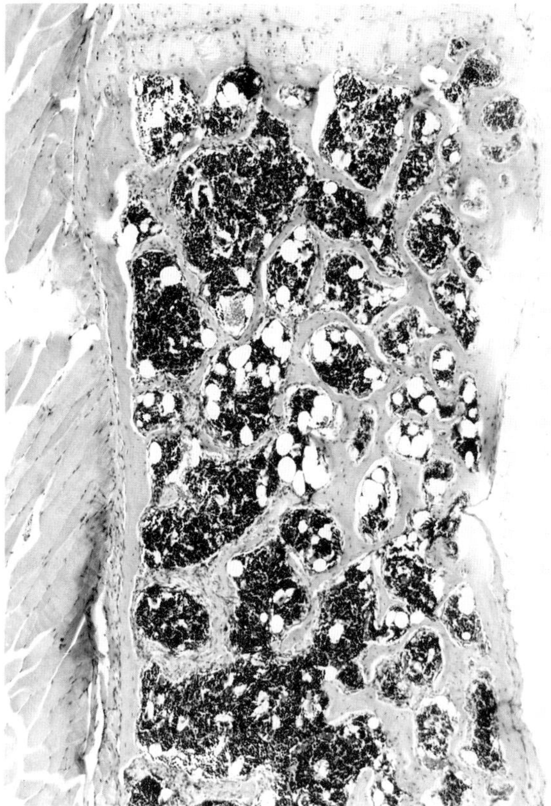

Fig. 88. Osteosclerosis, mouse, sternebra. Meshwork of normal trabecular bone extends into marrow cavity. H and E, × 125

long bones and sternebrae of mice were termed fibro-osseous lesions (Sass and Montali 1980).

Osteopetrosis, a hereditary disease of mice and dogs, may be difficult to differentiate histologically from osteosclerosis (Woodard and Montgomery 1978).

In osteopetrosis the entire skeleton is affected at an earlier age than in osteosclerosis which affects only a few bones. In osteopetrosis, the clubbed shape of the fetal long bones is maintained throughout adult life (Teitelbaum 1977), whereas the bones of mice with osteosclerosis retain their adult shape.

Biologic Features

Histogenesis

The histogenesis of myelofibrosis is as yet incompletely elucidated. Based upon the experimental induction of the lesion in female mice by estradiol (Rudali and Juliard 1962; Gaunt and Pierce 1985), female sex hormones appear to play a role in the spontaneous occurrence of myelofibrosis and osteosclerosis.

There are four main theories of the pathogenesis of myelofibrosis (Martin 1972).

1. Necrosis of the marrow is a necessary precursor.
2. It develops in the myeloproliferative syndrome.
3. and 4. Myelofibrosis develops independently of necrosis and the myeloproliferative syndrome.

A high incidence of myelofibrosis occurred in both control and treated female (C57BL/6N × C3H/HeN)F$_1$ mice that were the subjects of two long-term bioassays: daminozide (NCI Tech. Report Series 83, 1978 a) and 3-(chloromethyl)pyridine hydrochloride (NCI Tech. Report Series 95, 1978 b). In both studies there was evidence of estrogen stimulation manifested by uterine and ovarian cysts and metritis.

Studies (Gaunt and Pierce 1985) have revealed that 8 to 12-week-old female mice of strain C57Bl/6J which received subcutaneously 0.1 mg 17 β-estradiol-cyclopentyl propionate and were killed at 1 and 4 weeks later had loss in marrow cellularity and replacement of marrow cavities of proximal tibial metaphyses by bony trabeculae. There was concomitant metritis. The authors postulate that the decrease in numbers of thymic and marrow lymphocytes observed by them and others (Boorman et al. 1980; Dougherty 1952) which occurs following estradiol administration may be critical in causing a depression of myelopoiesis and resultant anemia.

Cellular Mechanisms of Pathogenesis

There is increasing evidence that progenitor or stem cells known as colony forming units (CFU), including those of macrophage (CFU-gm), erythroid, myeloid (granuloid) cells (CFU-c), fibroblast (CFU-f) and pluripotent (CFU-s) precursors, play an important role in the pathogenesis of myelofibrosis. Administration of estrogens decreased the number of CFU-s as assayed in CF$_1$ or BDF$_1$ female mice (Fried et al. 1974) or CFU-c in (BALB/c × A/He)F$_1$ female mice (Adler and Trobaugh 1978). Boorman et al. (1980) treated female (C57BL/6N × C3H)F$_1$ mice with diethylstilbestrol. A decrease in both CFU-s and CFU-gm using in vitro and in vivo assays was noted. Gaunt and Pierce (1985) demonstrated a decrease of CFU-f and CFU-gm in estradiol-treated female C57BL/6J mice.

Other findings in estradiol-treated mice with myelofibrosis or osteosclerosis included a decrease in marrow lymphoid cells, granulocytes, and erythroid cells. Neutropenia and thymic cortical atrophy were also noted (Gaunt and Pierce 1985); the latter change was also pronounced in the diethylstilbestrol-treated mice (Boorman et al. 1980).

Osteopetrotic (op) mice and (ia) rats serve as useful models for the study of abnormal bone deposition as it occurs in both osteopetrosis and osteofibrosis/osteosclerosis. In (op) mice (Raisz et al. 1977; Marks 1982) and (ia) rats (Schneider 1982) defective osteoclasts have lost their ability to absorb bone at the normal rate. The defective osteoclasts are believed to be derived from defective myelopoietic stem cells (Ko and Bernard 1981). It is possible that the decrease in myelopoietic cells (Gaunt and Pierce 1985) of estrogen-treated mice and the decreased number of marrow lymphocytes can affect the remodeling of bone.

Further, thymic lymphocytes, which play an important role in cell-mediated immunity, may also play a direct role in hemopoiesis or act indirectly in modifying the behavior of monocytes and macrophages (Gordon and Gordon-Smith 1981). The indirect role is believed to be through the release of macrophage factors.

Serial transplantation by spleen cells from strain RF mice with a disease characterized by anemia, splenomegaly, and myelosclerosis has been described (Upton and Furth 1955). The bones of the donor animal, a female, were not examined. The recipients developed myelosclerosis in addition to splenomegaly and anemia, the incidence of myelosclerosis was not stated.

Etiology

Radioisotopes of lead, uranium, plutonium, and radium induce myelofibrosis or osteomas in mice (Finkel and Biskis 1968; Stanton 1979). Polyomavirus induces lesions that are indistinguishable from myelosclerosis (Stanton et al. 1959; Dawe et al. 1959; Sjogren and Ringertz 1962) (see under Differential Diagnosis). FBJ virus (Finkel and Biskis 1968) and sarcoma 37 virus (Merwin and Redmon 1969), C Type RNA oncornaviruses, induce similar lesions (see Differential Diagnosis).

In the Registry of Experimental Cancers there are 14 cases of "marble bone disease" in BALB/c mice induced by estrogens alone or in combination with Maloney sarcomavirus. These lesions are identical with myelofibrosis. Female B6C3F$_1$ mice exposed to the chemicals daminozide and 3-(chloromethyl)pyridine hydrochloride developed myelofibrosis and osteosclerosis, but in both studies the lesions occurred in both the control and treated groups, suggesting that the feed may have contained substances with an estrogenic effect, since the historical controls in a number of bioassays had only a 1% incidence of the lesion (Ward et al. 1979).

Administration of gold thioglucose with and without estradiol to thymectomized male and female strain AKR and (AKR × RIII)F$_1$ hybrids resulted in intracranial osteomas (Rudali 1968) (see Differential Diagnosis). Chemicals that induce necrosis and fibrosis of the marrow in species other than the mouse are benzene (humans) (Mallory et al. 1939; Wyatt and Summers 1950) and saponin (rabbit) (Firket and Campos 1922; Argano et al. 1969; Hoshi and Weiss 1978). Lead acetate, given intravenously to Holtzman rat (Selye et al. 1963) or to inbred rats of unknown strain (Takacsi-Nagy and Juhasz 1971), induced myelofibrosis.

Frequency

The frequency of occurrence of both spontaneous and induced myelofibrosis in female B6C3F$_1$ mice is shown in Table 14. The lesions were originally diagnosed as fibrous osteodystrophy, but Sass and Montali (1980) examined representative sections from the sternebra and long bones of female mice from the two bioassays and described them as fibro-osseous lesions since they were unrelated to any renal or parathyroid lesions and thus were not lesions of fibrous osteodystrophy.

The high frequencies of myelofibrosis/myelosclerosis in both the control and treated animals in the two long-term (24 months) bioassays are difficult to explain (see Etiology).

The work of Urist et al. (1950) is remarkable in that endosteal lesions of the long bones were induced by estrogens in mice of strains CFI, IF, and CHI in a short time span (Table 15). Others (Silberberg and Silberberg 1970) treated strain C57BL female mice with weekly doses of 30 µg estradiol benzoate in sesame oil starting at 1, 6, or 12 months of age and continuing for a total of 5 months. A high incidence of myelofibrosis of both the tibias and femurs resulted (Table 15).

Table 14. Incidence of myelofibrosis in female (C57BL × C3HeN)F$_1$ (B6C3F$_1$) mice

Treatment/dose	No.	No. with lesions	Percentage	Reference
None(controls)	2522	25	1.0	Ward et al. (1979)
Controls in daminozide bioassays	20	13	65.0	NCI Carcinogenesis Bioassay Tech Rep no. 83 (1978 a)
Daminozide 5000 ppm in feed	41	19	46.5	NCI Carcinogenesis Bioassay Tech Rep no. 83 (1978 a)
Daminozide 10000 ppm in feed	48	21	44.0	NCI Carcinogenesis Bioassay Tech Rep no. 83 (1978 a)
3-(chloromethyl)-pyridine hydrochloride vehicle controls	20	7	35.0	NCI Carcinogenesis Bioassay Tech Rep no. 95 (1978 b)
3-(chloromethyl)-pyridine hydrochloride 100 mg/kg body weight by gavage	50	23	46.0	NCI Carcinogenesis Bioassay Tech Rep no. 95 (1978 b)
3-(chloromethyl-pyridine hydrochloride 200 mg/kg body weight by gavage	49	18	37.0	NCI Carcinogenesis Bioassay Tech Rep no. 95 (1978 b)

Comparison with Other Species

Myelofibrosis was induced experimentally in a few splenectomized Osborne-Mendel rats which received Rauscher virus at 3 days of age (van Gorp and Swaen 1969). Selye et al. (1963) used the term osteomyelosclerosis for the bone disease induced in Holtzman rats which received intravenous lead acetate.

The intravenous administration of lead acetate in 5-mg doses to rats of an unknown strain (Takacsi-Nagy and Juhasz 1971) resulted (within 14 days) in profound anemia, splenic and lymphoid atrophy with myeloid metaplasia in both the liver and spleen. Necrosis and fibrosis of the marrow was a prominent feature.

Myelofibrosis was induced in Wistar and Sprague-Dawley rats by whole body irradiation (Stodtmeister and Fliedner 1973). Some 34 of 516 (6.5%) rats developed myelofibrosis at intervals of 4–110 days following 750 R of whole-body X-irradiation and injection of allogeneic marrow cells. The development of myelofibrosis was characterized by necrosis followed by regeneration of lymphoid and myeloid cells. Destruction of these cells was followed by fibrosis.

Myelosclerosis occurred in 33% and myelofibrosis in 4% of 205 strain Fischer 344 rats with mononuclear cell leukemia (Stromberg and Vogtsberger 1983). The incidence of myelosclerosis and myelofibrosis in nonleukemia controls was 5.3% and 0%, respectively.

A woolly monkey which had multiple fibrosarcomas also developed myelofibrosis and myeloid metaplasia (Theilen et al. 1971). Twelve of 17 rabbits developed myelofibrosis with myeloid metaplasia following the intravenous administration of 1.2 mg/kg saponin every 4 days (Argano et al. 1969).

Myelosclerosis and osteosclerosis are most frequently reported in dogs of the Basenji breed which have a high incidence of anemia related to pyruvic kinase deficiency (Bannerman et al. 1973). A single case of myelofibrosis occurred in a male beagle aged 15 years. The animal was anemic and deficient in pyruvate kinase (Prasse et al. 1975). In a more recent publication, three additional canine cases are documented and the pertinent literature reviewed (Weiss and Armstrong 1985).

Myelofibrosis occurred in approximately 4% of beagle dogs exposed to low level gamma irradiation (10 gamma/day) (Seed et al. 1982). The authors, on the basis of an ultrastructural analysis, postulate that pathogenetically there was a failure to terminate early osteogenic-dependent repair sequences.

The sequence of necrosis, overgrowth of reticulum cells, and fibrosis can be reproduced in rabbits administered saponin (Hoshi and Weiss 1978).

In studying a model of granulopoiesis in cats, a single animal, age and sex not given, developed myelofibrosis (Prasse et al. 1973). The bone marrow of the cat was hyperplastic with increased

Table 15. Incidence of myelofibrosis or myelosclerosis in estrogen-treated mice

Treatment/dose		Strain	No.	No. with lesions	Percentage	Reference
Estradiol benzoate 0.5–2.0 mg 1–14 daily doses		CF1, IF CHI	65	not given	30[a] 100[b]	Urist et al. 1950
Thymectomized + estradiol	(m)	AKR	12	8	66	Rudali and Juliard 1962
Castration + estradiol	(m)	(AKR × RIII)F$_1$	11	3	27	
Uninoculated						
Controls	(f)	AKR	38	2	5	Rudali 1968
	(m)	AKR	0	0	0	
Thymectomy	(f)	AKR	23		4	
	(m)	AKR	0	0	0	
Thymectomized + gold thioglucose + estradiol[c]	(m)	AKR	11	8	70	
Thymectomized + gold thioglucose	(f)	AKR	12	5	41	
Thymectomized + gold thioglucose	(m)	AKR	9	1	11	
Thymectomized + estradiol[d]	(m)	AKR	31	14	42	
Untreated	(f)	C57BL	25	0	0	Silberberg and
Group 1[e]		C57BL	16	12	75	Silberberg 1970
Group 2[g]		C57BL	15	14	93.5	
Group 3[h]		C57BL	15	14	93.5	

[a] Incidence at 7–9 days post administration
[b] Incidence at 10–15 days post administration
[c] Injected at 2.5 months of age with gold thioglucose 750 mg/kg
[d] Implanted at 3.5 months of age with pellets composed of 10% estradiol +90% cholesterol
[e] Received 30 µg estradiol benzoate in sesame oil weekly for total of 5 months beginning at 1 months of age.
[g] Received 30 µg estradiol benzoate in sesame oil weekly for total of 5 months beginning at 6 months of age.
[h] Received 30 µg estradiol benzoate in sesame oil weekly for total of 5 months beginning at 6 months of age.
f, females.
m, males.

numbers of granulocytic, megakaryocytic, and erythrocytic precursors. Twelve of 13 cats inoculated intraperitoneally with feline leukemia virus (FeLV) developed anemia with medullary osteosclerosis. Type C particles compatible with FeLV were associated with osteocytes, osteoblasts, and megakaryocytes (Hoover and Kociba 1974). Thus, myelofibrosis in cats is now known to be caused by FeLV or occurs in FeLV-related disease.

A second spontaneously occurring case of myelofibrosis occurred in a 2.5-year-old, neutered, male, domestic, short hair cat (Flecknell et al. 1978). The disease was manifest by cranial hyper-ostoses and an increase in femoral endosteal bone; FeLV was isolated from the blood of this cat.

In humans, the histogenesis of myelofibrosis with accompanying myeloid metaplasia is unclear. First reported by Heuck (1879), it is classified as a component of the myeloproliferative syndrome (Rappaport 1966). Bone marrow necrosis is considered to be an important precursor of myelofibrosis (Wyatt and Summers 1950; Conrad and Carpenter 1979). The necrosis, preceded by vascular occlusion, may be associated with sickle cell anemia or malignant neoplasms. Infection, pregnancy with disseminated intravascular coagulation, or the myxoid degeneration of fat seen in starvation are also associated with marrow necrosis (Conrad and Carpenter 1979). Following necrosis, fibrosis (Conrad and Carpenter 1979) or overgrowth of reticulum cells followed by fibrosis (Wyatt and Summers 1950; Quesenberry and Levitt 1979) occurs, which in turn may result in osteosclerosis and extramedullary hemopoiesis.

In animals, as in humans, myelofibrosis and osteosclerosis are consistently associated with both megakaryotic hyperplasia and progressive reticulin sclerosis (Valli 1985). The role played by megakaryocytes in the pathogenesis of myelofibrosis is not clear.

References

Adler SS, Trobaugh FE, Jr (1978) Effects of estrogen on erythropoiesis and granuloid progenitor cell (CFU-C) proliferation in mice. J Lab Clin Med 91: 960–968

Argano SAP, Tobin MS, Spain DM (1969) Experimental induction of myelofibrosis with myeloid metaplasia. Blood 33: 851–858

Bannerman RM, Edwards JA, Pinkerton PH (1973) Hereditary disorders of the red cell in animals. In: Brown EB (ed) Progress in hematology, vol VIII. Grune and Stratton, New York, pp 131–179

Boorman GA, Luster MI, Dean JH, Wilson RE (1980) The effect of adult exposure to diethylstilbestrol in the mouse on macrophage function and numbers. J Reticuloendothel Soc 28: 547–560

Conrad ME, Carpenter JT (1979) Bone marrow necrosis. Am J Hematol 7: 181–189

Dawe CJ, Law LW, Dunn TB (1959) Studies of parotid-tumor agent in cultures of leukemic tissues of mice. JNCI 23: 717–797

Dougherty TF (1952) Effect of hormones on lymphatic tissue. Physiol Rev 32: 379–401

Finkel MP, Biskis BO (1968) Experimental induction of osteosarcomas. Prog Exp Tumor Res 10: 72–111

Firket J, Campos ES (1922) Generalized megalocaryocytic reaction to saponin poisoning. Bull Johns Hopkins Hosp 33: 271–283

Flecknell PA, Gibbs C, Kelly DF (1978) Myelosclerosis in a cat. J Comp Pathol 88: 627–631

Fried W, Tichler T, Dennenberg I, Barone J, Wang F (1974) Effects of estrogens on hematopoietic stem cells and on hematopoiesis of mice. J Lab Clin Med 83: 807–815

Gaunt SD, Pierce KR (1985) Myelopoiesis and marrow adherent cells in estradiol-treated mice. Vet Pathol 22: 403–408

Gordon MY, Gordon-Smith EC (1981) Annotation-lymphocytes and haemopoiesis. Br J Haematol 47: 163–169

Heuck G (1879) Zwei Falle von Leukemie mit eigenthumlichem Blutresp. Knochenmarksbefund. Virchows Arch Pathol Anat 78: 475–496

Hoover EA, Kociba GJ (1974) Bone lesions in cats with anemia induced by feline leukemia virus. JNCI 53: 1277–1284

Hoshi H, Weiss L (1978) Rabbit bone marrow after administration of saponin. An electron microscopic study. Lab Invest 38: 67–80

Ko JS, Bernard GW (1981) Osteoclast formation in vitro from bone marrow mononuclear cells in osteoclast free bone. Am J Anat 161: 415–425

Mallory TB, Gall EA, Brickley WJ (1939) Chronic exposure to benzene (benzol). III. The pathologic results. J Ind Hyg Toxicol 21: 355–393

Marks SC (1982) Morphological evidence of reduced bone resorption in osteopetrotic (op) mice. Am J Anat 163: 157–167

Martin H (1972) Tierexperimentelle Myelofibrosen und Hyperostosen im Vergleich zur Osteomyelosklerose des Menschen. Zentrabl Allg Pathol 116: 244–256

Merwin RM, Redmon LW (1969) Skeletal and reticular tissue disorders produced in mice by agent (s) from sarcoma 37. JNCI 43: 365–376

National Cancer Institute (1978 a) Carcinogenesis bioassay of daminozide for possible carcinogenicity (in F344 rats and B6C3F$_1$ mice). US Dept HEW, PHS, NIH, Washington DC (Technical report series 83)

National Cancer Institute (1978 b) Carcinogenesis bioassay of 3-(chloromethyl)pyridine hydrochloride for possible carcinogenicity (in F344 rats and B6C3F$_1$ mice). US Dept HEW, PHS, NIH, Washington DC (Technical report series 95)

Prasse KW, Crouser D, Beutler E, Walker M, Schall WD (1975) Pyruvate kinase deficiency anemia with terminal myelofibrosis and osteosclerosis in a beagle. J Am Vet Met Assoc 166: 1170–1175

Prasse KW, Seagrave RC, Kaeberle ML, Ramsey FK (1973) A model of granulopoiesis in cats. Lab Invest 28: 292–299

Quesenberry P, Levitt L (1979) Hematopoietic stem cells. (3rd of three parts) N Engl J Med 301: 868–872

Raisz LG, Simmons HA, Gworek SC, Eilon G (1977) Studies on congenital osteopetrosis in microphthalmic mice using organ cultures: impairment of bone resorption in response to physiologic stimulators. J Exp Med 145: 857–865

Rappaport H (1966) Tumors of the hematopoietic system. In: Atlas of tumor pathology, sect III, fascicle 8. Armed Forces Institute of Pathology, Washington DC

Rudali G (1968) Apparition d'osteomes intracraniens chez des souris injectees avec du thioglucose d'or. Rev Fr Etud Clin Biol 13: 40–8

Rudali G, Juliard L (1962) Production d'hyperostoses frontales internes chez les souris a l'aide d'estradiol. CR Acad Sci (Paris) 254: 3457–3458

Sass B, Montali RJ (1980) Spontaneous fibro-osseous lesions in aging female mice. Lab Anim Sci 30: 907–909

Schneider GB (1982) An evaluation of the phagocytic cells in the ia (osteopetrotic) rat: oxidative metabolism in monocytes and macrophages. J Reticuloendothel Soc 31: 225–232

Seed TM, Chubb GT, Tolle DV, Fritz TE, Poole CM, Doyle DE, Lombard LS, Kaspar LV (1982) The ultrastructure of radiationinduced endosteal myelofibrosis in the dog. Scan Electron Microsc 1: 377–391

Selye H, Gabbiani G, Tuchweber B (1963) An experimental model of osteomyelosclerosis. Acta Haematol 29: 51–62

Silberberg M, Silberberg R (1970) Age-linked modification of the effect of estrogen on joints and cortical bone of female mice. Gerontologia 16: 201–211

Sjogren HO, Ringertz N (1962) Histopathology and transplantability of polyoma-induced tumors in strain A/Sn and three coisogenic resistant (IR) substrains. JNCI 28: 859–895

Stanton MF (1979) Tumours of the bone. In: VS Turosov (ed) Pathology of tumours in laboratory animals. II. Tumours of the mouse. IARC Sci Publ 23: 577–610

Stanton MF, Stewart SE, Eddy BE, Blackwell RH (1959) Oncogenic effect of tissue-culture preparations of polyoma virus on fetal mice. JNCI 23: 1441–1475

Stodtmeister R, Fliedner TM (1973) Morphological aspects of myelofibrosis, observed in rats following sublethal whole body irradiation and subsequent allogeneic bone marrow cell transfusion. Folia Haematol (Leipz) 100: 23–50

Stromberg PC, Vogtsberger LM (1983) Pathology of the mononuclear cell leukemia of Fischer rats. I. Morphologic studies. Vet Pathol 20: 698–708

Takacsi-Nagy L, Juhasz J (1971) Experimental myelosclerosis. Haematologia 5: 283–291

Teitelbaum SL (1977) Metabolic and other nontumorous disorders of bone. In: Anderson WAD, Kissane JM (eds) Pathology, vol 2. Mosby, St Louis, chap 44

Theilen GH, Gould D, Fowler M, Dungworth DL (1971) C-type virus in tumor tissues of a woolly monkey (Lagothrix spp.) with fibrosarcoma. JNCI 47: 881–889

Upton AC, Furth J (1955) A transmissible disease of mice characterized by anemia, leukopenia, splenomegaly and myelosclerosis. Acta Haematol 13: 65–76

Urist MR, Budy BS, McLean FC (1950) Endosteal-bone formation in estrogen treated mice. J Bone Joint Surg (An) 32: 143–162

Valli VEO (1985) The hematopoietic system. In: Jubb KVF, Kennedy PC, Palmer N (eds) Pathology of domestic animals, vol 3. Academic, Orlando, pp 102–104

van Gorp LHM, Swaen GJV (1969) Myelofibrosis in rats experimentally infected with a murine leukemia virus. J Pathol 97: 235–240

Ward JM, Goodman DG, Squire RA, Chu KC, Linhart MS (1979) Neoplastic and nonneoplastic lesions in aging (C57BL/6N × C3H/HeN)F_1 (B6C3F_1) mice. JNCI 63: 849–854

Weiss DJ, Armstrong PJ (1985) Secondary myelofibrosis in three dogs. J Am Vet Med Assoc 187: 423–425

Woodard JC, Montgomery CA (1978) Musculoskeletal system, bones. In: Benirschke K, Garner FM, Jones TC (eds) Pathology of laboratory animals. Springer, Berlin Heidelberg New York, chap 10

Wyatt JP, Summers SC (1950) Chronic marrow failure, myelosclerosis and extramedullary hematopoiesis. Blood 5: 329–347

Chédiak-Higashi Syndrome, Mouse

David J. Prieur

Synonym. Beige mouse.

Gross Appearance

Mice of the C57BL/6 strain with the Chédiak-Higashi syndrome (CHS) have a dark gray (charcoal gray) coat color. No other abnormalities are apparent grossly.

Microscopic Features

The microscopic hallmark of CHS is an enlargement of cytoplasmic granules in most but not all granule-containing cells. Many of these enlarged cytoplasmic granules have been identified as lysosomes; however, not all lysosomes are enlarged, and not all enlarged granules are considered to be lysosomes. Enlarged granules have been identified as melanin granules in integumentary and ocular structures (Pierro and Chase 1963; Lutzner et al. 1967). Other enlarged granules have been observed in leukocytes, renal epithelial cells, liver parenchymal cells, pancreatic islet cells, osteoclasts, cells of adrenal glands, cerebral cortex, cerebellum, spinal cord, submaxillary gland, lacrimal gland, stomach, thyroid, and jejunum (Prieur et al. 1972; Oliver and Essner 1973; Ash et al. 1980). Leukocytes with enlarged granules include neutrophils, lymphocytes, eosinophils, and monocytes (Lutzner et al. 1967; Oliver and Essner 1973; Oliver and Essner 1975). Large granular lymphocytes, generally believed to be natural killer (NK) cells, contain enlarged granules in beige mice (Itoh et al. 1982). Granules in beige mouse mast cells, peritoneal macrophages, and type III pneumocytes are also enlarged (Chi and Lagunoff 1975; Strausbauch et al. 1982; Chi et al. 1976). These granules in neutrophils of affected mice range up to 10 μm in diameter and are often irregular in shape. They are azurophilic and positive by periodic acid-Schiff, Sudan black B, acid phosphatase, and myeloperoxidase in histochemical staining methods. Neutrophils of control mice contain numerous small acid phosphatase and myeloper-oxidase-positive granules, in contrast to the neu-trophils of affected mice which contain only a few, often greatly enlarged, granules.

Ultrastructure

The ultrastructural lesion in most cells of affected mice is the presence of enlarged cytoplasmic granules. Many of the enlarged granules are of normal composition: They are similar to the gran-ules in a particular normal cell type but are larger and sometimes irregular in shape. The enlarged granules arise by fusion, and often sections of cells contain evidence of the fusion process.

The enlarged granules in affected neutrophils consist of azurophil (primary) granules with many normal-sized specific (secondary) granules persisting throughout the cytoplasm (Figs. 89, 90). Peroxidase ultracytochemistry discloses few normal-sized azurophil granules remaining in mature neutrophils (Oliver and Essner 1975). The granules in eosinophils of normal mice contain one or two crystalloids. Eosinophils of beige mice contain fewer but larger granules, and the enlarged granules contain multiple crystalloids (Figs. 91, 92) (Oliver and Essner 1975). Bone marrow monocytes and peritoneal macrophages (Figs. 93, 94) of beige mice contain enlarged cyto-plasmic granules (Oliver and Essner 1975; Strausbauch et al. 1982). Elongated or dumbbell-shaped cytoplasmic granules are sometimes ob-served in macrophages and monocytes of affect-ed mice. Tissue (Chi and Lagunoff 1975) and peritoneal mast cells (Figs. 95, 96) of beige mice contain enlarged granules.

Enlarged cytoplasmic granules have also been observed in beige mouse renal epithelial cells (Prieur et al. 1972), hepatocytes (Essner and Oli-ver 1974), pulmonary type II pneumocytes (Chi et al. 1976), gastric chief and parietal cells (Sato and Spicer 1981), and other types of cells.

In platelets of beige mice, as well as in platelets of other species with CHS, the characteristic ul-trastructural lesion is the virtual absence of the "dense granule" (Holland 1976). Platelet alpha granules appear normal in platelets of affected mice.

Differential Diagnosis

The mutant mice termed pearl, maroon, pallid, ruby-eye, light ear, and pale ear share with beige mice a platelet storage pool deficiency and, at least, an anatomically restricted pigmentation al-teration (Novak et al. 1984). Additionally, abnor-malities of lysosomal enzyme secretion have ben reported with these mutants (Novak et al. 1984). However, no mutants with enlarged cytoplasmic granules similar to those in beige mice have been observed.

Biologic Features

Pathogenesis

The mechanisms by which some of the manifes-tations of CHS develop have been identified even though the underlying biochemical basis of the syndrome has not been elucidated. Enlarged granules result from the excessive, unregulated, and unexplained fusion of pre-existing and ap-parently morphologically normal granules.

The incomplete oculocutaneous albinism is the result of two phenomena: excessive fusion of melanin granules and excessive destruction of melanin in melanolysosomes. The percentage of unit area of hair, integumentary, and ocular tis-sue that contains melanin is less than that of the corresponding tissue of normal animals and thus appears "diluted." Increased susceptibility to in-fectious disease associated with the syndrome has been documented in beige mice (Lane and Murphy 1972; Elin et al. 1974) and is the result of dysfunction of leukocytes. The types of dys-function in neutrophils and macrophages include defective chemotaxis, abnormal cap formation, decreased bactericidal activity, increased mem-brane fluidity, and abnormal secretion (Gallin et al. 1974; Oliver et al. 1975; Morahan et al. 1980). Defects in NK cells (Roder and Duwe 1979; Tal-madge et al. 1980), T lymphocytes (Saxena et al. 1982), and mast cells (Chi and Lagunoff 1975) have also been documented. There is an obvious associated bleeding tendency, the basis for which is a platelet storage pool deficiency secondary to markedly decreased numbers of serotonin, ade-nine nucleotide, and bivalent cation-storing dense granules (Holland 1976; Novak et al. 1984).

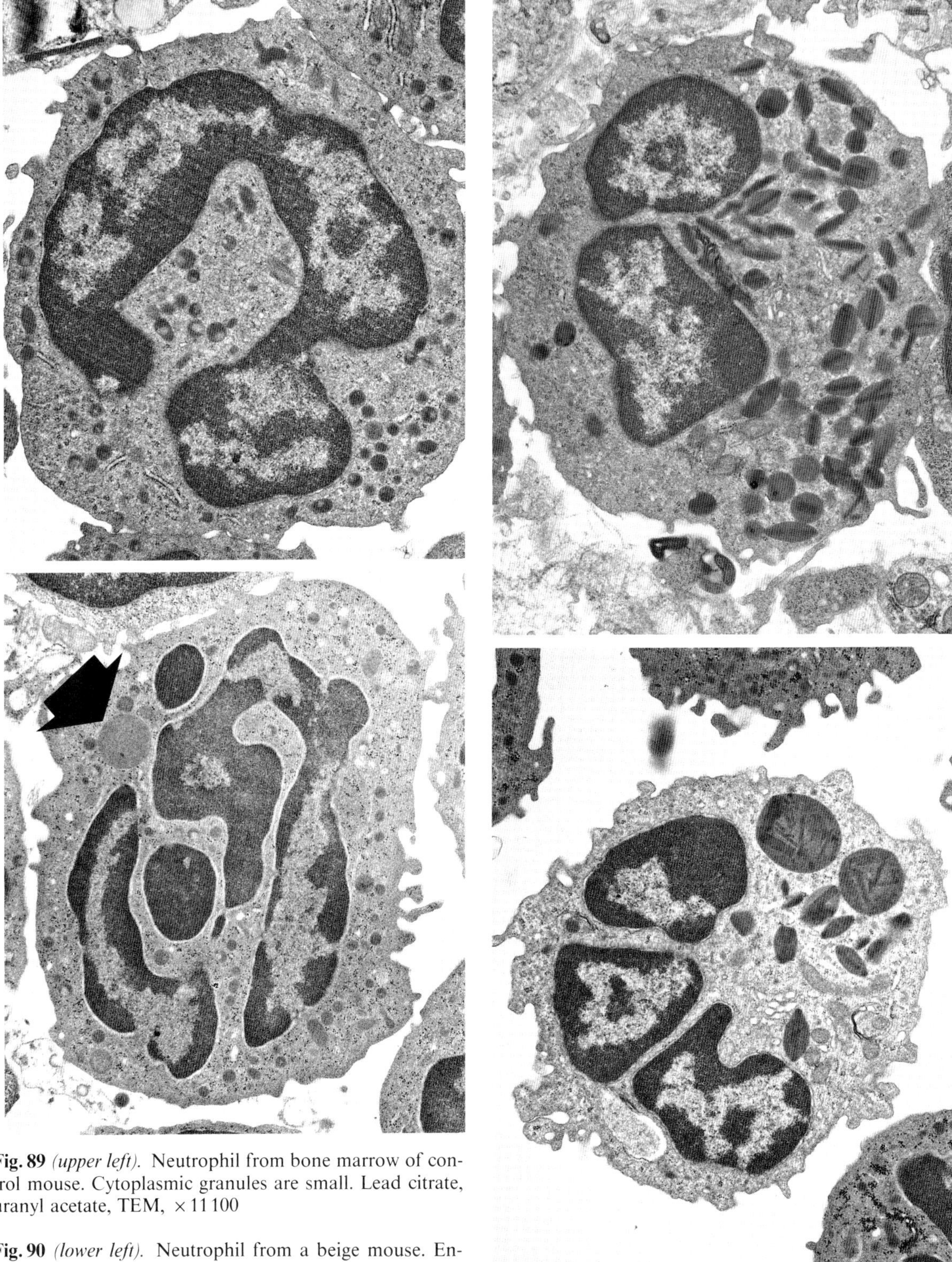

Fig. 89 *(upper left).* Neutrophil from bone marrow of control mouse. Cytoplasmic granules are small. Lead citrate, uranyl acetate, TEM, ×11100

Fig. 90 *(lower left).* Neutrophil from a beige mouse. Enlarged cytoplasmic granule *(arrow)* along with normal-sized granules. Lead citrate, uranyl acetate, TEM, ×11100

Fig. 91 *(upper right).* Eosinophil from bone marrow of control mouse. Numerous cytoplasmic granules, most of which contain a single crystalloid. Lead citrate, uranyl acetate, TEM, ×11300

Fig. 92 *(lower right).* Eosinophil from beige mouse. Decreased numbers of cytoplasmic granules in association with two large granules that contain multiple crystalloids. Lead citrate, uranyl acetate, TEM, ×11300

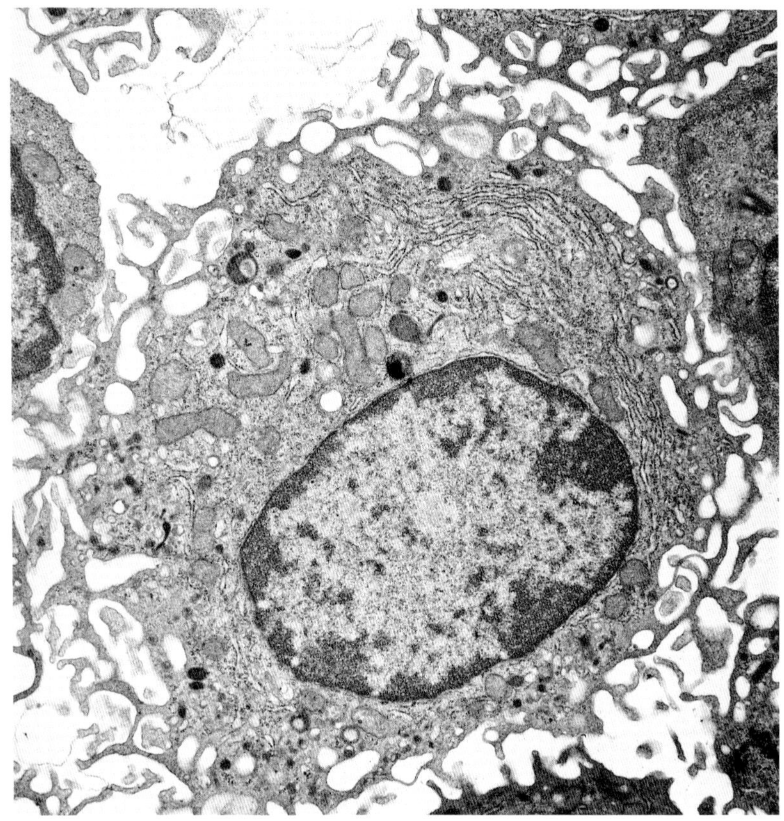

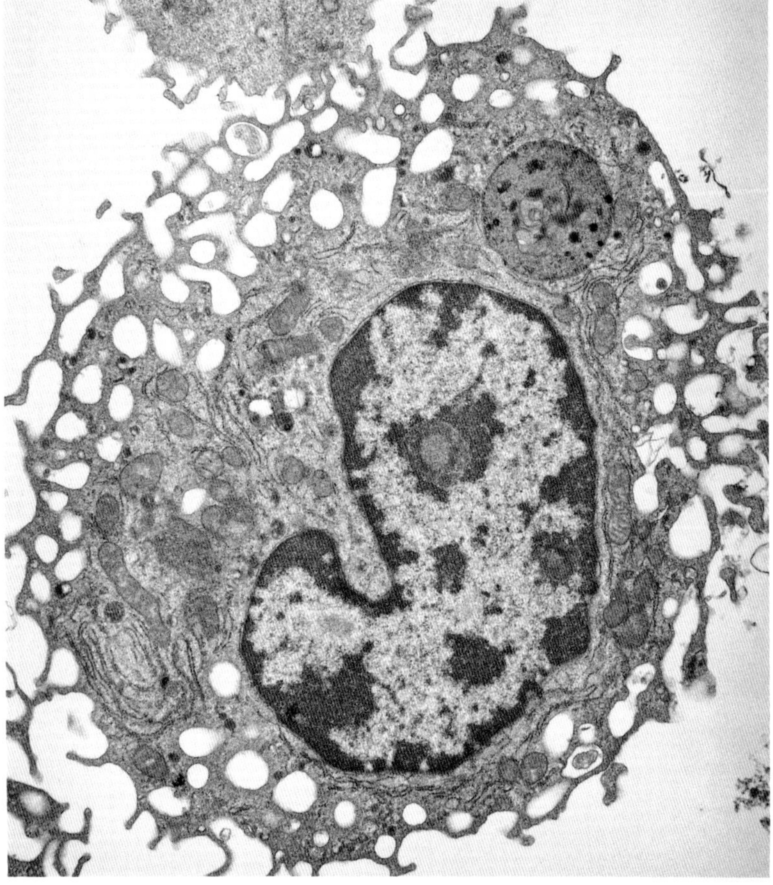

◄ **Fig. 93** *(above).* Peritoneal macrophage from normal mouse. Several small dense granules are present in the cytoplasm. Uranyl acetate, lead citrate, TEM, × 9600

Fig. 94 *(below).* Beige mouse macrophage. Several normal-sized granules are present along with one enlarged round granule with heterogeneous internal components. Uranyl acetate, lead citrate, TEM, × 9600

Fig. 95 *(above).* Peritoneal mast cell from a normal ► mouse. Numerous, regularly shaped, generally round, cytoplasmic granules. Uranyl acetate, lead citrate, TEM, × 7700

Fig. 96 *(below).* Mast cell from a beige mouse. A few massively enlarged cytoplasmic granules along with two normal-sized granules are present in the cytoplasm. One of the enlarged granules *(lower right)* is irregularly shaped with evidence that it had fused with a normal-sized granule. Uranyl acetate, lead citrate, TEM, × 7700

Etiology

The underlying biochemical defect in the syndrome is unknown. The fact that it is a recessive condition indicates that it is due to an enzyme deficiency, but the enzyme and even the biochemical pathways are unknwon. The condition is not a lysosomal storage disease in the classical concept of this group of diseases. Cellular metachromasia is corrected when fibroblasts from a human patient with a lysosomal storage disease are cultured with normal fibroblasts, affected fibroblasts, or fibroblasts of a patient with a different lysosomal storage disease. However, the cellular metachromasia of affected fibroblasts is not corrected by incubation with normal fibroblasts or fibroblasts of any of 11 types of lysosomal storage diseases (Danes and Bearn 1970). Even though CHS is not a lysosomal storage disease according to the commonly accepted definition, there is abnormal storage of glycosphinogolipids in some of the functionally deficient lysosomes. The lysosomes in cells of the kidneys of beige mice are functionally impaired in the catabolism of proteins (Prieur et al. 1972) and store markedly elevated amounts of glycolipids, particularly globotriglycosylceramides (Gross et al. 1985). Although deficiencies of the lysosomal proteases elastase and cathespin G have been documented in beige mice (Vassalli et al. 1978; Takeuchi et al. 1986), these deficiencies are not believed to be the primary genetic alterations in this syndrome.

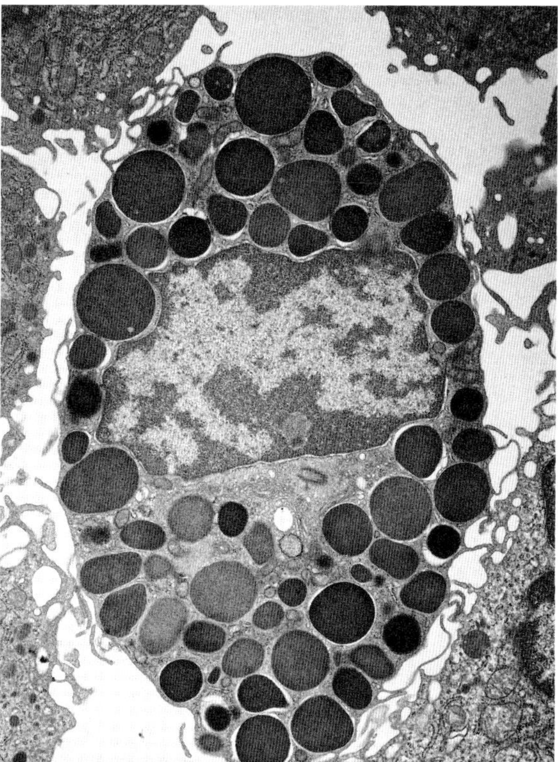

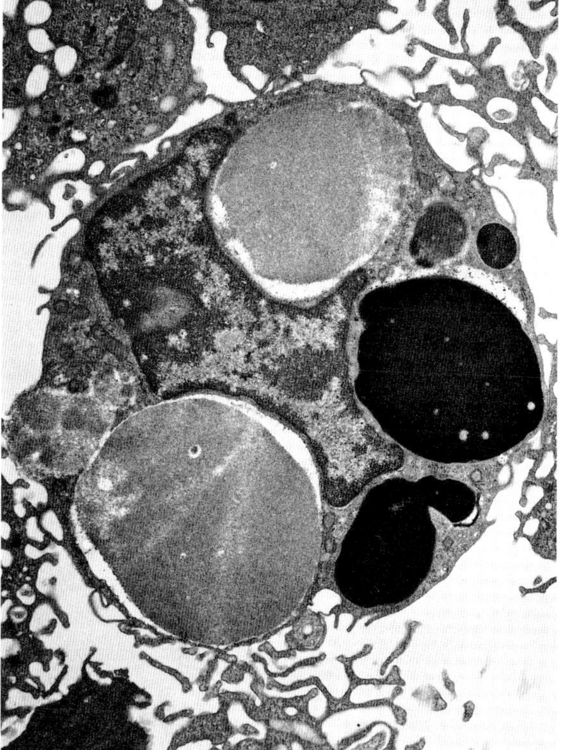

Frequency

The beige trait has arisen many times in mice. The Jackson Laboratory, for instance, has recorded new beige mutations eight times (Heiniger and Dorey 1980). The allelism of the bg^J (C57BL/6, bg^J/bg^J) and bg (SB/Le, bg/bg) mutations has been documented (Brandt and Swank 1976), whereas the allelism of the other beige mutations has been demonstrated but not published. Beige mice are frequently used in research. In a recent bibliography of CHS, many entries pertain to the syndrome in mice, and a total of 968 publications is listed (Prieur 1987). Because of the deficiency of NK cell activity, beige mice have been extensively used in studies of NK cells (Talmadge et al. 1980; Itoh et al. 1982).

Comparison with Other Species

Syndromes similar to that of the beige mouse have been described in humans (Beguez-Cesar 1943), cattle and mink (Padgett et al. 1964), killer whales (Taylor and Farrell 1973), cats (Kramer et al. 1977), blue foxes (Nes et al. 1983), and silver foxes (Nes et al. 1985). The syndromes in the various species have not been characterized to equal degrees; nevertheless, much homology has been documented. The similarities include: an incomplete oculocutaneous albinism; enlarged granules in leukocytes, melanocytes, and many types of cells; decreased resistance to infectious diseases; a bleeding tendency secondary to platelet dysfunction; and defects of leukocyte function There are differences in the degree of expression of some manifestations of the syndrome among various species, but these do not appear to be due to any intrinsic difference in the basic syndrome. Genetic complementation analysis after interspecific somatic cell hybridization indicates that the syndromes in humans, cats, and mink are homologous (Penner and Prieur 1987). The one significant difference among the species with the syndrome is the occurrence of a terminal lymphomatous condition in humans termed the "accelerated phase". A similar manifestation has not been documented in animals. Recent evidence suggests the accelerated phase may be due to Epstein-Barr virus infection (Rubin et al. 1985; Merino et al. 1986).

References

Ash P, Loutit JF, Townsend KMS (1980) Giant lysosomes, a cytoplasmic marker in osteoclasts of beige mice. J Pathol 130: 237–245

Beguez-Cesar A (1943) Neutropenia cronica maligna familiar con granulaciones atipicas de los leucocitos. Bol Soc Cubana Pediatr 15: 900–922

Brandt EJ, Swank RT (1976) The Chediak-Higashi (beige) mutation in two mouse strains: allelism and similarity in lysosomal dysfunction. Am J Pathol 82: 573–588

Chi EY, Lagunoff D (1975) Abnormal mast cell granules in the beige (Chediak-Higashi syndrome) mouse. J Histochem Cytochem 23: 117–122

Chi EY, Lagunoff D, Koehler JK (1976) Abnormally large lamellar bodies in type II pneumocytes in Chediak-Higashi syndrome in beige mice. Lab Invest 34: 166–173

Danes BS, Bearn AG (1970) Correction of cellular metachromasia in cultured fibroblasts in several inherited mucopolysaccharidoses. Proc Natl Acad Sci USA 67: 357–364

Elin RJ, Edelin JB, Wolff SM (1974) Infection and immunoglobulin concentrations in Chediak-Higashi mice. Infect Immun 10: 88–91

Essner E, Oliver C (1974) Lysosome formation in hepatocytes of mice with Chediak-Higashi syndrome. Lab Invest 30: 596–607

Gallin JI, Bujak JS, Patten E, Wolff SM (1974) Granulocyte function in the Chediak-Higashi syndrome of mice. Blood 43: 201–206

Gross SK, Shea TB, McCluer RH (1985) Altered secretion and accumulation of kidney glycosphingolipids by mouse pigmentation mutants with lysosomal dysfunctions. J Biol Chem 260: 5033–5039

Heiniger H-J, Dorey JJ (eds) (1980) Handbook of genetically standardized JAX mice, 3rd edn. Jackson Laboratory, Bar Harbor, p 5.35

Holland JM (1976) Serotonin deficiency and prolonged bleeding in beige mice. Proc Soc Exp Biol Med 151: 32–39

Itoh K, Suzuki K, Umezu Y, Hanaumi K, Kumagai K (1982) Studies of murine large granular lymphocytes. II. Tissue, strain, and age distributions of LGL and LAL. J Immunol 129: 395–405

Kramer JW, Davis WC, Prieur DJ (1977) The Chediak-Higashi syndrome of cats. Lab Invest 36: 554–562

Lane PW, Murphy ED (1972) Susceptibility to spontaneous pneumonitis in an inbred strain of beige and satin mice. Genetics 72: 451–460

Lutzner MA, Lowrie CT, Jordan HW (1967) Giant granules in leukocytes of the beige mouse. J Hered 58: 299–300

Merino F, Henle W, Ramirez-Duque P (1986) Chronic active Epstein-Barr virus infection in patients with Chediak-Higashi syndrome. J Clin Immunol 6: 299–305

Morahan PS, Morse SS, Mahoney KH (1980) The beige (Chediak-Higashi syndrome) mouse as a model for macrophage function studies. In: Skamene E, Kongshavn PA, Landy M (eds) Genetic control of natural resistance to infection and malignancy. Academic, New York, pp 575–582

Nes N, Lium B, Braend M, Sjaastad O (1983) A Chediak-Higashi-like syndrome in Arctic blue foxes. Finsk Veterinaertidsskr 89: 313

Nes N, Lium B, Sjaastad O, Blom A (1985) Norsk perlerev-mutant med Chediak-Higashi-liknende syndrom. Nor Pelsdyrbl 59: 325–328

Novak EK, Hui S-W, Swank RT (1984) Platelet storage pool deficiency in mouse pigment mutations associated with seven distinct genetic loci. Blood 63: 536–544

Oliver C, Essner E (1973) Distribution of anomalous lysosomes in the beige mouse: a homologue of Chediak-Higashi syndrome. J Histochem Cytochem 21: 218–228

Oliver C, Essner E (1975) Formation of anomalous lysosomes in monocytes, neutrophils, and eosinophils from bone marrow of mice with Chediak-Higashi syndrome. Lab Invest 32: 17–27

Oliver JM, Zurier RB, Berlin RD (1975) Concanavalin A cap formation on polymorphonuclear leukocytes of normal and beige (Chediak-Higashi) mice. Nature 253: 471–473

Padgett GA, Leader RW, Gorham JR, O'Mary CC (1964) The familial occurrence of the Chediak-Higashi syndrome in mink and cattle. Genetics 49: 505–512

Penner JD, Prieur DJ (1987) Interspecific genetic complementation analysis with fibroblasts from humans and four species of animals with Chediak-Higashi syndrome. Am J Med Genet 28: 455–470

Pierro LJ, Chase HB (1963) Slate – a new coat color mutant in the mouse. J Hered 54: 47–50

Prieur DJ (1987) An updated bibliography of the Chediak-Higashi syndrome of man and animals – 1987. Washington State University, Pullman, Washington, pp 1–75

Prieur DJ, Davis WC, Padgett GA (1972) Defective function of renal lysosomes in mice with the Chediak-Higashi syndrome. Am J Pathol 67: 227–236

Roder J, Duwe A (1979) The beige mutation in the mouse selectively impairs natural killer cell function. Nature 278: 451–453

Rubin CM, Burke BA, McKenna RW, McClain KL, White JG, Nesbit ME, Filipovich AH (1985) The accelerated phase of Chediak-Higashi syndrome: an expression of the virus-associated hemophagocytic syndrome? Cancer 56: 524–530

Sato A, Spicer SS (1981) An ultrastructural and cytochemical investigation of the development of inclusions in gastric chief cells and parietal cells of mice with the Chediak-Higashi syndrome. Lab Invest 44: 288–299

Saxena RK, Saxena QB, Adler WH (1982) Defective T-cell response in beige mutant mice. Nature 295: 240–241

Strausbauch P, Sawyer R, Volkman A (1982) Ultrastructure of beige mouse peritoneal macrophage lysosomes. J Reticuloendothel Soc 31: 361–365

Takeuchi K, Wood H, Swank RT (1986) Lysosomal elastase and cathepsin G in beige mice: neutrophils of beige (Chediak-Higashi) mice selectively lack lysosomal elastase and cathepsin G. J Exp Med 163: 665–677

Talmadge JE, Meyers KM, Prieur DJ, Starkey JR (1980) Role of NK cells in tumour growth and metastasis in beige mice. Nature 284: 622–624

Taylor RF, Farrell RK (1973) Light and electron microscopy of peripheral blood neutrophils in a killer whale affected with Chediak-Higashi syndrome. Fed Proc 32: 822 (abstract)

Vassalli JD, Granelli-Piperno A, Griscelli C, Reich E (1978) Specific protease deficiency in polymorphonuclear leukocytes of Chediak-Higashi syndrome and beige mice. J Exp Med 147: 1285–1290

Assessment of Toxicologic Effects upon Bone Marrow and Related Tissues

Richard J. Kociba and Gary J. Kociba

Introduction and Objectives

The hemopoietic system is a highly integrated and widely dispersed organ system that includes the bone marrow, spleen, blood, and related tissues. The mature erythrocytes, granulocytes, macrophages, platelets, and lymphocytes that provide diverse funtions to the organism are derived from a single pluripotential stem cell. The process of hemopoiesis is a very dynamic one and is dependent on the continued self-renewal and differentiation of the stem cells in the bone marrow. Hemopoietic cells are capable of rapid proliferation and thus are quite sensitive to certain toxicologic agents. Toxicity to the blood and bone marrow can affect the circulating mature cells and/or their precursor cells within the bone marrow.

The objective of this paper is to describe (a) the conventional parameters routinely used to evaluate the potential for bone marrow toxicity and (b) the more specialized supplemental tests, such as clonal assay techniques that can be used as adjunct tests to define more specifically the individual hemopoietic cellular components that may be affected by various toxicologic agents.

Assessment of Hemopoietic Toxicity During Conduct of Toxicologic Studies

As currently conducted, toxicologic studies for the purposes of safety assessment utilize several mammalian species. This generates a broader data base that facilitates extrapolation from animal studies to humans. In general, most of the commonly used laboratory animal species have been used effectively in these types of studies. The use of a larger animal such as the dog does allow a more comprehensive and temporal assessment of certain parameters.

The route of exposure used in these toxicologic studies typically simulates the route by which humans will be exposed to the agent. This may involve inhalation, ingestion, dermal contact, intravenous or other parenteral routes of administration. The toxicity studies are sequentially staged via acute (single dose), subacute, subchronic, and chronic durations of exposure. These time intervals cover the durations of exposure likely to be encountered by humans. Multiple dose levels of the test substance are studied concurrently with the control group(s), and a broad spectrum of methods are used to evaluate all organ systems of the body. The dose levels utilized should be chosen to evaluate a higher dose group wherein potential target organ toxicity can be defined qualitatively as well as intermediate and lower dose groups that will quantitatively define the dose-response pattern for the target organ. The lower dose levels also should define a lowest-observed-effect level (LOEL) as well as a no-observed-effect level (NOEL) for organ toxicity. The LOEL and NOEL values will quantitatively serve as the points of reference to which a safety factor is applied during the extrapolation process which will define that level of exposure deemed safe for humans. The concept in the term "no adverse effect level" (NOAEL) needs to be introduced here. NOAEL is considered to be a dose level associated with some adaptive or other physiologic response that is considered to be not an adverse effect. Scientific judgment is required to recognize the relevance of both statistical and biological assessments during the interpretation of results.

The highly integrated interrelationship of the hemopoietic system with all other organ systems of the body requires that its evaluation during toxicity studies be an integral part of the full complement of parameters that can be used to monitor all the organ systems of the body. The bone marrow and other components of the hemo-

Table 16. Effect of food restriction on hemologic parameters (4-week study in rats)

Parameter	Control unrestricted food intake (22–23 g/day)	Restricted food intake (g/day)		
		15	10	5
Body weight gain (g)	190	120	50	−20
Daily water intake (ml)	32	25	20	10
Thymus wt.				
Absolute (g)	0.72	0.53	0.36	0.10
Relative (% bw)	0.23	0.23	0.20	0.10
Spleen wt.				
Absolute (g)	0.76	0.51	0.39	0.21
Relative (% bw)	0.24	0.22	0.22	0.20
Leukocytes ($10^3/\mu l$)	4.81	3.55	2.57	1.40
Erythrocytes ($10^6/\mu l$)	5.13	5.73	5.72	5.52
HGB (g/dl)	10.8	12.1	11.8	11.5
PCV (%)	29.5	32.3	31.2	30.2

After Oishi et al. 1979.

poietic system must not be considered isolated from the rest of the body. It must also be kept in mind that the hemopoietic system is dynamic and can be sensitive and responsive to either the direct toxic effects of a test substance or the indirect/secondary effects associated with dehydration, inanition, or other nonspecific factors that can be encountered frequently during the conduct of a toxicity study. Table 16 depicts the substantial effects observed in a 4-week study wherein rats were maintained on a restricted dietary intake (Oishi et al. 1979). This simple restriction of food intake caused substantial decreases in body weight gain, water intake, weight of thymus, weight of spleen, and leukocyte concentration. It also caused minor and variable degrees of hemoconcentration.

Table 17 depicts the changes in hematologic parameters in rabbits maintained on a starvation diet for 2 weeks (Bathija et al. 1979). The data in Tables 16 and 17 represent the type of significant alterations that are frequently encountered during the conduct of toxicity studies wherein secondary or nonspecific factors can cause substantial effects that need to be carefully evaluated during the interpretation of the toxicologic effects of the test substance. To allow the investigator to delineate those effects directly attributable

Table 17. Changes in body weight, packed cell volume, and reticulocytes following 2 weeks' starvation (rabbits)

Body weight (kg)		Packed cell volume (%)		Reticulocytes (%)	
Initial	Final	Initial	Final	Initial	Final
3.23 ± 0.3	2.34 ± 0.2	38.5 ± 4.3	31.7 ± 0.9	1.4 ± 0.9	0.1 ± 0.2

After Bathija et al. 1979.

to the test substance from those attributable to secondary or nonspecific causes (such as inanition), it is imperative that a full complement of parameters be monitored. The current concept is to design and conduct routine toxicity studies in such a manner that comprehensive data are generated for all organ systems of the body. These comprehensive whole animal studies create the best opportunity to interpret the results and evaluate the potential of the test substance to elicit either a direct toxic effect on the hemopoietic system or an indirect nonspecific effect that can be manifest in the form of changes in the hemopoietic system.

The measurements that can readily be used in routine toxicity studies for evaluation of effects upon the hemopoietic system are listed in Table 18. The parameter listed in this table include both hematologic and morphologic data that are best interpreted as a package by the pathologist to assure that the most valid interpretation is given. Although statistical evaluations of the data are routinely conducted, final toxicologic interpretation of the data is dependent on a comprehensive assessment of all relevant findings, including whether the findings being attributed to the test substance appear biologically plausible and consistent.

Toxicity Mediated Principally Via Effect on Bone Marrow Production

The bone marrow is one of the largest organs of the body, comprising up to 4.8% of the adult body weight (Chanarin 1985). This makes it comparable in size to the liver. As hemopoietic activity in the bone marrow changes with age, it is important to have adequate concurrent control animals for comparative assessment. In laboratory animals typically used in toxicity studies, the long bones, sternum, ribs, vertebral bodies, pelvic girdle, skull bones, and spleen are sites of active hemopoietic activity. The pluripotential stem cell (PSC) is considered to be the common source of

Table 18. Parameters used in routine toxicity studies for evaluation of potential for effects upon the hemopoietic system

- Clinical observations
- Serial assays of peripheral blood elements
- Heinz bodies, methemoglobin, carboxyhemoglobin, eryhtrocyte fragility
- Clotting parameters
- Bone marrow biopsies and smears
- Autopsy examination
- Gravimetric evaluation of thymus, spleen, lymph nodes, etc.
- Histopathologic examination of all tissues (hemopoietic as well as all other organ systems)
- More specific supplemental tests if indicated by results:
  - Iron isotopes for study of marrow activity
  - Total nucleated cell counts of femur
  - Clonal assays of stem cells and precursors cell lines
  - Immunologic parameters

all blood cells (Schofield 1979). This stem cell has the key attributes whereby it maintains its own numbers by self renewal and differentiates into mature functional cells under appropriate stimulation.

Figure 97 depicts the schematic pathways whereby the self-renewing stem cell gives rise to two major multipotential precursor cells: (1) the common lymphoid progenitor cell which gives rise to T and B lymphocytes and other subsets and (2) a common myeloid progenitor cell which gives rise to megakaryocytes, red blood cells, granulocytes (neutrophils, eosinophils, and basophils), and monocytes.

A histologic section of bone marrow reveals a heterogeneous population of cells, including fat, small, dark-staining cells that are erythroid precursors and the granulocytic cells characterized by more abundant granular cytoplasm and nuclei which may be lobed or convoluted. The bone marrow provides a hemopoietic inductive microenvironment that is a necessary prerequisite for the process of hemopoiesis (Bentley 1982). This microenvironment can be considered on a morphologic basis when referring to the elements

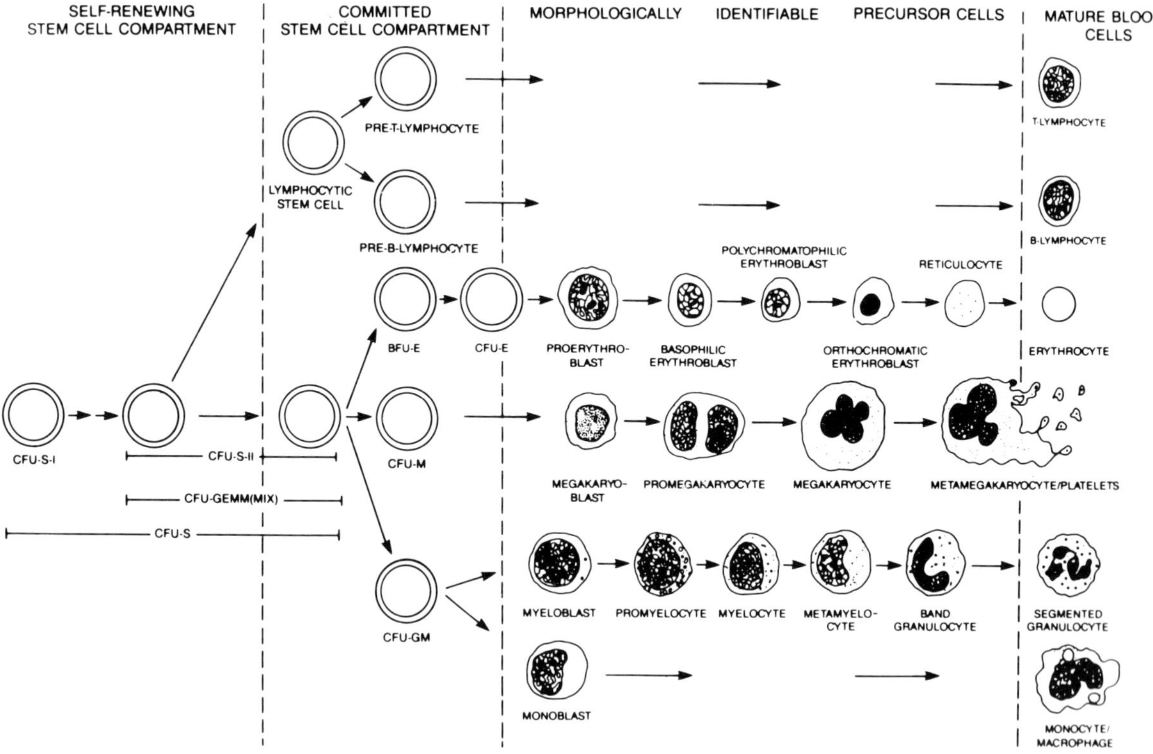

Fig. 97. Schematic diagram of hemopoiesis. For abbreviations see Table 1 p. 6 and text

that provide mechanical support for developing hemopoietic cells as well as on a functional basis, including those local factors that stimulate cells to develop along particular lines. Important morphologic components include the marrow vasculature, reticular cells (adventitial surface of the venous sinuses), adipocytes (marrow fat cells), marrow fibroblasts, nerve fibers, macrophages, and lymphocytes.

The morphologic elements, as well as specific regulating factors including multilineage colony stimulating factor, CSF (interleukin 3), other glycoprotein hormones which act as lineage-specific CSFs, or factors which alter responses to other cytokines, influence and regulate the process of hemopoiesis. Figure 97 depicts those precursors cells and mature blood cells which are morphologically identifiable as part of the hemopoietic maturation process.

In toxicologic studies, the most useful and readily accessible tool for assessment of potential hemopoietic toxicity is the periodic examination of peripheral blood components. The multiple quantitative and qualitative evaluations that can be conducted on serial peripheral blood samples allow investigators to monitor for toxicity affecting either hemopoietic precursors or circulating mature blood cells. If the examination of the peripheral blood gives indications of a possible effect, supplemental tests can be selected.

Excluding nutritional disturbances, the principal causes of bone marrow toxicity can be generally placed into two categories of toxicologic agents:

1. Cytotoxic agents, sometimes referred to as general cell poisons. These include alkylating type compounds and ionizing radiation. They typically cause a consistent and predictable injury that can be correlated with dose or duration of exposure to the material. For these cytotoxic agents, the animal models are usually predictive and have been very useful in preclinical safety assessment studies (Marsh 1976).

2. Agents associated with a unique sensitivity or idiosyncratic reaction in certain subjects. This group includes substances such as phenylbutazone, streptomycin, organic arsenicals, chlorpromazine, chloramphenicol, cephalosporine, and certain other antibiotics (Robbins and Cotran 1979; Bloom et al. 1987a). The role of an immunologic basis has been proposed for certain of these cases of unique sensitivity. This leads to a bone marrow toxicity that is

Table 19. Hemotoxicity induced by cephalosporin in the dog

- Peripheral blood changes
  - Nonregenerative anemia
  - Spherocytosis
  - Erythroblastemia
  - Increased osmotic fragility
  - Reticulocytopenia
  - Neutropenia, with toxic neutrophils
  - Thrombocytopenia with macroplatelets
- Bone marrow changes
  - Erythroid hypoplasia (cefonicid) or hyperplasia (cefazedone)
  - Granulocytic hypoplasia
  - Necrosis, hemophagocytosis, and hemosiderin deposits
  - Decreased CFU-GM
- Spleen and liver
  - Extramedullary hemopoiesis
  - Hemosiderin
  - Hemophagocytosis

After Bloom et al. 1987b.

Table 20. Estrogen-induced bone marrow depression in ferrets

Parameter (Blood)	Estrogen treated	Reference values
Packed cell volume (%)	24	42–55
Leukocytes/µl	2500	4000–18200
Platelets/µl	40500	310000–910000

After Bernard et al. 1983.

Table 21. Effect of 26-week benzene exposure on peripheral blood, bone marrow, and spleen

	Benzene concentration (ppm)	
	0	302
Peripheral blood		
Total leukocytes/µl	14406 ± 2016	6839 ± 1630
Neutrophils/µl	3080 ± 431	5212 ± 1365
Lymphocytes/µl	10213 ± 1848	1309 ± 247
RBC $\times 10^6$/µl	9.93 ± 0.32	6.23 ± 0.68
HCT (%)	50.5 ± 1.2	38.2 ± 3.8
Bone marrow		
Nucleated cells/femur $\times 10^{-6}$	21.8 ± 1.1	7.0 ± 3.1
Granulocytes/femur $\times 10^{-6}$	8.7 ± 1.8	2.6 ± 1.7
Nucleated RBC/femur $\times 10^{-6}$	4.6 ± 0.8	3.2 ± 0.9
Lymphocytes/femur $\times 10^{-6}$	6.5 ± 0.4	0.7 ± 0.4
Spleen		
Nucleated cells/spleen $\times 10^{-6}$	116.8 ± 3.8	19.3 ± 4.6
Granulocytes/spleen $\times 10^{-6}$	7.0 ± 0.4	3.2 ± 2.0
Nucleated RBC/spleen $\times 10^{-6}$	10.4 ± 2.3	10.1 ± 4.5
Lymphocytes/spleen $\times 10^{-6}$	95.5 ± 2.8	5.1 ± 1.8
Spleen weight (mg)	161.7 ± 4.5	109.0 ± 15.7

After Green et al. 1981.

unpredictable and typically is identified only after the drug is in widespread use in humans. The effect is not usually correlated with dose or duration. The animal models available for assessing bone marrow toxicity are of limited use in predicting this type of unique sensitivity or idiosyncratic response which is observed in an occasional human subject. It may sometimes be the result of a genetic trait (Haak 1980), and one proposal states that this idiosyncratic type of drug-associated aplastic anemia should be further differentiated to include a "conditional" drug-associated aplastic anemia that is conditional on the presence of a known metabolic deficiency, such as glucose-6-phosphate dehydrogenase deficiency.

The recent studies of Bloom et al. (1987a, b) have given indications that the dog can serve as a useful model for studying the mechanisms whereby the cephalosporin antibiotics cause a variety of blood dyscrasias. Table 19 summarizes the type of changes that can be induced by certain cephalosporin antibiotics in the dog.

Table 20 depicts some of the changes noted in the peripheral blood of ferrets as a result of estrogen toxicity (Bernard et al. 1983; Kociba and Caputo 1981). These findings point to bone marrow depression as indicated by the decreased values for both erythroid and myeloid cell lines. Figures 98 and 99 depict the effects of high doses of benzene in the peripheral leukocyte counts and nucleated cells in the bone marrow of the femur of mice. Benzene is one of the better characterized bone marrow toxicants. Table 21 lists various effects of repeated exposure to a toxic level of benzene (Green et al. 1981). Benzene caused changes in the peripheral blood, including decreases in total leukocytes, lymphocytes, erythrocytes, and packed cell volume. In the bone marrow decreases are seen the number of nucleated cells, granulocytes, nucleated erythroid

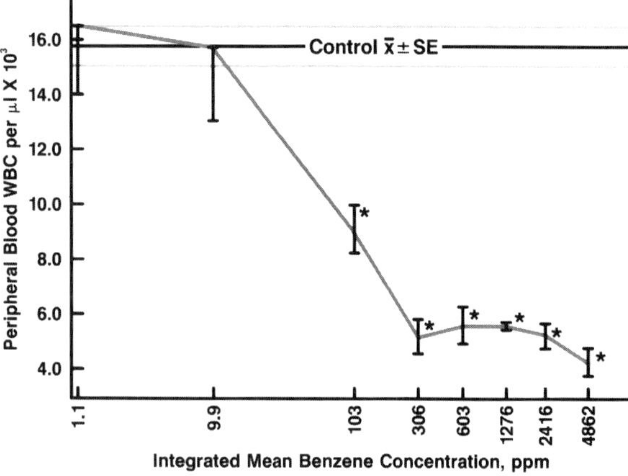

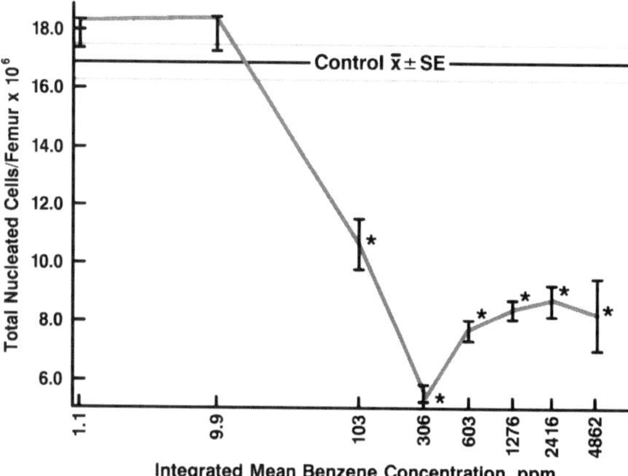

Fig. 98 *(above)*. Effect of benzene on peripheral blood of CD-1 mice. (After Green et al. 1981)

Fig. 99 *(below)*. Effect of benzene on bone marrow of CD-1 mice. (After Green et al. 1981)

cells, and lymphocytes. The weight of the spleen was decreased, with corresponding losses of its cellular constituents.

The rapid turnover of leukocytes in the blood and bone marrow may allow early recognition of toxic effects on hemopoietic cells. The temporal pattern of changes in the number of cells in the bone marrow of mice given a single dose of a cytotoxic agent such as the cancer chemotherapeutic drug *cis*-diamino-dichloroplatinum II is depicted in Table 22 (Zak et al. 1972; Kociba and Sleight 1971). Within 1 h of dosing, there was a decrease of approximately 8% in bone marrow cellularity. Maximal depression was noted 1–2 days post exposure, and recovery was noted 6 days post exposure. After detection of these types of toxic effects upon circulating mature

Table 22. Changes in number of cells in bone marrow of femurs of mice given a single dose of cis Pt II (cancer chemotherapy)

Time after treatment	Relative no. of cells present in bone marrow (%)
0	100
1 h	92.1
3 h	86.5
6 h	87.6
1 day	68.1
3 days	60.7
6 days	77.2
10 days	83.1

After Zak et al. 1972.

blood cells or bone marrow, supplemental testing with specialized clonal assays may be used to characterize more specifically the effects on hemopoietic cells of various lineages.

Table 23 tabulates some of the clonal assays that have been used in the assessment of hemopoietic stem cells and progenitor cell lines (Wilson 1985). Boorman et al. (1982) have proposed the routine use of clonal marrow assays to screen for potential myelotoxicity of test substances. In this scheme, after the test animals have been exposed to the test substance, a suspension of single cells is made of bone marrow flushed from an entire femur. The marrow concentration is measured to determine total nucleated cells per femur as a sensitive index of cellularity. Aliquots of the cell suspension are injected into irradiated recipients to measure colony forming units-spleen (CFU-S) and plated in cultures in semisolid media to which has been added granulocytes/macrophage CSF (GM-CSF), erythropoietin, interleukin 3, or other sources of CSFs. These assays allow the quantification of granulocyte-macrophage progenitors (CFU-GM), erythroid progenitors (BFU-E and CFU-E), megakaryocyte progenitors (CFU-M), and multilineage progenitors (CFU-S and CFU-GEMM). Table 24 depicts results generated by Boorman et al. (1982) using clonal assays with studies of diethylstilbestrol and indomethacin. Diethylstilbestrol caused dose-related decreases in bone marrow cellularity, pluripotent stem cells (CFU-S), and granulocyte-macrophage progenitors (CFU-GM). Indomethacin had no significant effects on bone marrow cellularity or CFU-S but produced an apparent enhancement of CFU-GM.

These types of specialized tests are most appropriately used as follow-up tests after the conven-

Table 23. Summary of assays for measurement of hemopoietic stem and progenitor cells

Potentiality of stem cells	Type of stem cell	Method	Stimulant
Pluripotent hemopoietic	CFU-S	In vivo spleen colony formation by reconstitution of irradiated mice	Mouse environment
		In vitro growth of CFU-S suspension cultures	Adherent stromal cells
Pluripotent stem cells with limited self-renewal	CFU-Mix	Formation of mixed hemopoietic colonies in agar or plasma clots	Growth factors from mitogen-stimulated lymphocytes or IL-3
Primitive erythrocytic committed stem cells	BFU-E	Plasma clot or agar and methylcellulose	Erythropoietin, erythroid burst-promoting factor
		Long-term suspension cultures	Adherent stromal cells
Committed erythrocytic progenitor cells	CFU-E	Plasma clot or methylcellulose semisolid culture systems	Erythropoietin
Granulocytic primitive committed stem cells	CFU-D	Diffusion chamber with agar	Mouse environment
Committed monocyte-granulocytic and/or macrophage progenitor cells	CFU-GM	Semisolid agar or methylcellulose culture systems	CSF-GM conditioned media
		Long-term suspension cultures	Adherent stromal cells
Committed megakaryocytic progenitor cells	CFU-Meg	Semisolid agar cultures, plasma clot	PHA-LyCM erythropoietin preparation
Committed lymphocytic progenitor cells	CFU-BL	Semisolid agar culture systems	PHA-LyCM, PWM, 2 ME, protein A
	CFU-TL	Semisolid agar or methylcellulose cultures	PHA and PWM alloantigens, T-dependent soluble antigens and T-cell growth factor
		T-cell suspension long-term suspension cultures	T-cell growth factor
Multipotential stromal stem cells and hemopoietic microenvironment		Inoculation of fibroblasts isolated from hemopoietic tissues into IP implanted diffusion chambers or directly into the renal capsule	In vivo mouse
Fibroblast progenitor cells	CFU-F	Formation of adherent fibroblast colonies in suspension or semisolid culture systems	Fibroblast growth factor (?)

After Wilson 1985, which should be consulted for specific details.

Table 24. Examples of in vivo and in vitro clonal assays for hemopoietic progenitor cells

Chemical	Dose (mg/kg daily)	Cell or colony numbers (% of controls)		
		Bone marrow cellularity	Pluripotent stem cells (CFU-S)	Granulocyte-macrophage progenitors (CFU-GM)
Diethylstilbestrol	0.2	84	97	16
	2	74	88	65
	8	68	59	63
	(5 days)			
Indomethacin	1	112	108	118
	2	88	ND	122
	4	96	81	120
	(6 days)			

After Boorman et al. 1982.

tional toxicity studies have given some indication for the potential of the test substance to cause an effect on the hemopoietic system. The application of these specialized tests on a selective follow-up basis allows a more informed and judicious use and design of these supplemental tests.

Toxicity Mediated Principally Via Effect on Integrity of Hemoglobin Content or Cellular Membrane of Peripheral Blood Cells

Toxicologic studies are also necessary to assess the potential for agents to cause an adverse effect upon the various types of circulating blood cells. In this regard, periodic evaluations of peripheral blood should include both quantitative and qualitative parameters that are useful in assessing the integrity of the circulating blood cells. Special attention should be given to evaluating whether the agent being studied has the potential to affect adversely the integrity of the cellular membrane or the hemoglobin content.

It is known that certain toxicologic agents can exert an adverse effect directly on the circulating blood cells. Phenylhydrazine, saponins, arsine, naphthalene, etc. can cause direct hemolysis of red blood cells. Other agents, such as primaquine may produce red blood cell hemolysis in cells inherently deficient in glucose-6-phosphate dehydrogenase. Peripheral blood cells may also be affected via an immunologic type of hypersensitization (Pisciotta 1973). Acetanilid has been associated with an autoimmune hemolytic anemia involving lysis of circulating blood cells (Smith 1975).

Autoimmune thrombocytopenia has been associated with certain drugs such as quinidine and acetophenetidin. Other toxicologic agents have the potential for adversely affecting the hemoglobin content of peripheral red blood cells. Carbon monoxide can interact with the hemoglobin of red blood cells to cause the classic cherry red color characteristic of carboxyhemoglobin formation. Hemoglobin can also undergo oxidation to methemoglobin upon exposure to compounds such as sodium nitrite, aniline, hydroxylamine, and nitrobenzene (Smith and Olson 1973).

The formation of Heinz bodies in red blood cells is a well-characterized result of exposure to certain agents (Fertman and Fertman 1955). A large number of aromatic amines (including aniline, toluidine, *p*-aminophenol, phenacetin, phenylhydrazine), aromatic nitroderivatives (such as nitrobenzene, nitrotoluene), complex aromatic amino-derivatives (such as Nile blue sulfate, methylene blue, phenothiazine, and colchicine), as well as inorganic compounds (such as hydroxylamine, sodium azide, sodium nitrate/nitrite, chlorates, and arsine) have been implicated in Heinz body formation in the red blood cells of humans and animals. Heinz bodies form under certain conditions in which oxidant stress exceeds the reductive capacity of the red blood cells. They are composed of denatured hemoglobin and cellular membrane proteins via oxidation of internal sulfhydryl groups or formation of hemichromes. The macromolecular complex is recognized morphologically as a Heinz body through the use of supravital stains, such as brilliant cresyl violet or Nile blue sulfate. As they protrude from the surface of the cell, they serve as a recognition site for premature degradation by macrophages within the reticuloendothelial tissues of the body. Many of the compounds that cause Heinz body formation also cause oxidation of hemoglobin to methemoglobin or hemolytic anemia (O'Donoghue 1986). Thus, the recognition of either effect should be interpreted as an indication that a thorough evaluation is warranted.

If the toxicologic studies have identified the potential for an adverse effect on the circulating blood cells or their components (such as intravascular hemolysis) the pertinent organs and tissues, such as the spleen, reticuloendothelial tissue, urinary system, and bone marrow, should be closely examined for the anticipated secondary and compensatory responses. This underscores the absolute need to evaluate hemopoietic toxicity as part of a cohesive and comprehensive pathologic evaluation of all organ systems of the body.

Conclusion

The potential for hemopoietic toxicity should be evaluated as an integral component of well-designed, comprehensive studies in multiple species of laboratory animals. As the bone marrow and other components of the hemopoietic system are highly dynamic and interrelated with the entire body, they must be evaluated as an integral part of the body as a whole.

Toxicologic studies must be conducted with full knowledge that the hemopoietic system can respond to direct toxic effects of the test substance or to the indirect/nonspecific effects associated with dehydration, inanition, or other nonspecific factors that can be encountered during toxicity studies. Toxicologic studies in laboratory animals have proved to be quite predictive in identifying the potential for hemopoietic effects of the type that have a cytotoxic basis of action. However, animal studies have been less predictive and of more limited value in identifying effects with an immunologic (or idiosyncratic) basis. The use of conventional parameters to assess the potential for hemotoxicity can now be supplemented with more specific tests, such as clonal assays to aid in the further delineation of adverse effects upon individual components of the hemopoietic system. While it is generally accepted that the conventional toxicologic studies in laboratory animal studies will identify most of the above effects that have a cytotoxic mechanism of action, it must be kept in mind that historical experience has indicated that certain of those effects with an immunologic (or idiosyncratic) basis may not be necessarily identified in the preclinical animal studies and thus will be identified only after human clinical usage. This underscores the need for a comprehensive assessment during the preclinical toxicity studies to maximize their usefulness as tools in identifying agents that are suspect relative to the potential for adversely affecting the hemopoietic system.

References

Bathija A, Davis S, Trubowitz S (1979) Bone marrow adipose tissue: response to acute starvation. Am J Hematol 6: 191–198

Bentley SA (1982) Bone marrow connective tissue and the hematopoietic microenvironment. Br J Haematol 50: 1–6

Bernard SL, Leathers CW, Brobst DF, Borham JR (1983) Estrogen-induced bone marrow depression in ferrets. Am J Vet Res 44: 657–661

Bloom JC, Lewis HB, Seller TS, Deldar A (1987a) The hematologic effects of cefonicid and cefazedone in the dog: a potential model of cephalosporin hematotoxicity in man. Toxicol Appl Pharmacol 90: 135–142

Bloom JC, Lewis HB, Seller TS, Deldar A, Morgan DG (1987b) The hematopathology of cefonicid- and cefazedone-induced blood dyscrasias in the dog. Toxicol Appl Pharmacol 90: 143–155

Boorman GA, Luster MI, Dean JH, Campbell ML (1982) Assessment of myelotoxicity caused by environmental chemicals. Environ Health Perspect 43: 129–135

Chanarin I (1985) Structure and function of the bone marrow. In: Irons R (ed) Toxicology of the blood and bone marrow. Raven, New York, pp 1–16

Fertman MH, Fertman MB (1955) Toxic anemias and Heinz bodies. Medicine 34: 131–192

Green JD, Snyder CA, LoBue J, Goldstein BD, Albert RE (1981) Acute and chronic dose/response effects of benzene inhalation on the peripheral blood, bone marrow and spleen cells of CD-1 male mice. Toxicol Appl Pharmacol 59: 204–214

Haak HL (1980) Experimental drug-induced aplastic anaemia. Clin Haematol 9: 621–639

Kociba GJ, Caputo CA (1981) Aplastic anemia associated with estrus in pet ferrets. J Am Vet Med Assoc 178: 1293–1294

Kociba RJ, Sleight SD (1971) Acute toxicologic and pathologic effects of cisdiamminedichloroplatinum (NSC119875) in the male rat. Cancer Chemother Rep 54: 325–329

Marsh JC (1976) The effects of cancer chemotherapeutic agents on normal hematopoietic precursor cells: a review. Cancer Res 36: 1853–1882

O'Donoghue JL (1986) Subchronic oral toxicology of 4-chloro-3-nitroaniline in the rat. Fundam Appl Toxicol 6: 551–558

Oishi S, Oishi H, Hiraga K (1979) The effect of food restriction for 4 weeks on common toxicity parameters in male rats. Toxicol Appl Pharmacol 47: 15–22

Pisciotta AV (1973) Immune and toxic mechanisms in drug-induced agranulocytosis. Semin Hematol 10: 279–310

Robbins SL, Cotran RS (1979) Pathologic basis of disease, 2nd edn. Saunders, Philadelphia, pp 712–756

Schofield R (1979) The pluripotent stem cell. Clin Hematol 8: 221–237

Smith RP (1975) Toxicology of the formed elements of the blood. In: Cassarett LJ, Doull J (eds) Toxicology: the basic science of poisons. MacMillan, New York, pp 225–243

Smith RP, Olson MV (1973) Drug-induced methemoglobinemia. Semin Hematol 10: 253–268

Wilson FD (1985) Clonogenic stem and progenitor cell assays for the evaluation of chemically induced myelotoxicity. In: Irons R (ed) Toxicology of the blood and bone marrow. Raven, New York, pp 65–100

Zak M, Drobnik J, Rezny Z (1972) The effect of cis-platinum (II) diamminodichloride on bone marrow. Cancer Res 32: 595–599.

Hemobartonellosis and Eperythrozoonosis

Henry J. Baker

Synonym. Eperythrozoon spp. and Hemobartonella spp. of the order Rickettsiales, family Anaplasmataceae, are small (350 μm), pleomorphic, extracellular parasites infecting a wide variety of mammalian hosts (Moulder 1974).

Gross Appearance

The phagocytic elements of the spleen, liver, lymph nodes, and other organs appear to be primarily responsible for limiting the multiplication of these parasites. Splenic macrophages are especially important in suppressing the infections, and splenomegaly is often the first and only readily apparent gross pathologic lesion of latent infection. Following experimental injection with *E. coccoides* (Baker et al. 1971), peak splenic enlargement of 3–4 times normal occurs approximately 7 days after infection but diminishes rapidly during the enusing week and reaches a plateau at 1.5–2 times normal by 21 days. This level of splenomegaly persisted for the remainder of a 42-day observation period. Splenomegaly is also a prominent gross pathologic sign of *H. muris* infection in rats; however, quantitative data are lacking.

Microscopic Features

E. coccoides has an annular or ring appearance in Romanowsky-stained blood smears (Fig. 100), and although this is known to be an artifact of fixation and staining, it remains a useful distinguishing feature of the organism. Extra-erythrocytic forms are seen frequently in the blood of infected mice (Fig. 100). In contrast, *H. muris* appears as solid coccoid elements arranged in clusters, chains, or singly on erythrocytes and is rarely seen free in plasma (Fig. 101). Both *Hemobartonella* and *Eperythrozoon* stain blue to polychromatophilic in Giemsa or Wright's stained blood smears. Acridine orange staining increases the sensitivity of parasite identification, especially when their concentration is low (Cassell et al. 1979). When examined by dark-field fluorescence microscopy, stained organisms fluoresce yellow-green to red-orange, depending on the procedure of acridine orange staining used. Fluorescing structures such as Howell-Jolly bodies, reticulocytes, and platelet fragments may be confused with organisms. Positive identification of these organisms in peripheral blood smears is made difficult by their small size and resemblance to other erythrocyte inclusions unless massive parasitemias are induced. For example, basophilic stippled erythrocytes, which occasionally reach high concentrations in the peripheral blood of normal young rodents, are easily confused with these organisms.

The morphologic changes that occur in the spleens of pathogen-free mice infected with *E. coccoides* are dramatic. By post inoculation day 4 or 5, the splenic follicles are transformed into massive sheets of blasts and stem cells in which are scattered large macrophages containing cellular debris. These large sheets become rather diffuse, often extending into the splenic cords and thus obliterating the normal pattern of spleen morphology. By the 6th or 7th day, the normal pattern is partially reestablished as many of the actively dividing cells have differentiated into erythroid series cells and populate the cords in large numbers. By 10–14 days and later, little or no microscopic evidence of infection remains in the spleen except for an increased number of plasma cells. Increased numbers of Kupffer's cells in the liver are noted early on, but after the 2nd week of infection their concentration is no greater than in normal liver (Baker et al. 1971; Cassell et al. 1979).

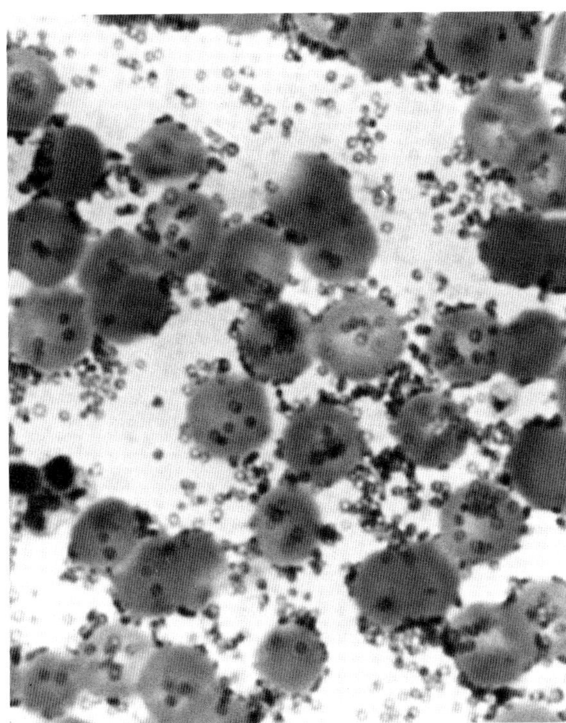

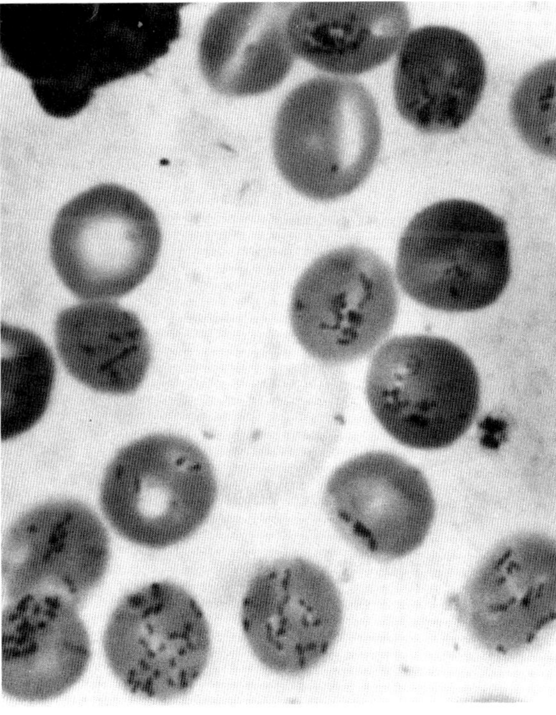

Fig. 100 *(above).* Blood of a mouse infected experimentally with *Eperythrozoon coccoides.* Ring-shaped organisms are attached to erythrocytes and free in plasma. The massive parasitemia illustrated occurs only in splenectomized mice given a substantial inoculum of virulent organisms. Giemsa stain, × 1500

Fig. 101 *(below).* Blood of rat infected experimentally with *Hemobartonella muris.* Organisms are solid coccoid bodies arranged in chains on the surface of erythrocytes. Giemsa stain, × 1500

Ultrastructure

SEM and TEM examination of these organisms reveals that they are spherical, approximately 350–700 µm in diameter, without distinguishing internal structure, and are closely associated with indentations of the erythrocyte plasmalemma but discretely separated from it (Moulder 1974; Baker et al. 1971; Cassell et al. 1979; Tanaka et al. 1965).

Differential Diagnosis

Disease activation with subsequent detection of organisms in the peripheral blood has provided the most reliable procedure for detecting latent infections, and surgical splenectomy is the most consistent and potent activator of these infections. Mice infected with *E. coccoides* frequently develop massive parasitemias 2–4 days after splenectomy, but peak parasitemias are of short duration (12–24 h) and regress rapidly to undetectable levels. Mice usually develop only modest anemia and rarely die as the result of activation of the disease. In contrast, *H. muris* parasitemias occur 5–10 days after splenectomy of infected rats and do not reach the extreme magnitudes commonly seen in active *E. coccoides* infections. Infected adult rats frequently experience severe hemolytic episodes which may terminate fatally.

Uninfected, splenectomized animals provide the most sensitive test subjects for detecting these agents in various biological materials. The incubation period and intensity of parasitemias are dose-dependent, and occasionally serial animal passage is necessary to raise the concentration of organisms to levels that are readily detectable. Uninfected mice, with spleens intact, will develop patent parasitemias if sufficient numbers of *E. coccoides* are given, while latently infected mice frequently fail to show patent parasitemia even when reinfected with a large number of organisms. In contrast, unless they are splenectomized, infected rats virtually never develop patent parasitemia, even when enormous numbers of *H. muris* organisms are given.

A variety of procedures, in addition to splenectomy, that compromise the reticuloendothelial system result in activation of latent *Hemobartonella* and *Eperythrozoon* infections. These include: chemical suppression of reticuloendothelial function (Stuart 1962), polonium injury of the spleen (Scott and Stannard 1954), and whole body irradiation (Scott and Stannard 1954; Bekers 1951).

Cortisone treatment, which is used as a diagnostic aid in unmasking other clinically silent infections of laboratory rats and mice, is ineffective in activating latent *H. muris* or *E. coccoides* infections and may actually inhibit the activating effect of splenectomy (Thurston 1955). Other immunosuppressive drugs, such as antilymphocytic serum and cyclophosphamide, also are ineffective in activating *H. muris* and *E. coccoides* infections (Baker et al. 1971).

Although little is known about the immunologic response of animals to these infection or the role of antibodies in maintaining the latent state, serum levels of immunoglobulins, IgG1, IgG2, IgM, and IgA, have been measured in ex-germfree mice infected experimentally with *E. coccoides* (Baker et al. 1971). Experimental mice were infected with washed parasitized erythrocytes while control mice were injected with equal volumes of washed normal mouse erythrocytes. Quantitative determinations of serum immunoglobulins performed by immunodiffusion showed a marked and sustained elevation of IgG2 in infected mice, with peak elevations reached 14 days after inoculation. Serum IgG2 levels in infected mice reached levels 5–20 times those in normal mice. Of the other classes of immunoglobulin, only IgM reached levels substantially above control values.

Several serologic methods have been evaluated for potential use in large scale testing of laboratory animal stocks for detection of these latent infections. The most promising of these employs an indirect fluorescent antibody reaction for detecting eperythrozoonosis (Baker et al. 1971).

Ample evidence indicates that measures such as ectoparasite control and caesarean derivation of laboratory rodents have reduced the incidence of these infections. However, periodic reports implicating these agents as complicating factors in research argue that the problem is not completely solved.

Biologic Features

Importance as an Experimental Variable

Infections of experimental animals that do not cause clinically apparent disease but induce subtle and profound alterations in experimental results create the most important and perplexing variables in animal experimentation. Agents of the genera *Hemobartonella* and *Eperythrozoon* represent some of the best defined examples of such inapparent disease complications (Baker et al. 1971; Cassell et al. 1979).

Transmission

Natural transmission of these organisms is by blood-sucking parasites. However, since such parasites have been eliminated from virtually all experimental animal production colonies, the most important source of infection currently is accidental transmission by in vivo passage of blood or blood-laden tissues. Inadvertent transmission via transplantable tumor tissue is of particular concern since some experimental tumor lines may be contaminated with these agents (Sacks and Egdahl 1960), and the methods used to preserve tumor tissues also preserve these agents. Present evidence indicates that transmission of *Hemobartonella* and *Eperythrozoon* spp. in tumor transplants probably represents nothing more than mechanical transfer of infected blood entrapped in tumor tissue, but the presence of these agents may influence tumor growth patterns and recipient susceptibility to implanted tumors, as well as host response to the pathogens (Sacks et al. 1960; Sacks and Egdahl 1960).

Transmission of these infections is readily accomplished by all parenteral routes of administration, and some workers have even demonstrated transmissions by ingestion and inhalation (Thurston 1955). The likelihood of fortuitous transmission is enhanced markedly by the exceptionally high infectivity and small size of these organisms. Stansly and Nelson (1965) estimated that only four to five organisms comprise an infectious unit of *E. coccoides*, while Wigand (1958) concluded that one parasitized erythrocyte is capable of establishing *H. muris* infection. Ultrastructural studies have shown that both *E. coccoides* and *H. muris* range in size from 350–700 µm (Tanaka et al. 1965). These data agree well with filtration studies which have shown that both agents readily pass filters having a pore size of 360–480 µm (Tanaka et al. 1965).

An additional characteristic of these organisms that is of potential importance in accidental transmission is their usually low specific gravity. Stansly and Neilson (1966) were unable to sediment *E. coccoides* completely by centrifugation of infected plasma at $100\,000 \times g$ for 1 h, and Moore et al. (1965) reported similar results in ultracentrifugation studies of *H. muris*. It has been observed that, after a single freeze and thaw, *E. coccoides* particles aggregate and sediment readily at $5000 \times g$ for 1 h (Stansly and Neilson 1966). Thus, it is apparent that these organisms are likely to be present in the usual "cell-free filtrates" of tissues from infected animals when either ultracentrifugation or filtration techniques are used without freezing. Neither *Hemobartonella* nor *Eperythrozoon* spp. grow on cell-free culture media.

Hemobartonella and *Eperythrozoon* spp. have been shown to be quite unstable in vitro. They are inactivated rapidly by drying or exposure to disinfectants. Whole blood is rendered noninfectious after incubation for 3 h at $37\,^{\circ}$C. Whole blood or plasma frozen at $-3\,^{\circ}$C remains infectious for 7-10 days, while freezing at $-70\,^{\circ}$C preserves infectivity for several months (Thurston 1955).

Interactions with Other Microorganisms

Many reports describe interactions between *Hemobartonella* spp. or *Eperythrozoon* spp. and a wide variety of other microorganisms. Unfortunately, most of these were discovered unwittingly by investigators who found an unusual response to experimental infection to be caused by concurrent hemobartonellosis or eperythrozoonosis. The interrelationships between *Hemobartonella, Eperythrozoon,* and other microorganisms are complex and difficult to reduce to common denominators; however, it is clear that the profound effect of these parasites on reticuloendothelial function exerts a strong influence on host response to other pathogens. Three pathogenic viruses of mice, lactic dehydrogenase virus (LDH), mouse hepatitis virus (MHV), and lymphocytic choriomeningitis virus (LCM), have a common pathogenetic pathway of replication in Kupffer's cells prior to invasion of liver parenchyma (Baker et al. 1971). The effect of these viruses on the functional capacity of Kupffer's cells can be observed by measuring the phagocytic index of mice infected with these agents. In each case, infection produces a severe reduction in phagocytosis. An additional feature common to the three viruses is a striking potentiation of their virulence by concurrent *E. coccoides* infection. Since *E. coccoides* causes profound alteration of phagocytosis, it can be reasoned that this agent may in some way increase the susceptibility of Kupffer's cells to the viruses. This viewpoint is strengthened by the observation that avirulent strains of MHV which have no depressing effect on phagocytosis are uniformly elevated to high virulence by *E. coccoides,* with the net effect of the dual infection being expressed clearly in depressed phagocytic function.

Experimental plasmodial infections of laboratory rats and mice are important animal models used in malaria research. Early in the development of this model, Hsu and Geiman (1952) and others (Ott and Stauber 1967; Peters 1965; Marmorston-Gottesman and Perla 1930) discovered that latent *H. muris* and *E. coccoides* infections are potentiated by concurrent plasmodium infection, and, furthermore, the course of malaria in such animals is altered markedly by active hemobartonellosis and eperythrozoonosis. Some stock inocula of *Plasmodium berghei, P. chabaudi,* and other rodent malaria species may be contaminated with *H. muris* or *E. coccoides,* and unfortunately it is difficult to substantiate the contaminated status of most of these inocula. In addition, when an inoculum known to be free of contamination is passed in rats or mice whose carrier status with reference to *H. muris* or *E. coccoides* is not defined, the possibility of contamination is raised once again.

Comparison with Other Species

Naturally occurring infections with similar host-specific agents occur in most laboratory animal species. Therefore, even though most of the scientific literature describes infections of rats and mice, investigators must be alert to the possible presence of these agents in other species. For example, recent reports document research complications due to these agents in squirrel monkeys (Adams et al. 1984) and sheep (Martin et al. 1988).

References

Adams MR, Lewis JC, Bullock BC (1984) Hemobartonellosis in squirrel monkeys *(Saimiri sciureus)* in a domestic breeding colony: case report and preliminary study. Lab Anim Sci 34: 82-85

Baker HJ, Cassell GH, Lindsey JR (1971) Research complications due to *Haemobartonella* and *Eperythrozoon* infections in experimental animals. Am J Pathol 64: 625-656

Bekers PE (1951) The effect of x-irradiation on rats with and without *Bartonella muris*. J Infect Dis 88: 224-229

Cassell GH, Lindsey JR, Baker HJ, Davis JK (1979) Mycoplasma and rickettsial diseases. In: Baker HJ, Lindsey JR, Weisbroth SH (eds) The laboratory rat, vol I. Academic, New York, pp 259–269

Hsu DVM, Geiman QM (1952) Synergistic effect of *Hemobartonella muris* on *P. berghei* in white rats. Am J Trop Med Hyg 1: 747–760

Marmorston-Gottesman J, Perla D (1930) Studies on *Bartonella muris* anemia of albino rats. I. *Trypanosoma lewisi* infection in normal albino rats associated with *Bartonella muris* anemia. And II. Latent infection in adult normal rats. J Exp Med 52: 121–129

Martin BJ, Chrisp CE, Averill DR Jr, Ringler DH (1988) The identification of *Eperythrozoon ovis* in anemic sheep. Lab Anim Sci 38: 173–177

Moore DH, Arison RN, Tanaka H, Hall WT, Chanowitz M (1965) Identity of the filterable hemolytic anemia agent of Sacks with *Hemobartonella muris*. J Bacteriol 90: 1669–1674

Moulder JW (1974) The rickettsias. In: Buchanan RE, Gibbons NE (eds) Bergey's manual of determinative bacteriology, 8th edn. Williams and Wilkins, Baltimore, pp 882–925

Ott KJ, Stauber LA (1967) *Eperythrozoon coccoides:* influence on course of infection of *Plasmodium chabaudi* in mouse. Science 155: 1546–1548

Peters W (1965) Competitive relationship between *Eperythrozoon coccoides* and *Plasmodium berghei* in the mouse. Exp Parasitol 16: 158–166

Sacks JH, Egdahl RH (1960) Protective effects of immunity and immune serum on the development of hemolytic anemia and cancer in rats. Surg Forum 10: 22–25

Sacks JH, Clark RF, Egdahl RH (1960) The induction of tumor immunity with a new filterable agent. Surgery 48: 244–260

Scott JK, Stannard JN (1954) Relationship between *Bartonella muris* infection and acute radiation effects in the rat. J Infect Dis 95: 302–308

Stansly PG, Neilson CF (1965) Relationship between spleen weight increase factor (SWIF) of mice and *Eperythrozoon coccoides*. Proc Soc Exp Biol Med 119: 1059–1063

Stansly PG, Neilson CF (1966) Sedimentation of *Eperythrozoon coccoides*. Proc Soc Exp Biol Med 121: 363–365

Stuart AE (1962) Experimental necrosis of spleen. J Pathol Bacteriol 84: 193–200

Tanaka H, Hall WT, Sheffield JB, Moore DH (1965) Fine structure of *Hemobartonella muris* as compared with *Eperythrozoon coccoides* and *Mycoplasma pulmonis*. J Bacteriol 90: 1735–1749

Thurston JP (1955) Observations on the course of *Eperythrozoon coccoides* infections in mice and the sensitivity of the parasite to external agents. Parasitology 45: 141–151

Wigand R (1958) Morphologische biologische und serologische Eigenschaften der Bartonellen. Thieme, Stuttgart

Trypanosoma Brucei Infection, Mouse

Jiro J. Kaneko and Victor O. Anosa

Synonym. Trypanosomiasis.

Gross Appearance

The bone marrow of infected mice is pale at 2 weeks post inoculation (Anosa 1975, 1980), and marrow nucleated cell counts decrease more markedly in splenectomized CFLP mice than in intact mice (Anosa 1980). Decreases in marrow nucleated cells counts are minimal in anemic deer mice (Anosa and Kaneko 1983a). However, marrow RBC counts decrease in both the CRLP mice and in deer mice (Anosa and Kaneko 1983a).

Deer mice with *Trypanosoma brucei* infection have decreased serum albumin and increased immunoglobulin concentrations (Anosa and Kaneko 1983a). Serum IgM is considerably increased (Amole et al. 1982; Poltera et al. 1980a; Stevens and Moulton 1978). Serum IgG1 decreases 10 days post inoculation but is 30% elevated between 15 to 30 days post inoculation (Stevens and Moulton 1978).

Spleen

Splenomegaly occurs consistently in *T. brucei*-infected mice, but the degree is variable. Spleens are enlarged 35 times in *T. brucei* TREU 667 infection of Swiss/Webster (S/W) mice (Amole et al. 1982), 10–15 times in TREU 67 infection of CFLP mice (Anosa 1975; Jennings et al. 1974), and 26–32 times in EATRO 110 infection of deer mice (Anosa and Kaneko 1983a; Moulton 1980). Death occurs in some mice due to the rupture of these enlarged spleens (Moulton 1980).

The marked splenomegaly which occurs in *T. brucei*-infected mice is related to three main functions of the spleen which become exaggerated: (a) trapping and phagocytosis of RBC (which increase approximately 21-fold and 23-fold in the Billroth's cords and sinuses of infected mice,

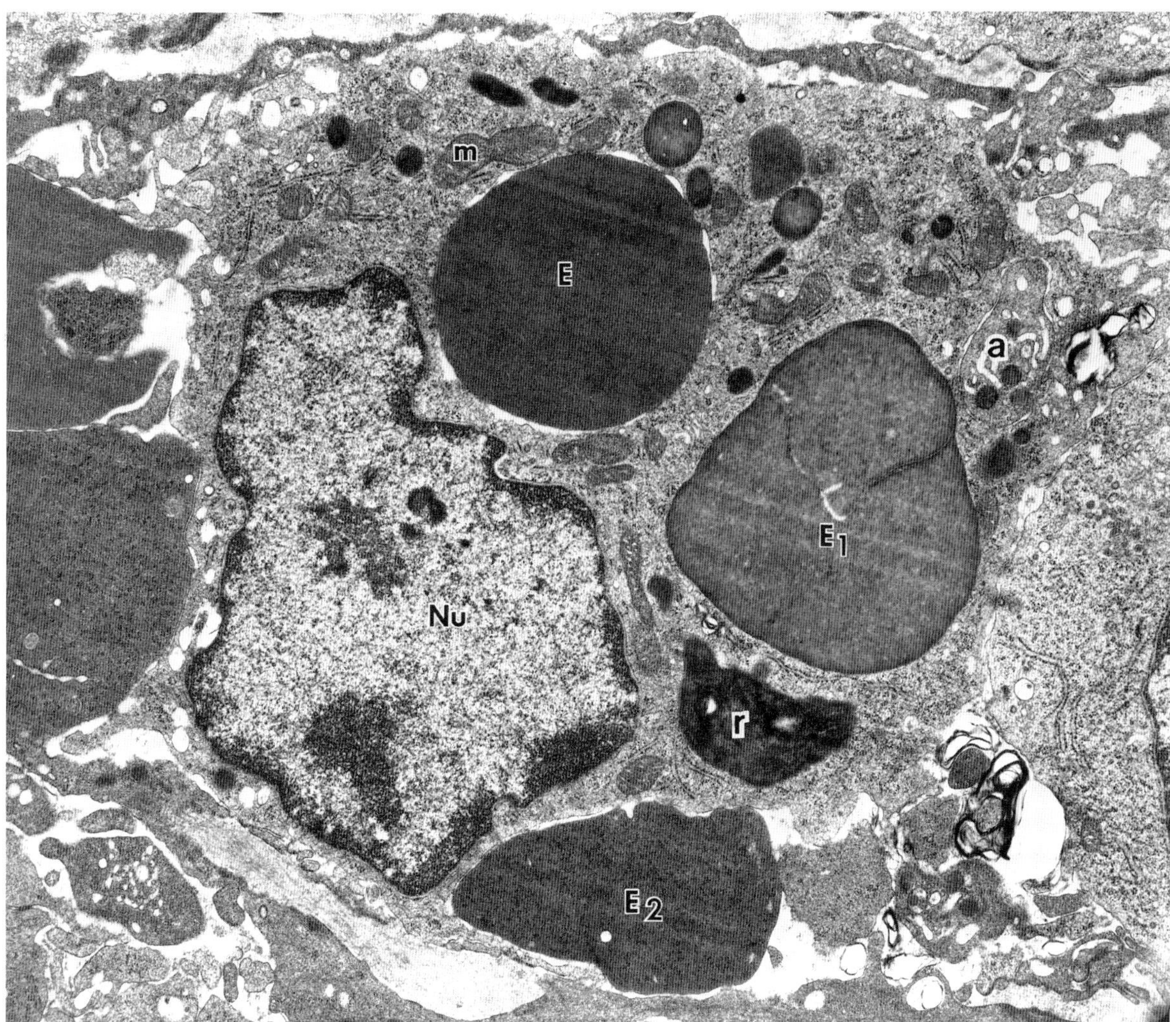

Fig. 102. Trypanosomiasis, mouse. Macrophage from spleen infected with *T. brucei*. Nucleus *(Nu)*, residual body *(r)*, mitochondrion *(m)*, freshly phagocytized RBC *(E)*, degenerating phagocytized RBD *(E₁)*, RBC being phagocytized *(E₂)*, and a phagocytized platelet *(a)*. TEM, ×10 700

respectively), leukocytes, and platelets; (b) enhancement of the immune response; and (c) accelerated hemopoiesis (particularly erythropoiesis). Hypersplenism (i.e., exaggerated splenic function) associated with splenomegaly probably contributes to anemia and leukopenia (Anosa and Kaneko 1984a).

Microscopic Features

As a result of its extravascularization, *T. brucei* invades virtually all tissues and induces some lesions in most, including the spleen, brain, heart, kidney, testes, and ovary.

Spleen

Histologically, there is hyperplasia of germinal centers and plasma cell infiltration with disruption of periarteriolar lymphocytic sheaths (Moulton 1980). The lymphoid follicles are prominent without cellular depletion, and there is marked proliferation of macrophages, plasma cells, and megakaryocytes, with erythrophagocytosis, hemosiderosis, and extramedullary hemopoiesis (Anosa 1975; Anosa et al. 1977).

Blood and Bone Marrow

Chronic *T. brucei* infection induces marked anemia in mice. Histologic electron microscopic and ^{51}Cr-labelled erythrocyte studies indicate that the anemia is primarily due to an accelerated destruction of erythrocytes (RBC) in the spleen (Fig. 102) and liver (Anosa 1975; Anosa et al. 1977; Anosa and Kaneko 1983b) and is accompanied by RBC fragmentation (Anosa and Kaneko 1983b) and IgM coating of RBC (Amole et al. 1982). There is a concomitant shortening of the RBC life span (Anosa et al. 1977). A hemolysin has also been identified in infected mice (Huan et al. 1975). The anemia is accompanied by intensive erythropoietic activity as evidenced by the marked reticulocytosis (Amole et al. 1982; Anosa 1975; Anosa et al. 1977; Anosa and Kaneko 1983a; Huan et al. 1975; Jennings et al. 1974), accelerated incorporation of ^{59}Fe in RBC (Jennings et al. 1974), and a decrease in the myeloid/erythroid ratio of the bone marrow (Anosa 1975; Anosa et al. 1977).

The anemia of *T. brucei* infection in mice is therefore hemolytic, although hemodilution contributes a minor part (Anosa 1980; Amole et al. 1982), and it is a responsive anemia as indicated by the marked reticulocytosis, decreased myeloid/erythroid ratio, and increased uptake of [59]Fe. On the other hand, the decline of bone marrow nucleated cell counts in infected mice between the 7th and 21st days postinfection (Anosa 1975, 1980) suggests that some degree of marrow cell destruction (ineffective erythropoiesis) also occurs. In fact, many marrow cells have evidence of degeneration on days 14 and 21 post infection (Anosa 1975, 1980). Both the bone marrow and the spleen function in erythropoiesis in normal mice, and splenic erythropoiesis is exaggerated in *T. brucei* infection of mice. After splenectomy, the loss of splenic erythropoiesis is apparently counterbalanced by a corresponding lack of splenic RBC removal so that splenectomy has no effect on the severity of the anemia in mice infected with *T. brucei* (Anosa et al. 1977).

Chronic *T. brucei* infection in mice also induces a leukopenia associated with lymphopenia, monocytosis, and eosinopenia (Anosa 1975, 1980), although in the deer mouse, leukocytosis associated with lymphocytosis, eosinopenia, and monocytosis develops (Anosa and Kaneko 1983a).

Testes

T. brucei produces testicular atrophy associated with necrosis and depopulation of cells of the seminiferous tubules, spermatid giant cell formation, and invasion of the intertubular tissue by many inflammatory cells, particularly lymphocytes, plasma cells, and macrophages (Anosa and Kaneko 1984b). The basal laminae of the seminiferous tubules acquire extra layers and are extensively folded. Trypanosomes and some inflammatory cells cross the myoid layer and occupy the space between the myoid layer and the basal laminae of the seminiferous tubules (Fig. 103), but the parasites do not invade the tubules proper. Inflammatory cells are not found within the tubules except for a few macrophages in the lumen. Although the Leydig's cells are slightly increased in number, there is evidence of cytopathology including small size, folded nuclear membranes, decreased mitochondrial size, and a sparsity of secretory material, suggesting decreased hormonal production.

Kidney

T. brucei infection increases the size and cellularity of the glomeruli (Anosa and Kaneko 1984a; Moulton 1980). TEM studies (Anosa and Kaneko 1984b) demonstrate that there is deposition of electron-dense material, probably immune complexes, in various parts of the glomerulus including the basement membranes, the visceral epithelium of Bowman's capsule, and less often the lumen of the peritubular vessels. In conjunction with a proliferation of mesangial cells, hypertrophy of podocytes, and invasion of the glomeruli by neutrophils, macrophages, and lymphocytes, these deposits cause enlargement of the glomeruli and a narrowing of Bowman's space and capillary lumen of the glomeruli (Fig. 104).

Heart

Pancarditis occurs in *T. brucei* infection of mice, affecting the epicardium, endocardium, and myocardium of all four chambers, as well as the valves (Anosa 1975; Anosa and Kaneko 1984a; Moulton 1980; Poltera 1980; Poltera et al. 1980a). The auricles are more severely affected than the ventricles (Anosa, personal observation; Moulton 1980), and the parasites are more numerous in the endocardium and epicardium than in the myocardium (Anosa 1975; Poltera et al. 1980a). Muscle fiber atrophy and necrosis occurs to a varying degree (Anosa 1975; Anosa and Kaneko 1984a; Poltera et al. 1980a), and under TEM study the degenerating muscle fibers lose most of their fibrils, have smaller mitochondria

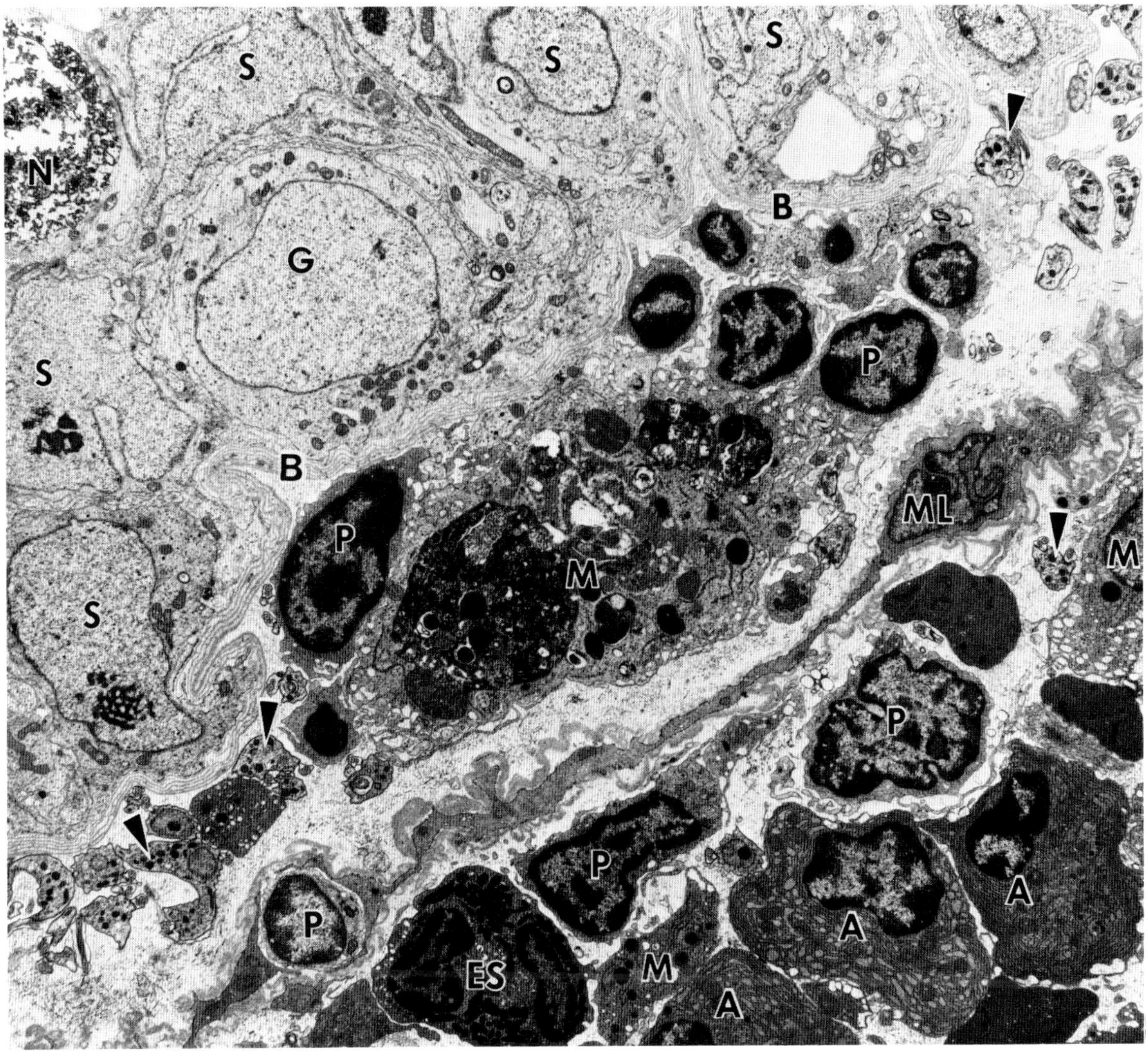

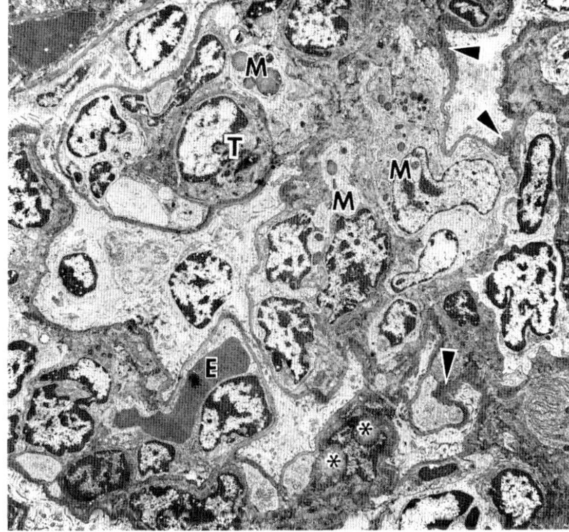

Fig. 103 *(above).* Trypanosomiasis, mouse. Testis of a mouse infected with *T. brucei.* Note loss of most cells of the seminiferous tubule except Sertoli cells *(S)* and a spermatogonium *(G).* Note also part of a necrotic cell *(N)* and the multilayered folded basal lamina *(B)* of the tubule. Many lymphocytes *(P),* an actively phagocytic macrophage *(M),* and trypanosomes *(arrowheads)* have crossed the myoid layer *(ML).* Lymphocytes *(P),* plasma cells *(A),* portion of macrophage *(M),* eosinophil *(ES),* and part of a trypanosome *(arrowhead)* are present in the intertubular tissue. TEM, ×4086

Fig. 104 *(below).* Trypanosomiasis, mouse. Part of a glomerulus of a mouse infected with *T. brucei.* Note uneven thickening of basement membranes *(arrowheads),* deposits in mesangial cell (*), invasion by macrophages *(M),* and neutrophils *(T).* Also note virtual obliteration of Bowman's space and capillary lumena. *E,* erythrocyte in capillary lumen. TEM, ×2826 and disorganized intercalated discs (Anosa and Kaneko 1984a). Macrophages, plasma cells, transformed T lymphocytes, and occasional giant and Mott cells are present between the fibers (Anosa 1975; Anosa and Kaneko 1984a; Moulton 1980; Poltera 1980; Poltera et al. 1980a). Epithelioid cells are present in some parts of the heart of infected mice, particularly beneath the endocardium. Associated with these lesions, IgM, IgG, and C3 deposits are widely dispersed in the heart of infected mice (Poltera et al. 1980a).

Central Nervous System

Cerebral lesions begin when the parasites first appear in the choroid plexus at 4 weeks postinfection and later spread to the perivascular region and meninges of the brain and spinal cord, resulting in an accumulation of plasma cells, lymphocytes, and macrophages (Moulton 1980; Poltera 1980; Poltera et al. 1980b). Demyelination occurs sporadically and only one of 38 mice had focal malacia in the basal ganglia with a microglial cell reaction (Moulton 1980). IgM, IgG, and C3 deposits were present in the choroid plexus at 3 and 4 weeks postinfection and later appeared in the meninges (Poltera 1980; Poltera et al. 1980b).

The cells involved in the inflammatory process induced by T. brucei are usually mononuclear cells: lymphocytes, plasma cells, Mott cells, transformed T lymphocytes, and macrophages including epithelioid cells. Granulocytes are seldom found, except for the few neutrophils and eosinophils in the testes (Anosa and Kaneko 1984b).

Ultrastructure

The macrophages from infected mice are activated in vivo (Anosa et al. 1983c; Fierer and Askonas 1982; Stevens and Moulton 1978). Activation results in marked increases in the size of the macrophages and their organelle content including mitochondria, lysosomes, rough endoplasmic reticulum (RER), and Golgi apparatus (Anosa and Kaneko 1983c). The average number of RER, mitochondria, and primary lysosomes per TEM section of splenic macrophages from control mice were 8.4 ± 1.0, 11.3 ± 1.4, and 6.0 ± 1.0, respectively, as compared with 33.9 ± 2.2, 23.8 ± 2.3, and 13.9 ± 1.8 in infected mice. The activated

macrophages engulf various materials in vivo including erythrocytes, trypanosomes, neutrophils, eosinophils, lymphocytes, nucleated erythrocytes, plasma cells, thrombocytes (Fig. 102), and heart muscle fibers at various locations (Anosa and Kaneko 1983b, c, 1984a). The presence of immune serum enhances in vitro phagocytosis of IgG- and C3-coated sheep RBC (Fierer and Askonas 1982) and trypanosomes (Stevens and Moulton 1978) by macrophages from T. brucei-infected mice.

Under TEM study (Anosa and Kaneko 1984a), there is a marked increase in the cellularity of the Billroth's cords and sinuses of the red pulp with increased contact between cells and dilatation of the sinuses (Fig. 105). Marked erythropoiesis is present. Therefore, while nucleated RBC form 4.7% of all cells (including RBC) in the Billroth's cords of spleens of control mice and are absent from the sinuses, they increase in the Billroth's cords of infected mice (21.7%) and invade the sinuses (4.6%), and this is matched by a marked increase in reticulocytes in both parts of the red pulp. Lymphocytes decrease from 49.9% in the Billroth's cords of the control mice to 16.4% in infected mice, and from 12.8% in the sinuses of control mice to 5.1% in infected mice. This is accompanied by increases in the numbers of plasma cells, transformed T lymphocytes, and Mott cells at these sites. Macrophages also increase in both areas of the red pulp, and erythrophagocytosis is common (Anosa and Kaneko 1983b, c, 1984a). When these cell increases are related to the 26-fold enlargement of infected mice spleens, the total increase in cell numbers is considerable. As a result, even though the lymphocyte percentage is decreased, there is an absolute 10-fold increase. The periarteriolar sheaths have marked plasma cell proliferation.

Summary

The pathological changes induced by T. brucei in mice are related to three main factors. Firstly, the massive recurrent parasitemias induce intense antigenic stimulation of the immune system with resulting marked proliferation of lymphocytes and their subsequent transformation to plasma cells and transformed T lymphocytes. Antibodies (more IgM than IgG) are produced in response to the stimulation and are deposited in tissues and on cells, contributing to tissue and cell destruction and anemia. Secondly, the anemia, whose pathogenesis is multifactorial, induces

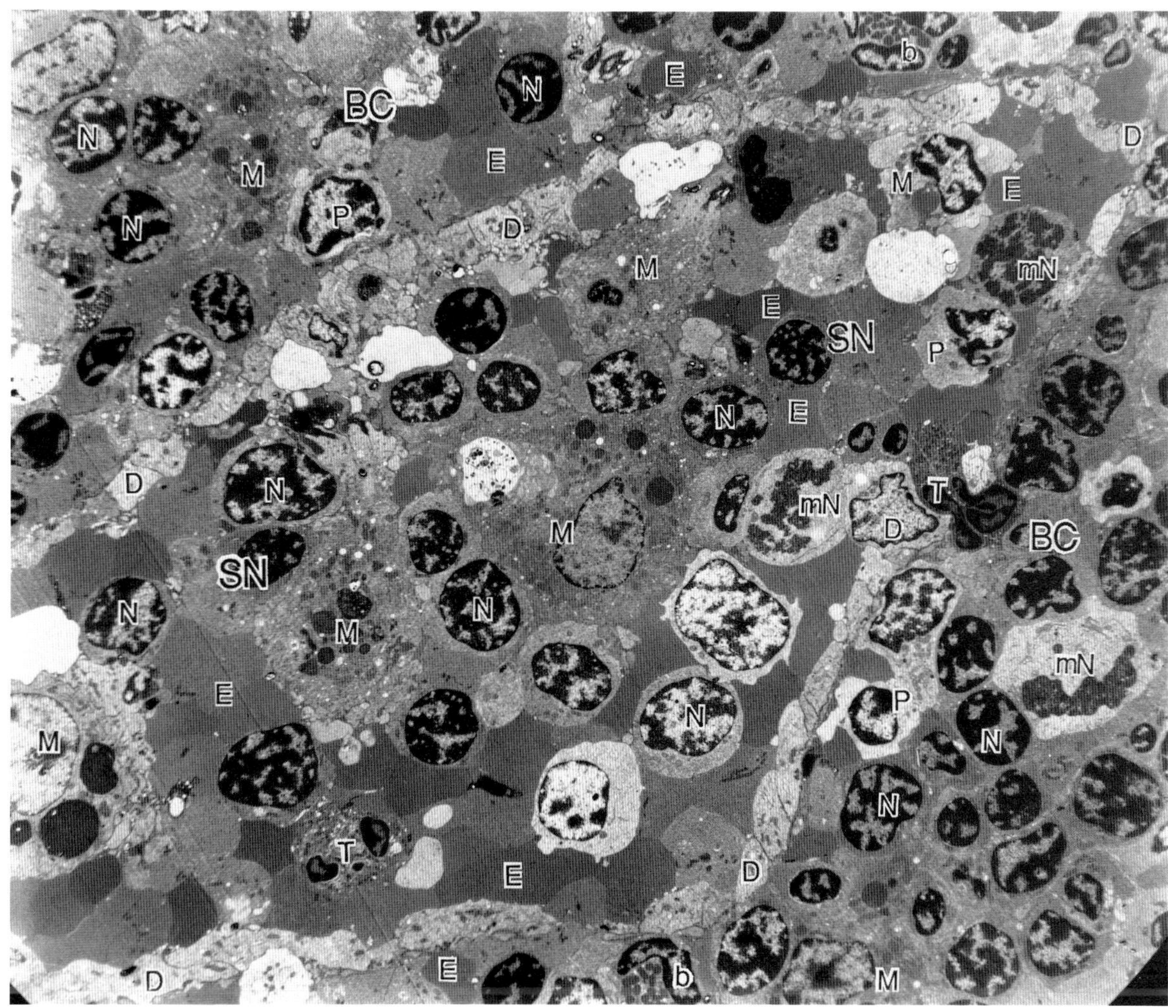

Fig. 105. Trypanosomiasis, mouse. Splenic red pulp of a mouse infected with *T. brucei*. Note hypercellularity of an enlarged sinus *(SN)* and Billroth's cord *(BC)*, separated by sinus endothelium *(D)*. SN and BC contain numerous red blood cells *(E)* and normoblasts *(N)*, several macrophages *(M)* and few lymphocytes *(P)*, two neutrophilic *(T)*, two basophils *(b)*, and three mitotic normoblasts *(mN)*. TEM, × 2091

marked splenic and hepatic erythroclasis and accelerated marrow and splenic erythropoiesis. Thirdly, there is extravascular localization of the parasites in tissues, with tissue destruction and marked mononuclear cell infiltration.

Biologic Features

Etiology

The pathogenic trypanosomes that affect human and domestic animals belong to two distinct groups (Losos and Ikede 1972). The hematogenous trypanosomes *(Trypanosoma vivax* and *T. congolense)* affect domestic animals and are essentially intravascular parasites. The humoral group *(T. brucei, T. gambiense, T. rhodesiense, T. evansi)* are also primarily intravascular, but in addition they spread into virtually all tissues and organs. *T. gambiense* and *T. rhodesiense,* which cause human sleeping sickness, are closely related to *T. brucei* and *T. evansi,* which cause animal disease. Except for *T. vivax,* which usually does not grow in mice, the other 5 species are infective for mice, and therefore the mouse is used extensively to study the pathogenesis and pathology of these parasites in the mammalian host. All reports have dealt mainly with the chronic infection, and none have specifically examined the acute forms.

Pathogenesis

The severity of the disease produced by *T. brucei* in mice varies from the hyperacute infection which kills mice within 1 week of infection to the chronic infection that lasts several months. The severity is determined by two factors: (a) the virulence of the strain of *T. brucei* and (b) the susceptibility of the mouse strain. Thus, while *T. brucei* EATRO 110 kills S/W mice in 4–5 days, deer mice *(Peromyscus maniculatus)* survive for an average of 63 days (35–83 days) (Anosa and Kaneko 1983a; Moulton and Stevens 1978). Similarly, the mean survival of three strains of mice (C3H/He, A/J, and C57BL/6J) to *T. brucei* strain Lister S42 were 29, 39, and 58 days, respectively (Clayton 1978).

After intraperitoneal infection of mice with *T. brucei*, parasitemia is evident within 2–4 days and reaches a peak at about the 7th day. Those animals that die of hyperacute infection die at about this time, and death is due to various perturbations such as hypoglycemia. In those that survive and develop chronic disease, repeated waves of parasitemia occur, and there is progressive invasion of various tissues by parasites.

Comparison with Other Species

Chronic *T. brucei* infection of mice closely resembles its infection of domestic animals (Ikede and Losos 1972) and *T. evansi* infection of horses (Ikede et al. 1983). It is a good animal model of human sleeping sickness (Moulton and Stevens 1978; Poltera 1980). Infections of domestic and laboratory animals with *T. congolense* and *T. vivax* usually precipitate more severe anemia than does *T. brucei* (Anosa and Kaneko 1984a). Since these two parasites do not invade tissues as does *T. brucei*, they do not produce significant organ damage (Anosa 1983) as compared with that caused by *T. brucei* or the human parasites *T. gambiense* and *T. rhodesiense.*

References

Amole BO, Clarkson AB Jr, Shear HL (1982) Pathogenesis of anemia in *T. brucei*-infected mice. Infect Immun 36: 1060–1068

Anosa VO (1975) The effect of splenectomy on the anemia and parasitemia of trypanosomiasis. MVM Thesis University of Glasgow

Anosa VO (1980) Studies on the parasitaemia, plasma volumes, leucocyte and bone marrow cell counts and the moribund state in *T. brucei* infection in splenectomized and intact mice. Zentralbl Veterinarmed [B] 27: 169–180

Anosa VO (1983) Diseases produced by *T. vivax* in ruminants, horses and rodents. Zentralbl Veterinarmed [B] 30: 717–741

Anosa VO, Kaneko JJ (1983a) Pathogenesis of *T. brucei* infection in deer mice *(P. maniculatus)*. Hematologic, erythrocyte biochemical and iron metabolic aspects. Am J Vet Res 44: 639–644

Anosa VO, Kaneko JJ (1983b) Pathogenesis of *T. brucei* infection in deer mice *(P. maniculatus)*. Light and electron microscopic studies on erythrocyte pathologic changes and phagocytosis. Am J Vet Res 44: 645–651

Anosa VO, Kaneko JJ (1983c) Pathogenesis of *T. brucei* infection in deer mice *(P. maniculatus)*. V. Macrophage ultrastructure and function. Vet Pathol 20: 617–631

Anosa VO, Kaneko JJ (1984a) Pathogenesis of *T. brucei* infection in deer mice *(P. maniculatus)*. Ultrastructural pathology of the spleen, liver, heart, and kidney. Vet Pathol 21: 229–237

Anosa VO, Kaneko JJ (1984b) Pathogenesis of *T. brucei* infection in deer mice *(P. maniculatus)*. Light and electron microscopic study of testicular lesions. Vet Pathol 21: 238–246

Anosa VO, Jennings FW, Urquhart GM (1977) The effect of splenectomy on anemia in *T. brucei* infection of mice. J Comp Pathol 87: 569–579

Clayton CE (1978) *T. brucei* influence of host strain and parasite antigenic type of infections in mice. Exp Parasitol 44: 202–208

Fierer J, Askonas BA (1982) *T. brucei* infection stimulates receptor-mediated phagocytosis by murine peritoneal macrophages. Infect Immun 37: 1282–1284

Huan CN, Webb L, Lambert PH, Miescher PA (1975) Pathogenesis of the anemia in African trypanosomiasis. Characterization and purification of a hemolytic factor. Schweiz Med Wochenschr 105: 1582–1583

Ikede BO, Losos GJ (1972) Pathological changes in cattle infected with *T. brucei*. Vet Pathol 9: 272–277

Ikede BO, Fatimah I, Sharifuddin W, Bongso TA (1983) Clinical and pathological features of a natural *T. evansi* infection in ponies in West Malaysia. Trop Vet 1: 151–157

Jennings FW, Murray PK, Murray M, Urquhart GM (1974) Anemia in trypanosomiasis: studies in rats and mice infected with *T. brucei*. Res Vet Sci 16: 70–76

Losos GJ, Ikede BO (1972) Review of the pathology of diseases in domestic and laboratory animals caused by *T. congolense, T. vivax, T. brucei, T. rhodesiense* and *T. gambiense* (abstr). Vet Pathol 9: 1–71

Moulton JE (1980) Experimental *T. brucei* infection in deer mice: splenic changes. Vet Pathol 17: 218–225

Moulton JE, Stevens DR (1978) Animal model of human disease: trypanosomiasis, sleeping sickness, in deer mice. Am J Pathol 91: 693–696

Poltera AA (1980) Immunological and chemotherapeutic studies in experimental trypanosomiasis with special reference to the heart and brain. Trans R Soc Trop Med Hyg 74: 706–715

Poltera AA, Hochmann A, Lambert PH (1980a) A model for cardiopathy induced by *T. brucei brucei* in mice. A histologic and amunopathologic study. Am J Pathol 99: 325–352

Poltera AA, Hochmann A, Rudin W, Lambert PH (1980b) *T. brucei brucei:* a model for cerebral trypanosomiasis in mice – an immunological, histological and electronmicroscopic study. Clin Exp Immunol 40: 496–507

Stevens DR, Moulton JE (1978) Ultrastructural and immunological aspects of the phagocytosis of *T. brucei* by mouse peritoneal macrophages. Infect Immun 19: 972–982

Lymph Nodes

STRUCTURE AND FUNCTION

Identification and Functional Characteristics of Lymphocytes with Natural Killer Activity

Craig W. Reynolds and Thomas J. Sayers

Synonyms. Natural killer cells; large granular lymphocytes (LGL); large granular cells (LGC); naturally cytotoxic (NC) cells; natural cell-mediated cytotoxicity (NCMC); spontaneous cell-mediated cytotoxicity (SCMC).

Introduction

For over 15 years, many laboratories have observed that lymphocytes from "normal" nonimmunized hosts are able to kill many tumor cells in vitro (Herberman 1982). This major histocompatibility complex (MHC)-unrestricted lysis of tumor cells has become known as natural killer (NK) activity. Although a variety of different cell types have been reported to have NK activity, it is now clear that most NK activity is mediated by a distinct population of cells known as large granular lymphocytes (LGL).

Microscopic Features

LGLs form a morphologically distinct population of lymphocytes characterized by a high cytoplasmic:nuclear ratio, prominent azurophilic granules in the cytoplasm, and a kidney-shaped nucleus (Timonen et al. 1981). These cells are generally of 10–12 µm in diameter and, therefore, of intermediate size between most lymphocytes (6–8 µm) and monocytes (12–20 µm). A comparison of LGL with other peripheral blood cells can be made from Fig. 106. In Wright-Giemsa stained cytocentrifuge preparations, LGL have a slightly basophilic (blue) cytoplasm,

Table 25. A comparison of some phenotypic characteristics of large granular lymphocytes (LGL) with those of other leukocytes

| | Cell type | | | | |
| | Lymphoid | | | Myeloid | |
	B cell	T cell	LGL	Monocytes	PMN
Morphology					
Size: mouse (µm)	6–10	6–10	8–10	12–20	10–14
rat (µm)	6–10	6–10	10–14	12–20	8–12
Nucleus	Round	Round	Kidney-shaped	Kidney-shaped	Multilobed
Granules	−	−	+ (Large)	−	+ (Fine)
Histochemistry					
Acid phosphatase	+	+	+	+	+
Nonspecific esterase	−	−	+/−	+	+
β-Glucuronidase	−	−	+	+	+
Peroxidase	−	−	−	+	+
Terminal deoxytransferase	+	−	−	−	−
Surface characteristics					
Plastic adherence	−	−	−	+	+
Phagocytosis	−	−	−	+	+

PMN, polymorphonuclear neutrophil leukocytes.

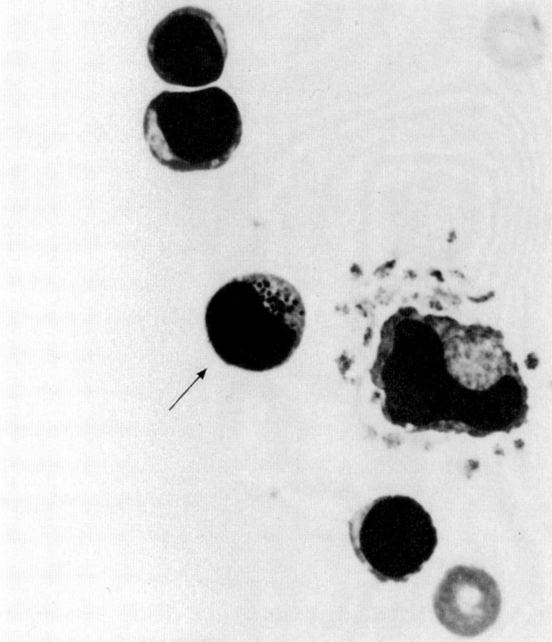

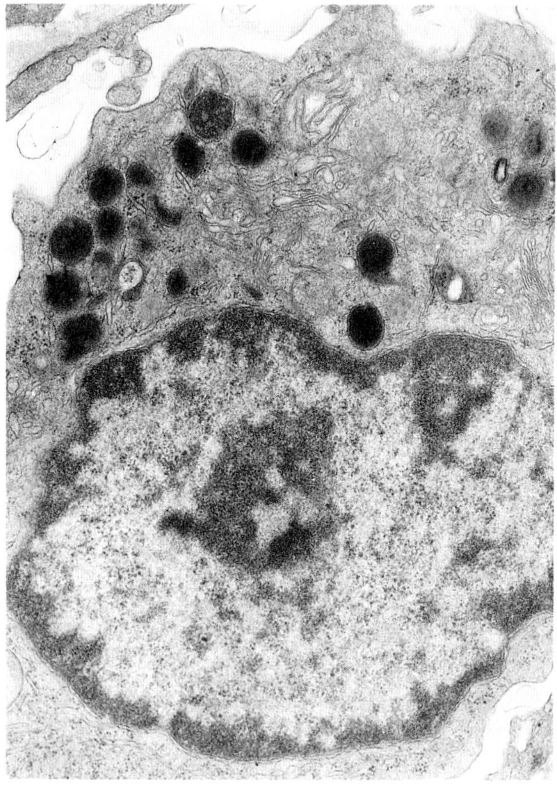

Fig. 106 *(above).* Peripheral blood cells, rat. Largest cell is a monocyte/macrophage; small lymphocytes are also present. Large granular lymphocyte indicated with an *arrow.* Giemsa stain, × 1500

Fig. 107 *(below).* Large granular lymphocyte *(LGL),* rat. TEM, × 1700

distinctly azurophilic (red) granules, and dense chromatin structure. In routine blood smears, LGL may be difficult to identify because the cytoplasmic characteristics of the cells prepared in this fashion are not easily observed. The histochemistry of LGL is similar to most other lymphocytes, i. e., they contain acid phosphatase and β-glucuronidase but lack large amounts of peroxidase and terminal deoxytransferase (Tdt). Like most other lymphocytes, LGL are nonadherent and nonphagocytic. A summary of these characteristics and comparisons with other lymphoid and myeloid cells can be found in Table 25.

Ultrastructure

The ultrastructure of a typical LGL can be seen in Fig. 107. This cell has irregular or kidney-shaped nuclear membranes with dense heterochromatin. Cytoplasmic granules appear as lysosomes in association with Golgi vesicles. Mitochondria are present but are not numerous. Aggregates of polysomes and rough endoplasmic reticulum are prevalent. The plasma membrane is smooth and regular with numerous microvilli. Viral particles are absent, although occasional parallel tubular arrays or coated vesicles can be found.

Antigenic Phenotype

Until recently, the cells responsible for NK activity could only be identified in a negative way, i. e., by distinguishing them from typical T cells, B cells, polymorphs, or monocytes. Recently, some surface antigens detected by specific antisera, or particularly by monoclonal antibodies (MoAb), have proved very useful in characterizing their phenotype (Table 26). In contrast to B cells, LGL of both the rat and mouse do not have surface immunoglobulin. Both rat and mouse LGL are strongly reactive with antibodies against asialo GM 1. However, appreciable numbers of monocytes and T cells also react with this antibody. Several MoAb with species-specific reactivity have also been used to determine the LGL surface characteristics. A significant number (about 50%) of murine LGL react with MoAb against Thy 1 (which also labels the majority of T cells). However, the MoAb used to define all T cells (CD3) and their subsets L3T4 (helper T cells) and Lyt 2 (cytotoxic/suppressor T cells) have no reactivity with LGL. Qa 5 is a

Table 26. A comparison of the surface antigen profiles of rat and mouse large granular lymphocytes (LGL) with those of other leukocytes

Antigens	Cell type				
	Lymphoid			Myeloid	
	B cell	T cell	LGL	Mono-cytes	PMN
Nonspecific-specific					
sIg	+++	−	−	−	−
asialo GM1	−	+	+++	+	−
Species-specific					
Mouse:					
Thy1	−	+++	++	−	−
L3T4	−	++	−	−	−
Lyt2	−	++	−	−	−
Qa5	−	++	+++	−	−
NK 1.1/1.2	−	−	+++	−	−
Ia	+++	−	−	−	−
Rat:					
CD2 (OX-34)	−	+++	+	−	−
CD8 (OX-8)	−	++	+++	−	−
Ia	+++	−	+	++	−

−, less than 10% of cells positive; +, 10%–30% of cells positive; ++, 30%–80% of cells positive; +++, >80% of cells positive.
PMN, polymorphonuclear neutrophil leukocytes.

Table 27. Large granular lymphocytes (LGL) frequency and organ distribution of natural killer activity in euthymic and athymic (nude) rats[a]

Organ	Percentage LGL	
	Euthymic	Athymic
Peripheral blood	7.0	22.0
Spleen	2.0	4.0
Peritoneal cavity	3.0	1.5
Bone marrow	<0.5	<1.0
Lymph nodes	1.0	2.0
Thymus	<0.5	not done
Lungs	7.0	not done

[a] Six to 12 weeks of age.

Table 28. Distribution of OX-8-positive cells in hemopoietic and nonhemopoietic tissues of the athymic (nude) rat

Tissue	Percentage OX-8-positive cells (mean ± SD)
I. Spleen white pulp	
PALS	6.4 ± 3.6
Follicle	0.8 ± 0.3
Marginal zone	2.9 ± 1.1
Red pulp	4.4 ± 3.6
II. Lymph node	
Paracortex	2.2 ± 1.3
Medullary cords/sinuses	4.7 ± 3.8
Cortex	1.1 ± 0.3
III. Peyer's patches	
Interfollicular zone	3.0 ± 1.3
Follicle	1.0 ± 0.2
IV. Lung (BALT)	5.2 ± 4.9
V. Bone marrow	0.6 ± 0.3

PALS, periarteriolar lymphocyte sheath; BALT, bronchial-associated lymphoid tissue.

cell surface determinant found on both LGL and a T cell subset. Murine and rat LGL appear to express few or no Ia antigens. The most specific MoAb for mouse LGL are the NK 1.1/1.2 antibodies which react with the LGL of different mouse strains but have no reactivity with any other leukocytes (Koo et al. 1986). To date, there is not a MoAb against rat LGL which has such a restricted specificity. In rats, antibodies against the CD8 structure (OX-8) bind to LGL but also to cytotoxic/suppressor T cells (Reynolds et al. 1981). Antibodies against CD2 (OX-34) which react strongly with all rat T cells also react with an appreciable number of rat LGL.

Tissue Distribution

In the mouse, LGL are present at relatively high levels in the peripheral blood, spleen, and lungs, lower levels in the lymph nodes, peritoneum, and bone marrow, and at undetectable levels in the thymus. The distribution in rats is very similar (Table 27), with the major difference being that rats tend to have higher levels of LGL in the peritoneal cavity. In both athymic and euthymic mice and rats, higher levels of LGL can be detected in virtually all organs, whereas there is an appreciable deficiency of T cells in these animals (Ward et al. 1983).

As previously mentioned, rats express the OX-8 antigen on LGL and on the cytotoxic/suppressor subpopulation of T cells. Since athymic rats have very low or undetectable levels of T cells, the OX-8 MoAb can be used in an immunoperoxidase staining technique to determine the histological distribution of LGL in athymic rats (Ward et al. 1983). A summary of the histological distribution of LGL from the hemopoietic and nonhemopoietic organs in athymic rats is presented in Table 28. In lymphoid organs, the highest percentage of LGL are found in the lymph node paracortex undergoing interdigitating cell hyperplasia, periarteriolar lymphoid sheath (PALS) area of the spleen, bronchial-associated lymphoid tissue (BALT), lymph node medulla, and splenic red pulp. A very few LGL ($<1\%$) are found scattered throughout virtually all nonlymphoid organs. These LGL in nonlymphoid parenchymal organs correlate with the presence of capillaries, sinuses, or sinusoids, a finding which should not be unexpected since LGL are found in appreciable numbers in the peripheral blood. Large numbers of LGL are also found at sites of inflammation (Ward et al. 1983). Their early appearance at inflammatory sites suggests that they play an important role in the first line of defense against infectious agents.

The relatively poor localization of LGL within the lymph node and spleen white pulp is highly suggestive that most LGL, unlike T and B cells, do not recirculate from blood to lymph. This has been confirmed by monitoring the appearance of i. v. injected, radiolabelled LGL and T cells in the thoracic duct lymph (TDL) of rats, followed by intermittent sampling from an indwelling thoracic duct cannula over an observation period of 6 days (Rolstad et al. 1986). In contrast to T cells, the majority of labelled LGL failed to enter the TDL over the complete observation period of 138 h. Furthermore, TDL collected over several days from both euthymic and athymic rats contains very few morphologically identifiable LGL. Similar results have been obtained in the mouse.

Lineage

Since LGL and T cells share a number of common surface antigens and functions, it has been suggested that LGL may be related to the T cell lineage. However, there is evidence in experimental animals to suggest that most LGL originate in the bone marrow, even in the absence of the thymus. Radioisotopes which destroy the bone marrow depress NK activity but leave T and B cell functions unaffected. Athymic mice and rats exhibit normal or enhanced levels of NK activity whereas numbers of T cells are severely depressed. Furthermore, it has been reported that mice with various immunodeficiency syndromes have an impaired T and B cell maturation, whereas myelopoiesis and LGL development remain unaffected.

Perhaps the most compelling evidence that LGL represent an entirely distinct lineage of lymphocytes is provided by recent data using molecular biological techniques. Human, mouse, and rat LGL do not transcribe functional length mRNA for the α-, β-, or γ-chains of the T-cell receptor (Young et al. 1986; Biron et al. 1987). Therefore, in contrast to T cells they express no T-cell receptor on their surface and must use a different target recognition system. These findings indicate that LGL belong to a distinct and separate lineage from both normal T or B lymphocytes and from normal macrophages or granulocytes.

Functions

It has recently become clear that LGL not only kill tumor cells but also participate in a number of other functional activities (Reynolds and Wiltrout 1988). The reported functions of cells with the phenotype of LGL are summarized in Table 29. LGL have been shown to produce a va-

Table 29. Reported functions of large granular lymphocytes

I.	Control of tumor cell growth
	A. Inhibit the development of primary tumors
	B. Control the development of metastases
II.	Involvement in the control of microbial infections
	A. Viral infections (CMV, influenza, HSV, MHV, HIV, etc.)
	B. Parasites (intercellular and extracellular)
	C. Fungi
	D. Bacteria
III.	Immunoregulatory properties
	A. Regulation of the antibody response
	B. Regulation of cell-mediated immunity
	C. Natural suppressor cells
IV.	Production of cytokines
V.	Control of hemopoietic stem cell growth and differentiation
VI.	Involvement in allograft rejection
	A. Bone marrow transplantation and hybrid resistance
	B. Organ transplantation
VII.	Disease states
	A. Involvement in the development of graft vs host disease
	B. Contribute to some forms of aplastic anemia/neutropenia
	C. Potentiate autoimmune and neurological disease
	D. Contribute to the development of some forms of diabetes

riety of lymphokines, augment or suppress the development of specific immune responses, regulate the rejection of organ allografts, as well as contribute to the pathogenesis of both chronic and acute graft vs. host diseases. Possibly most important, LGL have been shown to inhibit microbial colonization and growth, including intracellular and extracellular parasites, bacteria, fungi, and a wide variety of viral infections. These reports clearly suggest that LGL plays a crucial role in contributing to more than just the antitumor response of normal individuals.

Species Distribution

Although most of the work on LGL has been done in the mouse, rat or human, cells with these morphological and functional characteristics have been identified in a variety of other species including horses, cattle, miniature swine, hamsters, and guinea pigs (Kurloff's cells). A summary of the predominant characteristics in the major species studied can be found in Table 30.

Acknowledgment. This project has been funded at least in part with federal funds from the Department of Health and Human Services under contract number NO1-CO-74102. The content of this publication does not necessarily reflect the views or policies of the Department of Health and Human Services, nor does mention of trade names, commercial products, or organizations imply endorsement by the U. S. Government.

References

Biron CA, van den Elsen P, Tutt MM, Medveczky P, Kumar V, Terhorst C (1987) Murine natural killer cells stimulated in vivo do not express the T cell receptor alpha, beta, gamma, T3 delta, or T3 epsilon genes. J Immunol 139: 1704–1710

Herberman RB (ed) (1982) NK cells and other natural effector cells. Academic, New York

Koo GC, Dumont FJ, Tutt M, Hackett J Jr, Kumar V (1986) The NK-1.1 (−) mouse: a model to study differentiation of murine NK cells. J Immunol 137: 3742–3747

Reynolds CW, Wiltrout RH (1988) Functions of the natural immune system. Plenum, New York

Reynolds CW, Sharrow SO, Ortaldo JR, Herberman RB (1981) Natural killer (NK) activity in the rat. II. Analysis of surface antigens on LGL by flow cytometry. J Immunol 127: 2204–2208

Rolstad B, Herberman RB, Reynolds CW (1986) Natural killer cell activity in the rat. V. The circulation pattern

Table 30. Summary of similarities between rat, mouse, and human natural killer activity

Characteristic	Mouse	Rat	Human
Morphology	LGL	LGL	LGL
Effect of age	Absent at birth; peak 5–9 weeks; then low	Low at birth; remains relatively stable	Relatively stable
Organ distribution	Blood > spleen > PEC > lymph node > BM > thymus	Same as mouse	Same as mouse
Strain distribution	CBA and nudes high; SJL and A strains low	Nudes high; BN low	Some donors high; some low; with activity effected by HLA phenotype
Lymphokine augmentation	IFN, IL-2	IFN, IL-2	IFN, IL-2
Susceptible targets	Selected tumor cell lines; some primary tumors; virus-infected cells; normal thymocytes and BM cells	Same as mouse	Same as mouse
Effect of treatments	Radioresistant; sensitive to cyclophosphamide; ^{89}Sr and trypsin sensitive	Radioresistant; sensitive to cyclophosphamide	Radioresistant; sensitive to cyclophosphamide; trypsin sensitive
Inhibition of reactivity	PGE; phorbol esters; cAMP; suppressor cells; estrogens	PGE; suppressor cells; others not reported	PGE; suppressor cells; phorbol esters; cAMP; monomeric IgG
Factors promoting growth	IL-2	IL-2	IL-2

PEC, peritoneal exudate cells; BM, bone marrow; PGE, prostaglandin E; LGL, large granular lymphocytes.

and tissue localization of peripheral blood large granular lymphocytes (LGL). J Immunol 136: 2800–2808
Timonen T, Ortaldo JR, Herberman RB (1981) Characteristics of human large granular lymphocytes (LGL) and relationship to natural killer and K cells. J Exp Med 153: 569–582
Ward JM, Argilan F, Reynolds CW (1983) Immunoperoxidase localization of large granular lymphocytes in normal tissues and lesions of athymic nude rats. J Immunol 131: 132–139
Young HA, Ortaldo JR, Herberman RB, Reynolds CW (1986) Analysis of T cell receptors in highly purified human and rat large granular lymphocytes (LGL); lack of functional 1.3 kb beta-chain mRNA. J Immunol 136: 2701–2704

Identification and Functional Characteristics of T Lymphocytes

Norman L. Letvin

Introduction

The immune system is comprised of two limbs: the humoral and the cellular (Paul 1984). The humoral limb of the immune system is the antibody-mediated response to antigenic challenge. The cellular immune response includes delayed-type hypersensitivity reactions and cell-mediated killing of tumor and virus-infected target populations. The cells which constitute the immune system are members of three families: the macrophage, the B lymphocyte, and the T lymphocyte. Macrophages serve both as phagocytic and as antigen-presenting cells. In their role as antigen presenters, macrophages process antigen and display it to lymphocytes to initiate an immune response. B lymphocytes are the antibody-producing cells. T lymphocytes subserve a variety of very different functions. They are important as regulators of both cellular and humoral immunity and serve as effectors in delayed-type hypersensitivity responses and in the destruction of virus-infected cells.

Functions of T Lymphocytes

T lymphocytes act both as regulating and effector cells (Reinherz and Schlossman 1980). As regulating cells, they can increase or diminish immune responses. T lymphocytes which "up-regulate" the immune response are known as helper lymphocytes. Helper lymphocytes can be distinguished from other lymphocyte populations in that they express the CD4 molecule. The CD4 structure, a 55-kilodalton molecule expressed on the lymphocyte membrane, appears to play a crucial role in the ability of the cell to carry out the helper function. The initiation of virtually any humoral or cellular immune response requires the presence and participation of CD4-bearing lymphocytes. The CD4 lymphocyte serves to increase the magnitude of an antibody response, the intensity of a delayed-type hypersensitivity response, and the effectiveness of the T lymphocyte-mediated lysis of virus-infected cells. Recent studies have now clearly demonstrated that CD4 lymphocytes are comprised of two distinct subpopulations. One of those subpopulations includes the classic helper lymphocytes. The second is the inducer of suppression. The immunologic response which "down-regulates" both humoral and cellular immunity can only be initiated in the presence of this CD4-bearing inducer of suppression. Distinct and mutually exclusive cell surface markers in humans have recently been defined which subdivide the helper from the inducer of suppression within the CD4 lymphocyte population.

The importance in the immune system of the CD4 lymphocyte is underscored by the breakdown in host immune defenses in humans infected with the human immunodeficiency virus (HIV). The principal effect of HIV infection on the immune system appears to be a selective loss of CD4 lymphocytes. HIV-infected individuals develop profound immune deficiency and die from opportunistic infections and tumors.

The T lymphocyte which down-regulates the immune response is the suppressor T cell. This cell population expresses the 34-kilodalton CD8 molecule on its membrane. The mechanisms by which suppressor T lymphocytes down-regulate humoral and cellular responses are under active investigation at this time. They appear to do so through the production of soluble factors.

T lymphocytes are also cellular effectors in the immune system. They function as the mediators of delayed-type hypersensitivity and in the destruction of virus-infected cells. In a delayed-type hypersensitivity response, the T lymphocyte migrates to the site of the antigen and secretes lymphokines which recruit activated macrophages to assist in walling off the foreign antigen. In experimental settings, this response is seen as skin reactivity at the site of antigen deposition. The same cellular mechanisms are thought to occur in granuloma formation in diseases such as tuberculosis.

Cytotoxic T lymphocytes similarly perform an effector function in the immune response. These T lymphocytes recognize structures on the surface of target cells and lyse those target cells with remarkable specificity. These cytotoxic T cells control the spread of a viral infection within an organism. The delayed-type hypersensitivity T lymphocyte and usually the cytotoxic T lymphocyte express the CD8 molecule on its plasma membrane. As with the CD4 molecule and its association with helper/inducer T cell function, the CD8 molecule not only serves as a useful marker for effector T lymphocytes but is necessary for the functioning of those cells.

A second population of cells capable of killing targeted cells within a host are the NK cells. NK cells are probably, although not definitely, members of the T lymphocyte family. These cells are not antigen-specific but are capable of lysing tumor and virus-infected cells. They are important in the control of virus spread early after infection and are also critical for immune surveillance for tumor cells (see p. 103, this volume).

Specificity

A hallmark of the immune system is the exquisite specificity of the humoral and cell-mediated responses. This specificity is seen both in the recognition of antigen and in genetic restrictions which limit the interactions between immune cells. A T lymphocyte recognizes short sequences of amino acids with such specificity that a single amino acid change in such a sequence is readily recognized by it. The T lymphocyte also is restricted in its interactions with other cells of the immune system by major histocompatibility complex (MHC)-encoded cell surface structures (Klein 1986). Thus, MHC class I molecule recognition is required for a cytotoxic T lymphocyte to interact appropriately with and lyse target cells.

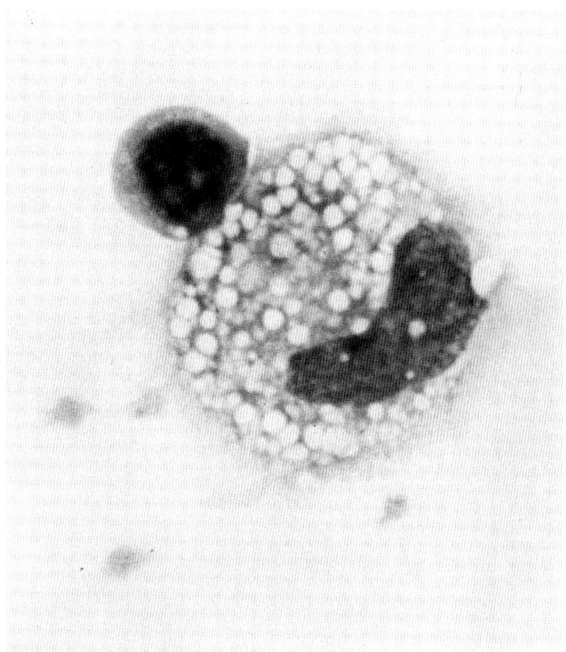

Fig. 108. A rhesus monkey macrophage opposed to a lymphocyte. Giemsa, × 1500. (Smear of peripheral blood leukocytes in culture kindly provided by Dr. Norval W. King)

Target cell lysis will only occur if the cytotoxic T cell and target cell are identical in their MHC class I phenotype. Similarly, the T lymphocyte recognizes the MHC class II-encoded structures on the surface of antigen-presenting macrophages. There must be identity between the T cell and the antigen-presenting cell at this class II genetic locus for a productive interaction to occur between the cell populations (Fig. 108).

The importance of MHC recognition and matching between immunologically active cells is dramatically illustrated by the events which follow transplantation of organs between MHC disparate individuals. In the absence of immunosuppression, a T lymphocyte-mediated destruction of a kidney graft occurs within 1 week of transplantation. If bone marrow progenitors contaminated with mature T lymphocytes are engrafted into an immunocompromised MHC-mismatched individual, the engrafted T lymphocytes mediate the destruction of host gastrointestinal, dermal, and hepatic parenchyma, a process known as graft-versus-host disease.

The ability of T lymphocytes to interact with such extraordinary specificity is conferred upon this cell by its T cell receptor complex (Marrack and Kappler 1986). This complex of molecules includes a disulfide-linked heterodimer, which

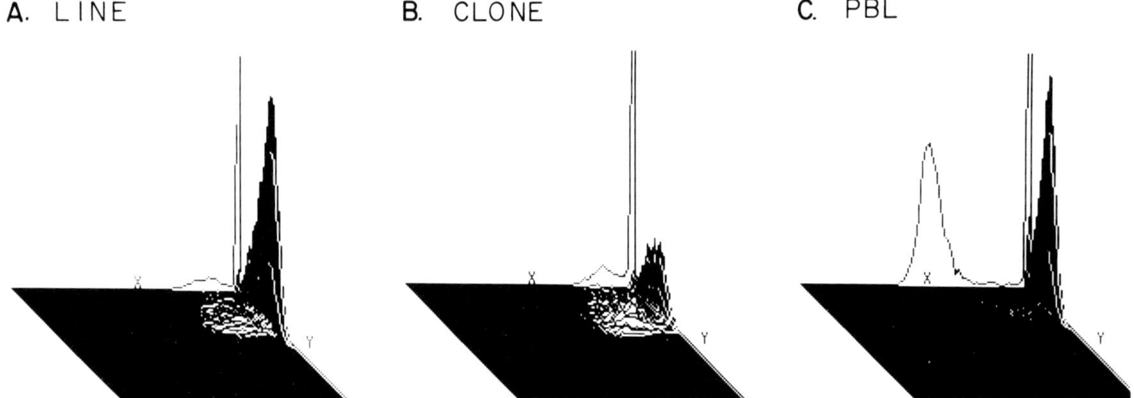

Fig. 109 A–C. Two-color immunofluorescence analysis by flow cytometry of **A** common marmoset lymphoid cell line as generated through in vitro immortalization with the T cell-tropic herpesvirus *H. ateles;* **B** clone AS-1 of that line; and **C** common marmoset peripheral blood lymphocytes *(PBL)*. Cells were stained with phycoery-thrin-conjugated anti-CD8 (gamma 1, x-axis), and anti-CD4 (gamma 2a, y-axis) followed by FITC-conjugated goat anti-mouse gamma 2a, antibody. Cells were then evaluated for expression of one, the other, or both surface antigens. The percentages of cells expressing each antigen were: **A** 70% CD4+, 22% CD4+ CD8+, 3% CD8+, and 6% CD4− CD8−; **B** 28% CD4+, 61% CD4+ CD8+, 4% CD8+, and 7% CD4− CD8−; **C** 59% CD4+, 3% CD4+ CD8+, 20% CD8+, and 19% CD4− CD8−

confers antigen specificity and the ability to interact in an MHC-restricted fashion, and the intimately related CD3 structure. The CD3 structure appears to be necessary for the triggering of the lymphocyte following antigen and MHC recognition.

Identification of T Lymphocytes

T lymphocytes and B lymphocytes are virtually indistinguishable by routine light microscopic examination. This surely accounts for the fact that these two populations have only been differentiated from each other in the past 20 years. New methods are now available to discriminate between these very different but histologically identical cell populations. In a normal lymph node, follicular cells are of mostly B lymphocyte lineage, and interfollicular or paracortical lymphocytes are T lymphocytes. Within the spleen, the T lymphocytes are found in the periarteriolar sheaths. However, in assessing peripheral blood lymphocyte populations or lymphocytes under pathologic conditions, we take advantage of the fact that lymphocytes express lineage-restricted cell surface structures. B lymphocytes can be assessed for surface immunoglobulin or various B cell-specific surface antigens. T lymphocytes can be differentiated from B lymphocytes not only by their absence of surface immunoglobulin, but their expression of the pan-T cell markers CD3 and CD2 (Kremsky and Clayberger 1985). Cells which react with antibodies to these structures can be visualized in situ in tissue by immunohistochemical techniques. When assessing distributions or in peripheral blood lymphocyte populations, fluorescence conjugated antibodies and flow cytometric technology is utilized (Fig. 109).

References

Klein J (1986) Natural history of the major histocompatibility complex. Wiley, New York

Krensky AM, Clayberger C (1985) Diagnostic and therapeutic implications of T cell surface antigens. Transplantation 39: 339–348

Marrack P, Kappler J (1986) The T cell and its receptor. Sci Am 254 (2): 36–45

Paul WE (1984) Fundamental immunology. Raven, New York

Reinherz EL, Schlossman SF (1980) Regulation of the immune response-inducer and suppressor T-lymphocyte subsets in human beings. N Engl J Med 303: 370–373

B-Cell Function and Ontogeny

Arnold S. Freedman

Introduction

The major function of B lymphocytes is the production of antibodies. These antibodies play a large role in the immune system as they are directed against antigens on microorganisms and other potential toxins. These antibodies facilitate the involvement of other defenses including the activation of complement and promotion of phagocytosis. The generation of immunoglobulin (Ig)-producing cells involves the interaction of B cells with T cells and accessory cells as well as a variety of cytokines. In addition to Ig production, B cells are involved in antigen presentation, and they appear to produce several growth and differentiation factors. This suggests that B cells are not simply passive recipients of exogenous signals, but also active participators in the generation and regulation of the immune response.

B Cell Ontogeny

The generation of antibody diversity has been extensively studied at the genetic level, especially in humans and mice. The rearrangement of Ig heavy chain V, D, J, and constant regions is followed by light chain rearrangement, all occurring independently of antigen. At the end of the pre-B cell stage, B cells subsequently express functional surface IgM. The regulation of pre-B cell differentiation is largely unknown. Recent studies with murine pre-B cells suggest that bone marrow stromal cells are important in the regulation of pre-B cell development. Several stromal cell line derived cytokines have been described, one of these, termed IL-7, drives murine pre-B cell differentiation. Studies with human normal and neoplastic pre-B cells suggest that both IL-2 and a low molecular weight BCGF are involved in pre-B cell proliferation (Kishimoto 1985).

The activation, proliferation, and differentiation of mature, resting B cells is better understood than pre-B cell development. Mature/resting sIgM+/D+ B cells are activated from the G_0 to the G_1 phase of the cell cycle following triggering with antigen or a variety of stimuli. In addition to antigen, human B cells can be activated by antibodies to surface Ig (anti-Ig), *Staphylococcus au-*

reus Cowan I, phorbol esters, Epstein-Barr virus (EBV), and monoclonal antibodies directed against the B cell-restricted antigen CD20. Murine B cells are also activated by IL-4, lipopolysaccharide, and dextran. Activation of B cells from G_0 to G_1 is characterized by a series of metabolic, biochemical, and molecular events. These include increases in intracellular Ca^{++} concentration and inositol phospholipid metabolism, expression of the proto-oncogene *c-myc*, cell enlargement, and RNA synthesis. With subsequent stimulation and interaction with a variety of growth factors, B cells enter S phase and proliferate.

Following the activation of resting B cells, the regulation of proliferation and differentiation, including Ig isotype switching, is controlled by a variety of T cell- and monocyte-derived cytokines. As stated previously, the T cell-derived polypeptide IL-4 can activate murine B cells from the G_0 to the G_1 phase of the cell cycle, hyperinduce MHC class II antigens, and induce cell enlargement. Moreover, resting B cells exposed in vitro to IL-4 have earlier entrance into S phase upon subsequent culture with anti-Ig. IL-4 also stimulates B cell proliferation with anti-Ig, and human B cells activated with anti-Ig are induced to proliferate by subsequent addition of IL-4. B cells which have been previously activated also proliferate in response to IL-2 and a variety of other cytokines including both low and high molecular weight B cell growth factor, interferon gamma (IN F-γ), and IL-1. Murine but not human B cells are also induced to proliferate by IL-5. The control of B cell Ig production is similarly under the control of various cytokines. Three of these factors can induce previously activated/proliferating B cells to secrete Ig including IL-2, IL-5, and IL-6. In addition, IN F-γ and IL-1 are reported to augment Ig synthesis but by themselves do not stimulate Ig production. Recent studies have demonstrated that several lymphokines are important in regulation of Ig class switching. IN F-γ stimulates the production of IgG2a isotype and inhibits the production of IgG3, IgG1, IgG2b, and IgE. In contrast, IL-4 induces IgG1 and IgE isotypes, suggesting that IL-4 and IN F-γ have reciprocal regulatory influences on B cells. More recently in both murine and human systems, it has been shown that IL-5

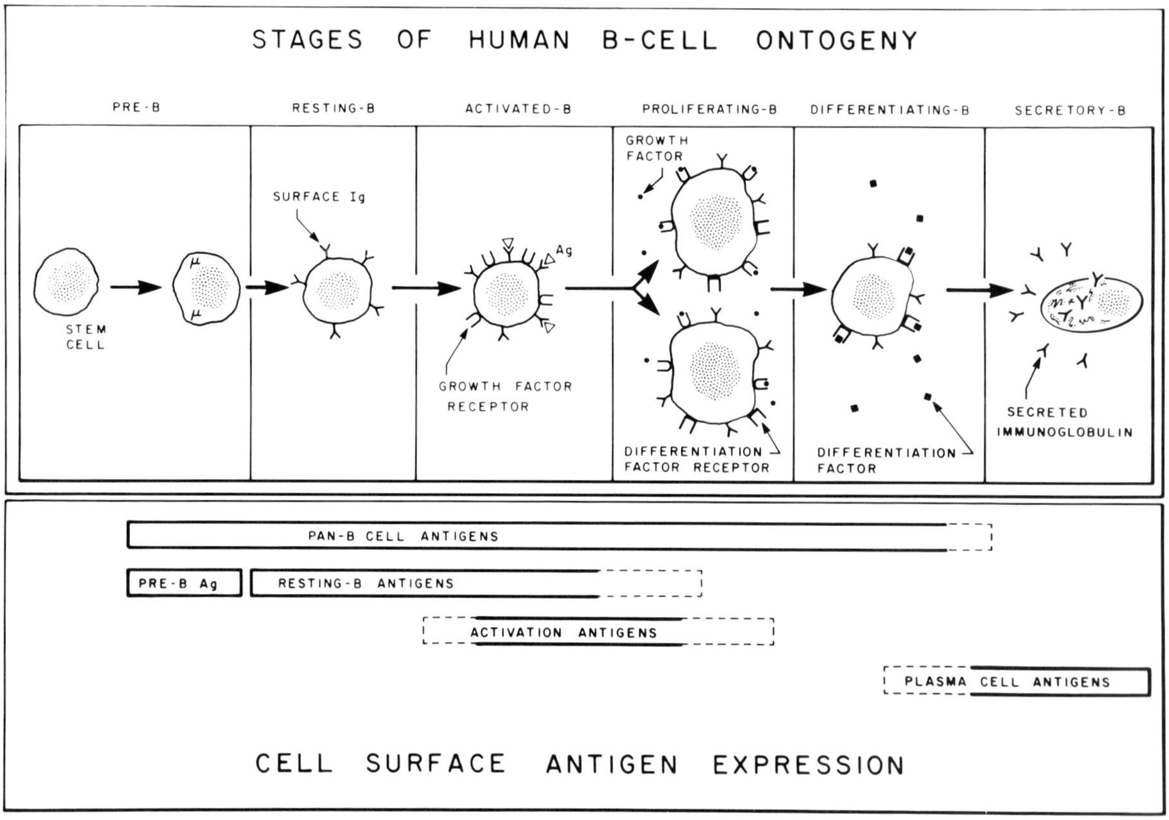

Fig. 110. Stages of normal B-cell differentiation in humans and the expression of B cell-restricted and -associated antigens. Similar stages have been found for mice

stimulates IgA production. The majority of these various B cell growth and differentiation factors are produced by activated T cells (IL-2, IL-4, IL-5, INF-γ) and monocytes (IL-1, IL-6). However, it has been reported that in vitro activated (either with *S. aureus* Cowan I or EBV) human B cells produce several polypeptides including a high molecular weight B cell growth factor, IL-6, and IL-1-like activity. These studies suggest that normal B cells are capable of proliferating and differentiating in an autocrine fashion. More importantly, the identification of low and high molecular weight B cell growth factors and IL-6 production by human malignant B cells suggests a role for these factors in neoplastic B cell proliferation (Cooper 1987; Howard and Paul 1983; Kishimoto 1985).

Expression of Cell Surface Antigens in Normal B-Cell Ontogeny

B-cell ontogeny begins with the migration of hemopoietic stem cells from the yolk sac to the fetal liver, at 8–9 weeks of gestation in humans. Later in fetal development, B cells populate the lymph nodes and spleen. It is only when hemopoiesis is established in the fetal bone marrow that pre-B cell development becomes primarily located there. During adult life the generation of B cells remains in the bone marrow.

B-cell ontogeny has been operationally divided into stages, including pre-B cell, mature/resting B cell, activated/proliferating B cell, differentiating B cell, and secretory or plasma cell (Fig. 110). These stages can be characterized by the expression of unique cytoplasmic and cell surface molecules. In this context, human B-cell antigens can be subgrouped into categories. These include: antigens that span ontogeny, the pan B cell antigens; antigens that appear at the mature/resting B cell stage, that are no longer expressed after B-cell activation; antigens that are not expressed on resting B cells but appear following activation; and antigens that appear at the terminal stages of differentiation. Many of these antigens have been characterized at the first, second, and third International Workshops on Human Leukocyte Differentiation Antigens. A CD (cluster designation) nomenclature has been adopted for these antigens, following extensive phenotypic and biochemical studies (Freedman and Nadler 1987; Clark and Ledbetter 1989). These designations, proposed for human antigens, have equivalents in the rat and mouse.

The earliest pre-B cells have been defined by their expression of cell surface antigens including HLA-DR (Ia) and the pan B cell antigen, CD19. By its lineage restriction, CD19 is the most reliable cell surface marker of B lineage at the pre-B cell level. Studies of non-T cell acute lymphocytic leukemia (ALL) and normal Epstein-Barr virus (EBV) transformed pre-B cells suggest that CD19 is expressed prior to Ig heavy chain rearrangement. Following the appearance of CD19, cells express CD10 (CALLA, the common ALL antigen), and finally they express the pan B cell antigen CD20. The expression of these antigens defines three stages of pre-B cell differentiation based on cell surface antigen expression: Ia+ CD19+CD10−CD20−, Ia+CD19+CD10+ CD20−, and Ia+CD19+CD10+CD20+. Another pan B cell antigen, CD22, is expressed early during pre-B cell development. However, CD22 is present in the cytoplasm and not on the cell surface until the mature sIgM/sIgD B cell stage. Finally, the last stage of pre-B cell ontogeny is defined by the expression of μ heavy chains in the cytoplasm. Two other pan B cell antigens, CD24 and CD45, are also expressed on pre-B cells, but their precise temporal appearance in human B-cell ontogeny has not been clarified (Kincade 1987).

In the adult, pre-B cell ontogeny resides in the bone marrow. As pre-B cells mature they are exported to the peripheral blood and lymphoid tissues where they reside until activated by antigen. Resting B cells express sIgM/D and continue to express Ia, CD19, CD20, and cell surface CD22. In addition, mature/resting B cells express C3b and Fcγ receptor as well as CD21, which has been shown to be the receptor for the C3d component of complement and Epstein-Barr virus.

Following binding with antigen or various mitogens, resting B cells are activated from G_0 to G_1 phase at the cell cycle. Depending on the stimulus, B cells demonstrate one or more events of activation, as previously described. The activation of mature/resting B cells is also accompanied by a sequence of cell surface antigenic changes. Within 24 h of activation, resting B cells begin to lose sIgD, CD21, and CD22. By 72–96 h cells will no longer express these antigens. As these antigens are lost, a large number of activation antigens sequentially appear. Most of these antigens demonstrate peak expression by 72 h and are no longer expressed by 120 h. These activation antigens can be divided into those which are B cell-restricted including CD23, B5, BB1, AB-1, Ba, Bac-1, and those that are B cell-associated such as IL-2 receptor (IL2R), CD23 transferrin receptor (T9), 4F2, and Blast-1. These activation antigens are excellent candidates for growth factor receptors, localization/adhesion molecules, and other regulatory structures.

The secretory or plasma cell stage is similarly characterized by the loss and acquisition of cell surface antigens. In addition to the above-mentioned loss of activation antigens, cells gradually lose the pan B cell antigens Ia, CD19, CD20, and CD24. This stage is also characterized by the appearance of other antigens including CD38 and PCA-1, which are expressed on plasma cells.

Murine B cells carry several of the cell surface antigens discussed above. In addition to sIg, mature murine B cells express C3b and C3d receptors, and activated murine B cells express IL2R and T9. Murine pre-B cells also express Ia, but it is present after cytoplasmic μ heavy chains are detected. The earliest marker of murine pre-B cells is the pan B cell antigen Ly-5 (B220) which is analogous to human CD45. Murine pre-B but not mature B cells express the BP-1 marker which to date has no human analogue. Another cell surface antigen on murine B cells which has not yet been identified on human ones is Lyb-2. This antigen is expressed on pre-B cells prior to the cytoplasmic μ stage as well as on mature B cells.

Morphology

By light microscopy with Giemsa staining, mature peripheral blood B cells and T cells are indistinguishable. Similarity by conventional TEM, B cells and T cells look alike. The majority of peripheral blood B cells are small, 5–8 mm in diameter, with a high nuclear to cytoplasmic ratio. The cytoplasm is scant and agranular, and the nucleus is dark on Giemsa staining with condensed chromatin but only rarely nucleoli. With TEM the nucleus contains electron-dense heterochromatin with nucleoli, and the cytoplasm may contain polyribosomes but little RER and small to moderate sized Golgi complex.

Following stimulation of B cells with antigen or mitogen, cells enlarge with an increased basophilic cytoplasm and an eccentric nucleus with prominent nucleoli and are termed "immunoblasts." By EM both smooth and rough ER are seen, and the Golgi complex increases in size. The terminally differentiated B cell or plasma cell has the characteristic basophilic cytoplasm, eccentric nucleus with clock-faced chromatin distribution, and prominent Golgi complex as seen by light microscopy. With TEM the most dramatic finding is parallel rays of RER consistent with the immunoglobulin-producing function of the plasma cell.

Conclusions

The understanding of normal B cell function and ontogeny has been tremendously advanced by the development of monoclonal antibodies directed against B cell surface antigens and the isolation and cloning of the various cytokines involved in B-cell differentiation. These tools have permitted the isolation and functional character-ization of homogeneous populations of B cells at various stages of development. More recently several of the B cell-restricted and -associated differentiation antigens have been cloned. This may facilitate the understanding of the function of these antigens and their natural ligands. More importantly, these studies may provide insights into controls of normal and neoplastic B cell growth and differentiation.

References

Clark EA, Ledbetter JA (1989) Structure, function, and genetics of human B cell associated surface molecules. Adv Cancer Res

Cooper MD (1987) B lymphocytes. Normal development and function. N Engl J Med 317: 1452–1456

Freedman AS, Nadler LM (1987) Cell surface markers in hematologic malignancies. Semin Oncol 14: 193–212

Howard M, Paul WE (1983) Regulation of B cell growth and differentiation by soluble factors. Annu Rev Immunol 1: 307–333

Kincade PW (1987) Experimental models for understanding B lymphocyte formation. Adv Immunol 41: 181–268

Kishimoto T (1985) Factors affecting B-cell growth and differentiation. Annu Rev Immunol 3: 133–157

Identification and Functional Characteristics of Monocytes/Macrophages

Luigi Varesio, M. Gonda, and Patricia S. Latham

Synonyms. The general denomination should be "mononuclear phagocytes". Other names have been improperly used as synonyms. For example, the term macrophage properly refers to mononuclear phagocytes located in the tissues and does not include monocytes which are in the circulation. The denomination of the various types of mononuclear phagocytes depends mainly on their anatomic compartmentalization, and this will be discussed in the tissue distribution section (Table 32).

Introduction

Macrophages arise from multipotential stem cells in the bone marrow, undergo a series of cell divisions, and differentiate into blood-borne monocytes that emigrate from the blood and develop into tissue macrophages. Heterogeneity within the macrophage population is largely determined by tissue localization, stage of differentiation, and the degree to which the macrophages have been stimulated by external substances and/or cytokines, a process termed activation. The primordial nature of these cells is exemplified by their ability to recognize and phagycytize microbial invaders such as bacteria, viruses, fungi, and parasites. By virtue of their phagocytic ability, macrophages serve as a vital first line of defense during infection by various microbes and parasites. This role of macrophages was first recognized by Metchnikoff who suggested in the late 1800s that phagocytes were the body's prime detectors of foreign invaders. Interest in this multifaceted cell has continued from that time with subsequent studies demonstrating that macrophages are rapidly mobilized to sites of injury and contribute substantially to inflammatory and antitumor responses.

Morphology

Mononuclear phagocytes have a diameter ranging from 12 to 20 µm. They have an abundant cytoplasm surrounding a central or slightly eccentric reniform nucleus (Fig. 111). A well-developed Golgi apparatus is present, as are large numbers of rod-shaped mitochondria and a complex cytoskeleton. The periphery of the cytoplasm and plasma membrane is irregular, with numerous ruffles and pseudopodia. Circulating monocytes are not usually called upon to be actively phagocytic, and so they contain relatively few secondary lysosomes in comparison with tissue macrophages. As monocytes emigrate into tissue, they acquire features characteristic of tissue macrophages. Since tissue macrophages are in contact with ground substance and other cells, they assume a variety of stellate and elongated shapes consistent with their adherent status (Fig. 112). Tissue macrophages evidence their role in clearance of foreign protein, organisms, and debris by their prominent phagocytic vacuoles, secondary lysosomes, and numerous pinocytotic vesicles (Figs. 113–117). The plasma membrane also reflects this increase in activity by an increase in elongated and tortuous pseudopodia (Figs. 115, 117). The plasma membrane may also develop labyrinthine invaginations, giving the appearance of "wormlike bodies" in Kupffer's cells of the liver or "zipperlike" inclusions (electron-dense core with 10-nm periodic striations) in Langerhans' cells of the skin. Surrounding the plasma membrane in tissue macrophages such as the Kupffer's cell is a fuzzy outer protein and mucosubstance coat, but this outer coating is frequently lost in tissue processing and requires special processing or staining with ruthenium red to be visualized.

Antigenic Phenotype

The main criteria to identify mononuclear phagocytes are based on morphologic, biologic, and biochemical features (Wiltrout and Varesio 1989). Surface antigens detected by specific antisera or by monoclonal antibodies have proved very useful in characterizing the phenotype of

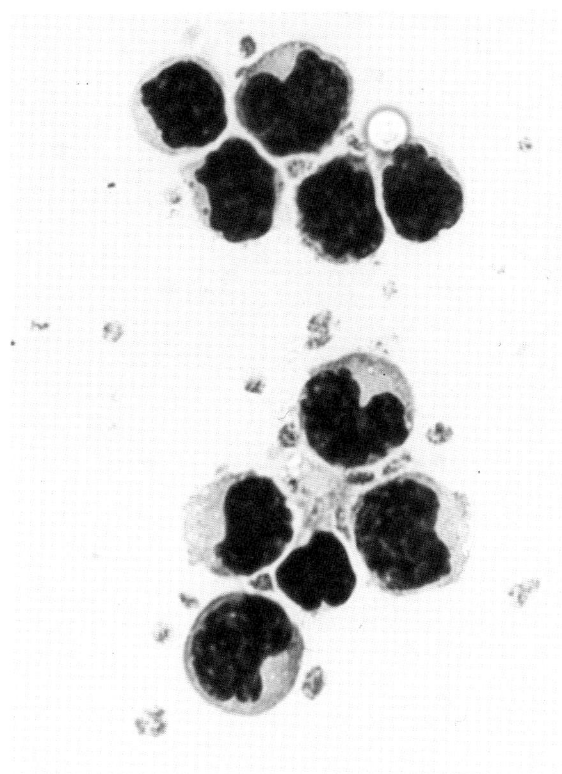

Fig. 111. Peripheral blood monocytes isolated from rat. The rounded contour and reniform nucleus are typical of the circulating monocyte. Whright-Giemsa stain, × 1386

macrophages. However, some biochemical and functional assays are still used in their identification. The most common functional markers are: (a) adherence to plastic (adherent macrophages cannot be detached by exposure to trypsin, and this feature is exploited to remove contaminating fibroblasts from macrophage cultures); (b) positive staining for nonspecific esterase; (c) positive staining for peroxidase; (d) production of lysozyme (this enzyme is produced by macrophages and monocytes as well as myeloid cells); and (e) phagocytosis (a property shared by polymorphonuclear cells). The antigens and receptors expressed on the surface of mononuclear phagocytes of mice and commonly used for their characterization are listed in Table 31 (Adams and Hamilton 1984; Wiltrout and Varesio 1989; Nathan 1987; Van Furth 1988; Springer and Unkeless 1984). Some markers such as the Mac-1, Mac-2, and CSF-1 receptor are relatively specific for myelomonocytic cells. However, there is no single reagent that can unequivocally identify a mononuclear phagocyte, and for this reason a panel of antibodies is generally used to identify

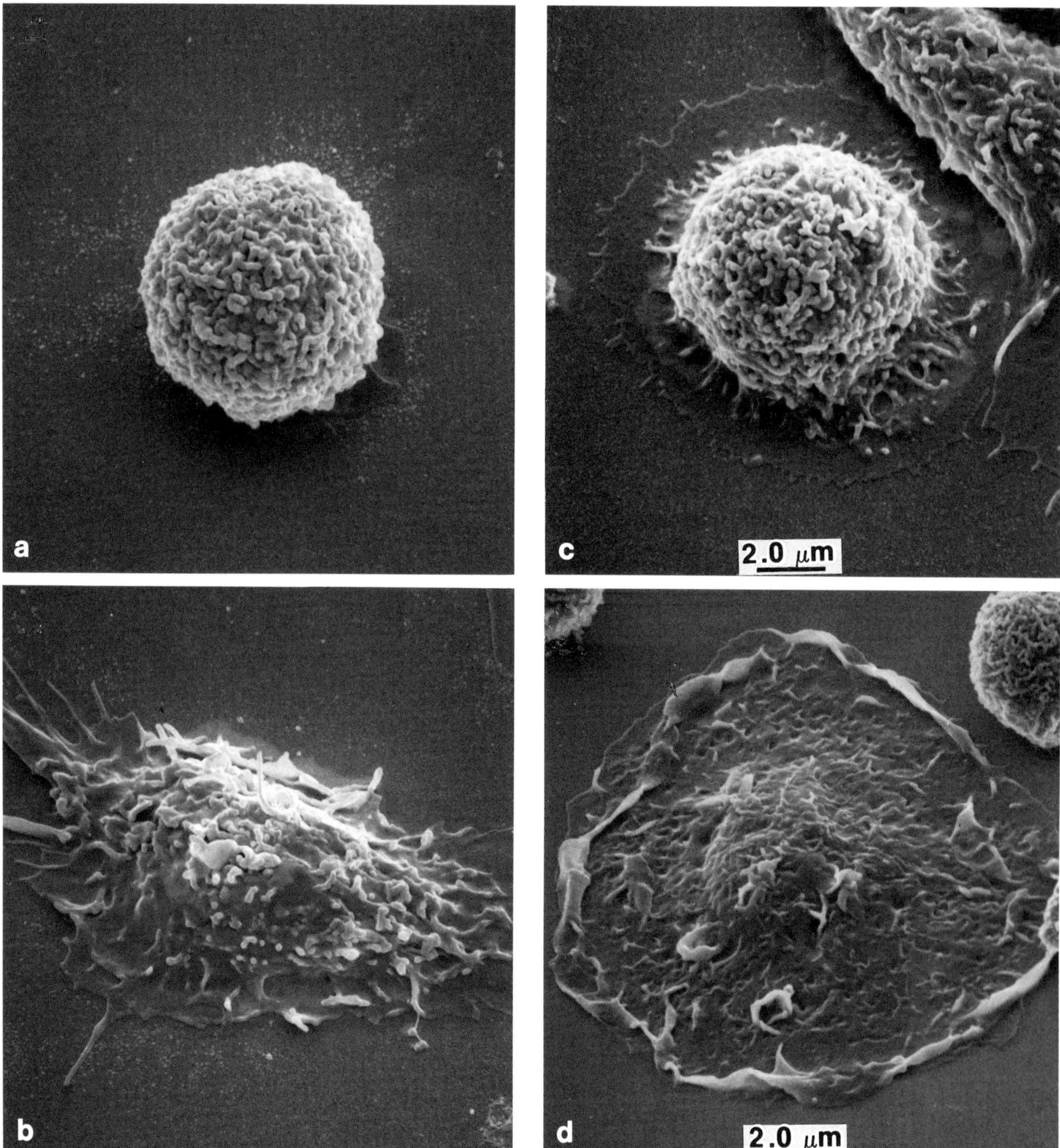

Fig. 112a-d. Peripheral blood monocytes isolated from a mouse and cultured in vitro on a glass substrate for up to 60 min. Sequential events of the monocyte and glass interaction from early attachment to spreading (**a→d,** respectively). Plasma membrane of the round cell loses its multiple microvilli and fenestrated lamellae (**a, b**) and acquires ruffles and pseudopodia (**c, d**) as it spreads out over the glass substrate. (SEM by Kunio Nagashima, Laboratory of Cell and Molecular Structure, National Cancer Institute, Frederick Cancer Research Facility)

these cells. The expression of some markers may vary in relationship to the type and/or activation state of the mononuclear phagocytes. For example, I a antigens are constitutively expressed on monocytes but are low or absent on resting tissue macrophages. The latter, however, may be induced to express high levels of Ia by IFN-γ. Fc receptors are constitutively present on mononuclear phagocytes, and their expression is also augmented by IFN-γ.

Fig. 113 *(above).* Peritoneal macrophages from mouse elicited by glycolate. The irregular shape of these cells, the generous cytoplasm, and the prominent phagocytic vacuoles are characteristic of the tissue macrophage. Giemsa stain, ×630

Fig. 114 *(below).* Resident peritoneal macrophage. Note the crescent-shaped nucleus, multiple mitochondria, rich population of endoplasmic reticulum, large (lipid-containing) and small heterophagocytic vacuoles, and abundance of pinocytotic vesicles that are characteristic of normal monocytes. The surface of the cell is covered by microvilli. TEM

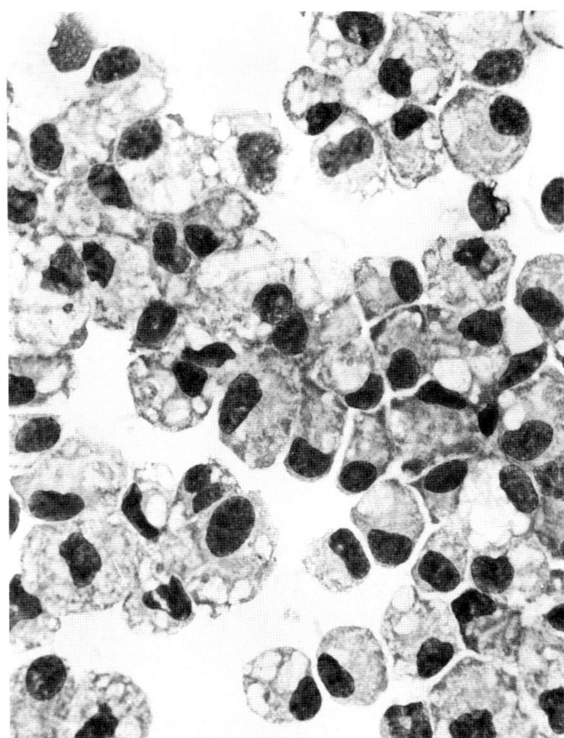

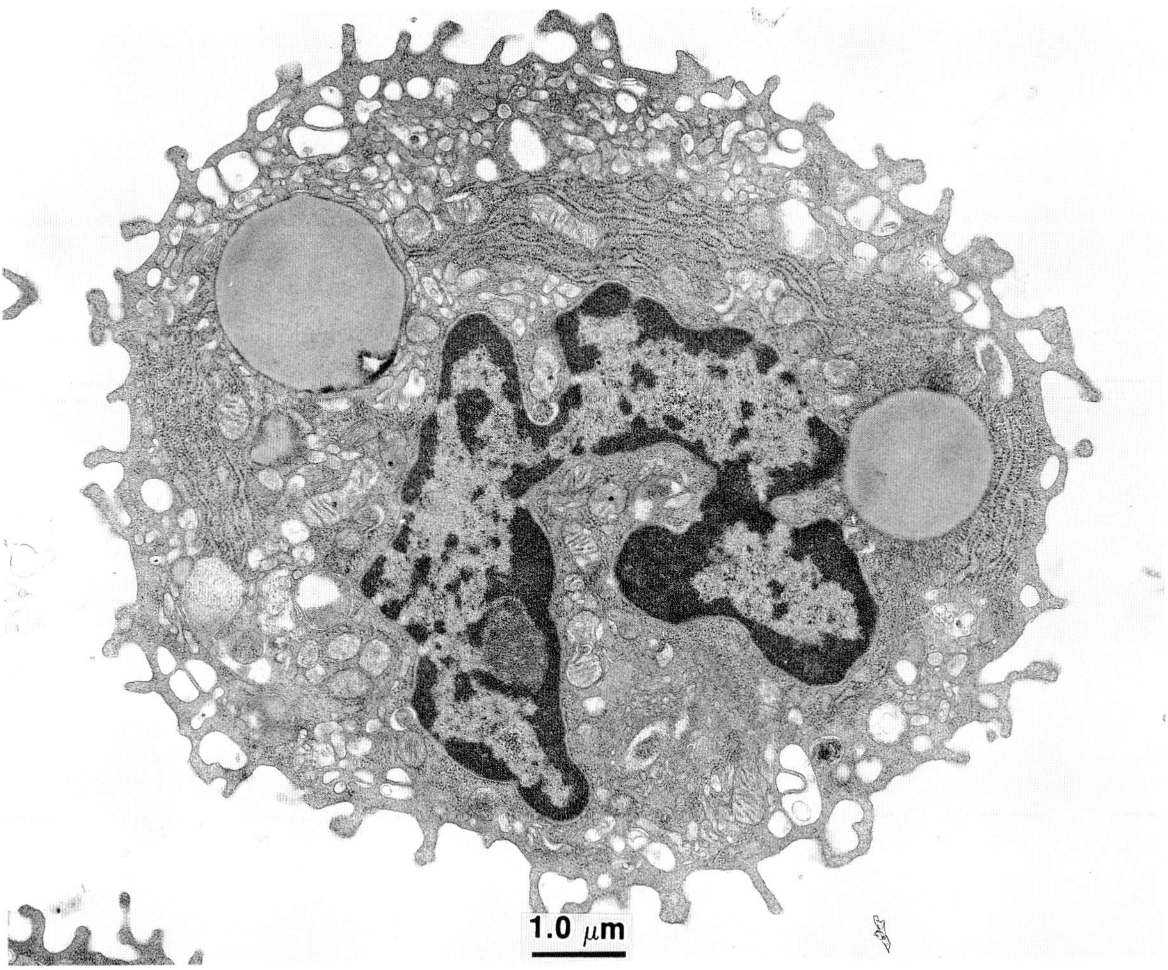

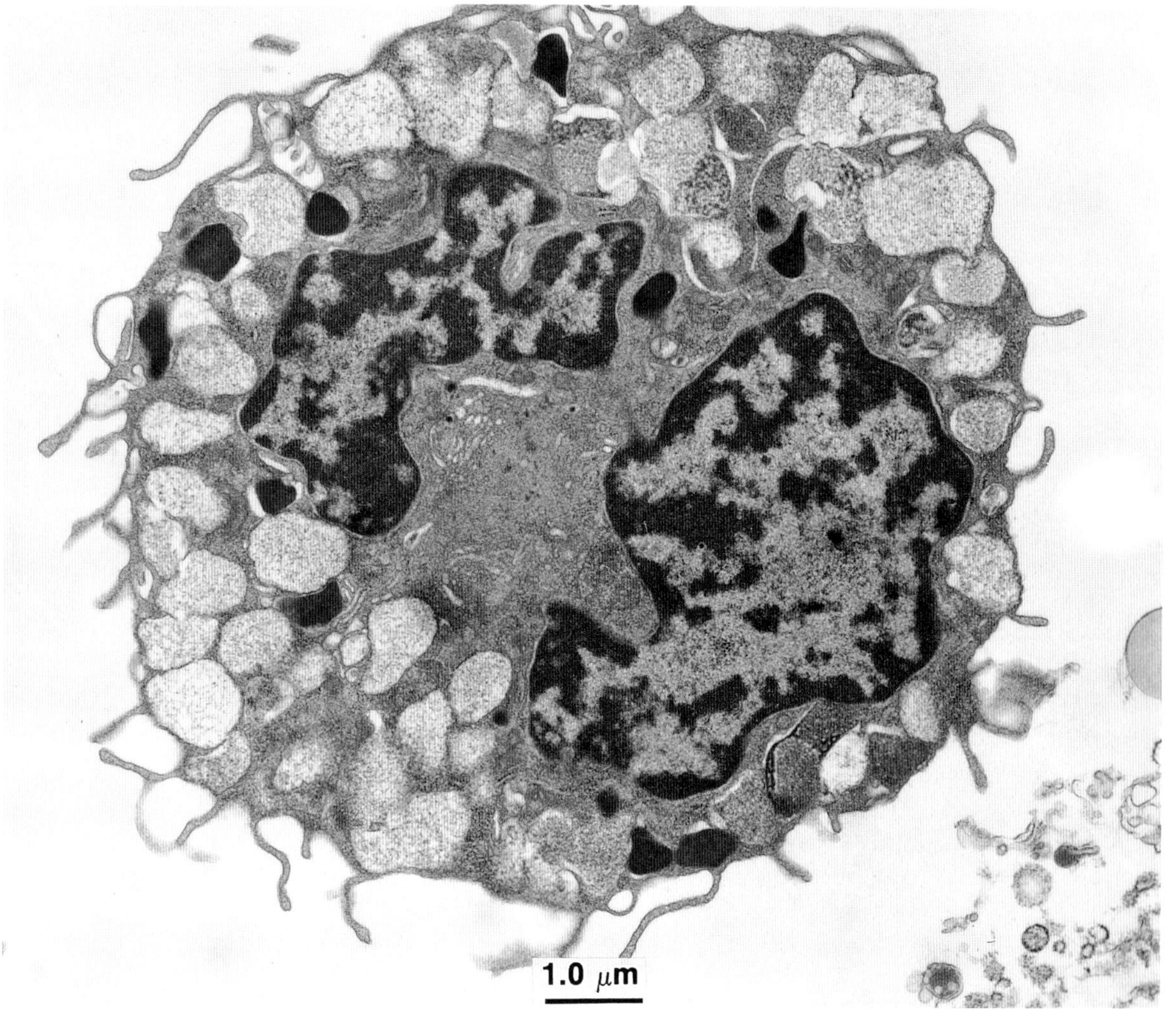

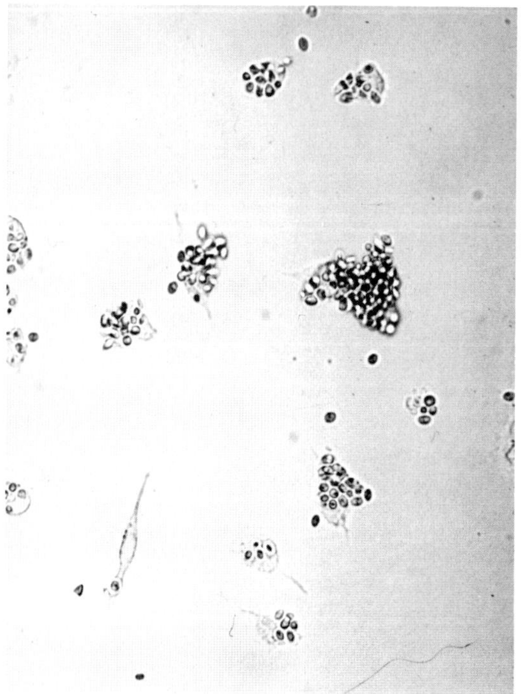

Fig. 115 *(above)*. Resident peritoneal macrophage from a mouse after activation by thioglycollate. Enhanced phagocytosis is indicated by the increase in size and number of intracellular vacuoles. Irregular nucleus is dissected by the plane of sectioning, Golgi complex, and a few mitochondria. Intracellular vacuoles represent electron-dense lysosomes and semi-electron-dense vacuoles, so-called secondary lysosomes, containing ingested material. Periphery of the cell is covered by ruffles cut in cross section. (TEM by Kunio Nagashima, Laboratory of Cell and Molecular Structure, National Cancer Institute, Frederick Cancer Research Facility)

Fig. 116 *(below)*. Phagocytosis of yeast organisms by peripheral blood monocytes isolated from mice and cultured in vitro. Wright-Giemsa stain, × 560

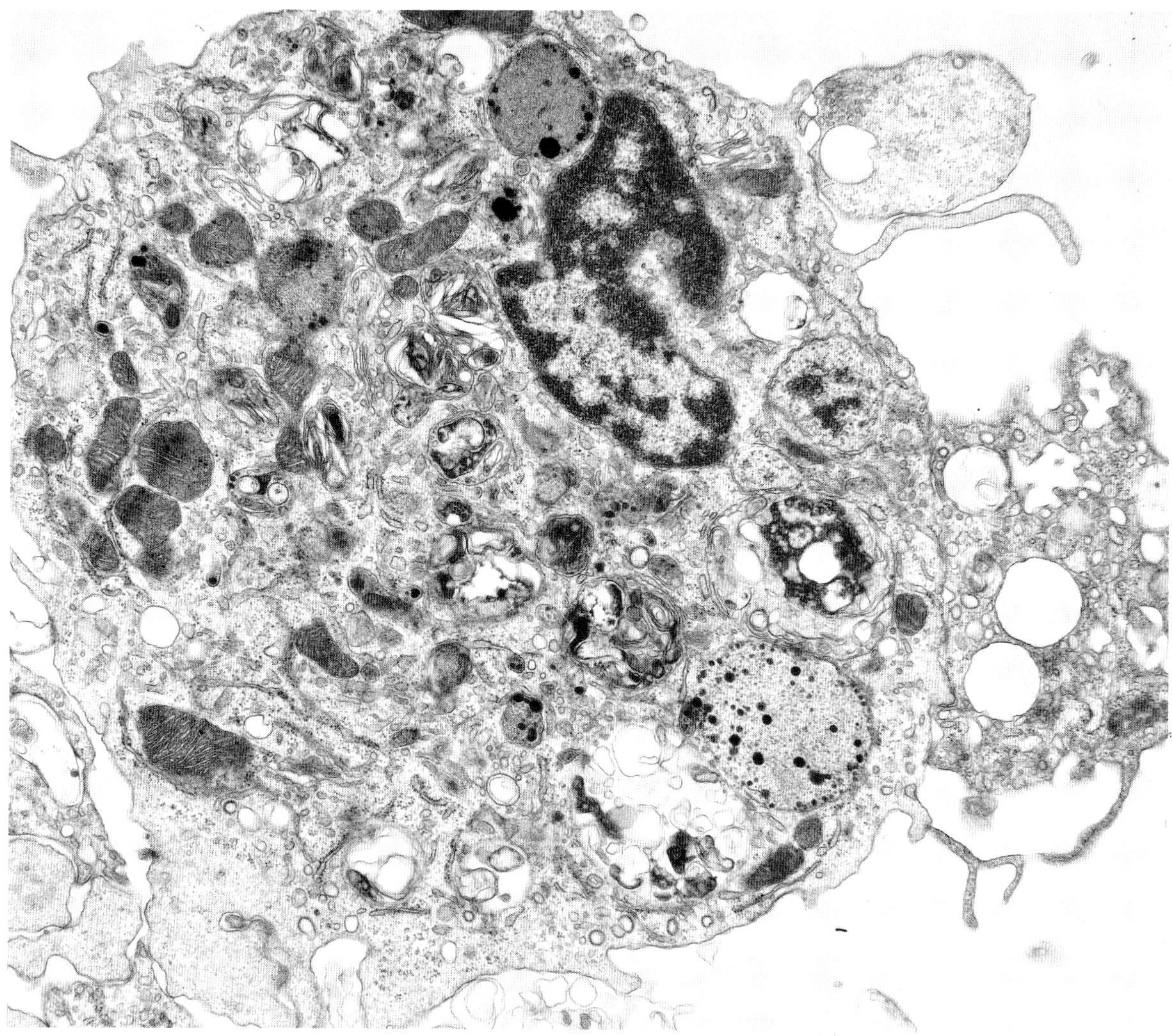

Fig. 117. Kupffer's cell after isolation from the liver of a mouse by collagenase perfusion and pronase digestion. Note pseudopodia with active phagocytosis of debris at the periphery of the cell and numerous phagocytic vacu- oles and secondary lysosomes within its cytoplasm. Abundant endoplasmic reticulum, well-developed Golgi apparatus, and numerous pinocytotic vesicles are seen in this macrophage. TEM, × 16000

Tissue Distribution

Mononuclear phagocytes are found in most body tissues. Table 32 indicates the relative de- nominations of the various mononuclear phago- cyte populations. The relative content of mono- nuclear phagocytes in each tissue may vary dramatically during inflammatory processes. For example, the peritoneal exudate of a 10 to 12-week-old mouse bred in a germ free environ- ment yields $1-2 \times 10^6$ cells of which 50%–60% are macrophages. Within 2–4 days following the injection of sterile irritants (mineral oil, thiogly- collate broth), the yield of peritoneal exudate cells may increase to $10-20 \times 10^6$ cells of which

80%–90% are macrophages. Redistribution and accumulation of macrophages in various tissues is not necessarily associated with a B- or T-cell response since it can be elicited in nude mice and rats. Under normal steady state conditions it has been calculated that the mean turnover time for murine macrophages is 4 days in the liver, 6 days in the spleen and lung, and 15 days in the perito- neal cavity (Van Furth 1988).

Lineage

Mature tissue macrophages have little or no pro- liferative capacity and are continuously replen-

Table 31. Surface markers/antigens on mononuclear phagocytes of mice

Marker	Cells with expression
Fc receptor	MP, B cells, PMN
C3 receptor	PMN, MP, erythrocytes, some B cells
Mannose-fucose receptor	MP, other
LPS receptor	MP, B cells, other
CSF1 receptor	MP (high levels), bone marrow cells
MAC-1 antigen	MP, bone marrow, PMN, NK cells
MAC-2 antigen	MP (not all)
Ia antigen	MP, B cells
Ly5	Leukocytes, stem cells
Asialo GM1 glycolipid	Some MP, NK cells, fetal thymocytes
Ly-6	Bone marrow, MP, leukocytes
Ly-5	MP, lymphocytes, bone marrow
LFA-1	PMN, MP, LGL

MP, mononuclear phagocyte; PMN, polymorphonuclear leukocyte; LGL, large granular leukocyte; NK, natural killer.

Table 32. Tissue distribution and types of mononuclear phagocytes

Tissue	Mononuclear phagocyte
Blood	Monocytes
Bone	Osteoclast
Bone marrow	Monoblast, promonocytes, monocytes
Connective tissue	Histiocytes
Lung	Alveolar macrophages
Liver	Kupffer's cells
Joints	Synovial macrophages
Nervous system	Microglial cells
Other (spleen, lymph nodes)	Tissue macrophages
Serous cavities (pleura, peritoneum)	Exudate macrophages
Skin	Langerhans' cells, histiocytes

ished by differentiated offspring of bone marrow precursors which in turn are derived from a pool of multipotent stem cells. The orderly development of tissue macrophages in the organism requires that a strict balance be maintained between self-renewal, differentiation, survival, and cell death. The self-renewal of macrophage precursors and the rate of differentiation are regulated by a complex network of growth and differentiation factors. Candidates for the induction of macrophage proliferation include M-CSF which is lineage-specific for macrophages, GM-CSF which works on both the granulocyte and macrophage lineages, and interleukin (IL) 3 which acts on myeloid, erythroid, and lymphoid precursors.

The two most developed differentiative stages are the circulating monocyte and more mature macrophages present in tissues. Most evidence suggests that resident tissue macrophage populations are derived from the emigration of blood-borne monocytes which then further differentiate into macrophages (Van Furth 1988). There is also evidence that at least a limited renewal of tissue macrophage populations occurs by proliferation in situ of extravasated monocytes, suggesting that a limited proportion of monocytes or poorly differentiated tissue macrophages retain the ability to divide.

Functions

Mononuclear phagocytes exert various functions that can be divided into two categories: immuno-modulatory and effector. As immunoregulatory cells, they can either augment or inhibit the immune response (Varesio 1983). Macrophages exert helper activity by presenting the antigen in association with class II major histocompatibility molecules to T and B lymphocytes. However, they can also inhibit the immune response by suppressing lymphoproliferation, lymphokine production, and protein synthesis. As effector cells, mononuclear phagocytes can exert microbicidal activity against intracellular and extracellular parasites (Nathan 1982) as well as antitumor activity (Varesio 1986). Macrophage secretory products (Nathan 1987) play an important role in the expression of mononuclear phagocyte functions. For example, IL-1 is a comitogenic factor for T lymphocytes as well as a growth inhibitory factor for certain tumors. Interferon and tumor necrosis factor are antiproliferative and involved in the resistance to viral infections. Reactive oxygen intermediates and lysozyme contribute to bactericidal activity. Transforming growth factors have antitumor and wound-healing properties. Colony stimulating factor promotes the proliferation/differentiation of macrophage precursors. Prostaglandins are important inflammatory mediators with immunosuppressive effects. Fortunately for the host, the various macrophage functions are not constitutively and simultaneously expressed by every mononuclear phagocyte. In the absence of stimulatory signals, immunomodulatory and effector functions are minimally expressed. Following stimulation by lymphokines (IFN-γ, IL-4, IL-2, etc.) or by microbial products (e. g., endotoxins), mononuclear phagocytes become activated and increase their secretory activities. The pattern of functions exerted by stimulated macrophages varies depending upon the nature of the stimulating agent and the length of stimulation. For example, IFN-γ induces microbicidal and tumoricidal macrophages as well as augmenting the helper activity of the cells by inducing class II antigens. However, IFN-γ will not induce immunosuppressive macrophages. On the other hand, endotoxins are poor inducers of helper activity, but they stimulate immunosuppressive and effector functions. The predominance of positive or negative effects of mononuclear phagocytes on the immune response are strongly dependent upon the proportion of mononuclear phagocytes and effector lymphocytes.

In fact, while 1%–2% of mononuclear phagocytes are sufficient to exert maximal helper activity on lymphocyte proliferation. 10% or more will begin to demonstrate substantial immunosuppressive effects. Such a dose-dependent effect is likely to be of importance in vivo since mononuclear phagocytes are mobile cells that can accumulate in inflammatory areas. For example, normal mouse macrophages make up 5%–7% of the total spleen cell population, but this can increase up to 15%–20% of the total cell population after a suspension of bacille Calmette Guérin (BCG) injection. In the latter situation, the immunosuppressive effect of the macrophages predominates. Macrophages can potentially damage the host tissue during the inflammatory process by the release of various monokines, reactive oxygen intermediates, and proteolytic enzymes. However, the damage of the host tissue is limited by a number of factors. First, the activated state is transient in the macrophages, and they return to a quiescent state upon removal of the stimulus. Second, as opposed to lymphocytes, the majority of tissue macrophages are terminally differentiated, and the activation process is not associated with proliferation and clonal expansion. Thus, the expression of the activated phenotype is limited in time and generally restricted to the inflammatory site. Third, some macrophage products can inhibit the development of the macrophage response via a feedback type of mechanism. For example, prostaglandins are secreted by mononuclear phagocytes and have inhibitory effects on the secretory as well as effector functions of macrophages, and thus prostaglandins can provide a negative regulatory signal on macrophage activation.

Acknowledgement. This project has been funded at least in part with federal funds from the Department of Health and Human Services under contract number NO1-CO-74102 with Program Resources, Inc. The content of this publication does not necessarily reflect the views or policies of the Department of Health and Human Services, nor does mention of trade names, commercial products, or organizations imply endorsement by the U. S. Government.

References

Adams DO, Hamilton TA (1984) The cell biology of macrophage activation. Annu Rev Immunol 2: 283–318

Nathan CF (1982) Secretion of oxygen intermediates: role in effector functions of activated macrophages. Fed Proc 41: 2206–2211

Nathan CF (1987) Secretory products of macrophages. J Clin Invest 79: 319–326

Springer TA, Unkeless JC (1984) Analysis of macrophage differentiation and function with monoclonal antibodies. Contemp Top Immunobiol 13: 1–31

Van Furth R (1988) Phagocytic cells: development and distribution of mononuclear phagocytes in normal steady state and inflammation. In: Gallin JI, Goldstein IM and Synderman R (eds) Inflammation basic principles and clinical correlates. Raven, New York, pp 281–295

Varesio L (1983) Suppressor cells and cancer: inhibition of immune functions by macrophages. In: Friedman H, Herberman RB, Escobar M, Reichard S (eds) The reticuloendothelial system, vol 5. Plenum, New York, pp 217–252

Varesio L (1986) Induction and expression of tumoricidal activity by macrophages. In: Dean RT, Jessup W (eds) Mononuclear phagocytes: physiology and pathology. Elsevier, Amsterdam, pp 381–407

Wiltrout RH, Varesio L (1989) Activation of macrophages for cytotoxic and suppressive effector functions. In: Oppenheim JJ, Shevach E (eds) Textbook of immunophysiology: role of cells and cytokines in immunity and inflammation. Oxford University Press, Oxford

Immunohistochemistry, Lymphoid Cells, Mouse

Paul K. Pattengale

Introduction

In the last decade, immunohistochemistry on fixed and frozen lymphoid tissues has become routine. With the advent of monoclonal antibody technology, lymphoid cells can be recognized using a battery of immunologically specific reagents. In contrast to tissue immunofluorescence in which morphological resolution is poor, it was soon learned that an antibody-coupled enzymatic label, such as horseradish peroxidase, could be applied to morphologically well defined tissues as viewed by conventional light microscopy. In this manner, it was possible to develop a colored reaction product visible by light microscopy, at the site of localization of the enzyme-labeled antibody in the tissue section. Although a number of enzymes, such as alkaline phosphatase and glucose oxidase, are potentially usable in such a system, horseradish peroxidase emerged as the most useful, since it was not only stable but was also available in a pure form. Furthermore, it could be easily demonstrated in tissues because of its accessibility to a wide range of chromogenic substrates (Sternberger 1979; Taylor 1978). Immunohistochemical techniques using immunoperoxidase methodology have been successfully applied to both fixed, paraffin-embedded tissues (Stein et al. 1980; Taylor 1980) and to fixed, frozen lymphoid tissues (Warnke and Levy 1980; Tubbs et al. 1980; Janossy et al. 1980). Although there are advantages in the immunomorphologic evaluation of paraffin-embedded tissues, such as good morphologic detail, permanent preparations, and high sensitivity, the main disadvantage continues to be possible antigen loss during tissue preparation. For this reason, it is more reliable to use frozen sections, especially if antigen loss is a practical problem. It is also clear that surface antigens, such as surface immunoglobulin, are best detected in cryostat (frozen) sections. Immunoperoxidase methodology can also be applied to cytocentrifuge and to imprint preparations.

Several variations of the immunoperoxidase methodology may be employed for different purposes in the immunohistochemical evaluation of various mouse lymphoid tissues (Taylor et al. 1985). First, horseradish peroxidase can be directly conjugated to the primary antibody; second, indirect conjugation can be achieved using peroxidase antiperoxidase methodology with the appropriate bridging antibody; third, primary or secondary antibodies can be biotinylated or biotin labeled, and then reacted with horseradish peroxidase bound either to avidin or to avidin-biotin complexes (ABC); and fourth, protein A-bound horseradish peroxidase can be used as a bridge to the primary detecting antibody. In my experience, biotin-labeled antobodies reacted with peroxidase ABC complexes form the method of choice in either frozen or paraffin-embedded mouse tissue sections. The peroxidase antiperoxidase methodology has also been successfully used in fixed, paraffin-embedded tissue sections.

Of particular importance in the mouse is the fact that the majority of monoclonal antibodies are, in fact, derived from the mouse or rat. For this reason, it is essential that the primary antibody be biotinylated to reduce background problems. This is not necessary with conventional polyclonal antibodies produced in other species such as rabbits or goats. Such primary antibodies can be used in indirect techniques which utilize secondary antibodies which are biotinylated.

Use of Immunohistochemistry with the Pattengale-Taylor Classification in Evaluating Spontaneous Lymphoid Cell Neoplasms Occurring in the Mouse

Table 33 documents the immunomorphological characterization of 601 spontaneously occurring lymphoid cell neoplasms from a wide variety of aged, inbred mouse strains and demonstrates that the majority of lymphomas were B cell-derived, follicular center cell lymphomas (408/601 = 68% total incidence). Although these lymphomas have characteristic B-cell morphology (see p. 147, this volume), it should be stressed that the demonstration of cytoplasmic immunoglobulin using conventional immunoperoxidase staining techniques on fixed, paraffin-embedded tissues is quite helpful in confirming the B-cell nature of these follicular center cell lymphomas (Figs. 118–121). To this end, we were able to demonstrate cytoplasmic immunoglobulin positivity in 252 of the 300 cases tested (84% positive)

Table 33. Immunomorphologic classification of 601 spontaneously occurring murine lymphoid cell neoplasms[a]

n	Morphologic diagnosis	No. of CIg$^+$/no. tested[b,c]	Percentage CIg$^+$	Percentage total incidence
408	Follicular center cell (FCC)[d]	252/300	84	68
77	Immunoblast	46/52	88	13
14	Plasma cell	8/8	100	2
70	Lymphoblast	24/40	60	12
32	Small lymphocyte	nt[e]	nt[e]	5
601		330/400	83	100

[a] Includes 100 Balb/c, 111 B6C3F$_1$s, 80 NZB, 102 NFS/N (V-congeneics), 35 *nu/nu* NIH(S), 69 B6CBAF$_1$s, 30 C57BL/6(B6), and 64 mice from miscellaneous imbred strains. With the exception of the NSF/N, V-congeneics, and *nu/nu* NIH(S), which developed spontaneous lymphomas at approximately 12–18 months of age, the vast majority (>95%) of the remaining strains were older than 18 months. With the exception of the NZB strain, with its preponderance of immunoblastic and plasma cell lymphomas, all of the remaining strains had a similar total incidence as depicted in the last column of this table.

[b] Positivity for cytoplasmic immunoglobulin (CIg) is determined by the presence of easily detectable cytoplasmic immunoglobulin in greater than 25% of the critical neoplastic cells using conventional immunoperoxidase staining on fixed, paraffin-embedded tissues.

[c] Not all animals were tested, primarily due to inadequate fixation of lymphoid tissues (see text).

[d] Of the 408 FCC lymphomas, 207 were large FCC type, 152 were mixed FCC type, and 49 were small FCC type.

[e] nt, not tested. Due to the scant amount of cytoplasm in the small lymphocyte type, cytoplasmic immunoglobulin cannot be properly evaluated.

using the peroxidase antiperoxidase staining method for either immunoglobulin heavy or light chain (Pattengale and Frith 1983; Taylor 1978). Since small follicular center cell cells do not have enough cytoplasm for proper evaluation, the majority of the cases negative for cytoplasmic immunoglobulin were found among the small cell types. It should also be emphasized that not all 408 cases of follicular center cell lymphoma were tested, primarily due to improper fixation of lymphoid tissues. For example, it was found that Carnoy's fixative is not optimal for immunoglobulin preservation in fixed tissues. In contrast, Bouin's solution, Tellyesniczky's, neutral buffered formalin, and B-5 fixatives allow adequate preservation.

The remaining 193 cases of nonfollicular center cell type were diagnosed as immunoblastic [77/601 = 13% total incidence with 46 of 52 tested (88%) being positive for cytoplasmic immunoglobulin], lymphoblastic [70/601 = 12% total incidence with 24 of 40 tested (60%) being positive for cytoplasmic immunoglobulin], plasma cell [14/601 = 2% total incidence with 8 of 8 tested (100%) being positive for cytoplasmic immunoglobulin], and small lymphocytic (32/601 = 5% total incidence with none tested for cytoplasmic immunoglobulin).

Although the vast majority of follicular center cell, immunoblastic, and plasma cell lymphomas were judged to be B cell-derived using a combined immunomorphologic approach, it should be emphasized that lymphoblastic and small lymphocytic lymphomas are not as easily evaluated using fixed, paraffin-embedded tissues. This problem relates to the observation that these morphologic types usually have a scant amount of cytoplasm, making evaluation of the cytoplasmic immunoglobulin troublesome. Furthermore, lymphoblastic and small lymphocytic proliferations do not have characteristic, morphologically identifiable, nuclear and/or cytoplasmic features attributable to either a B or T cell. For these reasons, it is important in these lymphoid cell types to combine additional methodologies with morphologic evaluation. This would include surface marker analysis using flow cytometry, detailed phenotyping using monoclonal antibodies on frozen tissue sections, and finally, genomic DNA analysis for B or T cell-specific gene rearrangements (Pattengale and Frith 1986). Since it is often difficult in flow cytometry to be certain that a positive cell is indeed the critical, neoplastic cell, it should be stressed that pathologists employ antibody staining techniques on frozen tissues from lymphomatous mice. This approach ensures the proper identification of the neoplastic cell as being either positive or negative for a particular antigenic marker. Figure 122 demonstrates unequivocal K light chain staining of a B cell-derived

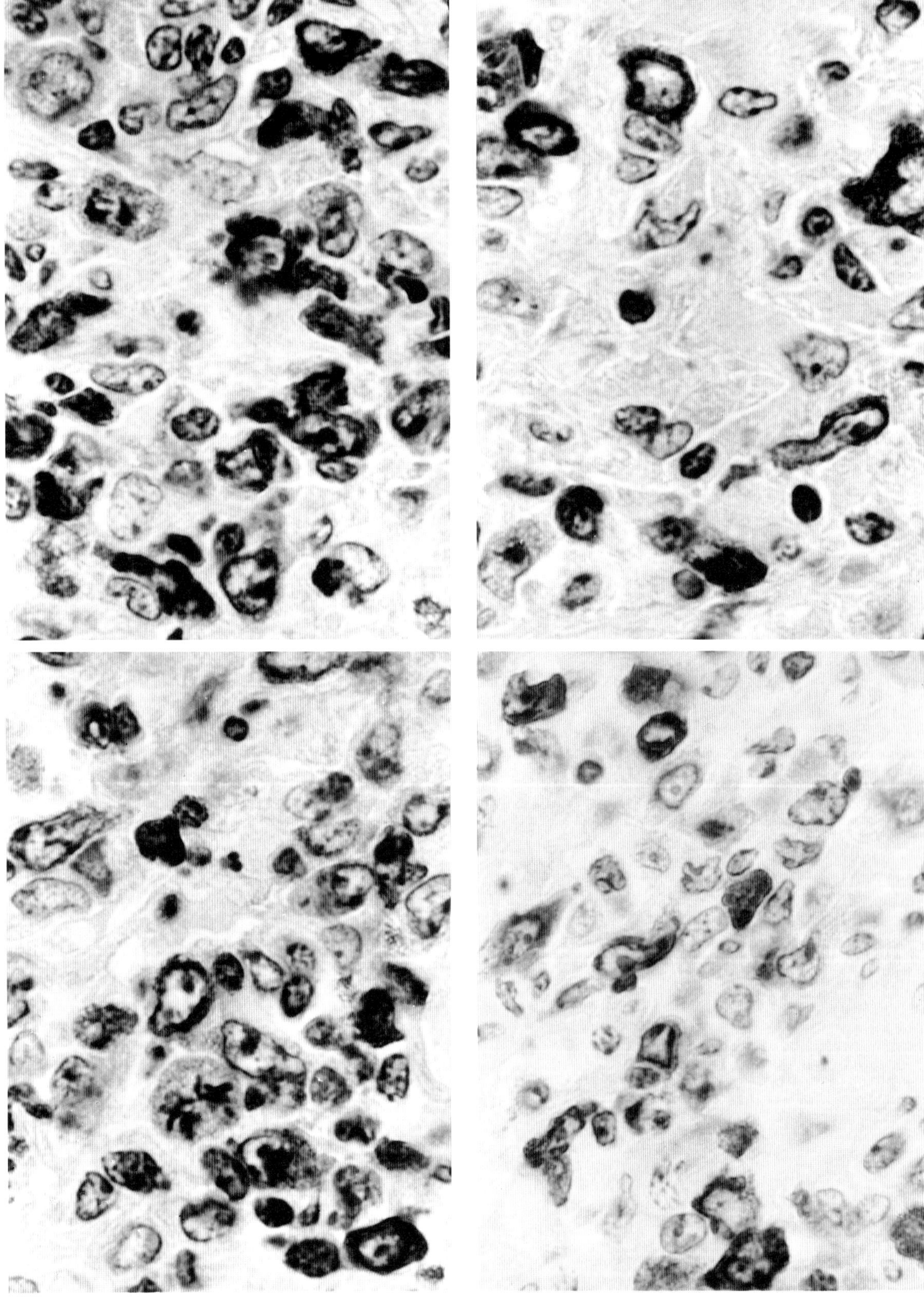

◀ **Fig. 118** *(upper left)*. Murine lymphoma of large follicular center cells (FCC lymphoma, large cleaved cell type), spleen, NFS/NV congeneic mouse. Note the predominance of intermediate to large, cohesive lymphoid cells with irregularly shaped, notched (cleaved) nuclei and moderate amounts of cytoplasm. In addition, note the positive (brown) staining for cytoplasmic immunoglobulin within the neoplastic follicular center cells using the peroxidase antiperoxidase immunoperoxidase technique. Immunoperoxidase stain, using a rabbit antibody to mouse IgA heavy chain, counterstained with hematoxylin, × 1000

Fig. 119 *(lower left)*. Murine lymphoma, large follicular center cells. Same case but different field as in Fig. 118. Immunoperoxidase stain, using rabbit antibody to mouse IgA heavy chain, counterstained with hematoxylin, × 1000

Fig. 120 *(upper right)*. Murine lymphoma, large follicular center cells. Same case but different field as in Fig. 118. Immunoperoxidase stain, using rabbit antibody to mouse kappa light chain, × 1000

Fig. 121 *(lower right)*. Murine lymphoma of large follicular center cells. Same case but different field as in Fig. 118. Immunoperoxidase stain, using rabbit antibody to mouse kappa light chain, × 800

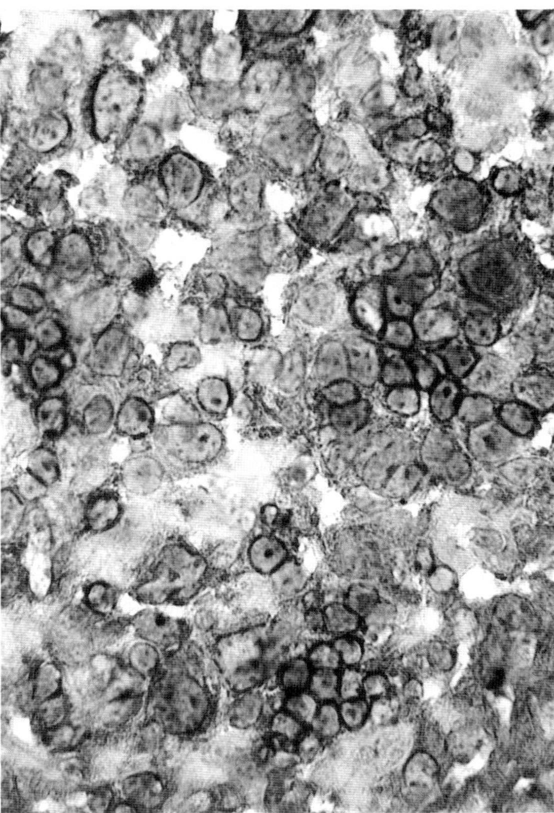

Fig. 122. Mouse immunoblastic lymphoma of B cell type, lymph node, NFS/NV congeneic mouse. Note the positive black staining with a biotinylated rat anti-kappa monoclonal antibody which was subsequently reacted with peroxidase avidin-biotin complexes. Frozen section, hematoxylin counter stain, × 580

immunoblastic lymphoma from a lymph node of an affected mouse. The details of this and other techniques are described elsewhere (Warnke and Levy 1981; Falini and Taylor 1983; Taylor et al. 1985).

Using the immunostaining approach on frozen sections with a panel of monoclonal antibodies, Pals et al. (in press) characterized 57 graft vs host induced lymphoid cell neoplasms occurring in (BALB/c × A)F₁ mice and correlated these findings with the morphologic types defined by Pattengale et al. (Pattengale and Taylor 1983; Pattengale and Frith 1983; Pattengale and Taylor 1981). Of the 54 lymphomas judged to be B cell-derived by positive immunostaining on frozen sections, 50 were morphologically designated as follicular center cell types, with the remaining 4 being of immunoblastic type. Of the 3 lymphomas judged to be T cell-derived by positive Thy-1 immunostaining on frozen sections, 2 were of lymphoblastic type, and one was of immunoblastic type.

Other antisera may be employed for demonstration of specific mouse B-cell antigens, other than immunoglobulin, even on paraffin-embedded tissues (Gendelman et al. 1983), such as T-cell antigens or monocyte/macrophage antigens (Thompson et al. 1982).

In summary, this approach is a valuable adjunct for the proper evaluation of lymphoid cell neoplasms and should be routinely employed by pathologists.

References

Falini B, Taylor CR (1983) New developments in immunoperoxidase techniques and their application. Arch Pathol Lab Med 107: 105–117

Gendelman HE, Moench TR, Narayan O, Griffin DE (1983) Selection of a fixative for identifying T cell subsets, B cells, and macrophages in paraffin-embedded mouse spleen. J Immunol Methods 65: 137–145

Janossy G, Thomas JA, Habeshaw JA (1980) Immunofluorescence analysis of normal and malignant lymphoid tissues with selected combination of antisera. J Histochem Cytochem 28: 1207–1214

Pals ST, Zijstra M, Radaszkiewicz T, Quint W, Cuypers HT, Shoenmakers HJ, Melief CJM, Berns A, Gleichmann E (1986) Immunological induction of malignant lymphoma graft versus host reaction induced B-cell lymphomas contain reintegrations of several types of murine leukemia virus sequences. J Immunol 136 (1): 331–339

Pattengale PK, Frith CH (1983) Immunomorphologic classification of spontaneous lymphoid cell neoplasms occurring in female BALB/c mice. JNCI 70: 169–179

Pattengale PK, Frith CH (1986) Contributions of recent reseach to the classification of spontaneous lymphoid cell neoplasms in mice. CRC Crit Rev Toxicol 16: 185–212

Pattengale PK, Taylor CR (1981) Immunomorphologic classification of murine lymphomas and related leukemias. In: Proceedings of the Rodent Lymphomas Workshop, March 4–5, 1981, Jefferson, Arkansas. Natl Cent Toxicol Res Press, Jefferson, pp 22–23

Pattengale PK, Taylor CR (1983) Experimental models of lymphoproliferative disease: the mouse as a model for human non-Hodgkin's lymphomas and related leukemias. Am J Pathol 113: 237–265

Stein H, Bonk A, Tolksdorf G, Lennert K, Rodt H, Gerdes J (1980) Immunohistologic analysis of the organization of normal lymphoid tissue and non-Hodgkin's lymphomas. J Histochem Cytochem 28: 746–760

Sternberger LA (1979) Immunocytochemistry, 2nd edn. Wiley, New York, pp 104–169

Taylor CR (1978) Immunoperoxidase techniques: practical and theoretical aspects. Arch Pathol Lab med 102: 113–121

Taylor CR (1980) Immunohistologic studies of lymphoma: past, present and future. J Histochem Cytochem 28: 777–787

Taylor CR, Hofman FM, Sherrod AE, Epstein A (1985) Immunohistologic techniques: their impact in tumor diagnosis with particular reference to lymphomas. In: Pattengale PK, Lukes RJ, Taylor CR (eds) Lymphoproliferative diseases: pathogenesis, diagnosis, therapy. Nijhoff, Dordrecht, pp 86–106

Thompson WD, Jack AS, Richmond J, Patrick RS (1982) The mononuclear phagocyte system of the mouse as demonstrated by the immunoperoxidase technique using anti-mouse macrophage antiserum. Diagn Histopathol 5: 19–32

Tubbs RR, Sheibani K, Sebek BA, Weiss RA (1980) Immunohistochemistry versus immunofluorescence for non-Hodgkin lymphomas. Am J Clin Pathol 73: 144–145

Warnke R, Levy R (1980) Detection of T and B cell antigens with hybridoma monoclonal antibodies: a biotin-avidin-horseradish peroxidase method. J Histochem Cytochem 28: 771–776

Warnke R, Levy R (1981) Tissue section immunologic methods in lymphomas. In: DeLellis RA (ed) Diagnostic immunohistochemistry. Masson, New York, pp 203–211

Sources of Antibodies and Immunological Reagents Used for Immunohistochemistry

Jerrold M. Ward and Craig W. Reynolds

Numerous commercial suppliers offer the reagents used for immunohistochemistry, especially for hemopoietic tissues (Tables 34, 35). Selected companies are listed here with their telephone numbers in the U. S. A. Those listed are not necessarily the sole or best source of the reagents. Products of other companies are available in this fast-evolving field. Investigators often prefer specific sources because of their personal preferences and their success with a particular product. Scientific papers in the literature also indicate sources of their reagents. Often the reagents are from commercial sources (Fig. 123). Sometimes, new reagents are not available from commercial sources but are prepared at the researcher's institution. Investigators are often willing to share a new reagent with another interested researcher. It is well worth the telephone call to the author of a paper. An excellent source for suppliers of all immunological reagents is *Linscott's Directory of*

Table 34. Sources of antibodies and immunological reagents for immunohistochemistry

Immunohistochemical kits		
Accurate Chemical & Scientific	Westbury, NY	1-800-645-6264
Biogenex Labs.	Dublin, CA	1-800-421-4149
Dako Corp	Santa Barbara, CA	1-800-235-5743
ICN Biomedicals	Lisle, IL	1-800-348-7465
Lipshaw	Detroit, MI	1-800-LIPSHAW
Miles Scientific	Naperville, IL	1-800-348-7465
SPI	West Chester, PA	1-800-2424-SPI
Vector Laboratories	Burlingame, CA	1-800-227-6666

Table 34 *(continued)*

Antisera to mouse and rat lymphocyte antigens		
Accurate Chemical & Scientific	Westbury, NY	1-800-645-6264
Becton Dickinson	Sunnyvale, CA	1-800-223-8226
Boehringer Mannheim	Indianapolis, IN	1-800-428-5433
Chemicon	El Segundo, CA	1-800-437-7500
Cooper Biomedical	Malvern, PA	1-800-523-7620
Dupont NEN	Boston, MA	1-800-225-1572
Fisher	Pittsburgh, PA	412-562-8300
ICN Biomedicals	Lisle, IL	1-800-348-7465
Jackson Immuno Research Labs.	West Grobe, PA	1-800-367-5296
Kirkegaard & Perry Labs.	Gaithersburg, MD	1-800-638-3167
Miles Scientific	Naperville, IL	1-800-348-7465
Pel-Freed	Rogers, AR	1-800-643-3426
Sera-Lab Limited	Sussex, UK	(0342) 71 63 66

Antisera to cell and tissue specific antigens		
Accurate Chemical & Scientific	Westbury, NY	1-800-645-6264
Becton Dickinson	Mountain View, CA	1-800-223-8226
BioGenix Labs.	Dublin, CA	1-800-421-4149
Boehringer Mannheim	Indianapolis, IN	1-800-428-5433
Calbiochem	San Diego, CA	1-800-854-9256
Chemicon	El Segundo, CA	1-800-437-7500
Dako Corporation	Santa Barbara, CA	1-800-235-5743
E-Y Labs.	San Mateo, CA	1-800-821-0044
ICN Biomedicals	Lisle, IL	1-800-348-7465
Lipshaw	Detroit, MI	1-800-LIPSHAW
Miles Scientific	Naperville, IL	1-800-348-7465
Ortho Diagnostic	Raritan, NJ	1-800-631-5807
Polysciences	Warrington, PA	1-800-523-2575
Whittaker Bioproducts	Walkersville, MD	1-800-638-8174

Immunological and Biological Reagents, for sale from 40 Glen Drive, Mill Valley CA 9 49 41, USA (telephone 415-681-3344).

References

Gendelman HE, Moench TR, Narayan O, Griffin DE (1983) Selection of a fixative for identifying T cell subsets, B cells, and macrophages in paraffin-embedded mouse spleen. J Immunol Methods 65: (1–2) 137–145

Ishii Y, Matsuura A, Yussa H, Narita H, Takami T, Kikuchi K (1983) Two distinct antigenic markers for rat thymus and T cells defined by monoclonal antibodies. Immunology 48: 743–754

Ishii Y, Matsuura A, Iwaki H, Takami T, Kikuchi K (1984) Two closely related antigens expressed on granulocytes, macrophages and some reticular elements in rat lymphoid tissues: characterization by monoclonal antibodies. Immunology 51: 477–487

Jeffries WA (1988) Hemopoietic and T-lymphocyte marker antigens of the rat characterized with monoclonal antibodies. In: Miyasaka M and Trnka Z (eds) Differentiation antigens in lymphohemopoietic tissues. Dekker, New York, pp 173–247

Ward JM, Argilan F, Reynolds DW (1983) Immunoperoxidase localization of large granular lymphocytes in normal tissues and lesions of athymic nude rats. J Immunol 131: 132–139

Table 35. Examples of commercial and other antibodies to leukocyte cell surface and cytoplasmic antigens

Molecule[a]	Antibody to:		Cell types	Selected sources
	Rat	Mouse		
		antigens		
CD2	OX34	ND[b]	Pan-T	Accurate, Sera
CD3	ND	T3	Pan-T	Accurate, Sera
CD4	W3/25	L3T4	T helper/inducer	Accurate, Sera
CD5	OX19, R1-3B3	Lyt-1[c]	Pan-T	Accurate, Sera, Ishii[d]
CD8	OX8[c]	Lyt-2	NK (LGL), T-cytotoxic, suppressor	Accurate, Sera
CD15	R2-1A6	ND	Monocytes, granulocytes	Ishii[d]
CD45	OX1	Ly-5	Leukocytes	Accurate, Sera
UK[e]	OX7	Thy-1.1	Pan-T	Accurate, Sera
UK	W3/13[c]	ND	Pan-T	Accurate, Sera
UK	ND	M1/70.15	Macrophages/monocytes	Accurate, Sera
UK	Lysozyme[c]	Lysozyme	Macrophages/monocytes/ granulocytes	DAKO
UK	ED-1,2, or 3	ND	Macrophages/monocytes/ dendritic cells	Dijkstra unit, this chapter
UK	PMN[c]	ND	Granulocytes	Accurate
UK	Rat immunoglobulins[c,f] (IgA,G,M)	Mouse immunoglobulins[c,f] (IgA,G,M)	B cells	Cooper Biomedical

[a] For cell surface antigens, CD (cluster designation), modified from W. A. Jeffries (1988), antisera to these antigens are available from accurate Chemical & Scientific Corporation, Sera-Lab Ltd., and other suppliers. See units for normal histology and neoplastic lesions for other antisera specific for these and other cell types. There are numerous other monoclonal and polyclonal antisera for similar antigens and cell markers. Frozen sections are often required for the demonstration of cell surface antigens. Often these antisera immunoreact with other cell types, and one must characterize the immunoreactivity.

[b] ND, not detected.

[c] Fixed tissues may be used. Bouin's fixative is preferred. For OX-8, see Ward et al. (1983). For Lyt-1, see Gendelman et al. (1983).

[d] Dr. Y. Ishii, Department of Pathology, Sapporo Medical College, Chuo-ku, 060 Sapporo, Japan. See Ishii et al. (1983, 1984).

[e] Unknown or not cell surface antigen.

[f] Polyclonal antisera against IgA, IgG and IgM may be used to screen for B cells containing any of these immunoglobulins. Antisera against light or heavy chains or specific immunoglobulins subtypes can also be used.

CELL SURFACE PHENOTYPE OF RAT LEUKOCYTES

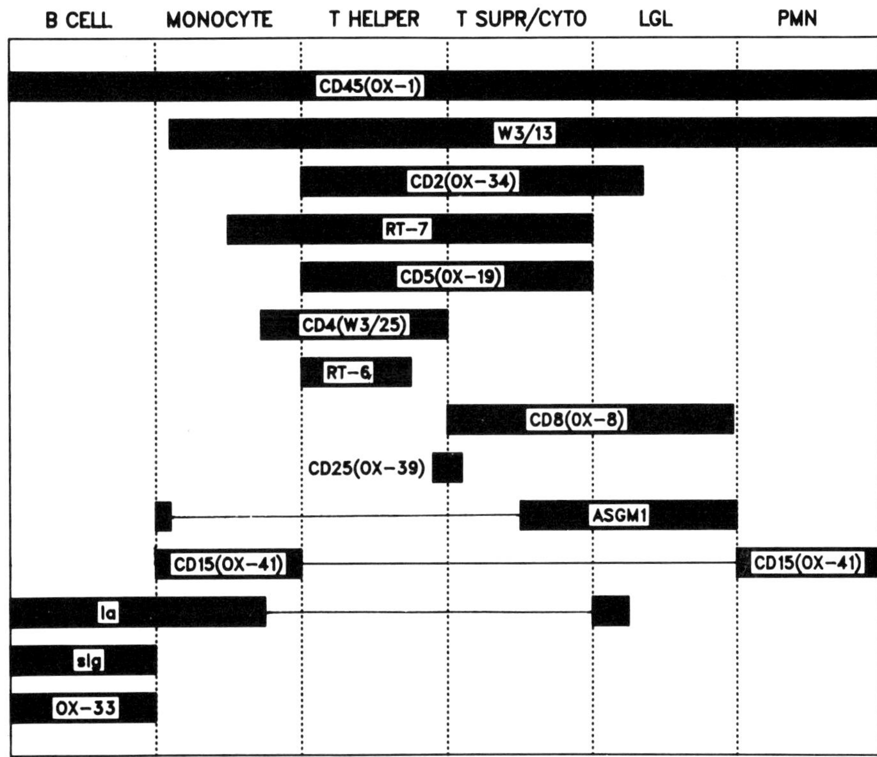

Fig. 123. Examples of antigens/monoclonal antibodies available for rat leukocytes. The designation *OX* indicates origin from hybridoma clones at Sera Laboratories and sold through other distributors (e. g., Accurate). *LGL*, large granular leukocyte; *PMN*, polymorphonuclear neutrophilic granulocyte

Normal Anatomy, Histology, Immunohistology, and Ultrastructure, Lymph Node, Rat

Christine D. Dijkstra, E. W. A. Kamperdijk, and A. J. P. Veerman

Gross Appearance

The lymph nodes of the rat are small, round, or kidney-shaped organs with a length of 3–5 mm which can be distinguished from the surrounding fat by their pearly gloss. They occur dispersed throughout the body, always connected with lymph vessels. Particularly in the axillar, inguinal, and cervical regions, along the larger arteries, and within the mesenterium, groups of nodes can be found (Fig. 124; Tilney 1971). The nodes are surrounded by a fibrous capsule from which trabeculae emerge. At the convex side thin afferent lymph vessels are recognizable, at the concave side (the hilus) small arteries and nerves supply the node, and the efferent lymph vessels and veins leave the node. The lymph vessels possess small valves to force the lymph stream in one direction. Though there are small variations between the different lymph nodes, in general the architecture is about the same. On cross section the cortex with small white nodules can be discriminated from the centrally located medulla. As an exception to the regular nodes, the renal nodes are reddish, due to the large numbers of red blood cells within the medullary region;

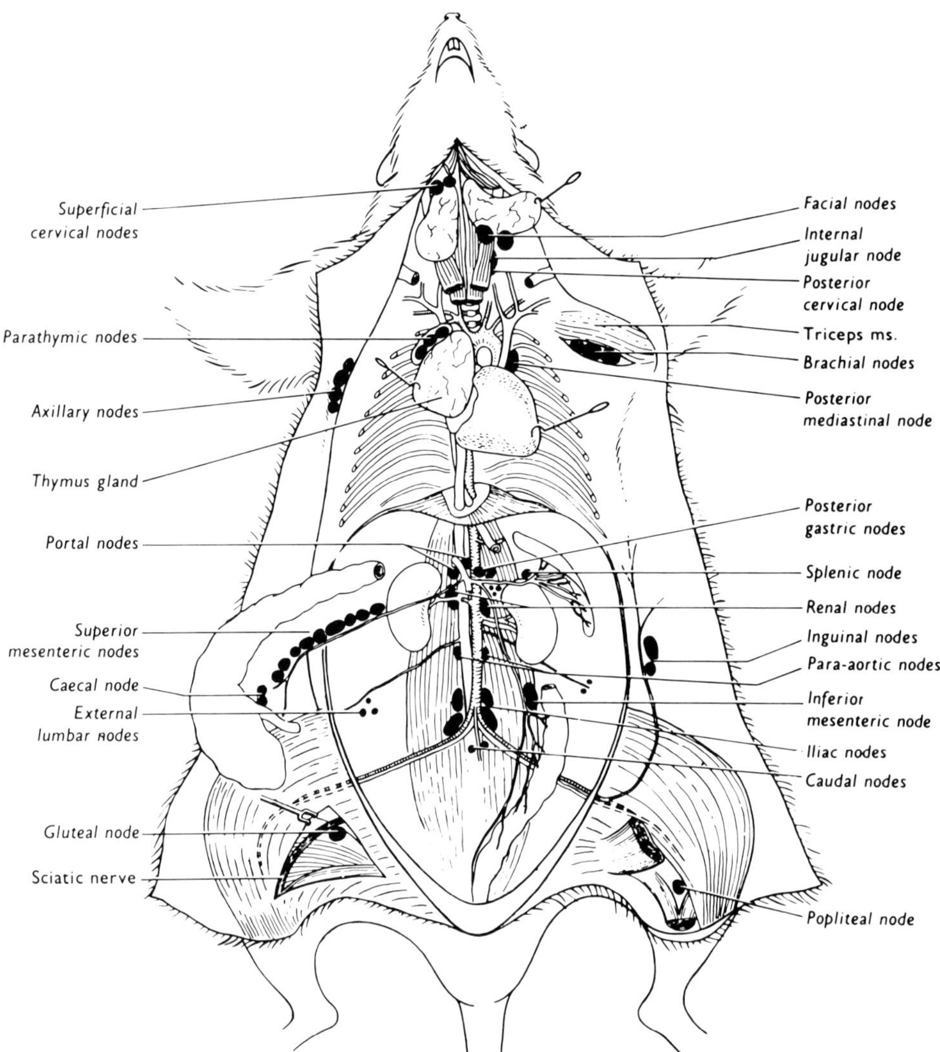

Fig. 124. Lymph nodes, adult rat. Nodes lying dorsally are demonstrated by reflecting muscles and viscera. (Courtesy of N. Tilney (1971), and *Journal of Anatomy*)

these nodes are designated as hemolymph nodes (Andreasen and Gottlieb 1946). Like all other lymph nodes these nodes are interposed in the lymphatic stream and thus possess normal afferent and efferent lymph vessels (Kazeem et al. 1982).

Microscopic Features

Under low magnification of a routine stained section, two major compartments of the lymph nodes can easily be recognized: the cortex at the convex side and the medulla at the side of the hilus (Fig. 125). The cortex is surrounded by the subcapsular sinus, which is connected with the afferent lymph vessels on the one hand and,

Fig. 125 *(upper left).* Mesenteric lymph node, rat. Different compartments of the lymph node: the outer cortex with lymphoid follicles *(F),* the paracortical area *(PA),* and the medulla *(M).* Glutaraldehyde fixed, embedded in epon, stained with toluidine blue, × 100

Fig. 126 *(lower left).* Mesenteric lymph node, rat. Subcapsular sinus *(SS)* containing a veiled cell *(arrow).* Glutaraldehyde fixed, embedded in epon, stained with toluidine blue, × 1810

Fig. 127 *(upper right).* Mesenteric lymph node, rat. Follicle with a lymphocyte corona *(LC)* and a follicle center *(FC).* × 400

Fig. 128 *(lower right).* Mesenteric lymph node, rat. A high endothelial venule in the paracortical area. *E,* endothelial cell; *L,* lymphocyte. Glutaraldehyde fixed, embedded in epon, stained with toluidine blue, × 1000

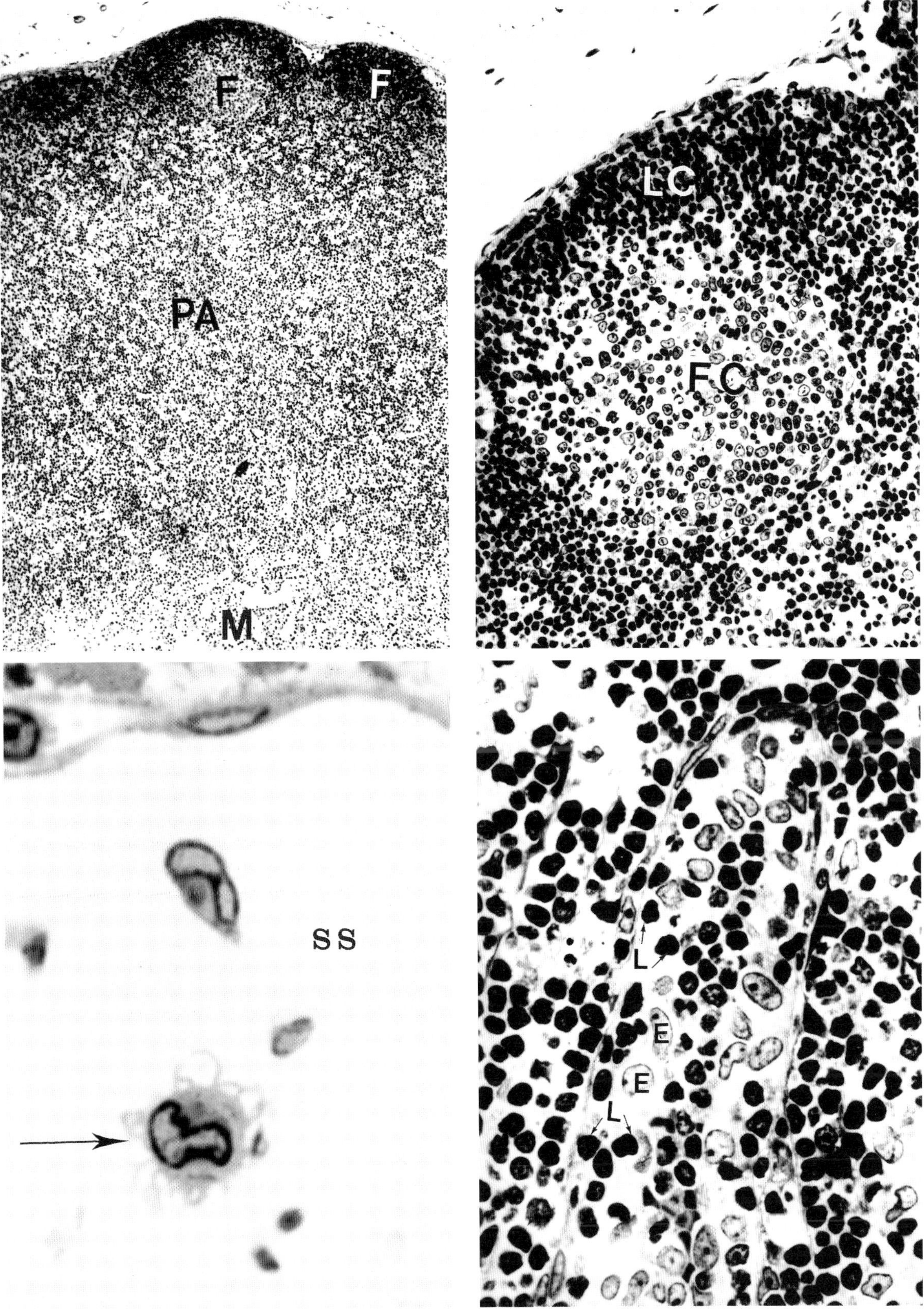
F
F
PA
M
LC
FC
SS
L
E
E
L

132   Christine D. Dijkstra, E. W. A. Kamperdijk, and A. J. P. Veerman

through the cortical (peritrabecular) sinuses, with the medullary sinuses on the other. The cortex is subdivided into an outer and an inner part. The outer cortex contains the lymph follicles and between them the interfollicular areas. The inner part is designated as paracortex (Gutman and Weissman 1972; Goldschneider and McGregor 1973), paracortical areas (Fossum 1980), or deep cortex (Belisle and Sainte-Marie 1981 a) and has been shown by careful tridimensional studies of Belisle and Sainte-Marie (1981 a) to consist of several basic "units." Each of these units is supplied by its own afferent lymph vessels (Belisle and Sainte-Marie 1981 b). Within the medulla, the medullary cords are visible as extensions of the cortical tissue between the medullary sinuses.

Immediately under the marginal sinus, the subsinus layer is comprised of a few superimposed layers of pale reticulum cells interspaced with lymphocytes and macrophages (Fig. 126; Sainte-Marie and Peng 1985). Follicles can be distinguished with small and medium sized lymphocytes in the lymphocyte corona, which surrounds the paler follicular center (Fig. 127). The pale color is due to the large size of the cells present in the center of the follicle. After antigenic stimulation the follicular center contains many blast cells, with pyrinophilic cytoplasm, as well as large macrophages filled with nuclear debris, the tingible body macrophages. Such an active follicle center is designated as a "germinal center". The deep cortex consists of areas with predominantly small lymphocytes. Within each of these fields or units central and peripheral parts can be distinguished by their different cellular composition. The center is characterized by a scarcity of reticular fibers and a high concentration of lymphocytes, whereas the periphery contains a dense reticular network with fewer lymphocytes than the center (Belisle and Sainte-Marie 1981 c). As a characteristic structure the high endothelial venule is present in predominantly the periphery of these fields (Fig. 128). This venule has a wall typically consisting of cuboid or even cylindric endothelial cells. In this endothelial wall, lymphocytes are often seen (Marchesi and Gowans 1964; Schoefl 1972). The medullary cords are compressed between the medullary sinuses as cell-rich strings. After antigenic stimulation of the node these cords contain many plasma cells in their network of reticulum cells. In the medullary sinuses, small lymphocytes and macrophages predominate (Fossum 1980).

Fig. 129 *(upper left).* Popliteal lymph node, rat. Ia-antigen, present on the B lymphocytes in the follicles *(F)* and on the interdigitating cells *(arrows)* in the paracortical area. Acetone-fixed cryostat section, stained in a two-step immunoperoxidase procedure, × 200

Fig. 130 *(lower left).* Popliteal lymph node, rat. Antimacrophage antibody ED3, identifying a rim of macrophages *(arrows)* under the subcapsular sinus as well as the macrophages present in the medulla, follicle *(F)*, and paracortical area *(PA)*. Acetone-fixed cryostat section, stained in a two-step immunoperoxidase procedure, × 200

Fig. 131 *(upper right).* Popliteal lymph node, rat. All T lymphocytes (W3/13) which are mainly confined to the paracortical area *(PA)* and follicle *(F)*. Acetone-fixed cryostat section, stained in a two-step immunoperoxidase procedure, × 200

Fig. 132 *(lower right).* Popliteal lymph node, rat. T suppressor/cytotoxic cells (OX8), present in the same area as clusters of positive cells. (*PA,* paracortical area; *F,* follicles). Acetone-fixed cryostat section, stained in a two-step immunoperoxidase procedure, × 200

Immunohistochemistry

The follicles of the lymph node consist predominantly of B cells (Fig. 129) but also contain a few T cells of the helper phenotype (Barclay 1981 a). The nonlymphocytic cell characteristic for the follicle, the follicular dendritic cell, can be recognized by the appropriate monoclonal antibodies (OX2, Barcley 1981 b; ED5, Jeurissen and Dijkstra 1986; Ki-M4R, Wacker et al. 1987) as a weblike structure within the follicles. Between the follicles T and B lymphocytes occur intermingled as do macrophages, which can be recognized by macrophage-specific monoclonal antibodies (Dijkstra et al. 1985).

Macrophages with a similar phenotype (ED3-positive, ED2-negative) as the marginal zone macrophages of the spleen lie immediately under the subcapsular sinus (subsinusoidal macrophages) extending their processes into the subcapsular area (Dijkstra et al. 1985) (Fig. 130). The paracortex consists predominantly of T cells (W3/13-positive; Fig. 131), the majority of the helper phenotype (W3/25-positive), a minority of the T suppressor/cytotoxic phenotype (OX8-positive; Fig. 132) (Barclay 1981 a). It should be noted that the monoclonal antibodies W3/13 and OX8 can be applied on paraffin-embedded tissues (Dijkstra et al. 1983; Ward et al. 1983). Among these T cells, nonlymphoid cells with extensive cell processes are present. They express high levels of the MHC class II or Ia-antigen

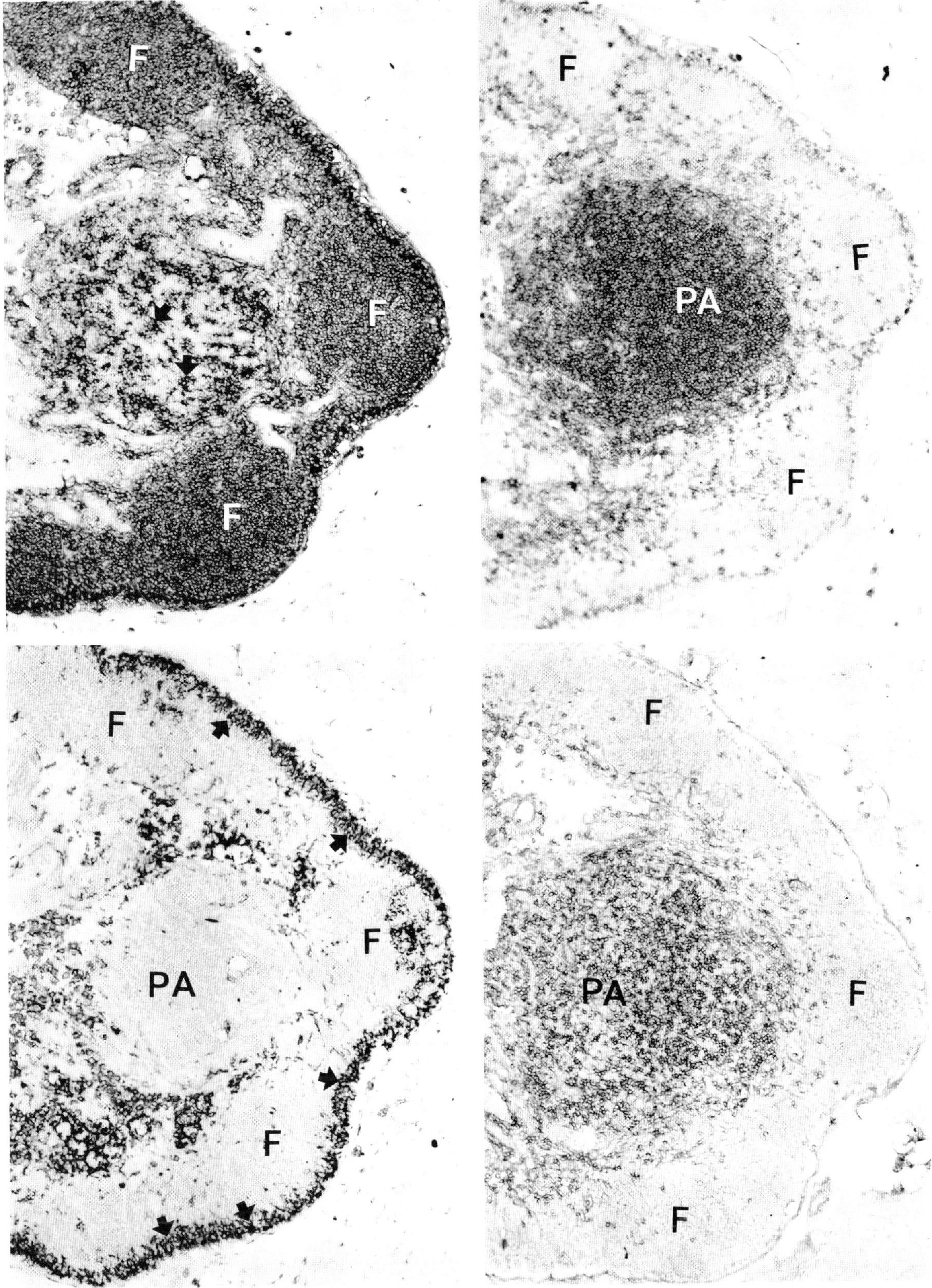

(Fig. 129; Barclay 1981 b). These cells represent the interdigitating cells which were first recognized at the ultrastructural level. In the medullary cords plasma cells and macrophages are the most conspicuous cell types. In the medullary sinuses all types of lymphocytes can be found among a large number of macrophages (ED1- and ED3-positive, a minority also ED2-positive) Dijkstra et al. 1985).

Ultrastructure

Ultrastructural studies are of great value in studying the differentiation of the nonlymphoid cell types of the lymphoid organs. Such investigations reveal that different sinuses contain different cell populations (Fossum 1980). The subcapsular sinus is covered with sinus lining cells and contains, in addition to monocytes and lymphocytes, nonlymphoid cells with an irregularly shaped nucleus and an electron-lucent cytoplasm with numerous cell processes, the so-called veiled cells (Balfour et al. 1981; Fig. 126) and macrophages. The deepley located sinuses contain predominantly small lymphocytes and macrophages (Fossum 1980).

Each of the compartments of the lymph node contains its own characteristic nonlymphoid cell type(s) (Hoefsmit et al. 1980; Fossum and Vaaland 1983). The characteristic nonlymphoid cell in the follicles is the follicular dendritic cell (Nossal et al. 1968). This cell has also been designated as the dendritic reticulum cell, but since the origin of this cell is still under discussion this name seems less appropriate. The follicular dendritic cell probably originates from the reticulum network (Humphrey et al. 1984; Dijkstra et al. 1985). It has characteristic morphological features, in particular extensive slender cell processes which are in intimate contact with the surrounding lymphoid cells (Fig. 133). In well-developed follicular centers these processes have many invaginations covered with electron-dense material (immune complexes; Nossal et al. 1968). The follicular dendritic cell has a quadrangular to multilobulated nucleus with finely dispersed heterochromatin, surrounded by a small rim of cytoplasm. Apart from this highly differentiated cell, the primary follicles (i. e., follicles which have not undergone any antigenic stimulation) contain less differentiated, fibroblastic reticulum cells. The germinal center is surrounded by a rim of flattened reticulum cells forming a sharp demarcation from the corona (Fossum 1980).

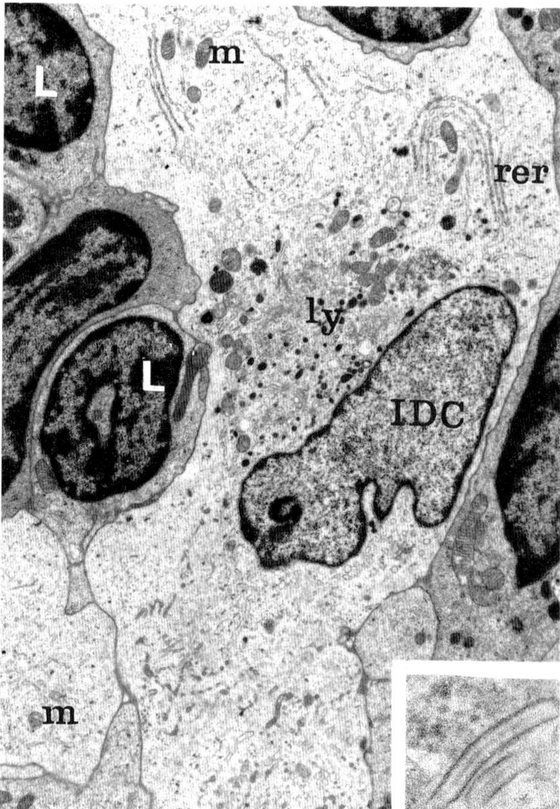

Fig. 133. Popliteal lymph node, rat. Interdigitating cell *(IDC)* in the paracortex. The cytoplasm is electron-lucent and contains mitochondria *(m)* and strands of rough endoplasmic reticulum *(rer)*. Lysosomes *(ly)* are only present in the central part of the cell. *L,* lymphocyte. TEM, ×7350. *Inset:* Birbeck granules, ×88600

In the paracortex the interdigitating cell is characteristic nonlymphoid cell (Veldman 1970). The veiled cells, present in the afferent lymph and in the marginal sinus, are likely to be the precursors of the interdigitating cell (Balfour et al. 1981). These interdigitating cells are considered to belong to the mononuclear phagocyte system (Van Furth et al. 1972) but differ from classic macrophages in many aspects. They have an irregularly shaped nucleus and typically an abundant, electron-lucent cytoplasm with fingerlike projections toward the surrounding lymphocytes (Veldman 1970; Kamperdijk et al. 1978, Hoefsmit et al. 1982; Fig. 134). In the center of the interdigitating cell a well-developed Golgi complex is usually present. The phagolysosomal apparatus is only poorly developed in comparison with macrophages and, in contrast to macrophages, is located in a central spot near the nucleus. In lymph nodes which drain epithelial tissue, the cytoplasm of some of the interdigitating cells con-

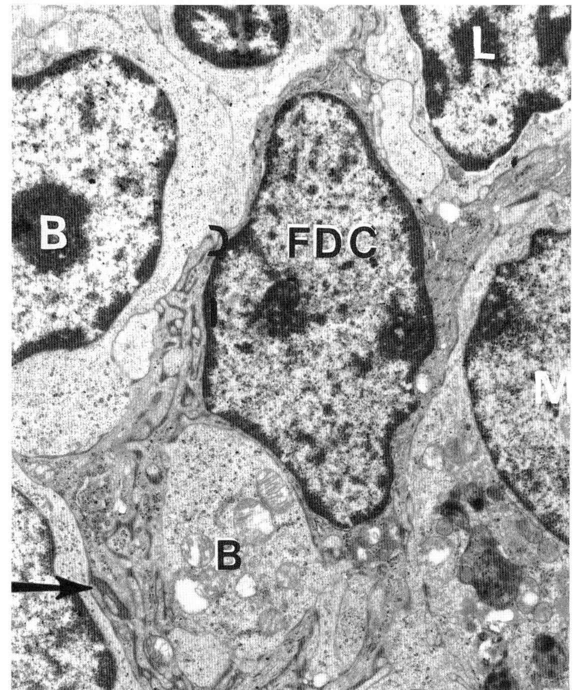

Fig. 134. Popliteal lymph node, rat. Follicular dendritic cell *(FDC)* in follicle center. The cytoplasm has many fine ramifications between lymphocytes *(L)* and lymphoblasts *(B)*. Electron-dense material, probably antigen-antibody complexes, is present in invaginations of the cell membrane *(arrow)*. *M,* macrophage. × 7520

tains so-called Birbeck granules, the characteristic cell organelles for Langerhans' cells (Birbeck et al. 1961).

The granules are especially evident shortly after stimulation of the lymph node (Kamperdijk et al. 1978). They are rod-shaped structures with rounded ends, limited by a membrane of approximately 6 nm thickness (Fig. 133, inset).

So-called dendritic cells, nonlymphoid cells with features of interdigitating and related cells, may be proportionately increased in cell suspensions of lymphoid organs by appropriate methods (Steinman and Cohn 1973; Kamperdijk et al. 1985).

The mode of migration of lymphocytes from the lumen of the high endothelial venule into the paracortex is still under discussion (Kraal et al. 1987). Some authors (Marchesi and Gowans 1964), using ultrastructural techniques, suggest that lymphocytes migrate through the cytoplasm of the endothelial cells. Others, using the same technique, describe migration of lymphocytes only between endothelial cells (Schoefl 1972).

Comparison with Other Species

Grossly, the architecture of the lymph nodes is similar in different mammalian species. Also the distribution of the different cell types in the lymph nodes of mice as assessed by immunohistochemical studies is very similar to that in the rat (Gutman and Weissman 1972; Hoffman-Fezer et al. 1976).

References

Andreasen E, Gottlieb O (1946) Haemolymph nodes of the rat. Danske Videnskabernes Selskal Biologishe Meddeleiser 19: 3–27

Balfour BM, Drexhage HA, Kamperdijk EWA, Hoefsmit ECM (1981) Antigen-presenting cells, including Langerhans cells, veiled cells and interdigitating cells. In: Microenvironments in haemopoietic and lymphoid differentiation. Ciba Found Symp 84: 281–301

Barclay AN (1981 a) The localization of populations of lymphozytes defined by monoclonal antibodies in rat lymphoid tissues. Immunology 42: 539–600

Barclay AN (1981 b) Different reticular elements in rat lymphoid tissue identified by localization of Ia, Thy-1 and MRC OX 2 antigens. Immunology 44: 727–736

Bélisle C, Sainte-Marie G (1981 a) Tridimensional study of the deep cortex of the rat lymph node. I. Topography of the deep cortex. Anat Rec 199: 45–59

Bélisle C, Sainte-Marie G (1981 b) Tridimensional study of the deep cortex of the rat lymph node. II. Relation of deep cortex units to afferent lymphatic vessels. Anat Rec 199: 61–72

Bélisle C, Sainte-Marie G (1981 c) Tridimensional study of the deep cortex of the rat lymph node. III. Morphology of the deep cortex units. Anat Rec 199: 213–226

Birbeck MS, Breathnach AS, Everall JD (1961) An electron microscope study of basal melanocytes and high-level clear cells (Langerhans cells) in vitiligo. J Invest Dermatol 37: 51–64

Dijkstra CD, Döpp EA, Langevoort HL (1983) Regeneration of splenic tissue after autologous implantation: homing of T- and B- and Ia-positive cells in the white pulp of the rat spleen. Cell Tissue Res 229: 97–107

Dijkstra CD, Döpp EA, Joling P, Kraal G (1985) The heterogeneity of mononuclear phagocytes in lymphoid organs: distinct macrophage subpopulations in the rat recognized by monoclonal antibodies ED1, ED2 and ED3. Immunology 54: 589–599

Fossum S (1980) The architecture of rat lymph nodes. II. Lymph node compartments. Scand J Immunol 12: 411–420

Fossum S, Vaaland JL (1983) The architecture of rat lymph nodes. I. Combined light and electron microscopy of lymph node cell types. Anat Embryol 167: 229–246

Goldschneider I, McGregor DD (1973) Anatomical distribution of T and B lymphocytes in the rat. J Exp Med 138: 1443–1465

Gutman GA, Weissman IL (1972) Lymphoid tissue architecture; experimental analysis of the origin and distribution of T-cells and B-cells. Immunology 23: 465–479

Hoefsmit ECM, Kamperdijk EWA, Hendriks HR, Beelen RHJ, Balfour BM (1980) Lymph node macrophages. In: Carr I, Daems WT (eds) The Reticuloendothelial System, vol I. Plenum, New York

Hoefsmit ECM, Duijvestijn AM, Kamperdijk EW (1982) Relation between Langerhans cells, veiled cells and interdigitating cells. Immunobiology 161: 255–265

Hoffman-Fezer G, Rodt H, Eulitz M, Thierfelder S (1976) Immunohistochemical identification of T and B cells delineated by unlabelled antibody enzyme method. I. Anatomical distribution of 0-positive and Ig-positive cells in lymphoid organs of mice. J Immunol Methods 13: 261–270

Humphrey JK, Grennan D, Sundarum V (1984) The origin of the follicular dendritic cells in the mouse and the mechanism of trapping immune complexes on them. Eur J Immunol 14: 859–864

Jeurissen SHM, Dijkstra CD (1986) Characteristics and functional aspects of non-lymphoid cells in rat germinal centers, recognized by two monoclonal antibodies ED5 and ED6. Eur J Immunol 16: 562–568

Kamperdijk EWA, Raaymakers EM, de Leeuw JH, Hoefsmit ED (1978) Lymph node macrophages and reticulum cells in the immune response. I. The primary response to paratyphoid vaccine. Cell Tissue Res 192: 1–23

Kamperdijk EWA, Kapsenberg ML, Van den Berg M, Hoefsmit ECM (1985) Characterization of dendritic cells, isolated from normal and stimulated lymph nodes of the rat. Cell Tissue Res 242: 469–474

Kazeem AA, Reid O, Scothorne RJ (1982) Studies on hemolymph nodes. I. Histology of the renal hemolymph node of the rat. J Anat 134 (Part 4): 677–683

Kraal G, Duijvestijn AM, Hendriks HR (1987) The endothelium of the high endothelial venule: a specialized endothelium with unique properties. Exp Cell Biol 55: 1–10

Marchesi VT, Gowans JL (1964) The migration of lymphocytes through the endothelium of venules in lymph nodes: an electron microscope study. Proc R Soc Ser B 159: 283–290

Nossal GJ, Abbot A, Mitchell J, Lummus Z (1968) Antigens in immunity. XV. Ultrastructural features of antigen capture in primary and secondary lymphoid follicles. J Exp Med 127: 277–290

Sainte-Marie G, Peng F-S (1985) Evidence for the existance of a subsinus layer of the peripheral cortex in the lymph node of the rat. Cell Tissue Res 239: 37–42

Schoefl GI (1972) The migration of lymphocytes across the vascular endothelium in lymphoid tissue. J Exp Med 136: 568–588

Steinman RM, Cohn ZA (1973) Identification of a novel cell type in peripheral lymphoid organs of mice. I. Morphology, quantitation, tissue distribution. J Exp Med 137: 1142–1162

Tilney NL (1971) Patterns of lymphatic drainage in the adult laboratory rat. J Anat 109: 369–383

Van Furth R, Cohn ZA, Hirsch JG, Humphrey JH, Spector WG, Langevoort HL (1972) The mononuclear phagocyte system: a new classification of macrophages, monocytes and their precursor cells. Bull WHO 46: 845–852

Veldman JE (1970) Histophysiology and electron microscopy of the immune response. Dijkstra Niemeyer, Groningen

Wacker H-H, Radzun HJ, Mielke V, Parwaresh MR (1987) Selective recognition of rat follicular dendritic cells (dendritic reticulum cells) by a new monoclonal antibody Ki-M4R in vitro and in vivo. J Leukocyte Biol 41: 70–77

Ward JM, Argilan F, Reynolds CW (1983) Immunoperoxidase localization of large granular lymphocytes in normal tissues and lesions of athymic nude rats. J Immunol 131: 132–139

Classification of Mouse Lymphoid Cell Neoplasms

Paul K. Pattengale

Pattengale-Taylor Classification

Following recent advances in the reclassification of human lymphoid cell neoplasms (Lukes and Collins 1975; Lennert et al. 1975), Pattengale and Taylor (1983) have reclassified murine lymphoid cell neoplasms using a newer immunomorphologic schema that is biologically and scientifically more accurate than previous classifications. This proposed classification can be easily taught, easily learned, is reproducible, and, because lymphoproliferative disease in the mouse closely resembles that of humans, it is clinically useful.

This classification is based on the concept that the immune system in the mouse, as in humans, is divided into T and B cell compartments, and that lymphoid cell neoplasms (lymphomas) represent neoplastic conversions of B or T cells. It is therefore logical to classify lymphomas and related leukemias in the mouse as either B- or T-cell type, with regard to their morphology, location, and functional characteristics. We attempted to correlate the morphology of the neoplastic lymphoid cells in the mouse with their B or T cell nature in a manner somewhat analogous to that proposed for the corresponding lymphomas in humans. This proposed immunomorphologic classification (Pattengale and Taylor 1981) (Table 36) presently lists five major morphologic cell types. It should be stressed that the diagnosis of lymphoma/leukemia is based first on morphologic criteria and is then subsequently combined with immunological phenotype. The B cell (lymphocyte) is defined as having easily detectable surface and/or cytoplasmic immunoglobulin (Ig); a T cell (lymphocyte) is defined as having easily detectable surface Thy-1; and a non-B, non-T cell is considered to be a phenotypically silent neoplastic lymphoid cell, which is defined as lacking both easily detectable surface Thy-1 and surface and/or cytoplasmic Ig. With regard to this latter and conceptually troublesome non-B, non-T category, it is becoming increasingly

Table 36. Immunomorphologic classification of murine lymphoma and related leukemias as proposed by Pattengale and Taylor (1981)[a]

Morphologic type[b] (lymphoid cell morphology)	Immunologic type[c]		
	B cell	T cell	Non-B, non-T cell
Follicular center cell[d]			
Small cell type	+	0	0
Large cell type	+	0	0
Large and small (mixed) type	+	0	0
Plasma cell	+	0	0
Immunoblast	+	+	+
Small lymphocyte	+	(+)	(+)
Lymphoblast	+[e]	+	+

[a] The proposed classification refers only to lymphoid cell, lymphocyte-derived neoplasms and therefore excludes those derived from the monocyte/macrophage/histiocyte series (i.e., true histiocytic lymphoma). It is also stressed that the diagnosis of lymphoma/leukemia is based primarily on morphologic criteria and is then subsequently combined with immunologically based parameters.

[b] The morphologic cell types listed are those which have been observed and documented to date. If this is analogous to humans, one would expect to observe additional cell types such as the cerebriform lymphocyte (i.e., Sézary-mycosis fungoides T cell) and the plasmacytoid B lymphocyte (i.e., Waldenström's macroglobulinemia).

[c] B cell is defined as having easily detectable surface and/or cytoplasmic Ig; T cell is defined as having easily detectable surface Thy-1 (i.e., theta antigen); non-B, non-T cell is defined as lacking both easily detectable Thy-1 and surface and/or cytoplasmic Ig. +, already observed and documented; (+), not yet observed, but expected; 0, not observed or expected.

[d] Follicular center cell (FCC) lymphomas with a marked lymph node follicular pattern analogous to those appearing in humans have not yet been well documented. FCC lymphomas may also contain equally prominent mixtures of both large and small FCC type [FCC lymphoma (mixed) large and small cell types].

[e] Lymphoblastic lymphoma of B cells is considered by some to be a follicular center cell (FCC) lymphoma and by others to be a separate category. In either event, it closely resembles the Burkitt's lymphoma spectrum.

clear, using newer Southern blotting techniques which detect T or B cell-specific gene rearrangements at the DNA level (Seidman et al. 1979; Arnold et al. 1983; Marx 1985), that this phenotypically silent group of lymphoid cell neoplasms may actually be designated or defined as T or B cell-derived based on genomic DNA analysis. Also, as seen in Table 36, follicular center cell ans plasma cell lymphomas are, by definition, B-cell proliferations that are morphologically distinct.

In contrast, lymphomas of small lymphocytes, immunoblasts, and lymphoblasts are often morphologically subtle and require immunologic confirmation as to their T-, B-, non-B-, or non-T-cell nature. It is believed that with time and experience, skilled morphologic evaluation will be predictive of the immunologic type. For example, if an immunoblastic proliferation contains large, transformed lymphocytes (i. e., immunoblasts) with prominent amphophilic cytoplasm and plasmacytoid features, it would be logical to classify the lesion presumptively as an immunoblastic lymphoma of B cells (see Fig. 140). Immunologic demonstration of cytoplasmic immunoglobulin (CIg) with the use of immunoperoxidase and/or immunofluorescence techniques would then confirm the lesion as a B-cell process (see p. 122, this volume).

The scientific accuracy of this neoplastic lymphoid cell classification has also allowed us to make definitive statements about lymphoid cell differentiation, particularly with regard to B cells. If one believes that lymphomas represent arrests or stops in the differentiation pathway, one can obtain reasonably homogenous populations of B cell types at various stages of differentiation. Lymphomas or lymphoid cell neoplasms have therefore been powerful tools in understanding the immunobiology of their normal B cell counterparts.

Lymphoid progenitor cells can go to either the B or T cell arm, depending on how the cell rearranges its DNA (Seidman et al. 1979; Marx 1985). If it goes to the B cell side, which starts with the pre-B series, it will rearrange its immunoglobulin genes (heavy μ followed by light followed by light) and express μ heavy chain in its cytoplasm. The earliest B cell to have an easily detectable surface Ig is an early or immature B cell which has surface IgM associated with one of the light chains. Lymphomas of early or immature B cells, which are called by some (Lennert et al. 1975) B cell lymphoblastic lymphomas and by others (Lukes and Collins 1975) small

noncleaved follicular cell lymphomas, are the Burkitt's lymphoma types. One can also observe lymphoblastic morphology in the pre-B series. Mature, virgin B cells have the morphology of small resting lymphocytes. Lymphomas of small lymphocytes [chronic lymphocyte leukemia (CLL) cells], similar to mature, virgin B cells, co-express surface IgM and IgD. FCC lymphomas are further along in B-cell differentiation and most often have class-switched to other Ig classes (usually IgG and IgA), which can now be easily detected in the cytoplasm. Lymphomas of B immunoblasts and plasma cells are characterized as postfollicular B cells, which are closer to terminal differentiation and are actively secreting Ig protein products.

Clearly, these B cell neoplasms have resulted in a more precise definition of morphologic B cell subtypes which has a direct application to B-cell differentiation. This has also been applied to frozen section methodology using monoclonal antibodies, which relates precise phenotypic characterization to intact histopathologic microanatomy (see p. 111, this volume).

Similar to human lymphoid cell neoplasms, neoplastic lymphocytic proliferations in the mouse may occur as a lymphoma (involving primarily lymph nodes and splenic white pulp) and/or a leukemia (involving primarily bone marrow, peripheral blood, and splenic red pulp). As with humans, this distinction can be, at times, rather difficult and somewhat arbitrary. I would prefer not to distinguish between lymphomas and leukemias in the mouse but simply to refer to them as lymphomas and designate them as either being leukemic or nonleukemic.

The cytologic and histologic features of the various murine lymphoid cell types are illustrated in Figs. 135–143. Using cell size, cytoplasmic and nuclear characteristics, mitotic activity, and pattern of tissue involvement, one can usually discriminate between the various cell types, provided that the tissue is adequately fixed and appropriately processed. In this context, mercury-containing fixatives (B-5) or Bouin's fixative and thin (1–3 μm) sections are essential for the proper evaluation of lymphoid cell proliferations (Bowling 1979) and demonstration of immunoglobulins. It should be further stressed that formalin fixation is less than optimal, since it induces both nuclear and cytoplasmic shrinkage artifacts. It may therefore be difficult in formalin-fixed tissues to distinguish a lymphoma of small lymphocytes from a lymphoma of lymphoblasts, both of which are noncohesive in tissue section, have

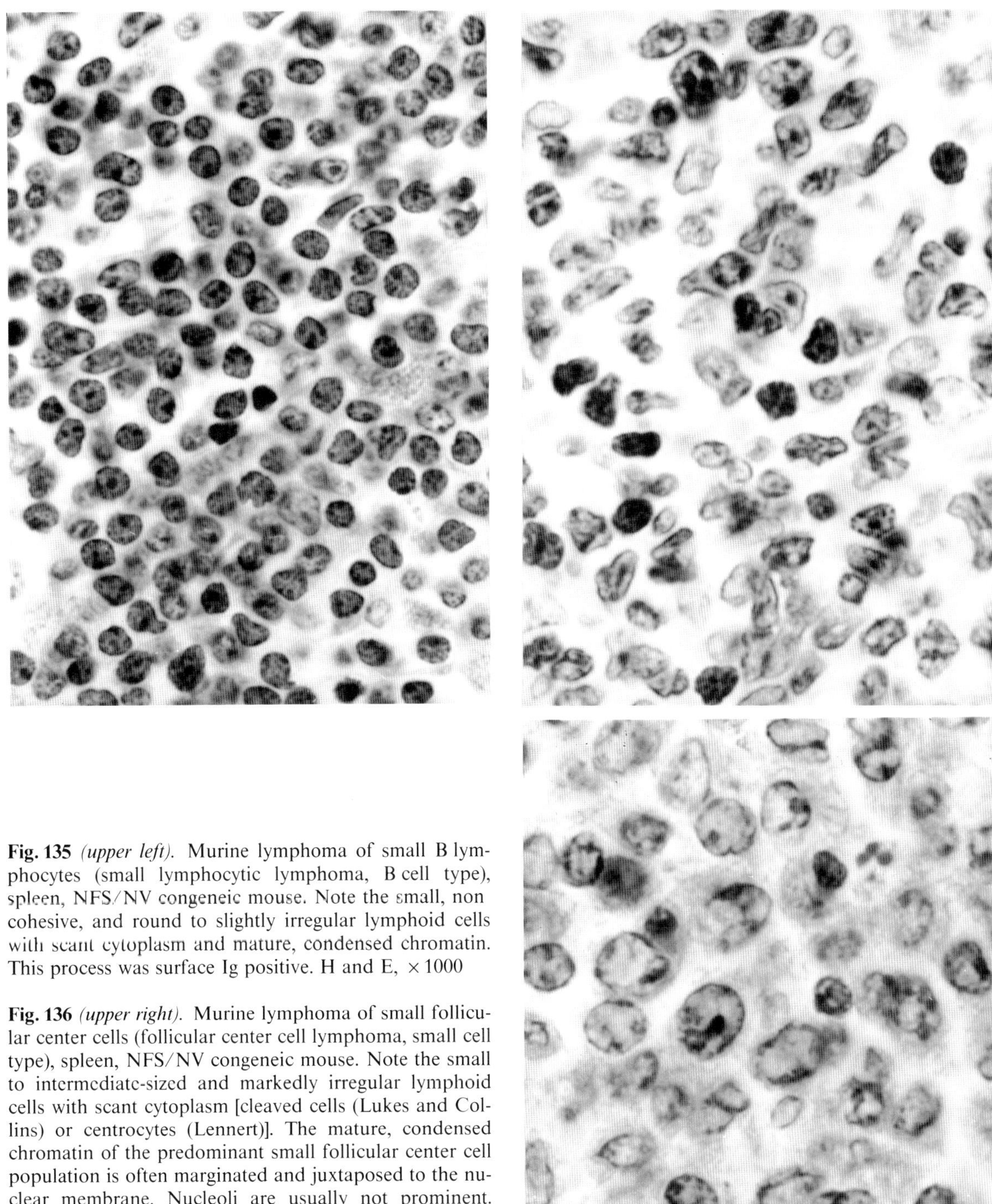

Fig. 135 *(upper left)*. Murine lymphoma of small B lymphocytes (small lymphocytic lymphoma, B cell type), spleen, NFS/NV congeneic mouse. Note the small, non cohesive, and round to slightly irregular lymphoid cells with scant cytoplasm and mature, condensed chromatin. This process was surface Ig positive. H and E, × 1000

Fig. 136 *(upper right)*. Murine lymphoma of small follicular center cells (follicular center cell lymphoma, small cell type), spleen, NFS/NV congeneic mouse. Note the small to intermediate-sized and markedly irregular lymphoid cells with scant cytoplasm [cleaved cells (Lukes and Collins) or centrocytes (Lennert)]. The mature, condensed chromatin of the predominant small follicular center cell population is often marginated and juxtaposed to the nuclear membrane. Nucleoli are usually not prominent. These cells were surface Ig positive. H and E, × 1000

Fig. 137 *(lower right)*. Murine lymphoma of large follicular center cells (follicular center cell lymphoma, large noncleaved cell type), lymph node, BALB/c mouse. Note the predominance of intermediate to large, cohesive lymphoid cells with rounded (noncleaved), vesicular nuclei. These cells stained positive for cytoplasmic immunoglobulin. H and E, × 1000

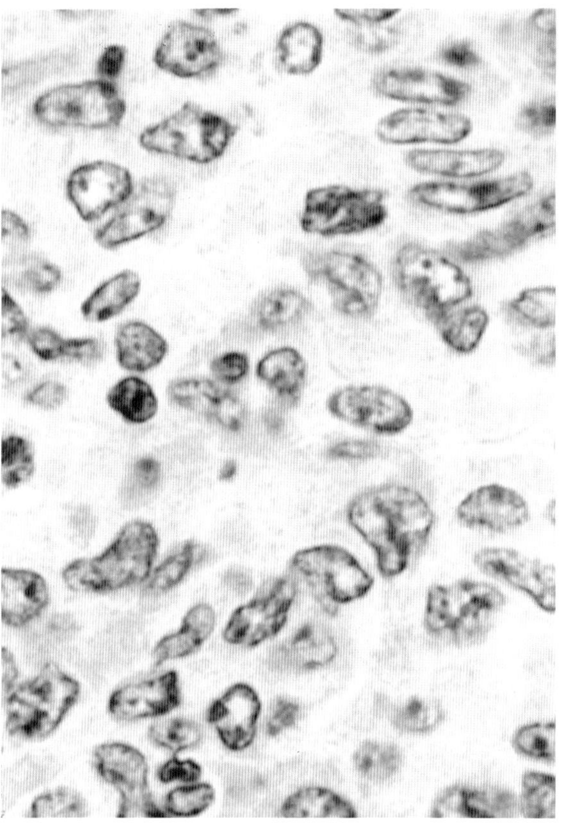

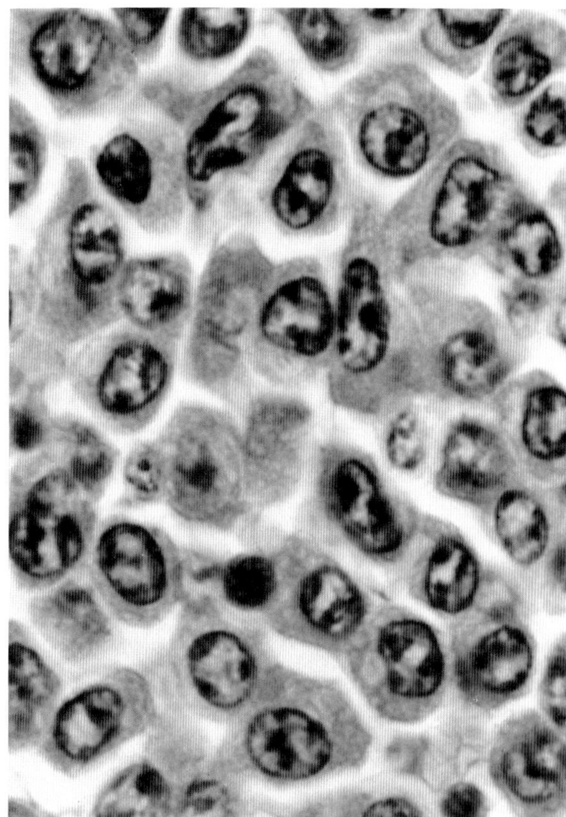

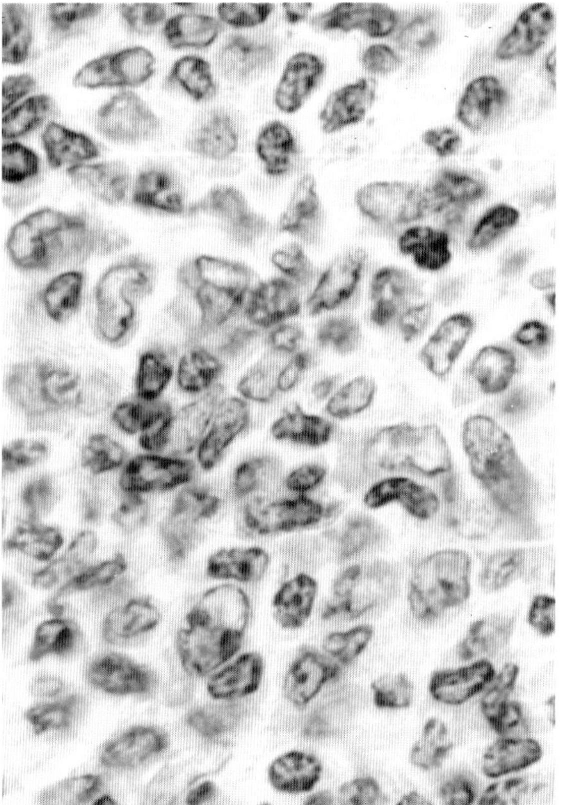

Fig. 138 *(upper left)*. Murine lymphoma of large follicular center cells (follicular center cell lymphoma, large cleaved cell type), spleen, NFS/NV congeneic mouse. Note the predominance of intermediate to large, cohesive lymphoid cells with irregularly shaped, notched (cleaved) nuclei and moderate amounts of cytoplasm. Similar to small follicular center cell populations, the chromatin is often condensed and marginated on the nuclear membrane. These cells stained positively for cytoplasmic immunoglobulin. H and E, × 1000

Fig. 139 *(lower left)*. Murine lymphoma of large and small (mixed) follicular center cells [follicular center cell lymphoma, large and small (mixed) cell type], spleen, NFS/NV congeneic mouse. Note the almost equal proportions of small and large follicular center cells. These cells stained positively for cytoplasmic Ig. H and E, × 1000

Fig. 140 *(upper right)*. Murine lymphoma of B immunoblasts [immunoblastic lymphoma (sarcoma), B cell type], BALB/c mouse. Note the monomorphous population of noncohesive, large lymphoid cells with round to oval, vesicular nuclei with prominent and distinct nucleoli and abundant, conspicuous cytoplasm. Also note the amphophilic cytoplasms and plasmacytoid features. These cells were positive for cytoplasmic Ig. H and E, × 900

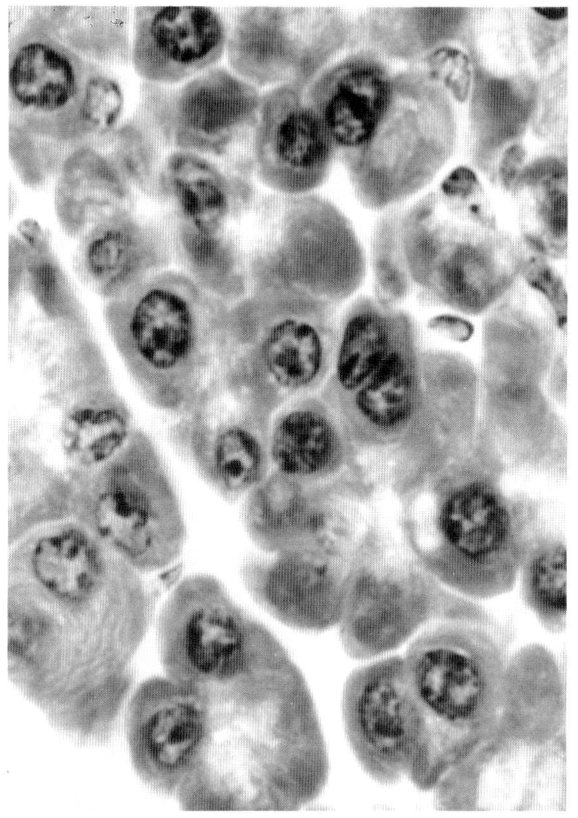

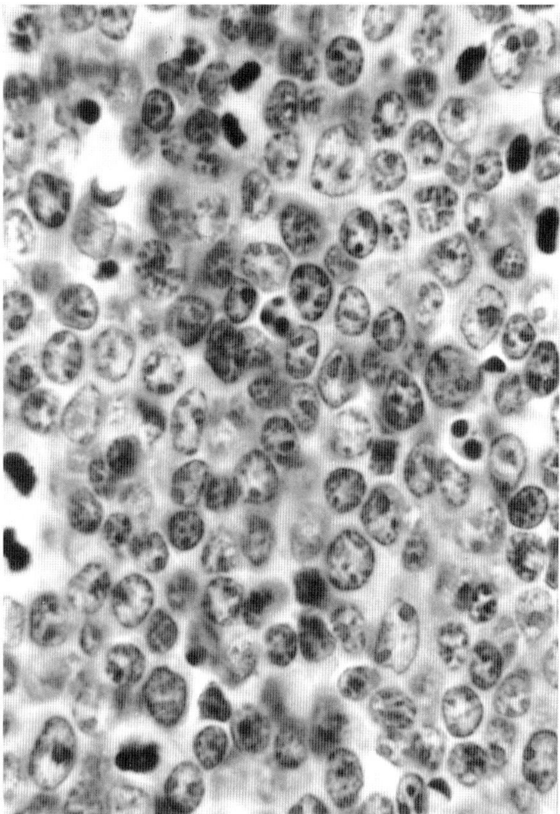

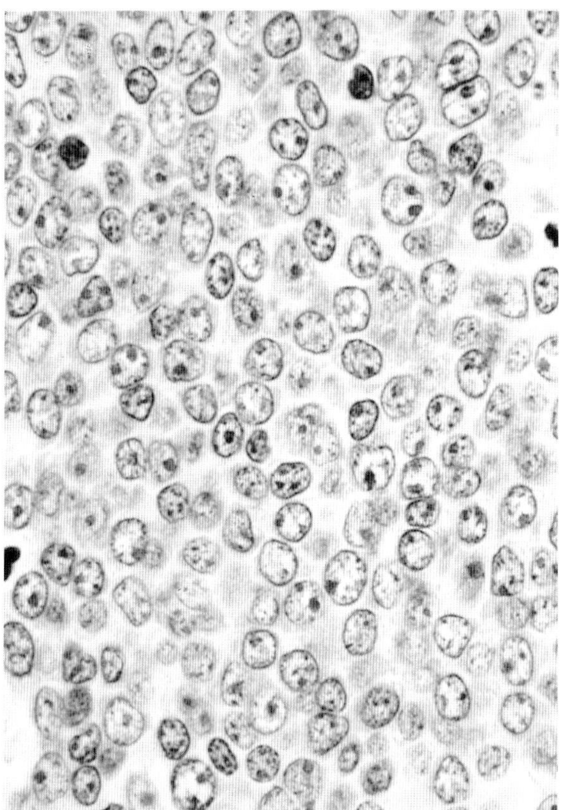

Fig. 141 *(upper left)*. Murine lymphoma of plasma cells (plasma cell lymphoma; plasmacytoma), BALB/c mouse. Note the population of plasma cells with dense, amphophilic cytoplasm and eccentric nuclei with clock-faced chromatin. Also note the presence of occasional prominent nucleoli. These cells stained positively for cytoplasmic Ig. H and E, × 1000

Figs. 142 *(upper right)*, **143** *(lower right)*. In both B and T cell types note the monomorphic, mitotically active, population of intermediate-sized lymphoblasts with rounded to oval nuclei and immature chromatin. B lymphoblasts often have conspicuous, multiple, often central nucleoli and stain positively for surface Ig. T lymphoblasts stain positively for Thy-1

Fig. 142. Murine lymphoma of lymphoblasts (lymphoblastic lymphoma) B cell type, spleen, NFS/NV congeneic mouse. These cells stained positively for Ig. H and E, × 1000

Fig. 143. Murine lymphoma of lymphoblasts, thymus, radiation-leukemia virus induced, C57BL/6 mouse. Lymphoblastic lymphoma, T cell type. These cells stained positively for Thy-1. H and E, × 900 scant cytoplasm, and a high nuclear to cytoplasmic ratio. With proper fixation, however, one can distinguish the primitive, rapidly dividing lymphoblast by its immature, finely dispersed nuclear chromatin (Figs. 142, 143) as compared with the slowly dividing small lymphocyte with its mature, clumped, and condensed nuclear chromatin (Fig. 135). Other pertinent examples include the distinction of large follicular center cells (Figs. 137, 138) from immunoblasts (Fig. 140) on cytoplasmic and nuclear to cytoplasmic ratio criteria, as well as the distinction of small lymphocytes (Fig. 135) from small follicular center cells (Fig. 136) on the basis of nuclear cleavage planes. For further details please refer to my previous publications (Pattengale and Frith 1983; Pattengale and Taylor 1983; Frith et al. 1985; Pattengale and Frith 1986).

Comparison of the Pattengale-Taylor Classification (1981) with Earlier Classifications

The *Dunn classification* (Dunn 1954, Table 37) compares the morphologic classification of Dunn (1954) with the neoplastic lymphoid cell types defined by Pattengale et al. (Pattengale and Taylor 1983; Pattengale and Frith 1983; Pattengale and Taylor 1981; Frederickson et al. 1985) and demonstrates that there is considerable heterogeneity within the "lymphocytic" and "reticulum cell neoplasm" categories of Dunn. Since this classification was based primarily on cell size, no distinction was made, for example, between lymphomas of lymphoblasts and small lymphocytes, each of which has a distinct and characteristic biological behavior. Small lymphocytic lymphomas are low-grade, mitotically inactive, lymphoid cell neoplasms occurring rarely in mice. In contrast, lymphoblastic lymphomas are high-grade, rapidly dividing, malignant, lymphoid cell neoplasms that occur frequently in mice. It should be noted that reticulum cell neoplasm (RCN) type B includes both lymphomatous (mixed follicular center cell and immunoblastic types) and prelymphomatous conditions of the non-Hodgkin's type (Pattengale and Taylor 1983), and that these conditions can occasionally bear a superficial resemblance to Hodgkin's disease (Taylor 1976). To the best of my knowledge, there is no available mouse model for Hodgkin's lymphoma at the present time.

It should also be emphasized that the vast majority of lesions designated as RCN type A by Dunn are actually true histiocytic sarcomas and

Table 37. Comparison of the Dunn and Pattengale-Taylor classifications for murine lymphomas and related leukemias[a]

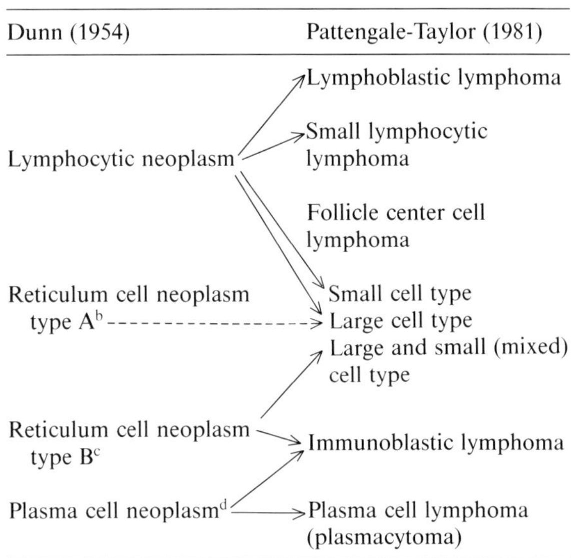

[a] As proposed by Dunn, lymphocytic neoplasms can be localized (i.e., lymphoma) or generalized (i.e., leukemia), involving the peripheral blood and bone marrow compartments. By comparison and direct analogy, lymphomas of lymphoblasts, small lymphocytes, and follicle center cells can manifest with leukemic phases (i.e., lymphoma/leukemias). Reticulum cell neoplasm (RCN) type C is considered by Dunn to be nonneoplastic and nonlymphoid in origin.

[b] The majority of RCN type A as proposed by Dunn are considered to be derived from true histiocytic cells (i.e., true nonlymphoid, phagocytic histiocytes) and can rarely present as a monocytic leukemia. The dotted line stresses the fact that a minority of tumors morphologically classified as RCN type A may represent large follicular center cell (FCC) lymphomas.

[c] Although RCN type B is now considered not to be representative of Hodgkin's disease, it can include both prelymphomatous, non-neoplastic lymphoproliferations and true lymphoid cell lymphomas (mixed FCC and immunoblastic cell types). A lymphoma is defined as a malignant lymphoid cell neoplasm (i.e., an autonomous monoclonal new growth, presumably derived from one cell). In contrast, a prelymphoma is defined as a conditioned, atypical, lymphoid cell hyperplasia derived from more than one cell (nonmonoclonal, oligoclonal, or polyclonal derivation) with a propensity to progress to a true lymphoid cell neoplasm with time.

[d] As stated by Dunn, a proportion of plasma cell neoplasms were formed by typical, well-differentiated plasma cells, while others were formed of a cell type resembling a reticulum cell (i.e., a B immunoblast with plasmacytoid features). This concept is in agreement with the Rask-Nielson classification of plasma cell neoplasms. It should be noted that the term plasma cell leukemia was used to denote a localized growth (lymphoma). True plasma cell leukemia with peripheral blood and bone marrow involvement is rare.

are derived from non-lymphoid, macrophage/histiocytic cells.

In the *Wogan (study group) classification* (1980; Wogan 1984) as depicted in Table 38 which compares the morphologic classification of Squire, Ward, Ferrell, and Grice in the Wogan study group with that of Pattengale et al. (Pattengale and Taylor 1983; Pattengale and Frith 1983; Pattengale and Taylor 1981), a similar spectrum of heterogeneity (as observed in the Dunn classification, Dunn 1954) exists among the lymphocytic and pleomorphic lymphoma designations. Although an attempt is made to update the Dunn classification along the lines of the Rappaport classification (Rappaport 1966) for human lymphomas (i. e., undifferentiated, well-differentiated, poorly differentiated, mixed, and histiocytic types), the Wogan classification (Wogan 1984) still relies primarily on cell size. This classification is commonly used in the USA by pathologists involved in rodent toxicology and carcinogenesis bioassays.

Although useful and somewhat easy to use, the Rappaport and Wogan classifications do not take into consideration the recent advances in our understanding of the two-armed immune system (B and T lymphocytes). For these reasons, the Lukes-Collins (1975) and Kiel (Lennert et al. 1975) classifications were proposed for humans, and the Pattengale-Taylor-Frith (Pattengale and Taylor 1983; Pattengale and Frith 1983; Pattengale and Taylor 1981) classification was proposed for the mouse.

References

Arnold A, Cossman J, Bakhshi A, Jaffe ES, Waldmann TA, Korsmeyer SJ (1983) Immunoglobulin-gene rearrangements as unique clonal markers in human lymphoid neoplasms. N Engl J Med 309: 1593–1599

Bowling MC (1979) Lymph node specimens: achieving technical excellence. Lab Med 10: 467–476

Dunn TB (1954) Normal and pathologic anatomy of the reticular tissue in laboratory mice, with a classification and discussion of neoplasms. JNCI 14: 1281–1433

Frederickson TN, Morse HC III, Yetter RA, Rowe WP, Hartley JW, Pattengale PK (1985) Multiparameter analysis of spontaneous non-thymic lymphomas occurring in NFS/N mice congenic for ecotropic murine leukemia viruses. Am J Pathol 121: 349–360

Frith CH, Pattengale PK, Ward JR (1985) A color atlas of hematopoietic pathology of mice. Toxicology Pathology Associates, Little Rock

Lennert K, Stein H, Kaiserling E (1975) Cytological and functional criteria for the classification of malignant lymphomata. Br J Cancer 31 (Suppl 2): 29–42

Lukes RJ, Collins RD (1975) New approaches to the classification of the lymphomata. Br J Cancer 31 (Suppl 2): 1–28

Table 38. Comparison of the Wogan study group and Pattengale-Taylor classifications for murine lymphoid cell neoplasms and related leukemias

Wogan (1984)[a]	Pattengale-Taylor (1981)
Lymphoma, undifferentiated cell type	→ Lymphoblastic lymphoma
Lymphoma, lymphocytic type	Small lymphocytic lymphoma Follicle center cell lymphoma → Small cell type → Large cell type Large and small (mixed) cell type
Lymphoma, pleomorphic type	→ Immunoblastic lymphoma Plasma cell lymphoma (plasmacytoma)

[a] This classification also lists two additional categories: lymphoma, not otherwise specified (NOS) and lymphocytic leukemia. Localized plasmacytomas are considered as a separate hemopoietic neoplasm and are not considered lymphoid neoplasms. In evaluating leukemic involvement of lymphoid cell neoplasms, please refer to footnote a in Table 37 and text.

Marx JL (1985) The T-cell receptor – the genes and beyond. Science 227: 733–735

Pattengale PK, Frith CH (1983) Immunomorphologic classification of spontaneous lymphoid cell neoplasms occurring in female BALB/c mice. JNCI 70: 169–179

Pattengale PK, Frith CH (1986) Contributions of recent research to the classification of spontaneous lymphoid cell neoplasms in mice. CRC Crit Rev Toxicol 16. 185–212

Pattengale PK, Taylor CR (1983) Experimental models of lymphoproliferative disease: the mouse as a model for human non-Hodgkin's lymphomas and related leukemias. Am J Pathol 113: 237–265

Pattengale PK, Taylor CR (1981) Immunomorphologic classification of murine lymphomas and related leukemias. Proceedings of the Rodent Lymphomas Workshop, March 4–5, 1981, Jefferson, Arkansas. Natl Cent Toxicol Res Press, Jefferson, pp 22–23

Rappaport H (1966) Tumors of the hematopoietic system. Atlas of tumor pathology, sect 3, fascicle 8, Armed Forces Institute of Pathology, Washington, DC

Seidman JG, Max EE, Leder P (1979) A kappa-immunoglobulin gene is formed by site specific recombination without further somatic mutation. Nature 280: 370–375

Taylor CR (1976) Immuno-histological observations upon the development of reticulum cell sarcoma in the mouse. J Pathol 118: 201–219

Wogan GN (1984) Tumors of the mouse hematopoietic system: their diagnosis and interpretation in safety evaluation tests. Report of a study group. CRC Crit Rev Toxicol 13: 161–81

Immunoblastic Lymphoma, Ileocecal Lymph Nodes, LOU/C Rat

Sabine Rehm, Kara Eberly, and Morris Pollard

Synonyms. Immunocytoma; IR-tumor; plasmacytoma; myeloma; lymphoblastic lymphosarcoma; malignant lymphoma; reticulum cell sarcoma; leukosarcoma.

Gross appearance

Immunoblastic lymphomas of LOU/C rats arise in the lymph nodes situated in the ileocecal mesentery and are rare in other rat strains. Clinically, these neoplasms can be palpated as solid, mobile masses. Necropsy findings depend on the extent of tumor growth. Initially, only one or more of the ileocecal lymph nodes are enlarged, but in later stages ascites-producing grayish masses with red-brown areas of necrosis may also spread to all abdominal viscera and involve the wall of the cecum (Bazin et al. 1972).

Microscopic Features

Histologically, LOU/C rat immunoblastic lymphomas (Figs. 144–146) originate from the B-lymphoblastic cell lineage, and 70% of these tumors synthesize and secrete monoclonal immunoglobulins (Figs. 145 and 146) including Bence Jones proteins (Bazin et al. 1978, 1988). The neoplasms can consist either of a uniform cell population or of a mixture of cells highly variable in size and shape (Figs. 144–146) and function, representing different stages of maturity (Bazin et al. 1972). The tumor may consist of large cells with abundant or sparse, mostly purplish cytoplasm and vesicular nuclei, usually with a prominent central nucleolus. Less frequent are small cells with features of mature plasma cells; cells of intermediate size are more often present. Nuclei are usually round or polygonal and occasionally display indentations. Mitotic figures are numerous. Characteristically, the neoplasms contain many capillaries, a scant reticular stroma without any particular organization, and large actively phagocytic macrophages. Areas of hemorrhage and necroses are frequent (Bazin et al. 1972; Burtonboy et al. 1978). Metastases occur in the spleen, liver, and mediastinal lymph nodes (Beckers and Bazin 1978).

Ultrastructure

Ultrastructurally, LOU/C rat immunoblastic lymphomas are seen to consist of large rounded cells among numerous small capillaries. The tumor cells have slightly eccentric vesicular nuclei with large nucleoli. Frequently, a ribbon-shaped deformation of the nuclear membrane surrounding a dense matrix may be seen as well as type A viral particles. The significance of both of these features is unknown. The cytoplasm usually contains many polyribosomes; however, the extent of rough endoplasmic reticulum varies from cell to cell and is unrelated to functional activity. Large Golgi complexes are regular features (Bazin et al. 1972; Burtonboy et al. 1978).

Differential Diagnosis

From the gross aspect of red-brown coloration, tumors of vascular origin have to be considered in establishing the diagnosis. Histologically, initial tumor formations need to be differentiated from reactive lymphoblastic B-cell hyperplasias that may be induced by bacterial toxins (Ward 1988). Immunoblastic lymphomas must be differentiated from all other hemopoietic neoplasms, in particular plasmacytoma, a rare tumor of fairly well-differentiated plasma cells. Besides various characteristic morphological and functional differences, lymphomas, myeloid neoplasms, and large granulocytic leukemias usually involve the liver, spleen, bone marrow, thymus, or multiple lymph nodes. In histiocytic sarcomas the pattern of metastatic spread may be similar to the immunoblastic lymphoma, but the cells of the histiocytic sarcoma are frequently spindle-shaped, form multinucleated giant cells, and often arise within the subcutis. Mesotheliomas and anaplastic intestinal adenocarcinomas should also be considered in the differential diagnosis and can be differentiated by their morphology under the light microscope.

Biologic Features

The rat ileocecal immunoblastic lymphoma has been most thoroughly studied in the LOU/C inbred rat derived from the outbred LOU/C/Wsl stock of Wistar origin (Beckers and Bazin 1978). These tumors can be detected in the living animal by palpation, laparotomy, and histologic study of biopsy specimens. The development of these tumors can effectively be prevented by early surgical removal of the ileocecal lymph nodes (Moriame et al. 1977). Most tumors develop in rats aged 12–15 months and progress rapidly, causing death of the animal within 4 weeks after clinical detection (Bazin et al. 1972, 1973).

Incidence

In LOU/C rats immunoblastic lymphomas arise in approximately 16% of the females and 32% of the males, whereas in histocompatible LOU/M rats the incidence is below 1% (Beckers and Bazin 1978; Bazin et al. 1980).

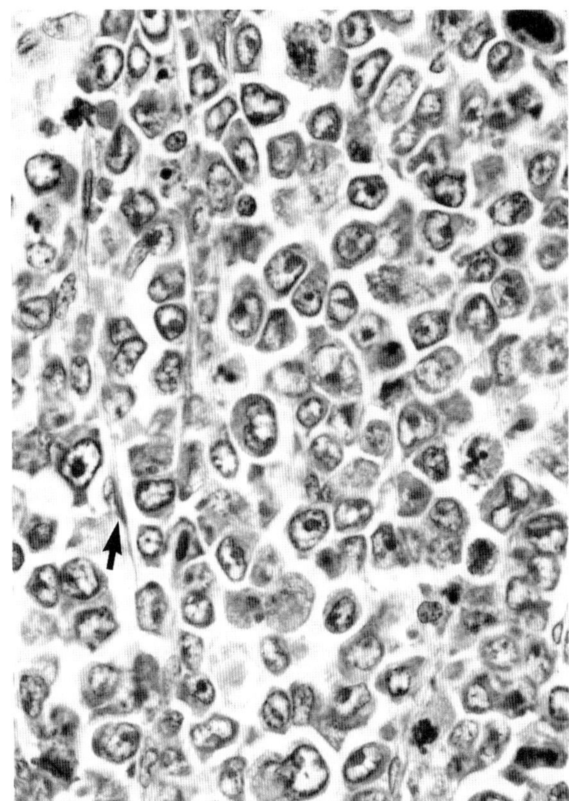

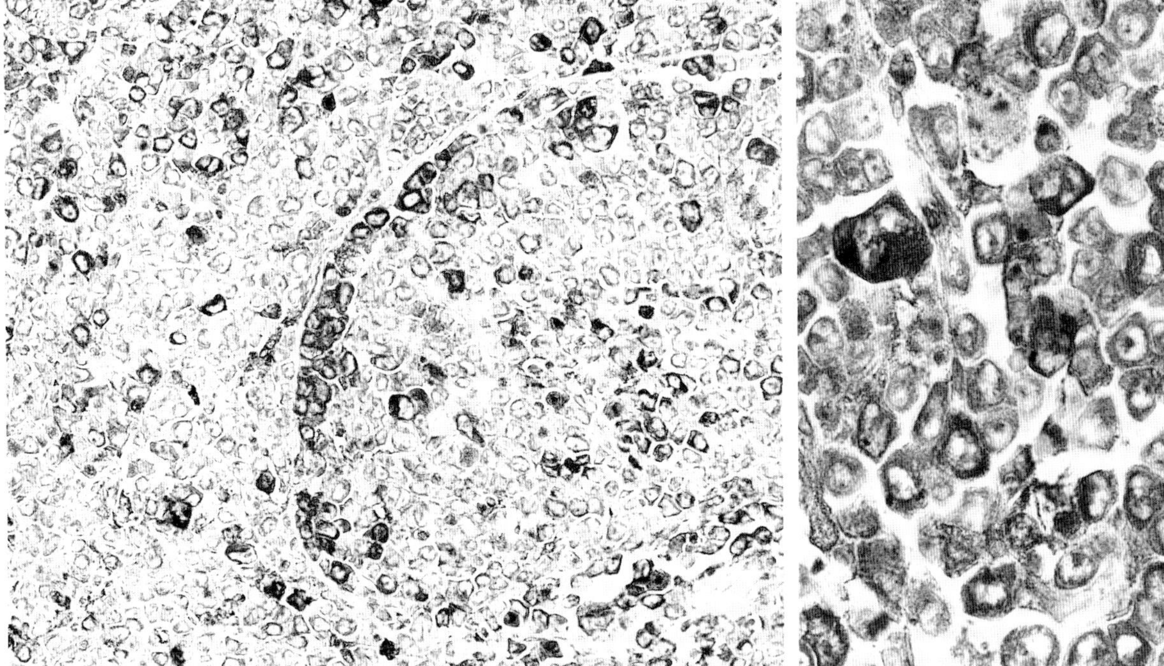

Fig. 144 *(upper right).* Ileocecal immunoblastic lymphoma, LOU/C rat. Note pleomorphic cytology, prominent central nucleolus, marginated nuclear chromatin, little cytoplasm, and scant reticular stroma *(arrow)*. H and E, ×630

Fig. 145 *(lower left).* Ileocal immunoblastic lymphoma, LOU/C rat. Note variable immunoreactive cytoplasmic staining for rat immunoglobulin light and heavy chains. Avidin-biotin complex immunocytochemistry, hematoxylin counterstain, ×250

Fig. 146 *(lower right).* Higher magnification of tumor in Fig. 145. ×630

Genetics

Mating experiments with LOU and OKA strain rats disclosed a genetically controlled susceptibility (dominant loci) or resistance (specific MHC locus) determining the development of ileocecal immunoblastic lymphomas (Beckers and Bazin 1978; Bazin et al. 1980, 1986, 1988). Chromosomal analysis indicates that rat immunoblastic lymphomas carry a reciprocal translocation between chromosomes 6 and 7 (Wiener et al. 1982). Immunoblastic lymphomas probably also develop in other rats (Bazin et al. 1972; Eberly 1978), based on tumor localization, age of the tumor bearer, and a comparable gross and light microscopic morphology. In most other rat stocks and strains it appears to be a rare tumor with an incidence of 0.3%–3% (Beckers and Bazin 1978). LOU/C rat immunoblastic lymphomas can be transplanted to and grown in syngeneic hosts or kept in culture as cell lines maintaining their functional properties over many successive passages (Bazin et al. 1972; Burtonboy et al. 1973; Eberly and Gavin 1979). Over 600 different monoclonal proteins produced by the LOU/C rat immunoblastic lymphomas have been studied, among which are IgG1, IgG2a, IgG2b, IgG2c, IgM, IgA, IgE, IgD, and Bence Jones proteins (Querinjean et al. 1972; Burtonboy et al. 1973; Bazin et al. 1973, 1974, 1978). These neoplasms are therefore very useful models for studying immunoglobulins that normally are present in only small quantities such as IgE and IgD (Eberly 1978). Furthermore, a cell line obtained from LOU/C immunoblastic lymphomas is available for cell fusion to produce hybridoma cells (Kearny 1984).

Comparison with Other Species

Tumors of the plasma cell lineage are rare spontaneous neoplasms in most other mammalian species and often represent well-differentiated plasma cell tumors (plasmacytomas, myelomas; Moulton and Dungworth 1978; Rywlin 1985). However, immature blastic (plasmablastic) variants that have a similar cytologic appearance to the LOU/C rat immunoblastic lymphoma are observed in humans, hamsters, and domestic animals (Rywlin 1985; Sträuli and Mettler 1982; Valli 1985). In the latter these neoplasms are referred to as secretory or non-secretory immunoblastic sarcomas. In humans, the nomenclature varies depending on the classification system used (Greaves et al. 1981; Rywlin 1985). Frequently, plasma cell neoplasms in humans, mice, hamsters, and dogs may be associated with bone destruction, amyloidosis, and cellular casts in the renal tubuli (myeloma kidney), lesions that have not been described to occur in affected LOU/C rats. In mice, rare, spontaneous, generalized (Rask-Nielsen and Gormsen 1951, 1956) and localized, transplantable plasma cell tumors arising in the ileocecal area have been described (Dunn 1957). Studies of plasmacytomas induced in BALB/c mice intraperitoneally by plastic disks, mineral oil, and pristane (Potter 1972, 1983) led to a tremendous increase of information on immunoglobulin structure and function (Morse et al. 1976; Kearny 1984). The tumors are widely used to establish hybridoma cells which, if transplanted intraperitoneally, frequently grow as immunoblastic lymphomas.

References

Bazin H, Deckers C, Beckers A, Heremans JF (1972) Transplantable immunoglobulin-secreting tumours in rats. I. General features of LOU/Wsl strain rat immunocytomas and their monoclonal proteins. Int J Cancer 10: 568–580

Bazin H, Beckers A, Deckers C, Moriame M (1973) Transplantable immunoglobulin-secreting tumors in rats. V. Monoclonal immunoglobulins secreted by 250 ileocecal immunocytomas in LOU/Wsl rats. JNCI 51: 1359–1361

Bazin H, Querinjean P, Beckers A, Heremans JF, Dessy F (1974) Transplantable immunoglobulin-secreting tumours in rats. IV. Sixty-three IgE-secreting immunocytoma tumours. Immunology 26: 713–723

Bazin H, Beckers A, Urbain-Vansanten G, Pauwels R, Bruyns C, Tilkin AF, Platteau B, Urbain J (1978) Transplantable IgD immunoglobulin-secreting tumors in rat. J Immunol 121: 2077–2082

Bazin H, Rousseaux J, Kints J-P, Herno J (1980) Studies on the incidence of rat ileocecal malignant immunocytoma: vertical transmission of the high tumour incidence. Cancer Lett 8: 353–357

Bazin H, Kints J-P, Rousseaux J (1986) Genetic control of the resistance to spontaneous immunocytoma (plasmacytoma – IR tumour) development in LOU/C rats. Anticancer Res 6: 45–48

Bazin H, Pear WS, Sumegi J (1988) Louvain rat immunocytomas. Adv Cancer Res 50: 279–310

Beckers A, Bazin H (1978) Incidence of spontaneous ileocecal immunocytomas in hybrids of LOU/C rats and rat strains with low spontaneous tumor incidence. JNCI 60: 1505–1508

Burtonboy G, Bazin H, Deckers C, Beckers A, Lamy ME, Heremans JF (1973) Transplantable immunoglobulin-secreting tumors in rats. III. Establishment of immunoglobulin-secreting cell lines from LOU/Wsl strain rats. Eur J Cancer Clin Oncol 9: 259–262

Burtonboy G, Beckers A, Rodhain J, Bazin H, Lamy ME (1978) Rat ileocecal immunocytoma. An ultrastructural study with special attention to the presence of viral particles. JNCI 61: 477–484

Dunn TB (1957) Plasma-cell neoplasms beginning in the ileocecal area in strain C3H mice. JNCI 19: 371–391

Eberly K (1978) Biological aspects of an immunoglobulin E producing rat immunocytoma. PhD Dissertation, University of Notre Dame, Notre Dame

Eberly K, Gavin JJ (1979) Propagation and characterization of a rat myeloma cell line producing immunoglobulin E in vitro. Proc Soc Exp Biol Med 160: 196–199

Greaves MF, Habeshaw JA, Stansfeld AG (1981) Lymphoproliferative disorders. In: Zucker-Franklin D, Greaves MF, Grossi CE, Marmont AM (eds) Atlas of blood cells, function and pathology, vol 2. Lea and Febiger, Philadelphia, pp 409–524

Kearny JF (1984) Hybridomas and monoclonal antibodies. In: Paul WE (ed) Fundamental immunology. Raven, New York, pp 751–766

Moriame M, Beckers A, Bazin H (1977) Decrease in the incidence of malignant ileo-caecal immunocytoma in LOU/C rats after surgical removal of the ileo-caecal lymph nodes. Cancer Lett 3: 139–143

Morse HC, Pumphrey JG, Potter M, Asofsky R (1976) Murine plasma cells secreting more than one class of immunoglobulin heavy chain. I. Frequency of two or more M-components in ascitic fluids from 788 primary plasmacytomas. J Immunol 117: 541–547

Moulton JE, Dungworth DL (1978) Tumors of the lymphoid and hemopoietic tissues. In: Moulton JE (ed) Tumors in domestic animals. University of California Press, Berkeley, pp 178–181

Potter M (1972) Immunoglobulin-producing tumors and myeloma proteins of mice. Physiol Rev 52: 631–719

Potter M, Wax JS (1983) Peritoneal plasmacytomagenesis in mice: comparison of different pristane dose regimens. JNCI 71: 391–395

Querinjean P, Bazin H, Beckers A, Deckers C, Heremans JF, Milstein C (1972) Transplantable immunoglobulin-secreting tumours in rats. II. Purification and chemical characterization of four kappa chains from LOU/Wsl rats. Eur J Biochem 31: 354–359

Rask-Nielsen R, Gormsen H (1951) Spontaneous and induced plasma-cell neoplasia in a strain of mice. Cancer 4: 387–397

Rask-Nielsen R, Gormsen H (1956) On the occurrence of plasma-cell leukemia in various strains of mice. JNCI 16: 1137–1147

Rywlin AM (1985) Hemopoietic system: reticuloendothelial system, spleen, lymph nodes, bone marrow, and blood. In: Kissane JM (ed) Anderson's pathology, vol 2. Mosby, St Louis, pp 1338–1340

Sträuli P, Mettler J (1982) Tumours of the haematopoietic system. In: Turusov VS (ed) Pathology of tumours in laboratory animals. III. Tumours of the hamster. IARC Sci Publ 34: 343–369

Valli VEO (1985) The hematopoietic system. In: Jubb KVF, Kennedy PC, Palmer N (eds) Pathology of domestic animals, vol 3. Academic, Orlando, pp 107–112

Ward JM (1988) Classification of reactive lesions of lymph nodes. In: Jones TC, Ward JM, Mohr U, Hunt RD (eds) Monographs on pathology of laboratory animals. Hemopoietic system. Springer, Heidelberg Berlin New York (in press this volume)

Wiener F, Babonits M, Spira J, Klein G, Bazin H (1982) Non-random chromosomal changes involving chromosomes 6 and 7 in spontaneous rat immunocytomas. Int J Cancer 29: 431–437

Follicular Center Cell Lymphoma, Mouse

Paul K. Pattengale

Synonyms. Reticulum cell sarcoma, type B; B cell lymphoma; follicular center cell lymphoma, large, small, or mixed cell; lymphoma, mixed or pleomorphic.

Gross Appearance

Early lesions are whitish in color and are confined initially to the white pulp of the spleen. With time the lesions progress to confluence, first in the spleen, and later in the lymph nodes, liver, lungs, and kidneys (Pattengale and Frith 1983; Pattengale and Taylor 1983; Pattengale and Frith 1986; see also p. 137, this volume).

Microscopic Features

Follicular center cell (FCC) lymphomas, as proposed in the Pattengale-Taylor classification of mouse lymphoid cell neoplasms (see p. 137, this volume), are composed of neoplastic, malignant, B cell-derived follicular (germinal) center cells. They are comprised of small and/or large FCCs. These lymphomas in the mouse can therefore be designated as large, small, or small and large (mixed). A useful guideline for the designation as mixed is a ratio of small to large FCCs in the range of 30:70 to 70:30 (i.e., small:large). Furthermore, lymphoid cell neoplasms with greater than 70% large or small follicular center cells would be designated either large or small. For purposes of this discussion, mixed or pleomorphic lymphomas (also called reticulum cell neoplasm, type B) are terms which have been used to describe FCC lymphomas in the mouse (Fig. 139). Although the term mixed lymphoma most often refers to a mixed FCC lymphoma, this term has also been used to describe either large or small FCC lymphomas. This overlap is based on the presence of both large and small FCCs in any such lesion.

The detailed microscopic and histologic features are illustrated in Figs. 136–139. Briefly, small FCCs are 6–10 μm in diameter, have scant cytoplasm, and have a high nuclear to cytoplasmic ratio (Fig. 136). They are cohesive, have an absent to low mitotic rate, possess mature condensed chromatin, and often have cleaved nuclei with inconspicuous nucleoli. Large FCCs are 8–16 μm in diameter, have scant to moderate amounts of cytoplasm, and have a moderate to high nuclear to cytoplasmic ratio (Figs. 137, 138). They are also cohesive, but, in contrast to small FCC lymphomas, they have a high mitotic rate and often prominent nucleoli juxtaposed to the nuclear membrane. Cells of large FCC lymphomas also have nuclear chromatin which is marginated and often condensed on the nuclear membrane.

Ultrastructure

Briefly, the ultrastructural features of FCC lymphomas are not diagnostic and therefore only complement the light microscopic features. These ultrastructural findings are illustrated in another publication (Fredrickson et al. 1985).

Differential Diagnosis

With proper fixation and thin sectioning (Pattengale and Taylor 1983), FCC lymphomas should be readily distinguishable from other morphologic types of lymphomas (Pattengale and Frith 1983; Pattengale and Frith 1986). It should be mentioned that the entity previously referred to as reticulum cell neoplasm or reticulum cell sarcoma type A by Dunn (Dunn 1954) is actually a nonlymphoid neoplasm composed of malignant histiocytic cells (i. e., a true histiocytic sarcoma). In poorly fixed tissues, the morphology of histiocytic sarcoma can sometimes be confused with a FCC lymphoma. Histiocytic sarcoma, unlike FCC lymphomas, diffusely involve the liver sinus-

oids and are composed of a monomorphous population of neoplastic histiocytes with a dark basophilic nucleus and abundant, distinctly eosinophilic cytoplasm (Pattengale and Frith 1986). Mast cell neoplasms are often composed of neoplastic cells with irregularly shaped nuclei which can be confused with a diagnosis of FCC lymphoma. Geimsa staining for metachromatic granules is definitive for mast cell neoplasms and quickly rules out a FCC lymphoma (Pattengale and Frith 1986).

Biologic Features

Reticulum cell sarcomas (neoplasm), type B, have been described in a variety of mouse strains and are reviewed in detail elsewhere (Dunn and Deringer 1968; Pattengale and Taylor 1983; Pattengale and Frith 1983; Fredrickson et al. 1985; Pattengale and Frith 1986). They have also been designated as pleomorphic lymphomas (Wogan 1984). It should be stressed that these designations refer to B cell-derived FCC lymphomas. In general, spontaneous FCC lymphomas arise in aged mice with a slight preponderance of females as compared with males. SJL/J, NZB, C57BL, C57L, B6C3F-1, C3H, DBA/2, and NFS/N V congeneics (Fredrickson et al. 1985) are some of the more common strains which spontaneously develop FCC lymphomas. Some strains of mice, such as BALB/c females over 18 months of age, exhibit a very high incidence (35%) of FCC lymphoma (Pattengale and Frith 1983). Since these lymphomas arise spontaneously in older mice and, at present, are causally *not* associated with murine retroviruses, it is difficult to provide any substantive information on their pathogenesis. Furthermore, spontaneous FCC lymphomas in the mouse are not associated with any significant structural changes in any of the known B cell lymphoma-associated oncogenes (i. e., *myc, myb, abl, mos, bc1-2*).

Comparison with Other Species

As previously described in detail (Pattengale and Taylor 1983), mouse FCC lymphomas closely resemble human FCC lymphomas. Other species such as rats, cats, dogs, etc. have not been as well defined using the newer immunomorphologic criteria. For these reasons, the mouse is an excellent immunopathologic model for human B cell-derived FCC lymphomas.

References

Dunn TB (1954) Normal and pathologic anatomy of the reticular tissue in laboratory mice, with a classification and discussion of neoplasms. JNCI 14: 1281–1433

Dunn TB, Deringer MK (1968) Reticulum cell neoplasm, type B, or the "Hodgkin's-like lesion" of the mouse. JNCI 40: 771–820

Fredrickson TN, Morse HC III, Yetter RA, Rowe WP, Hartley JW, Pattengale PK (1985) Multiparameter analyses of spontaneous nonthymic lymphomas occurring in NFS/N mice congeneic for ecotropic murine leukemia viruses. Am J Pathol 121: 349–360

Pattengale PK, Frith CH (1983) Immunomorphologic classification of spontaneous lymphoid cell neoplasms occurring in female BALB/c mice. JNCI 70: 169–179

Pattengale PK, Frith CH (1986) Contributions of recent research to the classification of lymphoid cell neoplasms in mice. CRC Crit Rev Toxicol 16: 185–212

Pattengale PK, Taylor CR (1983) Experimental models of lymphoproliferative disease: the mouse as a model for human non-Hodgkin's lymphomas and related leukemias. Am J Pathol 113: 237–265

Wogan GN (1984) Tumors of the mouse hematopoietic system: their diagnosis and interpretation in safety evaluation tests. Report of a study group. CRC Crit Rev Toxicol 13: 161–181

A Morphologic Classification of Hemopoietic Tumors, Rats

Johannes H. Harleman and Wolfgang Jahn

Introduction

This classification scheme was developed for a database of tumor incidences in control rats. Preliminary steps were taken in 1987, and in 1988 the database was set up under the guidance of Prof. Ulrich Mohr as a joint development between various German and Swiss companies and the Fraunhofer Gesellschaft. In setting up a lexicon or classification scheme for routine toxicologic pathology one needs to fulfill certain criteria:

1. The classification should be suitable for application to safety assessment or evaluation procedures in routine toxicity and oncogenicity testing and appraisal systems (formalin-fixed tissues, H and E staining).
2. It should have application and acceptance at the international level.
3. It should be based on histopathologic criteria and should be compatible with generally accepted classification systems currently in use in human and veterinary medicine.

Tumors of the lymphoreticular and hemopoietic tissues have a relatively low incidence in most common rat strains, except for the Fischer 344 strain. Incidences of these tumors have been reported ranging from 1% to 10% (Kroes et al. 1981; Chu et al. 1981; Burek 1978; Anver et al. 1982; Altmann and Goodman 1979). In the Fischer 344 rat strain a high incidence (10%–50%) of LGL leukemia occurs in aging rats

(Chu et al. 1981; Stromberg and Vogtsberger 1983; Losco and Ward 1984). Except for some experimental models and the Fischer leukemia, the characterization and classification of these tumors in rats is, for the most part, based on morphologic criteria, because methods used in human (Lukes and Collins 1975) and murine (Pattengale and Taylor 1983) classifications with specific immunologic and cytochemical markers are not generally available (Greaves and Faccini 1984; Swaen and van Heerde 1973; Pattengale and Taylor 1983; Frith et al. 1985). In toxicologic pathology it would be useful to have a classification scheme for formalin-fixed material for the two most frequently used rodent species (rats and mice). The following scheme for rats is a modification of a proposed classification for mice (Wogan et al. 1984).

Proposed Classification

The lymphoreticular and hemopoietic tumors in rats were divided into three main groups. These may be combined for statistical purposes in safety evaluations.

I. Lymphomatous Tumors

1. Malignant lymphoma, lymphocytic
2. Malignant lymphoma, lymphoblastic
3. Malignant lymphoma, pleomorphic
4. Malignant lymphoma, large granular cell

5. Malignant lymphoma, plasmacytic
6. Malignant lymphoma, NOS
To each tumor type may be added one or more of the following modifiers based on the primary site or distribution of the tumor: thymic, leukemic, multicentric, mesenteric, etc. No modifier is used when the primary site is unknown.

II. Thymomas

7. Thymoma
Each tumor may have one or more of the following modifiers: benign, malignant, epithelial.

III. Nonlymphomatous Hemopoietic Tumors

  8. Granulocytic leukemia
  9. Erythroid leukemia
10. Megakaryocytic leukemia
11. Mast cell tumor
12. Myeloproliferative disorder
13. Leukemia, NOS
NOS, Not otherwise specified. This term may be used if a more specific classification is not necessary or precluded by autolysis or fixation or other factor.

I. Lymphomatous Tumors (Kroes et al. 1981; Burek 1978; Stromberg and Vogtsberger 1983; Losco and Ward 1984; Greaves and Faccini 1981, 1984; Swaen and van Heerde 1973)

1. Preferred diagnostic term: Malignant lymphoma, lymphocytic

Synonyms. Lymphosarcoma; small cell lymphoma; lymphocytic lymphoma, well and intermediate differentiation.
This tumor consists of a proliferation of small to medium-sized well to intermediately differentiated lymphocytes. The tumor cells are relatively uniform. In the smaller cells the nuclear chromatin is densely clumped, and a narrow rim of cytoplasm is usually visible. They may differ little, if at all, from normal circulating lymphocytes. Lymphocytic lymphomas also may contain slightly larger cells with somewhat larger irregular nuclei, corresponding to the small cleaved follicular center cells (Fig. 147; see p. 147, this volume).

Differential Diagnosis. Lymphoid hyperplasia (see p. 155, this volume)

2. Preferred diagnostic term: Malignant lymphoma, lymphoblastic

Synonyms. Lymphosarcoma; undifferentiated lymphoma; lymphoma, poorly differentiated.
This tumor is composed principally of large lymphoblastic cells with a high nuclear to cytoplasmic ratio; the nucleus is round to ovoid and not indented or twisted and may contain prominent nucleoli. The nucleus is surrounded by a small rim of basophilic cytoplasm with few, if any, granules. This tumor generally has a high mitotic index (Fig. 148).

3. Preferred diagnostic term: Malignant lymphoma, pleomorphic

Synonyms. Reticulum cell sarcoma; lymphosarcoma; reticulum sarcoma; histiocytic malignant lymphoma (see p. 147, this volume).
These are tumors with fairly large cells. They may have a varying degree of pleomorphism ranging from uniform to considerable pleomorphism of cells and nuclei within the same tumor. These tumor cells resemble the large cells seen in germinal centers. Large irregular (cleaved or centroblastic) cells may be seen, as well as smaller cells with rounded nuclei and basophilic cytoplasm. The cells are usually mononuclear and may have prominent nucleoli, but occasional multinucleated cells occur. The multinucleated cells may resemble Reed-Sternberg cells (Fig. 149).

Differential Diagnosis. Fibrous histiocytic sarcoma, undifferentiated sarcoma.

Comment. This tumor may sometimes resemble a fibrous histiocytic sarcoma as described by Greaves and Faccini (1981).
The fibrous histiocytic sarcoma, however, tends to have a more fibrous structure and a different anatomic distribution pattern. The primary site may be in the subcutis of a rear leg, in the retroperitoneal tissue, or in the liver, and in most cases it is not distributed among lymph nodes.

4. Preferred diagnostic term: Malignant lymphoma, large granular cell

Synonyms. Mononuclear leukemia of Fischer rat; monocytoid leukemia; large granular lymphocytic (LGL) leukemia.
These tumors are made up of the large granular lymphocytes which are found in the peripheral blood of normal rats. The nuclei are round, oval, slightly irregular, and reniform and have clumped nuclear chromatin including nucleoli.

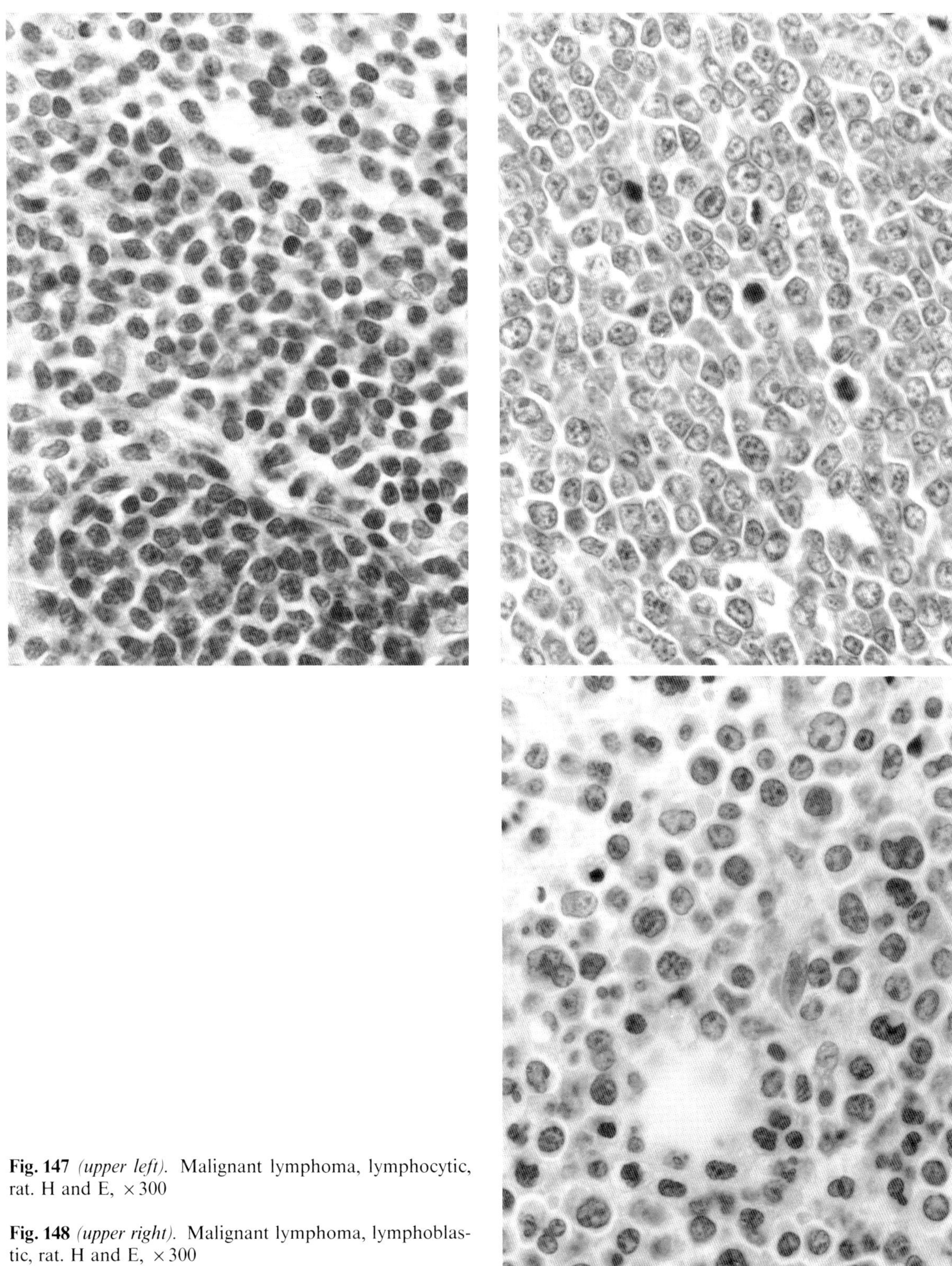

Fig. 147 *(upper left)*. Malignant lymphoma, lymphocytic, rat. H and E, ×300

Fig. 148 *(upper right)*. Malignant lymphoma, lymphoblastic, rat. H and E, ×300

Fig. 149 *(lower right)*. Malignant lymphoma, pleomorphic, rat. H and E, ×300

The basophilic cytoplasm has several reddish granules seen in peripheral blood smears stained with Giemsa but not in routine and E stained sections. These cells react positively with the OX-8 mouse monoclonal antibodies (Fig. 150). The primary organs involved are spleen and liver, but other organs may also be infiltrated (see p. 194, this volume).

Differential Diagnosis. Lymphoma, leukemic.

5. Preferred diagnostic term: Malignant lymphoma, plasma cell

Synonyms. Plasmacytoma; myeloma; plasma cell sarcoma.
This rare tumor consists primarily of plasma cells and/or cells with a clear plasmacytoid differentiation. The nuclei are round, often with a cartwheel appearance. The cytoplasm is basophilic and pyroninophilic, and a small perinuclear halo may be present (see p. 137, this volume).

Differential Diagnosis. Lymphoid hyperplasia, lymphoma lymphocytic, plasmocytosis.

6. Preferred diagnostic term: Malignant lymphoma NOS (not otherwise specified)

Synonym. Lymphosarcoma.
Lymphoma NOS is defined as a local or generalized tumor of cells of the lymphocytic type. This classification may be used if further classification is not necessary or precluded by the presence of autolysis, poor fixation, etc.

Differential Diagnosis. Lymphoid hyperplasia.

II. Thymomas (Kroes et al. 1981; Greaves and Faccini 1984; Kuper et al. 1986; Abbott and Cherry 1982; Naylor et al. 1988)

7. Thymomas are tumors with the involvement of thymic epithelial cells in the neoplastic process. They are localized tumors which generally are well-encapsulated, but they may invade locally. Metastases are rarely observed. Various levels of differentiation may be present, ranging from tumors with a predominantly normal thymic structure with medullary differentiation to those without medullary differentiation and composed of a mixture of epithelial cells and lymphocytes and to others composed exclusively of epithelial cells.

In Fig. 151 may be seen the spectrum of these tumors, varying from a well-differentiated thymoma with an abundance of lymphocytes to a purely epithelial thymoma.
The following modifiers may be used: benign for well-encapsulated, localized tumors; malignant for locally invasive and/or metastasizing tumors; epithelial, when the tumor consists almost exclusively (more than 80%) of thymic epithelial cells.

Differential Diagnosis. Malignant lymphoma of thymus.

III. Nonlymphomatous Hemopoietic Tumors (Kroes et al. 1981; Burek 1978; Greaves and Faccini 1984; Swaen and van Heerde 1973; Jarrett and Mackey 1974)

8. Preferred diagnostic term: Granulocytic leukemia

Synonyms. Myeloid leukemia; chloroleukemia.
Granulocytic leukemias are relatively common in old rats. Two different types have been described. One type is associated with variable but often very high white cell counts (up to 1 million cells/μl). The increased number of white blood cells in this case is mainly due to myelocytes and mature neutrophils; blast cells and promyelocytes are uncommon in the peripheral blood. The other form, also called myeloblastic leukemia, has a high white blood cell count, but the cells resemble normal myeloblasts and promyelocytes. These cells are a little more irregular and may have a more abundant cytoplasm. The nuclei have prominent nucleoli, and azurophilic granules are infrequently present. The most common form is neutrophilic granulocytic leukemia. Modifiers: neutrophilic, eosinophilic, or basophilic (Fig. 152).

Differential Diagnosis. Myeloid hyperplasia.

Comment. Myeloid hyperplasia does not produce the extremely high peripheral blood cell counts found in granulocytic leukemia and is generally a reaction, part of an inflammatory response to a chronically ulcerated tumor, for example.

9. Preferred diagnostic term: Erythroid leukemia.

Synonyms. Erythroleukemia.
Erythroid leukemia has not been described as a spontaneous lesion in the rat. The tumor is char-

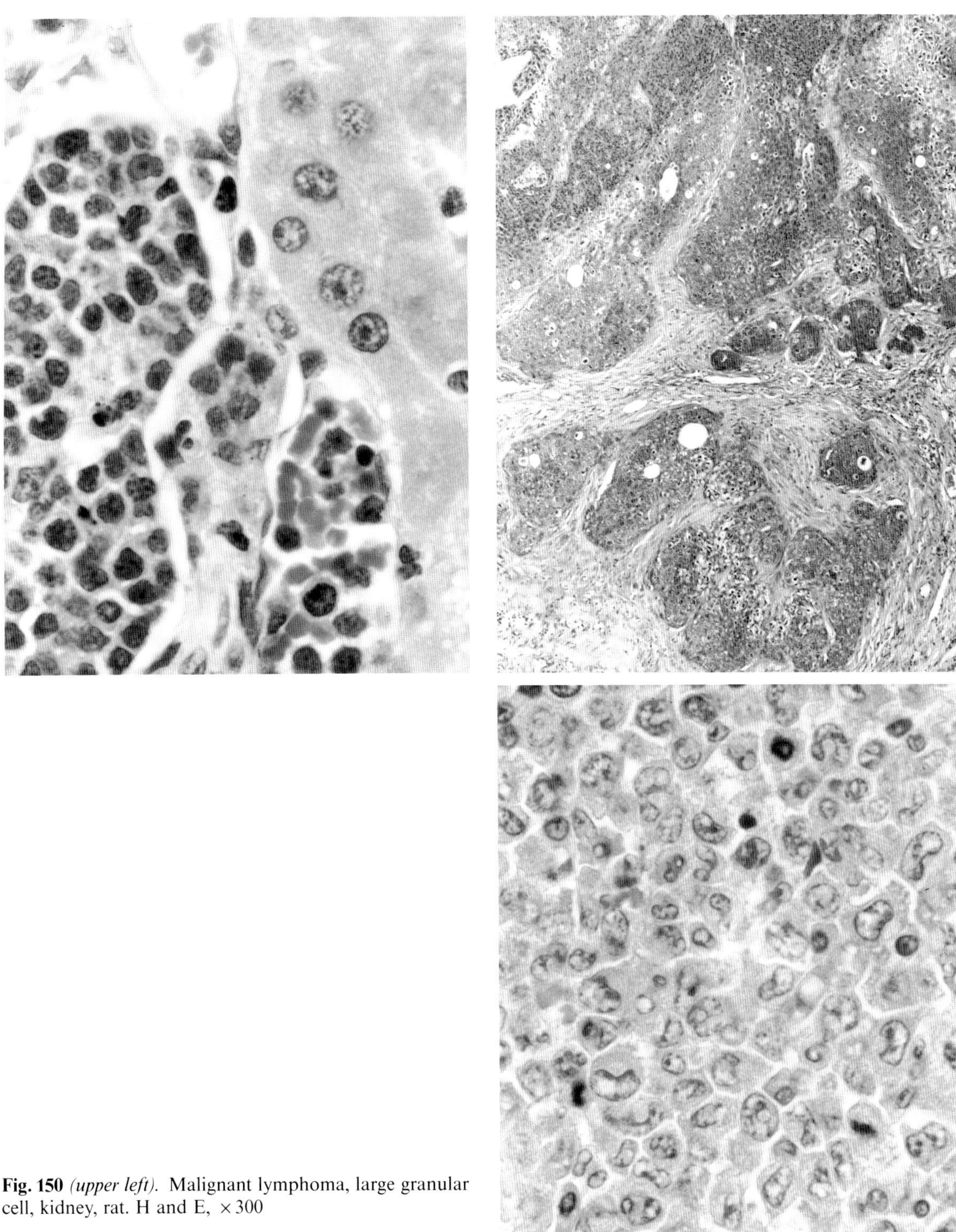

Fig. 150 *(upper left).* Malignant lymphoma, large granular cell, kidney, rat. H and E, ×300

Fig. 151 *(upper right).* Thymoma, epithelial, rat. H and E, ×100

Fig. 152 *(lower right).* Granulocytic leukemia, neutrophilic, rat. H and E, ×300 acterized by an excessive proliferation of erythro-blastic cells. This condition has been described in rats after radiation and trimethylbenz[*a*]anthracene treatment (Swaen and van Heerde 1973).

10. Preferred diagnostic term: Megakaryocytic leukemia.

This type is included although we are not aware of any report of this lesion in rats. In other species it is a tumor in which the neoplastic cells are mainly megakaryoblasts and promegakaryocytes. The latter are readily recognized by their large size and partially lobulated nuclei. The nuclei are not condensed and contain nucleoli. Abnormal forms and mitosis occur (Jarrett and Mackey 1974).

11. Preferred diagnostic term: Mast cell tumor.

Synonyms. Mastocytoma.
Again this term is included, but we are not aware of any spontaneous occurrence of this tumor in the rat. A "Retikulose mit reicher Mastzellbeteiligung" (reticulocytosis with prominent mast cells) has been described by Hunstein et al. (1963) after whole body irradiation in a Wistar rat.

12. Preferred diagnostic term: Myeloproliferative disorder.

Synonym. Panmyelosis.
This diagnosis is used when there is an obvious malignant proliferation of more than one cell line.

Differential Diagnosis. Bone marrow hyperplasia.

13. Preferred diagnostic term: Leukemia NOS (not otherwise specified).

This classification is used if no further classification is considered necessary or if the condition of the specimen (autolysis, poor fixation, etc.) precludes a more definitive diagnosis.

References

Abbott DP, Cherry CP (1982) Malignant mixed thymic tumor with metastasis in a rat. Vet Pathol 19: 721–723

Altmann NH, Goodman DG (1979) Neoplastic diseases. In: Baker HJ, Lindsey JR, Weisbroth SH (eds) The Laboratory Rat, vol I. Biology and Diseases. Academic, New York, chap 13

Anver MR, Cohen BJ, Lattuada CP, Foster SJ (1982) Age-associated lesions in barrier-reared male Sprague Dawley rats. A comparison between Hap (SD) and Crl: COBS[R]CD[R]SD stock. Exp Aging Res 8: 3–24

Burek JD (1978) Pathology of aging rats. CRC Press, Boca Raton

Chu KC, Cueto C Jr, Ward JM (1981) Factors in the evaluation of 200 National Cancer Institute carcinogen bioassays. J Toxicol Environ Health 8: 251–280

Frith CH, Pattengale PK, Ward JM (1985) A color atlas of hematopoietic pathology of mice. Toxicology Pathology Associates, Little Rock

Greaves P, Faccini JM (1981) Spontaneous fibrous histiocytic neoplasms in rats. Br J Cancer 43: 402–411

Greaves P, Faccini JM (1984) Rat histopathology. Elsevier, Amsterdam

Hunstein W, Stutz E, Reinecke U (1963) Strahlen-induzierte Leukämien bei Wistar-Ratten nach fraktionierter Ganzkörperbestrahlung. Blut 9: 389–404

Jarrett WFH, Mackey LJ (1974) Neoplastic diseases of the hematopoietic and lymphoid tissues. Bull WHO 50: 21–34

Kroes R, Garbis-Berkvens JM, de Vries T, van Nesselrooy HJ (1981) Histological profile of a Wistar rat stock including a survey of the literature. J Gerontol 36: 259–279

Kuper CF, Beems RB, Hollanders VMH (1986) Spontaneous pathology of the thymus in aging Wistar (Cpb: Wu) rats. Vet Pathol 23: 270–277

Losco PE, Ward JM (1984) The early stage of large granular lymphocytic leukemia in the F344 rat. Vet Pathol 21: 286–291

Lukes RJ, Collins RD (1975) New approaches to the classification of the lymphomata. Brit J Cancer 31: (suppl 2): 1–28

Naylor DC, Krinke GJ, Ruefenacht HJ (1988) Primary tumours of the thymus in the rat. J Comp Pathol 99: 187–203

Pattengale PK, Taylor CR (1983) Experimental models of lymphoproliferative disease. The mouse as a model for human non-Hodgkin's lymphomas and related leukemias. Am J Pathol 133: 237–265

Stromberg PC, Vogtsberger LM (1983) Pathology of the mononuclear cell leukemia of Fischer rats. I. Morphological studies. Vet Pathol 20: 698–708

Swaen GJV, van Heerde P (1973) Tumours of the haematopoietic system. In: Turusov VS (ed) Pathology of tumours in laboratory animals, vol I, part I. Tumours of the rat. IARC, Lyon, pp 185–201

Wogan GN, Clayson DB, Rapp F (1984) Tumors of the mouse hematopoietic system: Their diagnosis and interpretation in safety evaluation tests. Report of a study group. CRC Crit Rev Toxicol 13: 161–181

Classification of Reactive Lesions of Lymph Nodes

Jerrold M. Ward

Lymph nodes function as filters of tissues and tissue fluids and as sites of origin and production of lymphocytes for normal physiological functions, and they react to exogenous and endogenous stimulants. The various anatomical regions of the node respond to these stimulants to varying degrees and with specific morphological and functional patterns. These responses may be acute or chronic. Basic lesions, often found after exposure to toxins, include degeneration of specific cell types, necrosis, atrophy, and hyperplasia. These lesions have been documented in lymph nodes from human patients (Hartsock 1975; Ioachim 1982; Jaffe and Bennington 1985; Nathwani et al. 1986; Robb-Smith and Taylor 1981; Weissman et al. 1978) and in rodents (Frith and Wiley 1981; Frith et al. 1985; Van Rooijen 1987). Aging rodents often have hyperplastic cellular nodes, some of which may mimic lymphomas.

It is very important to evaluate a lymph node initially at low magnification to identify the anatomic substructure of the node and compare it with normal lymph nodes of the same anatomic location (Nathwani et al. 1986). The capsule, cortex, paracortex, and medulla can be readily examined and evaluated for cellular density, normal anatomic structure, and relationships to other substructures (Table 39). The reactive node may show complex changes involving several of its anatomic subunits which make it difficult to evaluate and understand. This review will attempt to simplify some of these changes. Since there is little published information on reactive lesions of lymph nodes of rodents, this classification is a provisional one. Specific morphologic diagnoses may be used in the future which might include types of reactive hyperplasia (follicular, diffuse, medullary, sinus, etc.) and specific lesions due to unique causes, i. e., vaccine lymphadenitis, radiation atrophy, etc.

The lymph node may be divided into reactive functional zones including the capsule, cortical

Table 39. A classification of reactive lesions of lymph nodes

Anatomic location	Reactive lesion
Capsule	Acute and chronic lymphadenitis
	Fibrosis
Cortex	
Follicles	Necrosis
	Atrophy
	Follicular hyperplasia
Paracortex	Necrosis
	Atrophy
	Lymphocyte hyperplasia
	Interdigitating dendritic cell hyperplasia
	Hyperplasia of "high endothelial venules"
Medulla	
Medullary cords	Plasmacytosis
	Myeloid metaplasia
	Pigmentation
	Mastocytosis
Sinuses	Sinus histiocytosis
	Pigmentation
	Erythrophagocytosis
	Lymphangiectasis
	Tumor emboli and metastases

B-cell zone (follicles, germinal centers), T-cell zone (paracortex), cortical and medullary sinuses, and medullary cords. Each may undergo a specific and characteristic morphologic change in response to a specific stimulant (antigen, microorganism, foreign material, etc.).

The *capsule* of the node is usually a thin connective tissue layer covering the subcapsular sinuses. In acute inflammation, the capsule may contain neutrophils, mast cells, edema fluid, and histiocytes. In chronic lesions, fibrosis may be evident along with chronic inflammatory cells including plasma cells and immature lymphocytes. A densely cellular node with a monotypic population of lymphocytes in the capsule and perinodal

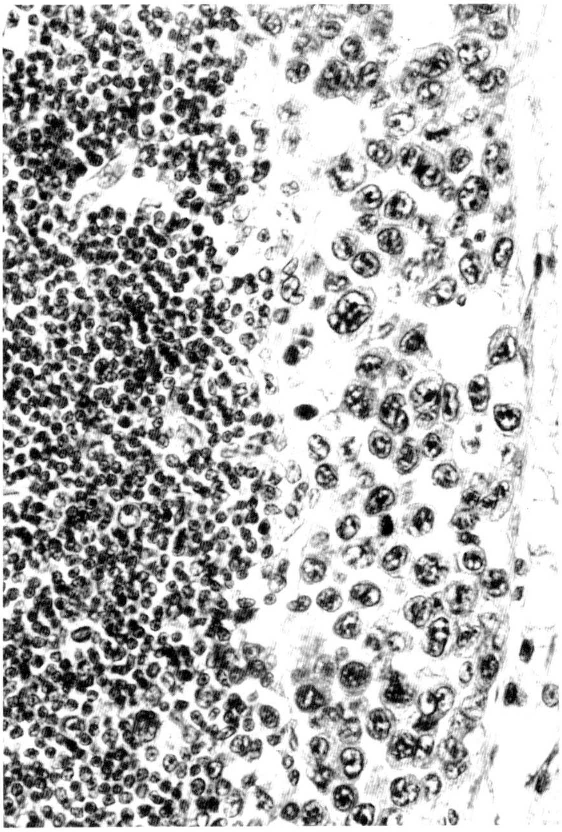

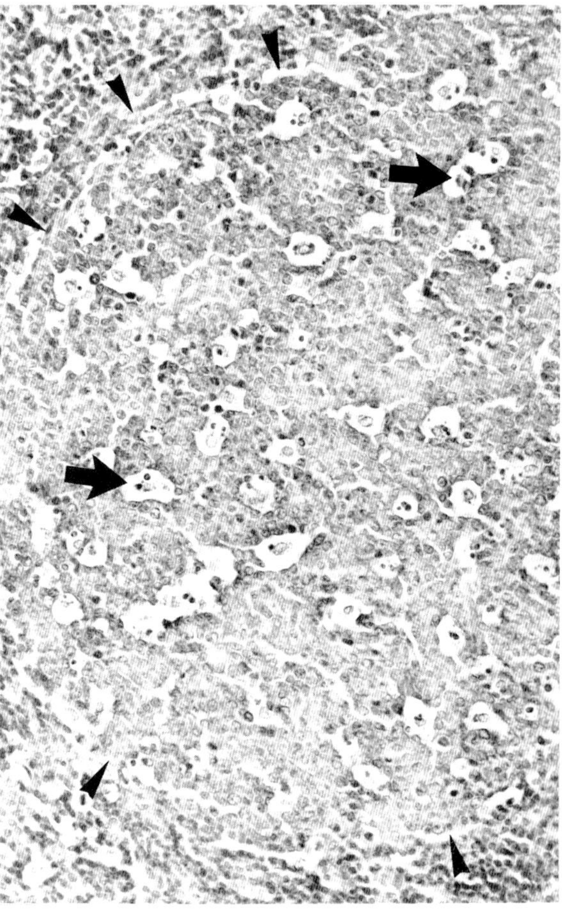

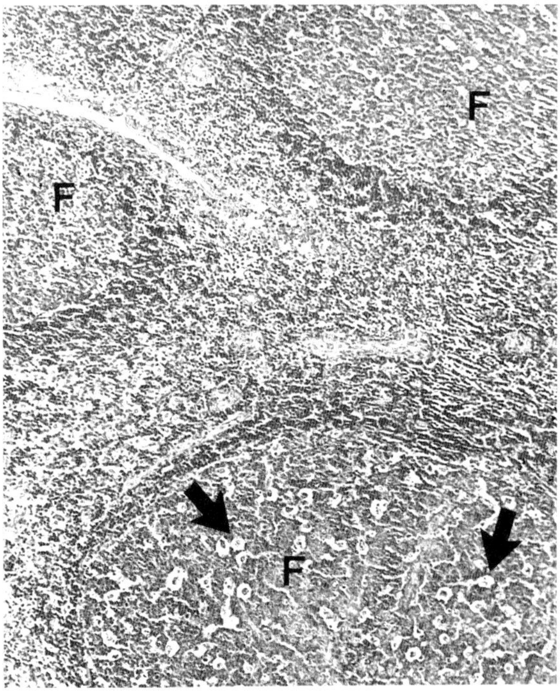

Fig. 153 *(upper left).* Tumor cells from intraperitoneally injected hybridoma (immunoblastic lymphoma) in the subcapsular sinus of mouse mesenteric lymph node. The peritoneal cavity had numerous tumor nodules and ascites. H and E, ×400

Fig. 154 *(lower left).* Three hyperplastic follicles *(F)* in rat lymph node. Note prominent tingible body macrophages *(arrows).* H and E, ×100

Fig. 155 *(upper right).* Hyperplastic follicle (germinal center), lymph node *(arrowheads).* Note prominent spaces occupied by follicular dendritic cells (tingible body macrophages) containing cell debris *(arrows).* H and E, ×250 adipose or connective tissue may be indicative of lymphoma or leukemia. The identification of lymphocytes in the capsule is not, however, pathognomonic for neoplasia. It is seen more commonly with reactive lesions in rodents.

In acute lymphadenitis, inflammatory cells including neutrophils and macrophages may be found in the capsule, subcapsular and medullary sinuses, and medullary cords. Often this occurs in nodes draining acute or chronic suppurative lesions or tumors with ulcerated epithelium (skin or GI tract). Tumor cells and their emboli often enter the subcapsular sinuses of a regional node through the afferent lymphatics (Fig. 153). In rodents, this is often seen in superficial nodes draining sites of induced cutaneous carcinomas and in cecal or mesenteric nodes regional to intestinal carcinomas.

The *cortex* of the lymph node contains the follicles. In normal rats, follicles may be evident to varying degrees, in part dependent on the plane of section of the node, the age of the animal, and its health status. In a normal response to antigens, the follicle develops a hyperplastic germinal center with immature B cells. The B-cell response is measured by the number and size of the follicles (Fig. 154), presence of germinal centers, activity of the cells in the follicles, and numbers of immunoglobulin-containing cells (immunoblasts, plasma cells) in the cortex and medullary cords. Cellular activity is indicated by the size of the cell, immaturity of the nucleus, and presence of mitotic figures and tingible body macrophages with cytoplasmic debris (Fig. 155). The latter cells are probably active follicular dendritic cells. The cells in the follicles can be stained for B-cell antigens. If any of these parameters of follicular activity is increased over normal for a particular lymph node or in comparison with controls in an experiment, *follicular hyperplasia* can be used as a descriptive or diagnostic term. *Follicular atrophy* describes the situation when few, small, or no follicles are observed. Necrosis may precede atrophy, especially after exposure to drugs or radiation.

The *paracortex* is composed of a thymus-dependent (T-cell) zone which contains many T cells, interdigitating dendritic cells (IDC), and high endothelial venules (HEV), the sites of lymphocyte migration from the blood into the lymph node. Atrophy of the paracortex can be seen as a consequence of necrosis of lymphocytes induced by radiation or drugs. There is loss of lymphocytes in the T-cell zone. Hyperplasia of lymphocytes in this zone may be simulated if the plane of section

through the node is not competely through the cortex and medulla. If proper sections are made, an increased density of lymphocytes in this zone may be due to a true hyperplasia of T and B lymphocytes. In aging rodents, a densely cellular paracortex is often found, composed of mature lymphocytes and plasma cells. Most often, plasmacytosis involving the medullary cords extends into this T-cell zone, giving the appearance of hyperplasia of lymphocytes in the T-cell zone. At high magnification, the typical morphology of plasma cells may be easily observed.

Hyperplasia of IDC occurs in nude rats in the T-cell zone (Figs. 156–159), in part in response to T-cell atrophy and hyperplasia of large granular lymphocytes in this zone (Ward et al. 1983). The IDC have large irregular vesicular nuclei and sparse or abundant cytoplasm (Fig. 159). They are present in normal nodes but may be difficult to see except for their characteristic nuclei. *Hyperplasia and hypertrophy of HEV* in the paracortex can be found sometimes in large reactive nodes, with lymphadenitis (Fig. 160) and in response to immunological adjuvants (Anderson 1985). We have seen HEV hyperplasia in subcutaneous nodes from SENCAR mice used in skin painting studies.

The *medulla* contains the medullary *sinuses* which extend from the subcapsular and cortical sinuses, draining lymph from adjacent tissues. The sinuses are lined by histiocytes/macrophages which react to materials within the draining sinus. These sinus histiocytes can phagocytize exogenous and endogenous pigments, i. e., from food, air, drugs, injected materials, erythrocytes, hemosiderin, microorganisms, etc. The mesenteric nodes of rats and mice are usually the site of various degrees of large pigmented macrophages in the sinuses and within the medullary cords. Multinucleated giant cells are sometimes seen. An increase in number or activity of the sinus histiocytes is *sinus histiocytosis* (Fig. 161). Pigmentation of sinus or medullary cord histiocytes is common in mesenteric nodes (Fig. 162). The reactive lesion can also originate from an immune response to vaccines, endotoxins, and allergic materials. *Lymphangiectasis* is seen in old rats, more commonly in some strains. It is characterized by focal or diffuse dilated sinuses in any part of the node, grossly visible as cysts filled with lymph. Erythrocytes are not present.

The *medullary cords* are often the site of the migration of differentiated B cells, the plasma cells (Van Rooijen 1987). The cords may become distended with plasma cells (Figs. 163–165) as the

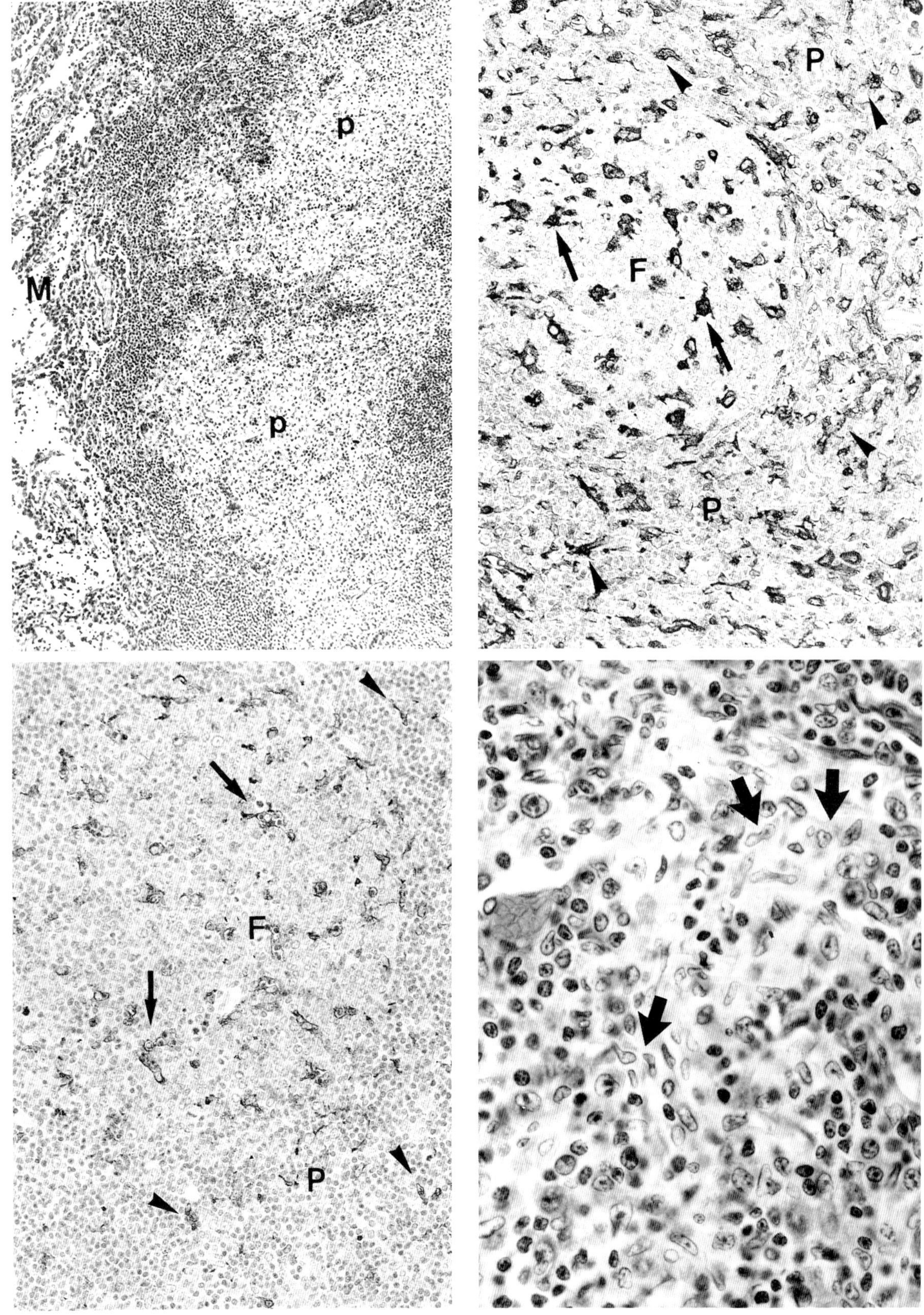

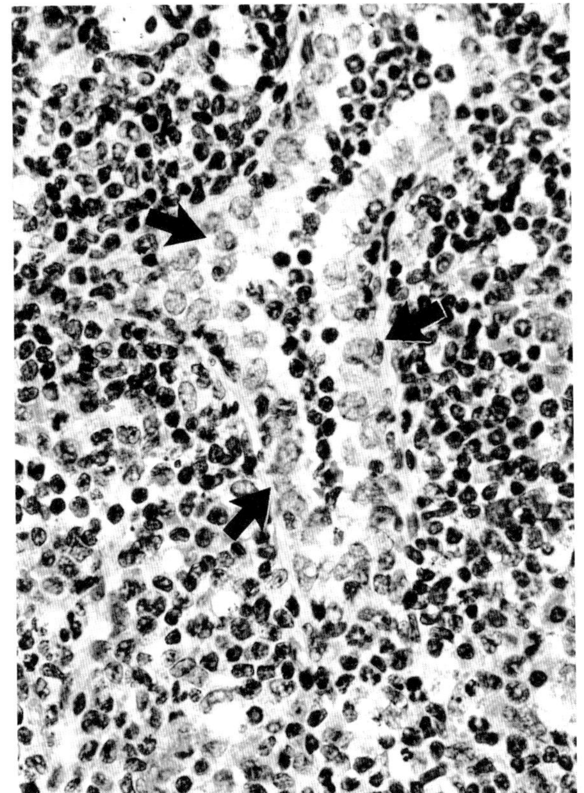

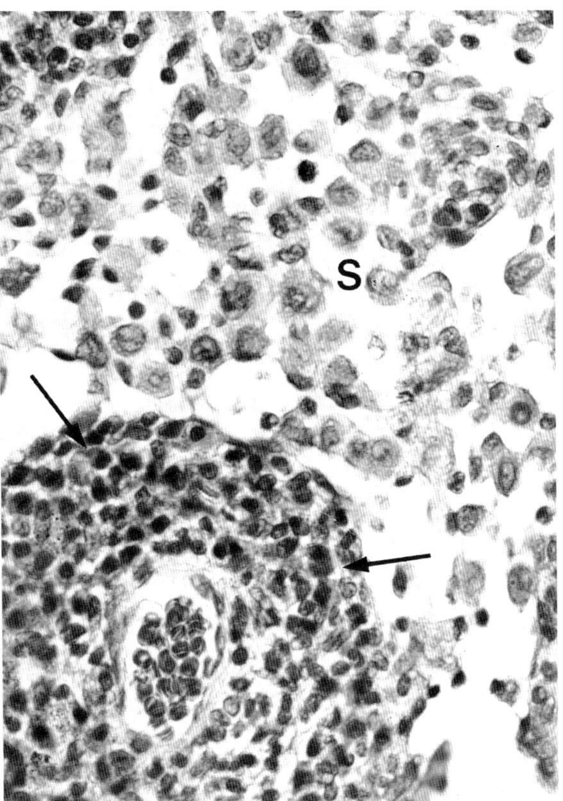

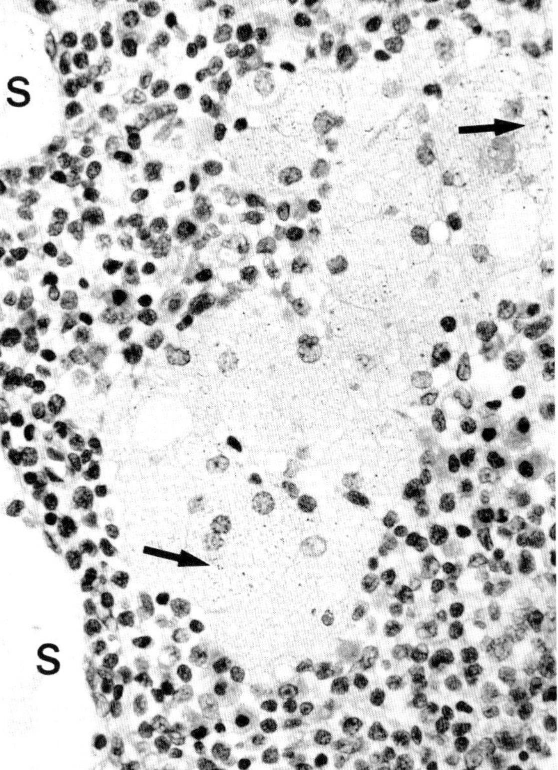

◀ **Fig. 156** *(upper left).* Lymph node, nude rat. Note pale zone of interdigitating dendritic cell hyperplasia *(p)* and depletion of T cells. *M,* medulla. H and E, × 100

Fig. 157 *(lower left).* Follicular dendritic cells *(arrows)* and interdigitating dendritic cells *(arrowheads)* in paracortex *(P)* of normal rat are demonstrated with polyclonal antibody to lysozomal enzymes, especially esterases. *F,* follicle center. Avidin-biotin complex immunoperoxidase, hematoxylin, × 250

Fig. 158 *(upper right).* Follicular dendritic cells *(arrows)* in pale follicle *(F)* and interdigitating dendritic cells *(arrowheads)* in paracortex *(P)* in lymph node of nude rat are greatly increased in number. Compare with normal node in Fig. 157. Avidin-biotin complex immunoperoxidase, hematoxylin, × 250

Fig. 159 *(lower right).* Hyperplasia of pleomorphic interdigitating dendritic cells *(arrows)* in paracortex of lymph node from nude rat. H and E, × 630

Fig. 160 *(upper left).* Hyperplasia and hypertrophy of high ▶ endothelial venule *(arrows)* in lymph node of mouse with chronic lymphadenitis. H and E, × 400

Fig. 161 *(upper right).* Sinus histiocytosis *(S)* in rat lymph node after exposure to a cytotoxic drug. Note plasmacytosis in medullary cord *(arrows).* H and E, × 400

Fig. 162 *(lower right).* Pigmentation *(arrows)* of foamy macrophages in medullary cord in mesenteric lymph node, rat. *S,* medullary sinus. H and E, × 400

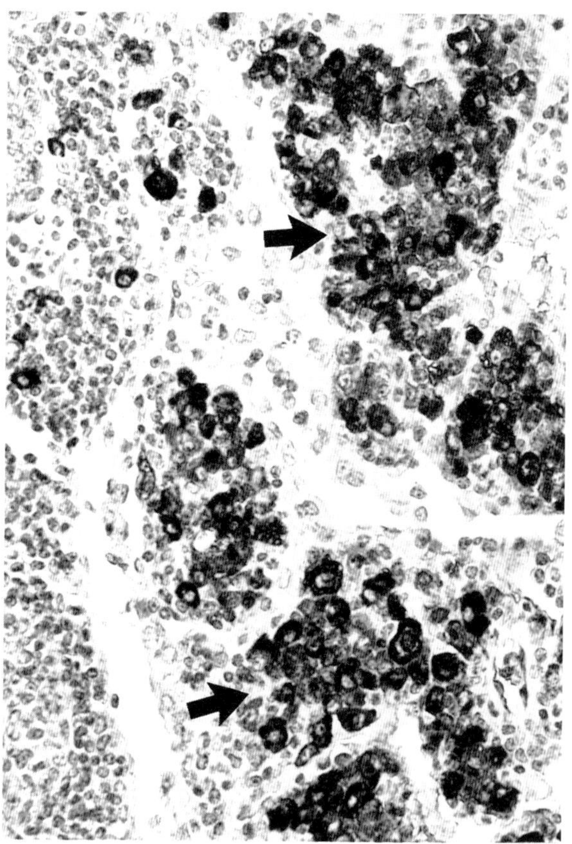

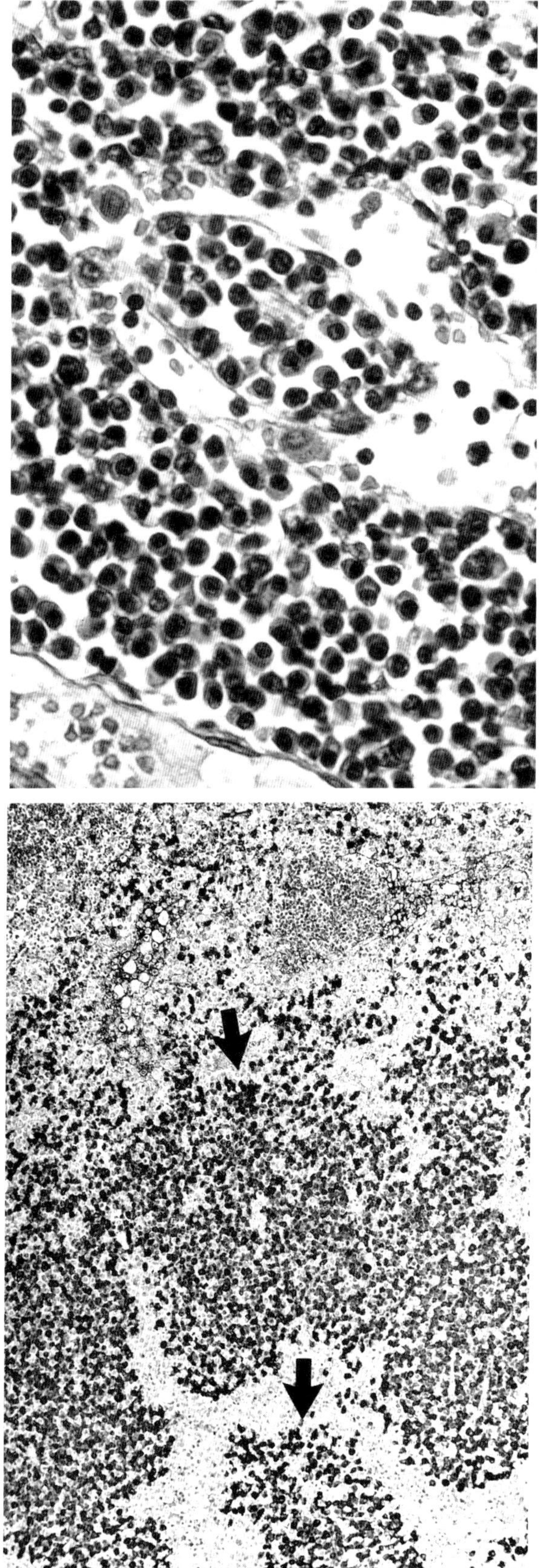

Fig. 163 *(upper left)*. Severe plasmacytosis in medullary cord of rat lymph node. Note mature plasma cells. H and E, ×630

Fig. 164 *(lower left)*. Immunoglobulins in moderate degree of medullary plasmacytosis *(arrows)*. Avidin-biotin complex immunoperoxidase for rat immunoglobulins, hematoxylin, ×100

Fig. 165 *(upper right)*. Plasma cells *(arrows)* in medullary cords of mouse. Avidin-biotin complex immunoperoxidase for mouse immunoglobulins. ×400 node responds intensely to antigens. A severe degree of plasma cell infiltration is termed *plasmacytosis*. Some plasma cells may contain Russell's bodies. Mature plasma cells have a characteristic purple to intensely eosinophilic cytoplasm, eccentrically placed nucleus, and a cartwheel nuclear chromatin pattern. In acute responses, immunoblasts may be seen among the mature plasma cells. These cells have less cytoplasm than plasma cells but have a large blast nucleus with a prominent nucleolus. Plasmacytosis is often seen in lymph nodes draining tissue with lesions caused by infectious agents (ulcerated skin tumor, pneumonia) and tumors (with abundant tumor antigens). The mandibular nodes of rats are the most frequent site of marked plasmacytosis. This lesion can be so severe as to suggest a diagnosis of lymphoma. The nodal architecture may be completely effaced. The pathologist should evaluate the node at low magnification, the possible source of antigens, and involvement of other nodes. Often a node with severe plasmacytosis has follicular atrophy and a cellular T-cell zone. In many species, marked follicular hyperplasia usually accompanies severe plasmacytosis. The occurrence of these two lesions concurrently is less common in rodents. Large numbers of mast cells are rarely seen in lymph nodes of rodents but may involve sinuses and other portions of the node.

The medullary cords can also be the site of extramedullary hemopoiesis (myeloid metaplasia), ordinarily in response to regional infectious lesions (i. e., infected ulcerated skin tumors). Pigmented macrophages are also seen in mesenteric nodes (Fig. 162).

Hyperplastic and atrophic lesions in different anatomic structures of nodes are often in reaction to inflammation or tumors. Frequently, follicular atrophy accompanies marked plasmacytosis. Sinus histiocytosis is also seen with follicular hyperplasia. Nodes draining suppurative lesions may undergo myeloid metaplasia and plasmacytosis. Viral infections can cause follicular atrophy, atrophy of the T-cell zone, and hyperplasia of interdigitating dendritic cells in the paracortex.

Early lymphomas are difficult to evaluate in lymph nodes, although the distribution and morphology of the tumor cells is usually very different from those of normal cells. Their cellular uniformity should be identical to obvious neoplastic cells in the primary tumor mass and other tissues. Early primary or metastatic lymphomatous lesions may occur in the medullary cords, T-cell areas, or cortical follicles.

References

Anderson AO (1985) Multiple effects of immunological adjuvants on lymphatic microenvironment. I. Role of immunologically-relevant angiogenesis in the mechanisms of action of CFA, MDP and Avridine. Int J Immunother 1: 185–195

Frith CG, Wiley LD (1981) Morphologic classification and correlation of incidence of hyperplastic and neoplastic hematopoietic lesions in mice with age. J Gerontol 36: 534–545

Frith CH, Pattengale PK, Ward JM (1985) A color atlas of hematopoietic pathology of mice. Toxicology Pathology Associates, Little Rock, pp 30, Abst 8326

Hartsock RJ (1975) Reactive lesions in lymph nodes. In: Rebuck JW, Berard CW, Abell AR (eds) The reticuloendothelial system. Williams and Wilkins, Baltimore, pp 152–183

Ioachim HL (1982) Lymph node biopsy. Lippincott, Philadelphia

Jaffe ES, Bennington JL (eds) (1985) Surgical pathology of the lymph nodes and related organs. Saunders, Philadelphia

Nathwani BN, Burke JS, Winberg CD (1986) Architectural features of normal, neoplastic and nonneoplastic lymph nodes: a practical approach. In: Murphy GF, Mihm MC, Jr (eds) Lymphoproliferative disorders of the skin. Butterworths, Stoneham, pp 73–119

Robb-Smith AHT, Taylor GB (1981) Lymph node biopsy: a diagnostic atlas. Oxford University Press, New York

Van Rooijen N (1987) The "in situ" immune response in lymph nodes: a review. Anat Rec 218: 359–364

Ward JM, Argilan F, Reynolds CW (1983) Immunoperoxidase localization of large granular lymphocytes in normal tissues and lesions of athymic nude rats. J Immunol 131: 132–139

Weissman IL, Warnke R, Butcher EC, Rouse R, Levy R (1978) The lymphoid system: its normal architecture and the potential for understanding the system through the study of lymphoproliferative diseases. Hum Pathol 9: 25–45

Autoimmune Hemolytic Anemia, NZB Mice

Robert M. Lewis and Catherine A. Picut

Synonyms. Hemolytic disease of NZB mice; autoimmune disease of NZB mice.

Gross Appearance

Splenomegaly is the most prominent lesion observed in moribund animals. Hepatomegaly and generalized lymphadenopathy are also usually present. All three of these lesions may develop initially at approximately 6 months of age, and increase in magnitude and frequency as the anemia becomes increasingly severe (Creighton et al. 1979). The thymus may or may not be grossly prominent.

Microscopic Features

Within the spleen, there is expansion of both the white and red pulp (Figs. 166, 167). Lymphoid follicles with large germinal centers and periarteriolar sheaths are prominent. An abundance of mature and immature plasma cells may also be present. The hyperplastic red pulp is characterized by extramedullary hematopoiesis, eryhtrophagocytosis, and hemosiderosis.

The liver lesion is characterized by Kupffer's cell hyperplasia, erythrocyte sequestration, hemosiderosis, and erythrophagocytosis (Fig. 168). Multifocal lymphoid infiltrates within centrilobular and portal areas are common. Pigmented choleliths and extensive focal zones of hepatocellular necrosis may accompany severe terminal hemolysis.

Reactive lymphoid hyperplasia of lymph nodes may be widespread, with diffuse cortical hyperplasia and expansion of the medullary cords (Figs. 169–171).

Lymphoproliferative lesions extend beyond the liver, spleen, and lymph nodes. Lymphoid hyperplasia is commonly prominent in a peribronchiolar distribution in the lung (Figs. 172–174) as perivascular aggregates in the kidney (Fig. 175) and diffusely throughout the bone marrow. Follicular aggregates of lymphocytes with germinal centers occur in the perivascular sheaths of the thymic medulla.

In addition to lymphoid hyperplasia, lymphoid tumors also occur in NZB mice. The incidence was reported to be 2.4% in the original NZB colony. Higher frequencies (10%–20%) have been reported in other satellite colonies; however, these discrepancies must be viewed carefully due to the difficulty in interpreting advanced lymphoid hyperplasia from overt lymphoid neoplasia in NZB mice solely on histologic grounds (Howie and Simpson 1974). The neoplastic cell types have seen reported as B type reticulum cell tumors, pleomorphic lymphomas, germinal center cell lymphomas, and thymomas.

Evidence of intravascular hemolysis may be observed in the kidney as hemosiderosis of the proximal tubular epithelium.

A second renal lesion encountered in some NZB mice is a membranous to membranoproliferative glomerulonephritis. The severity of the glomerular lesion varies widely but has been shown to reflect the characteristic features of immune complex-mediated glomerulonephritis (ICGN). The principal immunoreactants in the lesion are IgG_2 autoantibody with specificity for DNA and host complement. The ICGN which is encountered in limited numbers of aged NZB mice is similar to the renal lesion encountered in $NZB/NZWF_1$ hybrids, which serve as the murine model for systemic lupus erythematosus.

Gastroduodenal ulcers which arise from circumscribed plaques of hyperplastic glands may be observed in up to 50% of moribund NZB mice.

Differential Diagnosis

Given the presence of Coombs'-positive hemolytic anemia, hepatosplenomegaly, and generalized lymphoproliferative lesions in an NZB mouse, there is in reality no differential diagnosis.

Biologic Features

Mice of the inbred NZB strain regularly develop hemolytic anemia which leads to their premature death. The earliest indication of impending hemolytic disease appears in a small percentage of animals at 3 months of age, at which point they exhibit a positive direct antiglobulin test (Coombs' test) (Howie and Helyer 1968). The frequency of

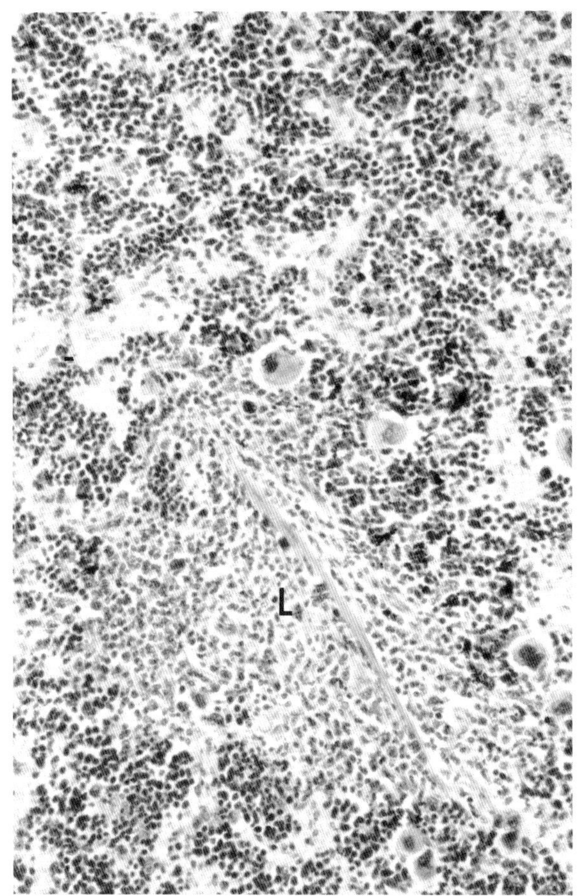

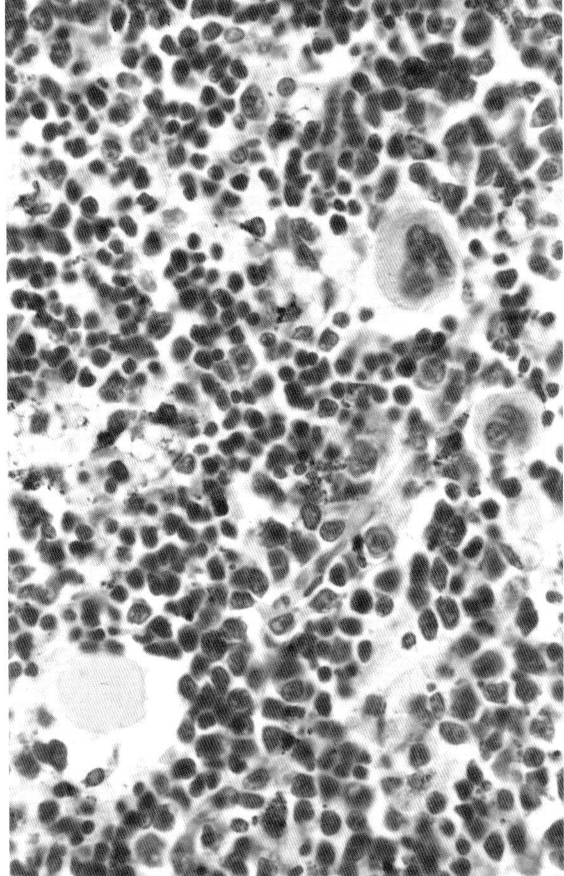

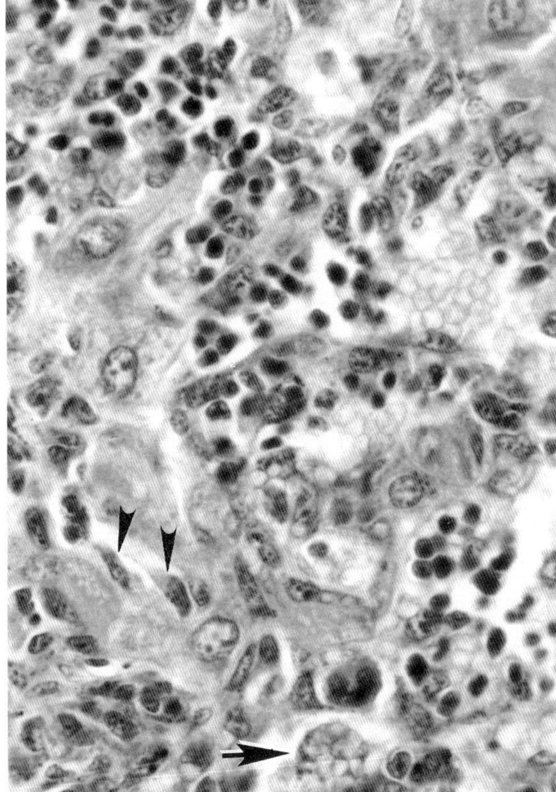

Fig. 166 *(upper left)*. Spleen, NZB mouse. The expanded red pulp contains numerous nests of erythroid precursor cells and megakaryocytes indicative of extramedullary hemopoiesis. A periarteriolar sheath of lymphocytes *(L)* representing T-cell hyperplasia courses diagonally through the field. H and E, × 250

Fig. 167 *(upper right)*. Spleen, NZB mouse. Splenic red pulp illustrating extramedullary hemopoiesis. H and E, × 400

Fig. 168 *(lower right)*. Liver, NZB mouse. Hyperplasia of Kupffer's cells *(arrowheads)*, sequestration of erythrocytes extramedullary hemopoiesis and erythrophagocytosis *(thin arrow)* characterize the changes in the liver associated with hemolytic disease. H and E, × 400

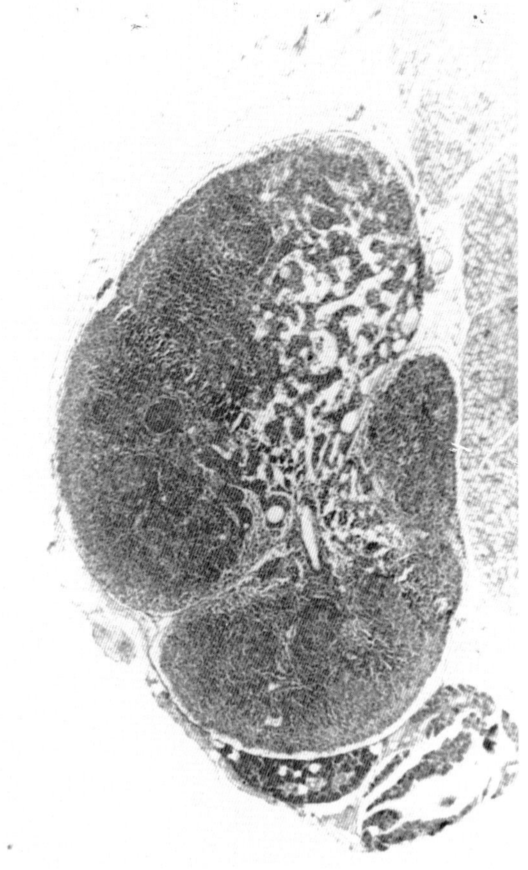

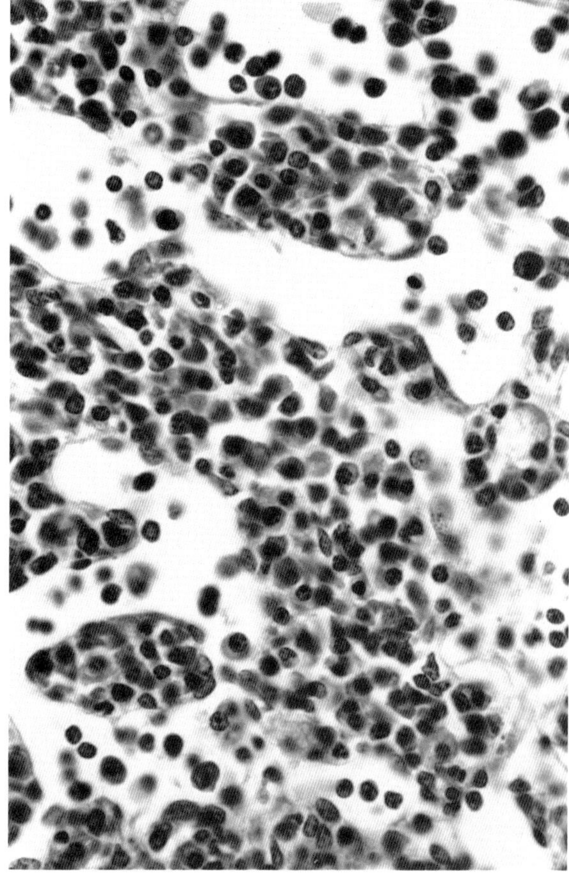

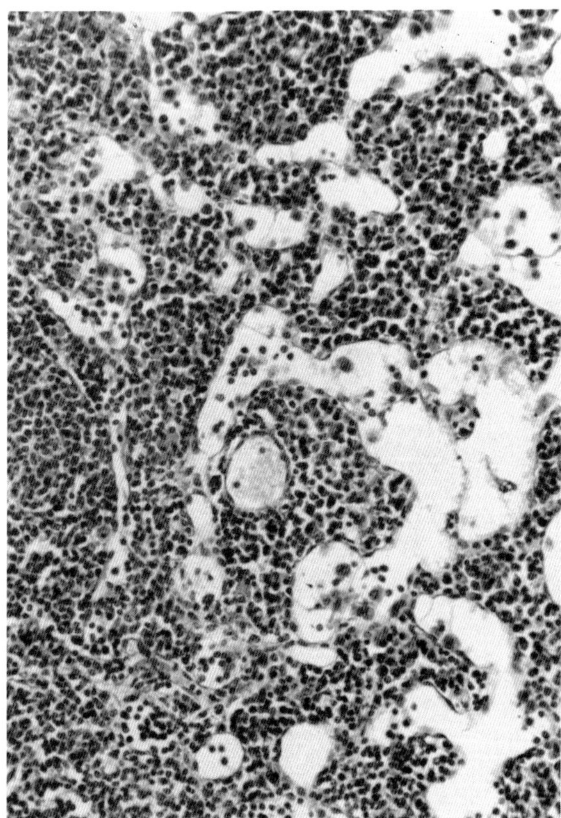

◄ **Fig. 169** *(upper left)*. Lymph node, NZB mouse. Cortical hyperplasia with prominent lymphoid follicles and expansion of the paracortex and medullary cords accompany the generalized lymphadenopathy. Note that the normal cytoarchitecture is preserved, and the medullary sinusoids are dilated and devoid of cells and exudate. H and E, × 14

Fig. 170 *(lower left)*. Lymph node, NZB mouse. Expanded medullary cords separated by sparsely populated sinusoids. H and E, × 250

Fig. 171 *(upper right)*. Lymph node, NZB mouse. Marked plasmacytosis of medullary cords. H and E, × 400

Fig. 172 *(upper left)*. Lung, NZB mouse. Peribronchiolar ▶ and perivascular lymphoid aggregates may be prominently disseminated throughout the lung. H and E, × 100

Fig. 173 *(lower left)*. Lung, NZB mouse. Segmental peribronchiolar lymphoid hyperplasia. H and E, × 250

Fig. 174 *(upper right)*. Lung, NZB mouse. Higher magnification of Fig. 173, further illustrating lymphoid hyperplasia. H and E, × 400

Fig. 175 *(lower right)*. Kidney, NZB mouse. Periarteriolar lymphoid hyperplasia is prominent at the corticomedullary junction. H and E, × 250

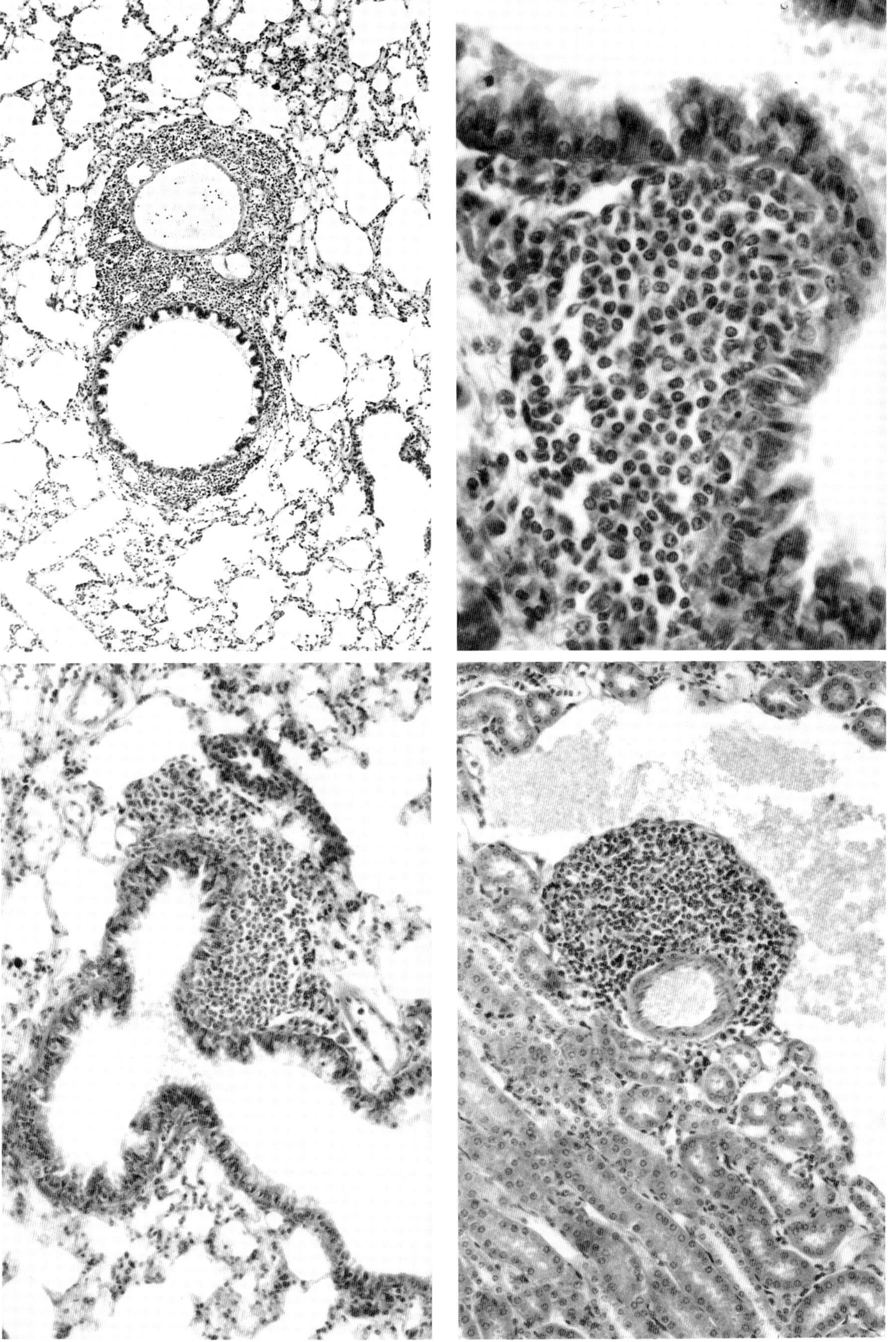

Coombs' test positively in NZB mice reaches 100% by 18 months of age in most colonies. Evidence of overt hemolysis usually follows this conversion to Coombs' positivity by 2–3 months. Variances in the time of onset, rate of progression, morbidity, and mortality of hemolytic disease are associated with three distinct classes of animals within NZB mouse colonies: males, virgin females, and breeder females. In general, the hemolytic disease is most florid in virgin females (Howie and Simpson 1974). Accompanying the signs of anemia are hepatosplenomegaly and occasionally jaundice. Depression, wasting, and intercurrent infections may be observed in chronically anemic mice. The average life span of NZB mice is 15–18 months, with males living approximately 1 month longer than females (Milich and Gershwin 1980).

Laboratory Findings

Anemia, indicated by hematocrit values below 40%, is accompanied by spherocytosis and increasingly severe reticulocytosis (Figs. 176, 177). The direct antiglobulin test (Coombs' test) becomes positive, usually several months prior to actual increased destruction of erythrocytes (hemolysis). Free circulation, unbound, erythrocyte-specific antibody may also be demonstrated in some mice by the indirect antiglobulin test. The erythrocyte-specific autoantibody is of the IgG_1 subclass, and it acts as an "incomplete" warm agglutinin with a thermal range of $18°–37°C$.

The pathogenic erythrocyte autoantibody of NZB mice primarily reacts with the exposed X surface autoantigen of murine red blood cells. Following its binding to X antigen, autoantibody may also exhibit specificity for a second "cryptic" erythrocyte autoantigen, designated HB (DeHeer and Edgington 1976). Rising concentrations of erythrocyte autoantibody correlate closely with increasingly severe anemia, reticulocytosis, and splenomegaly (Cohen 1980).

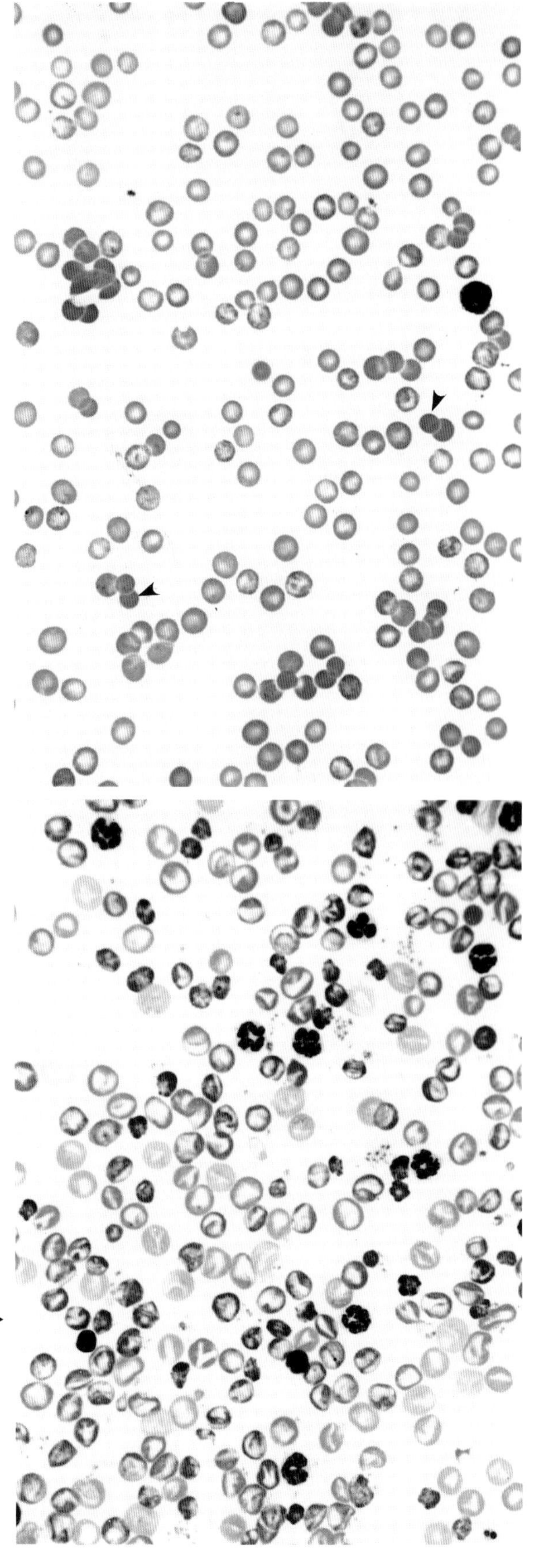

Fig. 176 *(above).* Blood film, NZB mouse. Marked ▶ spherocytosis characterizes the erythrocyte morphology during periods of severe hemolysis *(arrowheads).* May-Grünwald-Giemsa stain, × 400

Fig. 177 *(below).* Blood film, NZB mouse. Severe anisocytosis, poikilocytosis, and polychromatophilia characterize the erythrocyte morphology during the regenerative phase of chronic hemolytic anemia. May-Grünwald-Giemsa stain, × 400

Etiology and Pathogenesis

Since virtually all NZB mice develop a positive Coombs' test, hybridization experiments with nonautoimmune strains of mice have been conducted to clarify whether this autoimmune trait is genetically determined. These experiments demonstrated transmission of Coombs' positivity to the F_1 heterozygous hybrids, thus establishing the inheritance pattern as an autosomal dominant trait. Currently, three genes *(Aia-1, Aia-2,* and *Aem-1)* have been postulated to control erythrocyte-specific autoantibody production (Shirai et al. 1984).

Certain immunologic defects have also been shown to contribute to the development of autoimmune hemolytic disease in NZB mice. These involve T-cell abnormalities related to establishing and maintaining tolerance to endogenous and exogenous antigens, as well as immunoregulatory defects between T cells and B cells (Russell et al. 1981).

In the first instance, the development of autoantibody to X erythrocyte autoantigen results from the abrogation of immunologic tolerance of T cells with X specificity. Their subsequent interaction with X-specific B cells results in the production of X-specific autoantibody.

An alternative explanation involves a reduction in T suppressor cells which results in B cell hyperreactivity and excessive antibody production. During this process the clonal expansion of B cells with X specificity leads to erythrocyte-specific antibody and subsequent hemolytic disease (Cooke and Hutchings 1984). In addition, a primary B-cell defect resulting in hyperreactivity and excessive antibody production has been proposed.

The spontaneous production of thymocyte-specific autoantibody in NZB mice may also play a vital role in these immunologic aberrations. The possibility that oncogenic or nononcogenic viruses might be important causal or modifying factors in the autoimmune disease of NZB mice has been extensively investigated, since a small percentage of NZB mice develop lymphomas. However, to date the role played by viruses in the etiology of NZB hemolytic disease remains elusive (Milich and Gershwin 1980).

Comparison with Other Strains

Although the NZB strain serves as the prototype for murine autoimmune hemolytic anemia,

Table 40. Frequency of positive direct Coombs' tests in selected strains of autoimmune mice

Strain	Sex	Age	Frequency
NZB	Female	3 months	5%
	Female	6 months	32%
	Female	9 months	89%
NZB × NZW (BWf$_1$)	Female	6 months	11%
		9 months	78%
BXSB	Male	6 months	18%
MRL/1	Male	Adult	11%
	Female	Adult	4%

Coombs' test-positive hemolytic disease has been reported in several other inbred "autoimmune" mouse strains. These include the first generation hybrids of NZB × NZW parentage (BWf$_1$), BXSB, SJL/J, and MRL-Lpr. Although the specific events associated with hemolytic disease in these strains vary to some degree from those of NZB mice, many features of their hematologic disorder are similar to those of the prototype (NZB) strain (Quimby 1988). In these other strains, the predominant immunopathology is associated with a lupus-like syndrome, with Coombs' test-positive hemolytic disease (AIHA) contributing only a minor component to their systemic disorder. Table 40 lists the frequency of Coombs' test positive reactivity in several strains of these "autoimmune" mice. Although the frequency of Coombs' test positive reactivity is as high as 78% in female BWf$_1$ mice, clinical anemia per se is relatively rare.

References

Cohen PL (1980) Bone marrow as the major site of anti-erythrocyte autoantibody production in NZB mice. Arthritis Rheum 23: 1045–1048

Cooke A, Hutchings P (1984) Defective regulation of erythrocyte autoantibodies in SJL mice. Immunology 51: 489–492

Creighton WD, Zinkervagel RM, Dixon FJ (1979) T cell mediated immune responses of lupus prone BXSB mice and other murine strains. Clin Exp Immunol 37: 181–189

DeHeer DH, Edgington TS (1976) Specific antigen-binding and antibody-secreting lymphocytes associated with the erythrocyte autoantibody responses of NZB and genetically unrelated mice. J Immunol 116: 1051–1058

Howie JB, Helyer BJ (1968) The immunology and pathology of NZB mice. Adv Immunol 9: 215–264

Howie JB, Simpson LO (1974) Autoimmune haemolytic disease in NZB mice. Ser Haematol VII: 386–426

Milich DR, Gershwin ME (1980) The pathogenesis of autoimmunity in New Zealand mice. (Reviews). Semin Arthritis Rheum 10: 111–147
Quimby F (1988) Immunodeficient rodents: a guide to their immunobiology, husbandry and use. National Academy Press, Washington
Russell PJ, Cunningham J, Dunkley M, Wilkinson NM (1981) The role of suppressor T cells in the expression of autoimmune hemolytic anaemia in NZB mice. Clin Exp Immunol 45: 496–503
Shirai T, Hirose S, Ohta K, Maruyama N (1984) H-2-linked genes and autoimmune disease in New Zealand mice. In: Sasazuki T, Tada T (eds) Immunogenetics: its application to clinical medicine. Academic, New York, pp 75–84

Toxic Effects on the Immune System, Rat

J. G. Vos and Magda A. M. Krajnc-Franken

Introduction

Toxicologic research during the past decade has indicated that the immune system is a potential target for many foreign chemicals. In an international workshop held in Luxembourg in the fall of 1984 (IPCS, 1986) immunotoxicology was defined as the discipline that is concerned with the study of the events that can lead to undesired effects as a result of the interaction of xenobiotics with the immune system. These undesired effects may result from (a) the direct and/or indirect action of the xenobiotic and/or its biotransformation product on the immune system, or (b) an immunobiologically based host response to the compound and/or its metabolite(s) or to host antigens modified by the compound and/or its metabolites. The discipline of immunotoxicology can be subdivided into four main subdisciplines, i. e., (a) the study of the altered immunologic events associated with the exposure of humans or animals to xenobiotics, including drugs not originally intended for immunomodulatory purposes; (b) the study of altered immune events that may follow exposure to immunotherapeutic agents; (c) the study of allergy and autoimmunity resulting from exposure to xenobiotics (including drugs); and (d) the development and application of immunologic techniques and approaches in toxicology (Berlin et al. 1987).

This chapter is focussed on the histopathologic examination of lymphoid tissues of rats following exposure to xenobiotics. This assessment can be best performed in the context of conventional toxicology studies, in which high dose levels of toxic compounds are used and which are aimed at establishing the toxicologic profile and the target organs of toxicity (Vos and Van Loveren 1987; IPCS 1986). For a first tier screening, a set of general parameters of the specific and nonspecific defense potential is used. Important immunotoxicologic parameters for the screening of potential immunotoxic compounds are weight and histology of lymphoid organs. In routine toxicology studies, histopathologic examination consists mostly of H and E staining of paraffin-embedded tissue sections. In many studies, this routine histopathology has been useful for assessing the immunotoxicity of a chemical, in particular when the results are related to observations on changes in weight of the lymphoid organs. Because of the structural division of the spleen and lymphoid nodes into thymus-dependent and thymus-independent areas, indications regarding the relative effects of chemicals for T- and B-cell compartments can be obtained. Depending on the route of exposure to the test compounds, it may be necessary to examine bronchus-associated (BALT) or gut-associated lymphoid tissue (GALT); these tissues also show T/B-cell compartmentalization.

The potential immunotoxicity of a chemical can be confirmed or further analyzed by more sophisticated and sensitive techniques such as histochemistry. With regard to immunohistochemistry, the immunoperoxidase technique is of particular significance. Most cytoplasmic antigens, e. g., immunoglobulins in plasma cells or lysozyme in macrophages, can readily be demonstrated in fixed paraffin sections. Cell surface antigens, which are only present in small amounts, e. g., surface markers on macrophages, T helper, and T suppressor cells, can be better shown in preserved frozen sections. A difficulty for the toxicologic pathologist in the evaluation of often minor chemically induced lesions is designing objective classification. By randomizing and coding the slides, bias in reading can be avoided, and qualitative analysis is possible. Classification is improved by morphometric analysis since quantitative measurements on cells and tissues can be made by this method. In this context, it is of interest to mention that recent developments in monoclonal antibodies, computer processing, and cytometrical instrumentation has led to the new field of clinical flow cytometry. This field has already found specific applications in diagnostic immunopathology, including the study of congenital and acquired immune deficiency diseases (Lovett et al. 1984).

In this chapter, after a short description of the biologic and microscopic features of the thymus, spleen, lymph nodes, and Peyer's patches, examples of chemically induced lesions in these tissues will be described. In addition, tissues of so-called athymic nude rats will be shown to demonstrate clearly the compartmentalization into B- and T-cell areas.

Thymus

Biologic and Microscopic Features

The thymus derives embryologically from the endoderm of the third and fourth branchial pouches and reaches its maximum size during neonatal life, after which a gradual process of involution begins. Histologically, the thymus is a lymphoepithelial organ consisting of many lobules, each containing a cortex and medulla. Stem cells, which originate from the bone marrow, undergo extensive proliferation particularly in the periphery of the thymic cortex. Lymphocytes (thymocytes) of varying size are closely packed in the cortex together with epithelial cells and macrophages. Thymocytes migrate from the cortex to the medulla, where they further differentiate before they migrate to the peripheral lymphoid system as mature cells. Like the cortex, the medulla contains many epithelial cells. Epithelial cells play an active role in thymocyte differentiation: they secrete thymic hormones (humoral factors) promoting T-cell maturation, and they interact directly with thymocytes through cell-to-cell contacts and thereby influence their antigen specificity. Ultrastructurally, membrane contacts between the cytoplasmic processes of epithelial cells and thymocytes can be seen. The thymic hormones promote T-lymphocyte maturation in the thymus and at other sites in the body. Exam-

ples of these hormones are the nonapeptide thymulin and thymosin α_1. Medullary epithelium is also organized into Hassall's corpuscles, the precise function of which is not known. For a detailed description of the normal anatomy of the thymus, the reader is referred to Dijkstra and Sminia (see p. 249, this volume).

Chemically Induced Alterations

Pronounced effects on rat thymus morphology and thymus-dependent immune function are found in short-term toxicity experiments with the environmental contaminant bis(tri-n-butyltin)oxide (TBTO) (Krajnc et al. 1984; Vos et al. 1984). Dietary TBTO administration to rats for 6 weeks elicits remarkable atrophy of the thymic cortex, leading to absence of distinct corticomedullary junctions due to lymphocyte depletion (Fig. 178). This reduced cellularity can, at least in part, be explained as a result of thymocyte destruction (karyopyknosis and karyorrhexis), giving an indication of direct toxic action of TBTO on thymocytes (Fig. 179).

Depending on the thymotoxic action of the chemical, the atrophy of the thymic cortex may be reversible. Thus, thymic atrophy induced by single dose treatment of rats with di-n-butyltindichloride is restored in a few days by an increased proliferative activity of thymocytes (Penninks and Seinen 1987). On the other hand, thymic atrophy in the rat produced by perinatal maternal treatment with 2,3,7,8-tetrachlorodibenzo-p-dioxin persisted for at least 5 months (Faith and Moore 1977).

Spleen

Biologic and Microscopic Features

The spleen is the largest lymphoid organ in the circulation. Its function is to clear particulate materials from the blood by its abundant number of phagocytes and also to concentrate blood-borne antigens. It is also the site of erythrocyte storage and of the removal of effete erythrocytes and leukocytes. Histologically, the spleen is divided into the white pulp, the major lymphoid mass surrounding the small arteries and arterioles, and the red pulp containing cellular cords with many macrophages between erythrocyte-filled venous sinuses. In the spleen, T- and B-cell areas are segregated. The diffuse lymphoid tissue immedi-

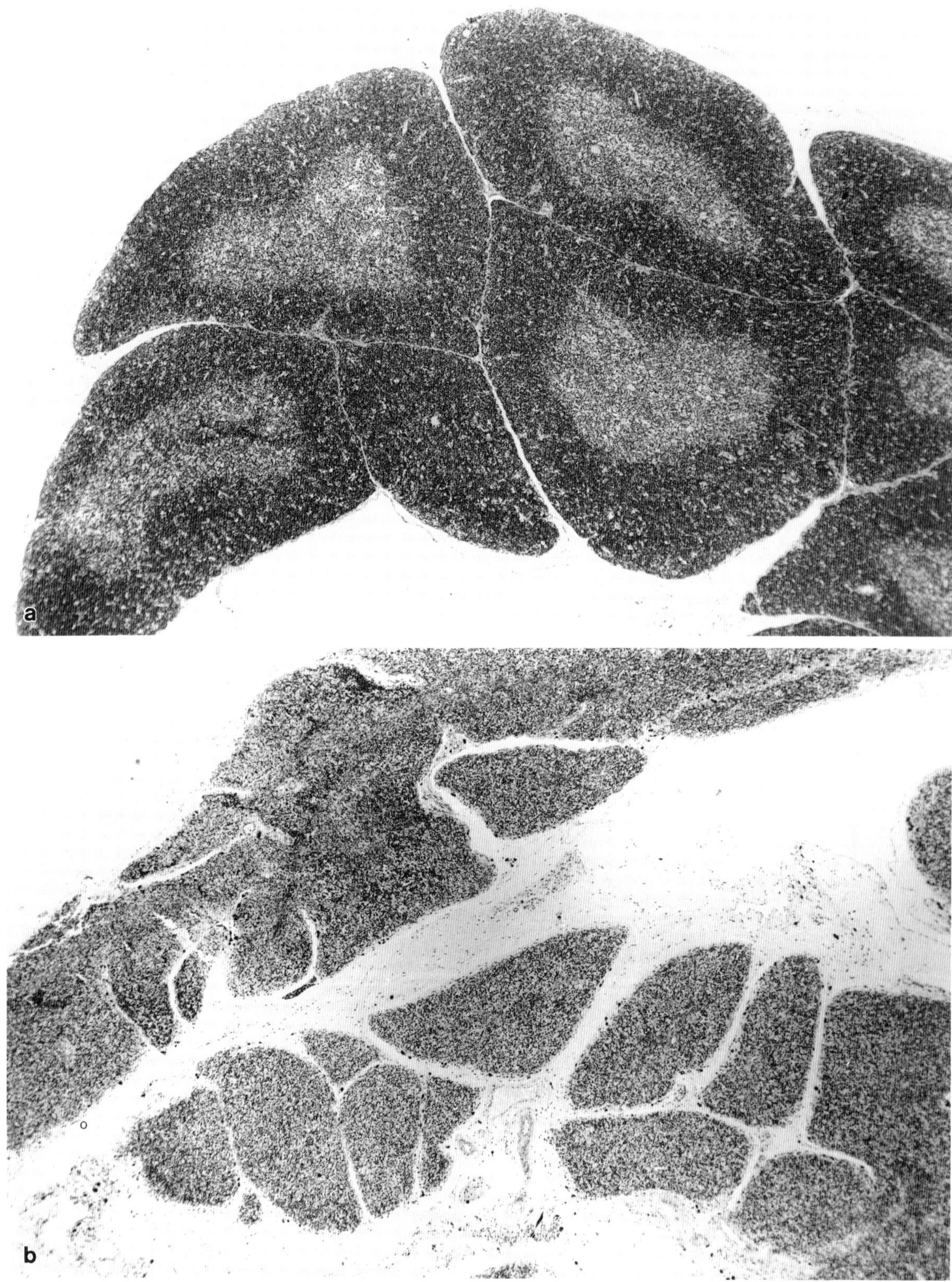

Fig. 178a, b. Thymus, (a) from control rat and (b) from rat fed 320 mg TBTO/kg diet for 4 weeks; note severe lympho-cyte depletion and atrophy of the cortex and absence of distinct corticomedullary junctions. Glycolmethacrylate embedding, Giemsa stain, ×45

Fig. 179 a, b. Thymus, (a) from control rat with densely ▶ populated thymic cortex and distinct corticomedullary junction and (b) from rat fed 320 mg TBTO/kg diet for 3 days showing evidence of thymocyte destruction (karyo-pyknosis and karyorrhexis). Glycolmethacrylate embedding, Giemsa stain, × 500

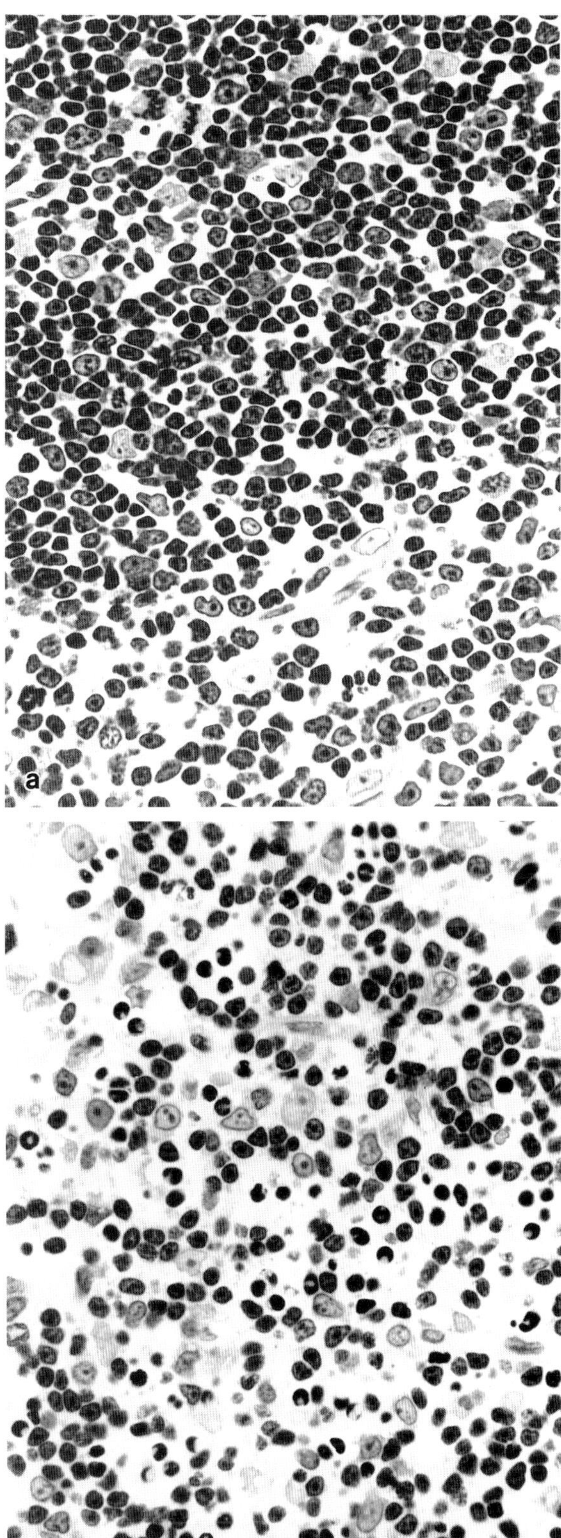

ately surrounding the arteriole, the periarteriolar lymphocyte sheath (PALS), is populated predominantly by recirculating small T cells. The adjacent B-cell area comprises the follicles with a germinal center. The marginal zone (MZ) contains B lymphocytes and some T lymphocytes and is separated from the PALS and follicles by a marginal sinus. It is seen as a broad band of medium-sized lymphocytes that also borders the red pulp. Plasma cells in the spleen are mainly found in the red pulp cords (see p. 226, this volume).

Compartmentalization of B- and T-cell areas in the spleen is clearly demonstrated in congenital athymic *rnu/rnu* rats as compared with their heterozygous thymus-bearing +/*rnu* littermates. The histologic appearance of the spleen of the +/*rnu* rats is consistent with that observed in other rat strains as it is composed of a normal red pulp and a white pulp with marginal zones, follicles, and the thymus-dependent PALS (Fig. 180a). In contrast with their thymus-bearing littermates, athymic nude rats have remarkably fewer lymphoid cells in the PALS (Fig. 180b). With the indirect peroxidase-labeled antibody method using monoclonal rat T cell-specific antibody, only in the PALS of the +/*rnu* rats can T lymphocytes be identified (Vos et al. 1983a).

Chemically Induced Alterations

Besides its effect on the thymus, the administration of TBTO to rats also causes morphologic alterations in the spleen. The effects observed are atrophy of the PALS and the follicles as well (Krajnc et al. 1984). Analogous to the histopathologically observed lymphocyte depletion in the PALS, a marked decrease in the number of immunoreactive T lymphocytes is noticed in the PALS of rats treated with TBTO (Fig. 181).

In contrast, a stimulatory effect on the lymphoid system in the rat is achieved with hexachlorobenzene correlating with the stimulatory effects on immune function (Vos et al. 1979, 1983b). In a 3-week feeding experiment, hexachlorobenzene caused an increase in the weight of the spleen and the lymph nodes. The splenomegaly is char-

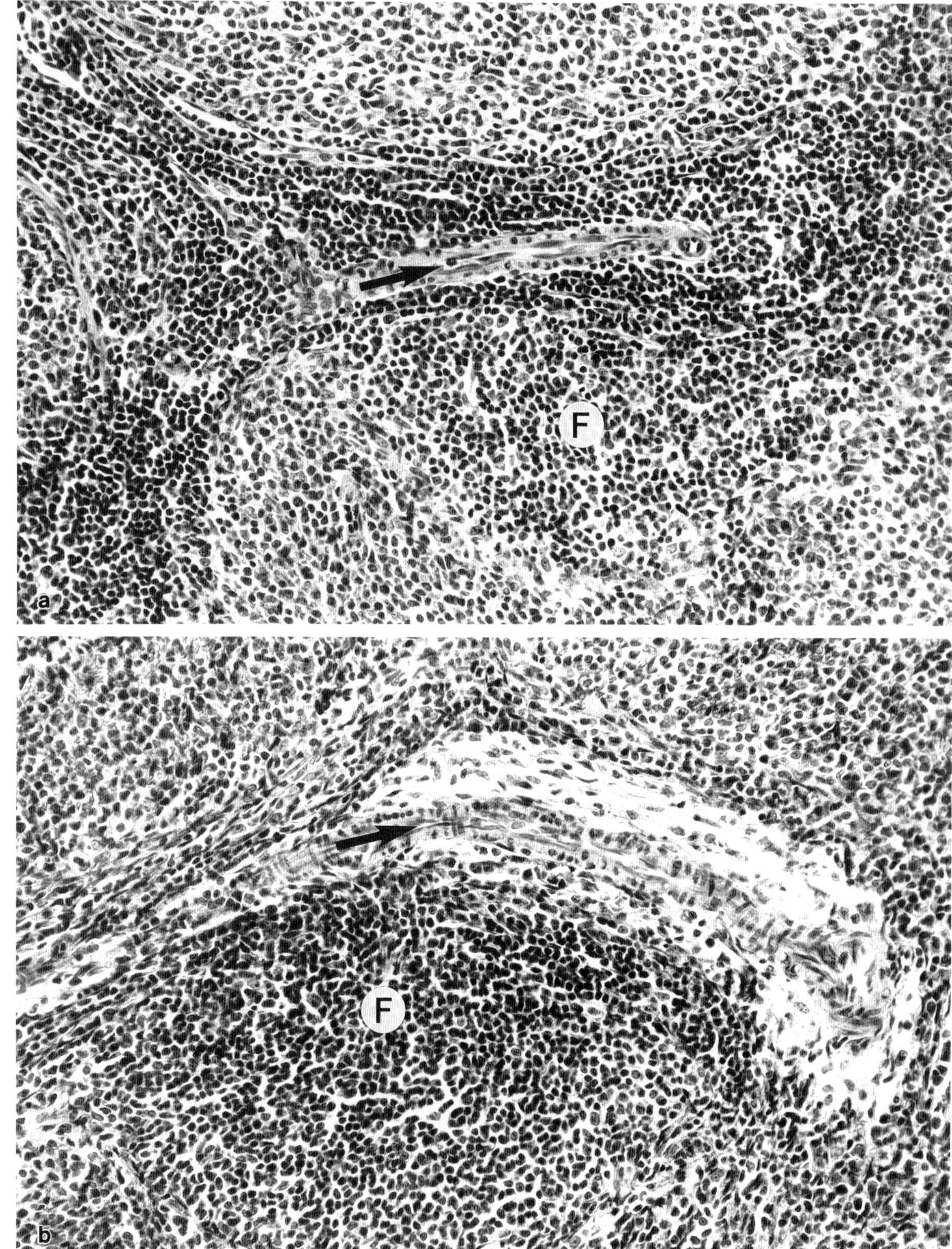

Fig. 180 a, b. Spleen, (**a**) from + / *rnu* rat with large numbers of small lymphocytes in the thymus-dependent area around the longitudinally sectioned central artery *(arrow)* (*F*, follicle) and (**b**) from *rnu/rnu* rat showing the reticular framework of the thymus-dependent area around the longitudinally sectioned central artery *(arrow)* that is virtually devoid of lymphocytes, and a normally developed follicle. H and E, ×270

Fig. 181 a, b. Immunocytochemical staining for T lymphocytes in the spleen using monoclonal W3/13 mouse anti-rat antibodies from (**a**) control rat showing immunoreactive cells in the periarteriolar lymphocyte sheaths and (**b**) from rat fed 320 mg TBTO/kg diet for 6 weeks; note severe atrophy. ×80

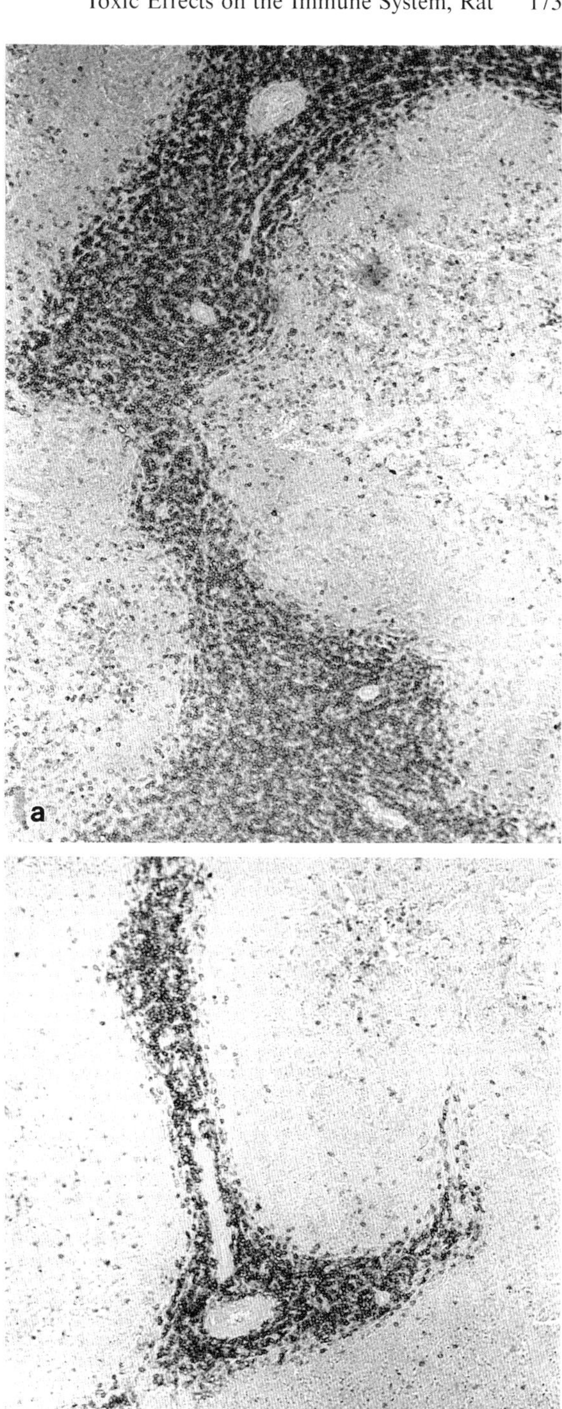

acterized by an increase in the size of the marginal zones, follicles, and possibly PALS, as a result of lymphocyte hyperplasia (Fig. 182).

Lymph nodes

Biologic and Microscopic Features

Lymph nodes are peripheral lymphoid organs that contain lymphocytes within a reticular stroma. They receive lymph from a neighboring region of the body by way of afferent lymphatics which enter the nodes at the subcapsular sinus. Within the nodes, lymph flows through the superficial and deep cortex and medullary sinuses towards the hilar efferent lymphatics.

As in the spleen, there is compartmentalization of B and T lymphocytes. The superficial cortex contains follicular aggregations made up predominantly of B cells. Following antigenic stimulation primary follicles enlarge to secondary follicles having a pale staining central area of macrophages and proliferating lymphocytes. In these so-called germinal centers B lymphocytes differentiate to plasmablasts and become antibody-producing plasma cells in the medullary cords which lie between the medullary sinuses. T lymphocytes are confined to the interfollicular and deep cortical regions, referred to as thymus-dependent or paracortical areas. Following stimulation with an antigen that evokes a T cell-mediated response, the paracortical area enlarges with lymphoblasts, making it evident. The paracortical area contains postcapillary venules lined by specialized high endothelium through which circulating lymphocytes enter the node. This is the main site at which lymphocytes in the blood enter the lymphatic circulation, enabling a continuous recirculation from blood to lymph and back to blood (see p. 129, this volume).

As in the spleen, in the mesenteric and popliteal lymph nodes no differences in morphology are observed between +/rnu rats and other rat strains (Vos et al. 1980). The lymph nodes are composed of an outer cortex with follicles, paracortex, and medulla. In the lymph nodes of athymic rnu/rnu rats, there is a striking lymphoid

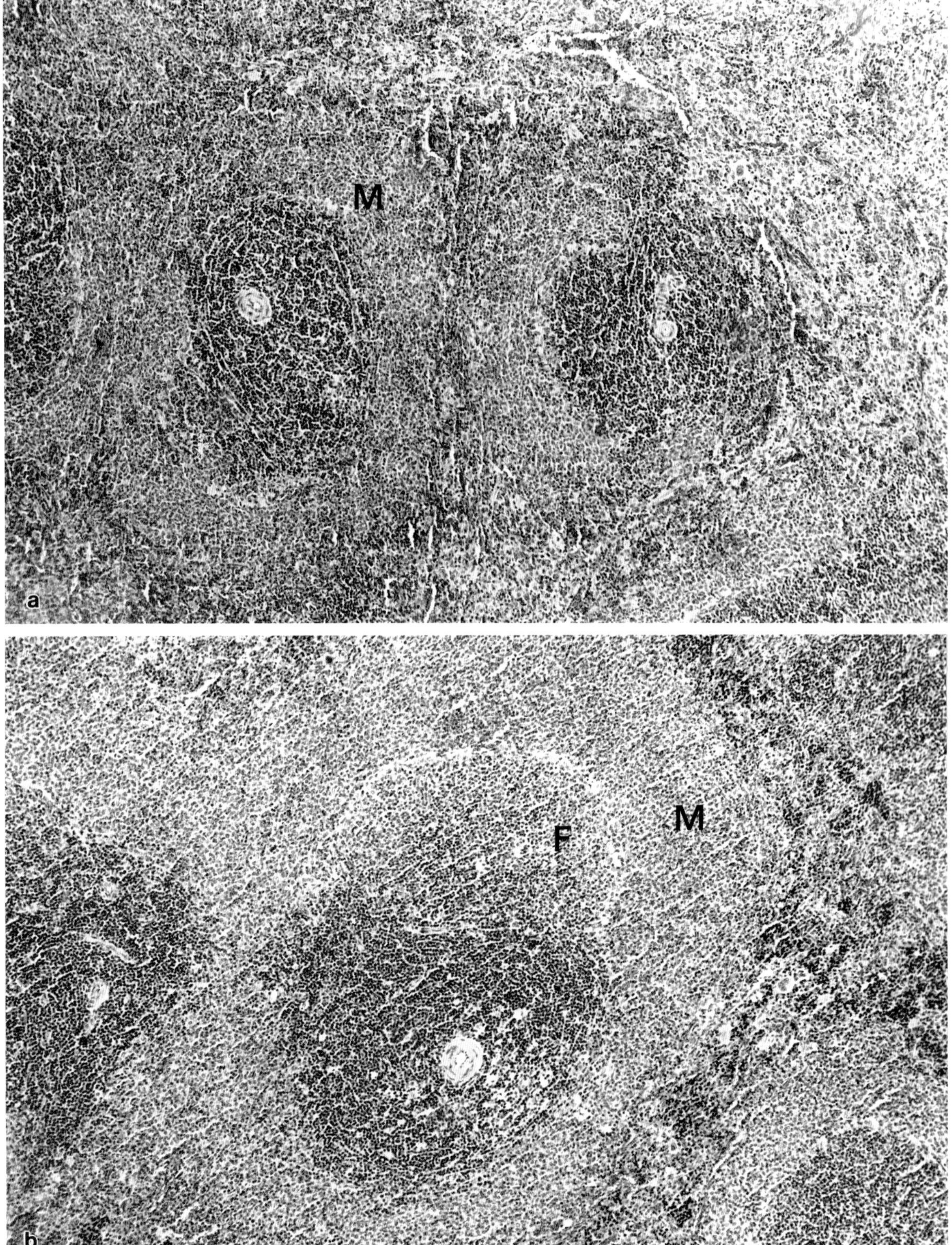

Fig. 182a, b. Spleen, (a) from control rat showing normally developed follicles *(F)* with marginal zones *(M)* and (b) from rat fed 1000 mg HCB/kg diet for 3 weeks. Note the enlargement of follicles and marginal zones. Perls' stain, × 110

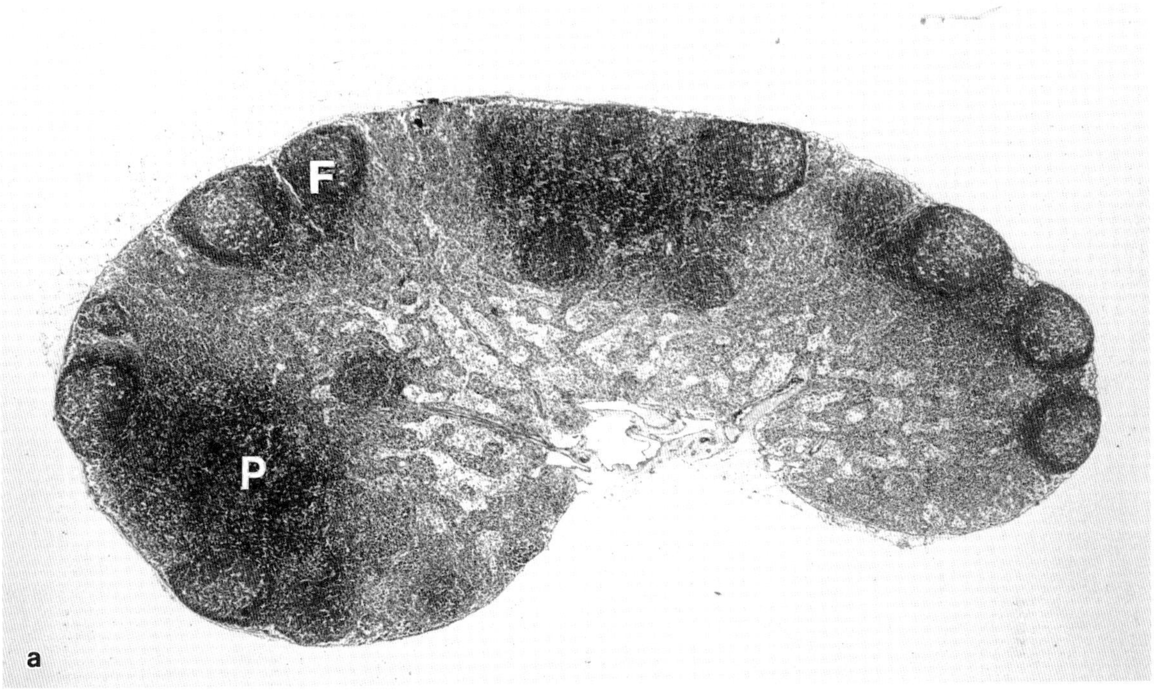

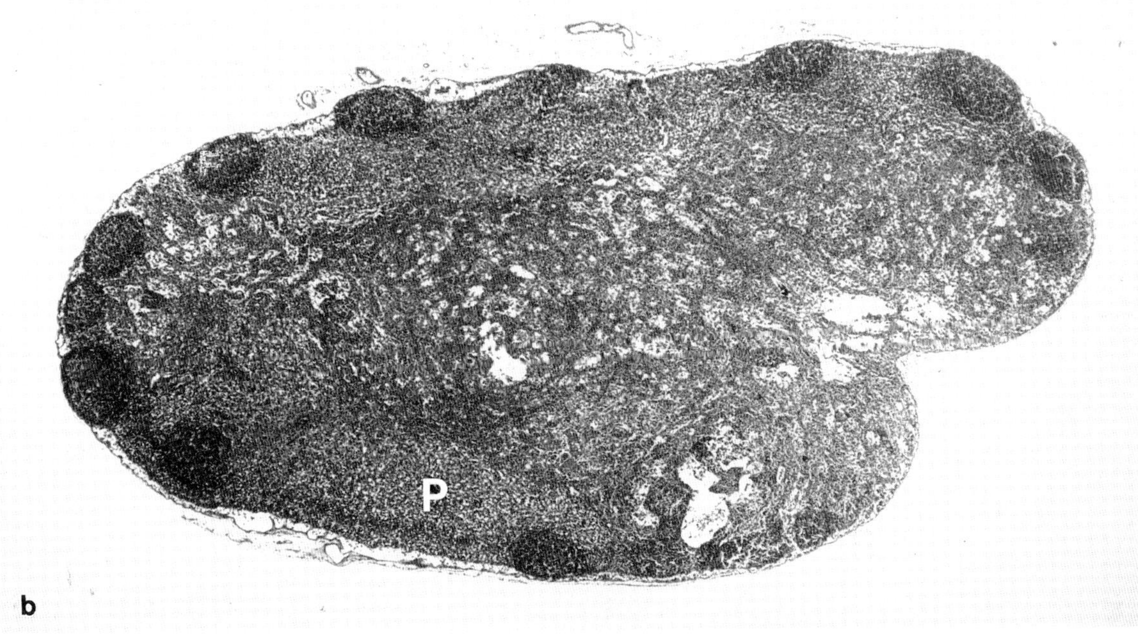

Fig. 183a, b. Mesenteric lymph node, (a) from +/*rnu* rat with normal paracortex *(P)* and follicles *(F)* with germinal center and (b) from *rnu/rnu* rat with profound lymphocyte depletion in the paracortex. H and E, ×25

hypocellularity in the paracortex. As this thymus-dependent area is conspicuously poor in lymphocytes, the reticular framework becomes prominent (Fig. 183). Moreover, in contrast to the presence of high endothelial venules in the paracortex of +/*rnu* rats with lymphocytes migrating through the walls, these venules are thin walled in nude *(rnu/rnu)* rats. Although no differences are observed in the number of follicles, germinal centers regularly encountered in thymus-bearing rats are only incidentally seen in athymic animals.

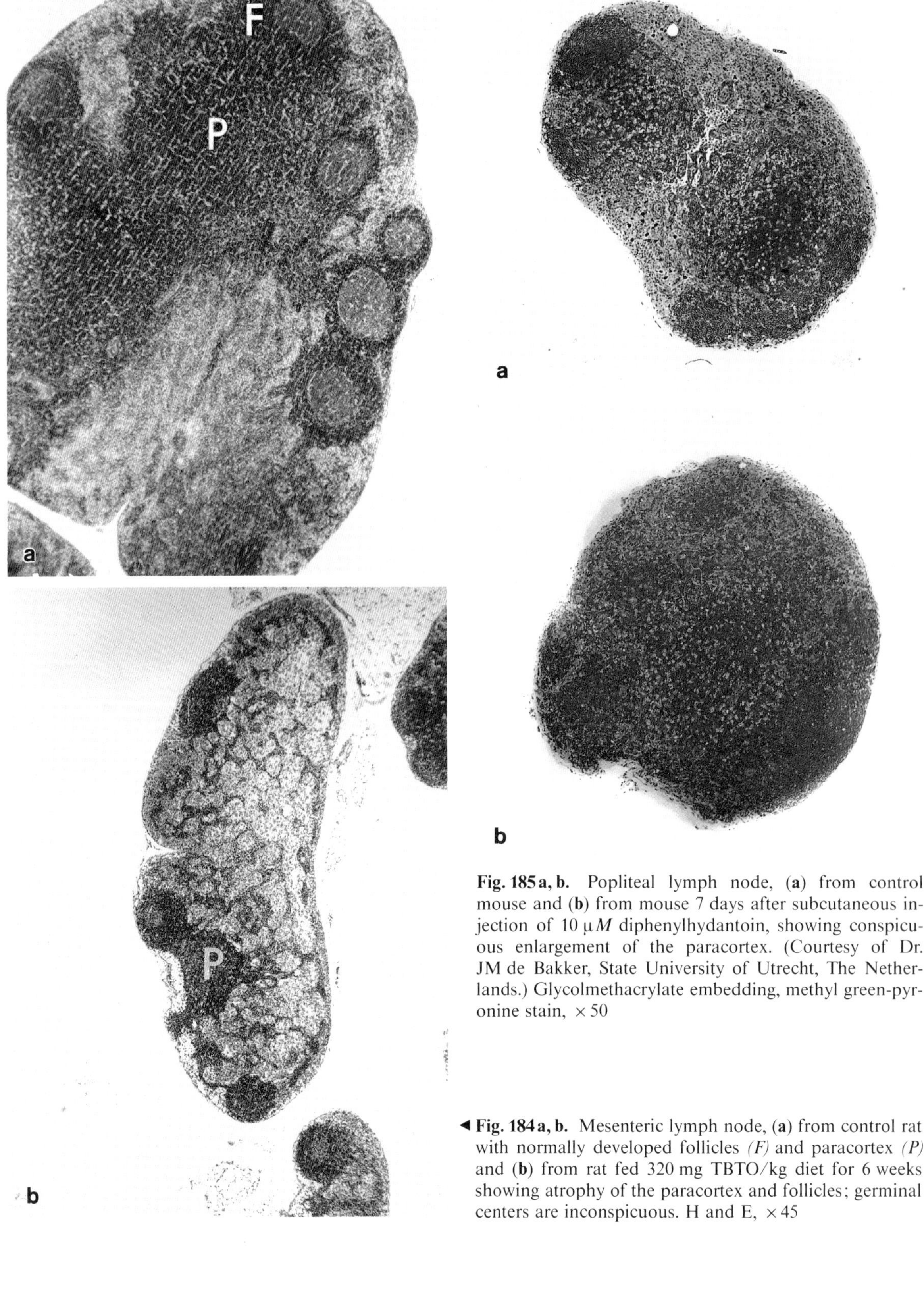

Fig. 185a, b. Popliteal lymph node, (a) from control mouse and (b) from mouse 7 days after subcutaneous injection of 10 μM diphenylhydantoin, showing conspicuous enlargement of the paracortex. (Courtesy of Dr. JM de Bakker, State University of Utrecht, The Netherlands.) Glycolmethacrylate embedding, methyl green-pyronine stain, × 50

◀ **Fig. 184a, b.** Mesenteric lymph node, (a) from control rat with normally developed follicles *(F)* and paracortex *(P)* and (b) from rat fed 320 mg TBTO/kg diet for 6 weeks showing atrophy of the paracortex and follicles; germinal centers are inconspicuous. H and E, × 45

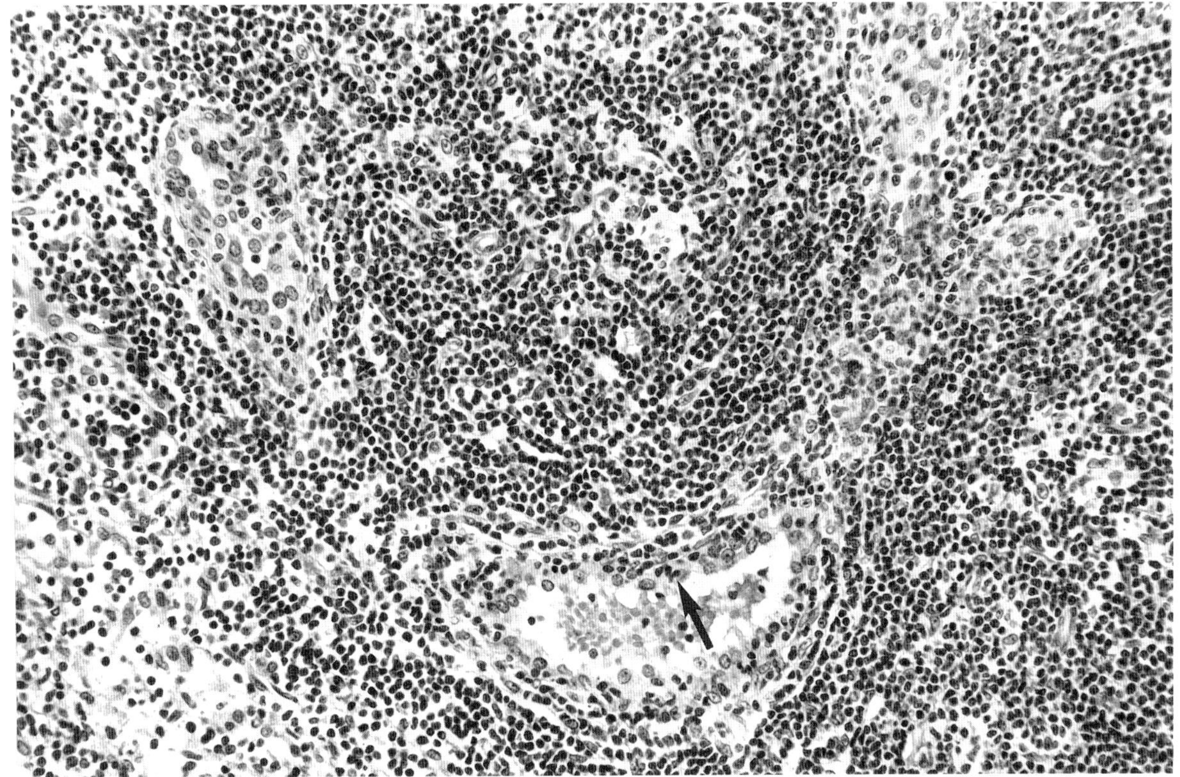

Fig. 186. Mesenteric lymph node from rat fed 500 mg HCB/kg diet for 3 weeks showing an increased number of high endothelial venules, with an increased number of recirculating lymphocytes migrating through the endothelium *(arrow)*. H and E, × 270

Chemically Induced Alterations

Lymphocyte depletion in the thymus-dependent area of the lymph nodes is induced by TBTO (Krajnc et al. 1984). Apart from an effect on the paracortex of the mesenteric lymph node, there is also atrophy of the medulla and a decrease in the number and size of the follicles. Germinal centers are inconspicuous (Fig. 184). By immunocytochemical staining a decrease in the number of immunoreactive T lymphocytes in the paracortex of the TBTO-treated animals has been demonstrated.

A striking alteration in lymph node morphology occurs when chemicals or drugs, which evoke (auto-)immune responses, are examined in the so-called popliteal lymph node assay with certain inbred mouse strains. Here, subcutaneous injection of diphenylhydantoin induces conspicuous hyperplasia of the paracortex, mimicking a graft versus most reaction (De Bakker et al., submitted) (Fig. 185).

An effect on the postcapillary venules in the paracortex of mesenteric and popliteal lymph nodes of rats is observed after dietary administration of hexachlorobenzene, consisting of proliferation of the high endothelial venules (Vos et al. 1979). Moreover, an increased number of recirculating lymphocytes migrating through the endothelium is seen (Fig. 186).

Enlargement of the medullary cords in the mesenteric lymph nodes in the rat is seen after oral exposure to the opiates methadone and, in particular, morphine (Fig. 187). The increased cellularity represents an increase in the number of plasma cells and may be indicative of an effect on humoral immunity.

Mucosa-Associated Lymphoid Tissues

Biologic and Microscopic Features

The digestive, respiratory, and genitourinary tracts contain lymphoid tissue which is organized into nonencapsulated accumulations or diffuse collections of lymphocytes. In the digestive tract these lymphoid structures are called Peyer's patches, which contain lymphocytes separated into B-cell (follicles) and T-cell areas. The latter

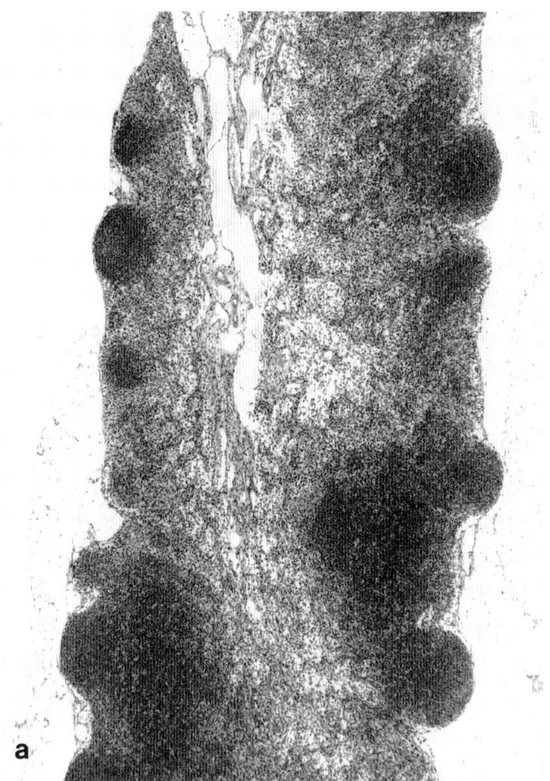

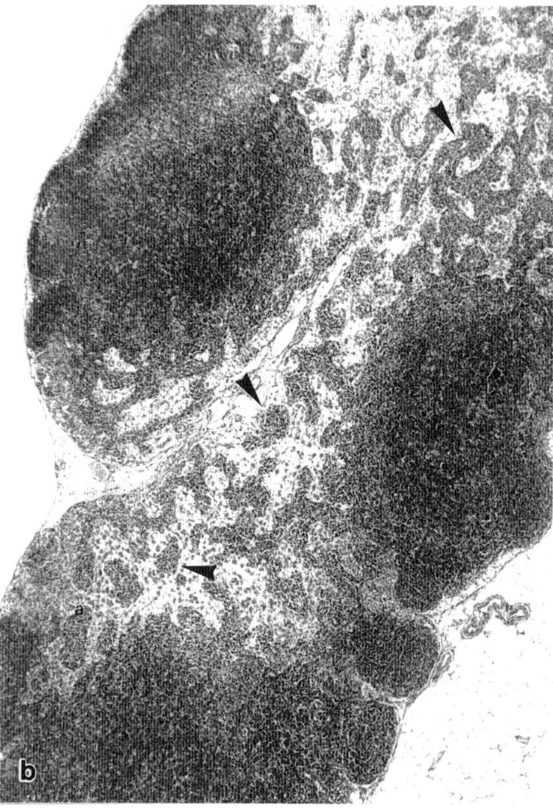

Fig. 187a, b. Mesenteric lymph node, (a) from control rat and (b) from rat fed 1 g morphine/kg diet for 6 weeks, showing increased cellularity of the medullary cords *(arrowheads)*. H and E, ×40

includes isolated follicles as well as lymphocytes, macrophages and plasma cells (mainly producing immunoglobulin A class antibodies) scattered in the loose connective tissue under the mucosal surfaces, or lymphocytes in the epithelium. A proper evaluation of intestinal lymphoid tissue can be facilitated by preparing so-called Swiss rolls of the intestinal tract (Moolenbeek and Ruitenberg 1981).

Mononuclear Phagocytes

Chemically Induced Alterations

After dietary administration of TBTO to rats, an effect on mononuclear phagocytes is found in the mesenteric lymph node. In the sinuses bordering the atrophic medullary cords the number of rosette arrangements (mononuclear cells surrounded by erythrocytes) is very high (Krajnc et al. 1984) (Fig. 188a). Under ultrastructural examination, it appears that many erythrocytes adhere to cytoplasmic projections of the macrophage without signs of erythrocyte uptake (Fig. 188b). Although the mechanism of rosette formation is as yet unclear, it may be a morphologic expression of deficient phagocytosis. This is supported by the finding of decreased bacterial clearance (Vos et al. 1984).

Hexachlorobenzene also seems to interact with the mononuclear phagocyte system. Following oral administration of hexachlorobenzene to rats, lung weight increases, and an accumulation of mononuclear cells in the alveolar lumina focally around the venules is observed microscopically (Vos et al. 1979, 1983b) (Fig. 189a). By use of immunocytochemistry with a polyclonal antibody against rat lysozyme, the macrophage nature of these cells is clearly demonstrated (Fig. 189b).

Exposure of rats to ozone results in a dose-dependent pulmonary response, morphologically characterized by an increase in the number of

Fig. 188a, b *(left).* Mesenteric lymph node from rat fed ▶ 80 mg TBTO/kg diet for 6 weeks; (a) dilated sinuses which are bordered by atrophic medullary cords and are crowded with rosettes *(arrowheads).* H and E, ×270; and (b) ultrastructural detail demonstrating the nature of rosettes: erythrocytes adhering to cytoplasmic processes of macrophages. ×2300

Fig. 189a, b *(right).* Lung, (a) from rat fed 100 mg HCB/ kg diet for 6 weeks with accumulation of mononuclear cells in alveolar lumina around venules. H and E, ×110; and (b) immunocytochemical staining for lysozyme showing the macrophage nature of these cells. ×270

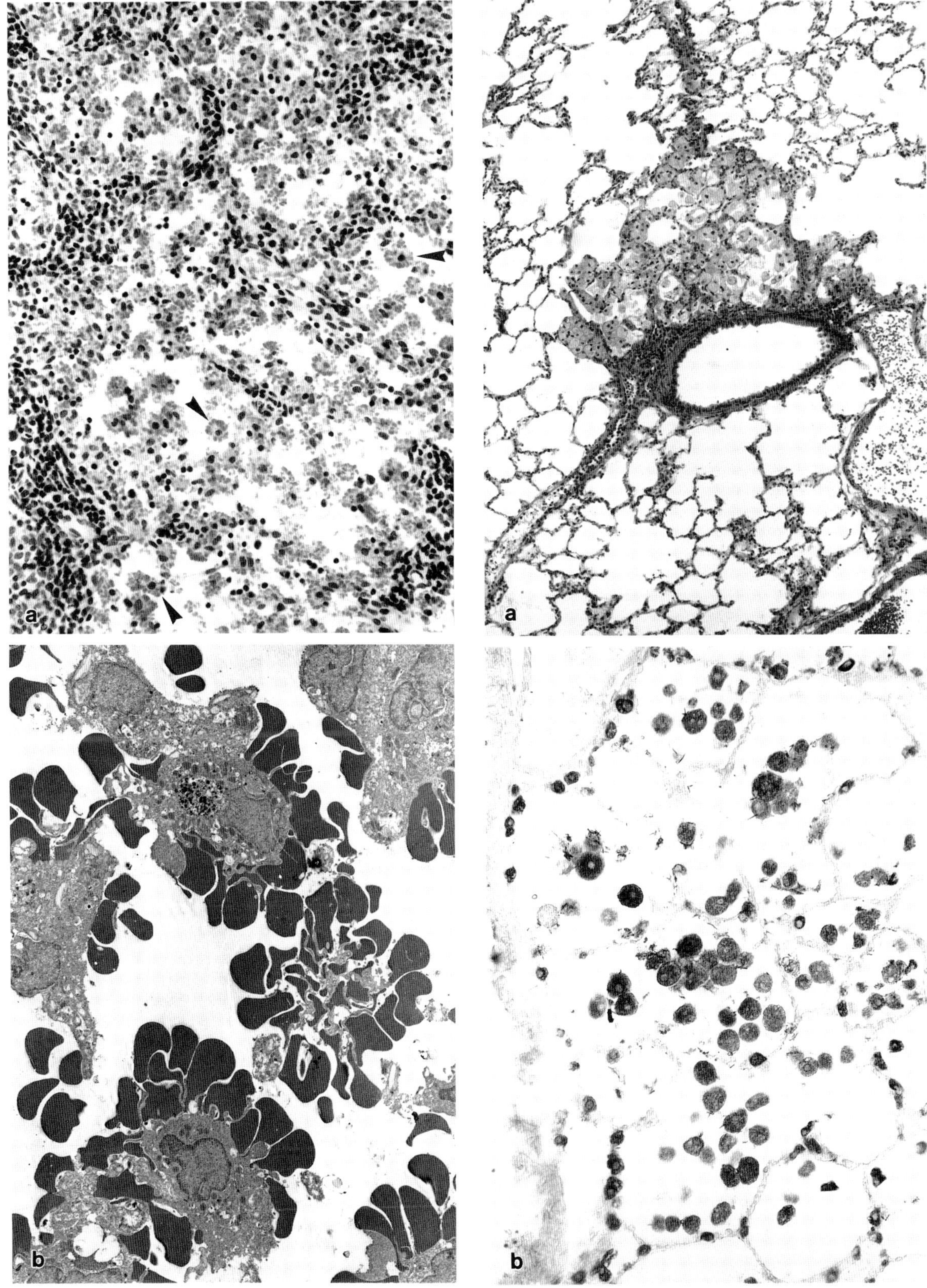

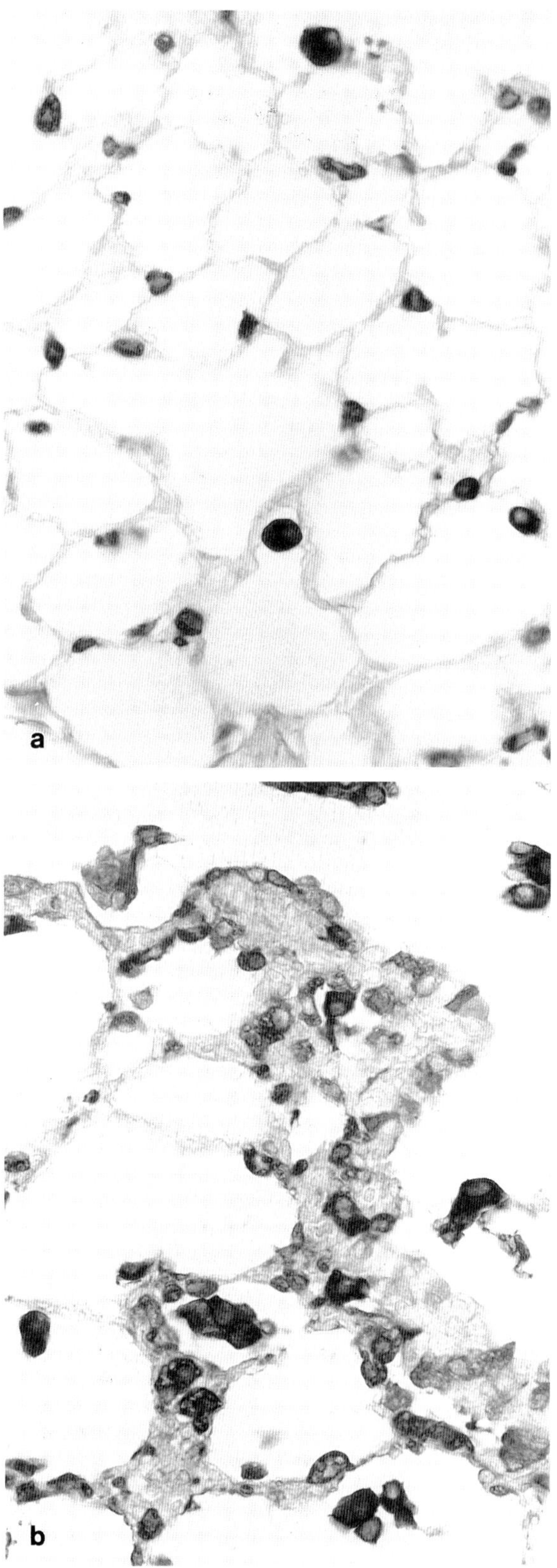

Fig. 190 a, b. Immunocytochemical staining for lysozyme in the lung (**a**) from control rat showing immunoreactive macrophages in the alveolar lumina and (**b**) from rat exposed to 0.75 ppm O_3 for 7 days with an accumulation of the macrophages in the centroacinar region. × 425

alveolar macrophages within the proximal alveoli of the alveolar ducts (Schwartz et al. 1976). Using the indirect peroxidase-labeled antibody method with polyclonal rat lysozyme-specific antibody, an accumulation of free alveolar lysozyme-containing cells is shown representing mainly macrophages and occasionally other inflammatory cells, particularly in the centroacinar region (Fig. 190). Suppression of specific cellular immune responses as well as nonspecific defense mechanisms has been shown by functional assessment in ozone-exposed rats (Van Loveren et al. 1988).

References

Berlin A, Dean J, Draper MH, Smith EMB, Spreafico F (1987) Immunotoxicology. Nijhoff, Dordrecht

De Bakker JM, Kammüller ME, Muller ESM, Lam AW, Seinen W, Bloksma N (submitted) Kinetics and morphology of chemically-induced popliteal lymph node reactions in comparison with antigen-, mitogen-, and graft versus host reaction induced responses. Am J Pathol

Faith RE, Moore JA (1977) Impairment of thymus-dependent immune functions by exposure of the developing immune system to 2,3,7,8-tetrachlorodibenzo-p-dioxin (TCDD). J Toxicol Environ Health 3: 451–464

IPCS (1986) Immunotoxicology. Development of predictive testing for determining the immunotoxic potential of chemicals. Report of a technical review meeting, International Programme on Chemical Safety, London, 2–5 Nov 1986

Krajnc EI, Wester PW, Loeber JG, van Leeuwen FXR, Vos JG, Vaessen HAMG, van der Heijden CA (1984) Toxicity of bis(tri-*n*-butyltin)oxide in the rat. I. Short-term effects on general parameters and on the endocrine and lymphoid systems. Toxicol Appl Pharmacol 75: 363–386

Lovett EJ III, Schnitzer B, Keren DF, Flint A, Hudson JL, McClatchey KD (1984) Application of flow cytometry to diagnostic pathology. Lab Invest 50: 115–140

Moolenbeek C, Ruitenberg EJ (1981) The "Swiss roll": a simple technique for histological studies of the rodent intestine. Lab Anim 15: 57–59

Penninks AH, Seinen W (1987) Immunotoxicity of organotin compounds. A cell biological approach to dialkyltin induced thymus atrophy. In: Berlin A, Dean J, Draper MH, Smith EMB, Spreafico F (eds) Immunotoxicology. Martinus Nijhoff, Dordrecht, pp 258–278

Schwartz LW, Dungworth DL, Mustafa MG, Tarkington BK, Tyler WS (1976) Pulmonary responses of rats to ambient levels of ozone. Lab Invest 34: 565–578

Van Loveren H, Rombout PJA, Wagenaar SjSc, Walvoort HC, Vos JG (1988) Effects of ozone on the defense to a respiratory *Listeria monocytogenes* infection in the rat. Suppression of macrophage function and cellular immunity and aggravation of histopathology in lung and liver during infection. Toxicol Appl Pharmacol 94: 374–393

Vos JG, Van Loveren H (1987) Immunotoxicity testing in the rat. In: Burger EJ, Tardiff RG, Bellanti FA (eds) Environmental chemical exposure, and immune system integrity, vol 13. Princeton Scientific, Princeton, pp 167–180

Vos JG, Van Logten MJ, Kreeftenberg JG, Kruizinga W (1979) Hexachlorobenzene-induced stimulation of the humoral immune response in rats. Ann NY Acad Sci 320: 535–550

Vos JG, Berkvens JM, Kruijt BC (1980) The athymic nude rat. I. Morphology of lymphoid and endocrine organs. Clin Immunol Immunopathol 15: 213–228

Vos JG, Ruitenberg EJ, Van Basten N, Buys J, Elgersma A, Kruizinga W (1983a) The athymic nude rat. IV. Immunocytochemical study to detect T-cells, and immunological and histopathological reactions against *Trichinella spiralis*. Parasite Immunol 5: 195–215

Vos JG, Brouwer GMJ, Van Leeuwen FXR, Wagenaar SJ (1983b) Toxicity of hexachlorobenzene in the rat following combined pre- and postnatal exposure: comparison of effects on immune system, liver, and lung. In: Gibson GG, Hubbard R, Parke DV (eds) Immunotoxicology. Academic, New York, pp 219–235

Vos JG, De Klerk A, Krajnc EI, Kruizinga W, Van Ommen B, Rozing J (1984) Toxicity of bis(tri-*n*-butyltin)oxide in the rat. II. Suppression of thymus-dependent immune responses and of parameters of nonspecific resistance after short-term exposure. Toxicol Appl Pharmacol 75: 387–408

Spleen

Normal Anatomy, Histology, Ultrastructure, Rat

Christine D. Dijkstra and A. J. P. Veerman

Gross Appearance

The spleen of the rat is a parenchymatous organ with the shape of an elongated bean. It is surrounded by a capsule from which fibrous trabeculae emerge. Five to seven arterial vessels accompanied by nerves reach the spleen at the hilus and enter the organ through the trabeculae. Veins collect the blood from the venous sinuses and leave the spleen at the hilus.

In cross section, white patches are recognizable with the naked eye within the deep reddish organ. These patches are designated the white pulp and represent the lymphoid compartment of the spleen. They are surrounded by the red pulp, the compartment of the spleen which deals with removal of foreign particles and aged erythrocytes.

For a good understanding of its microscopic features, some remarks on the vascularization of the spleen are necessary. At the point at which the splenic arteries leave the trabeculae, they become the central arteries which are surrounded by lymphocytes and concentric sheaths of flattened reticular cells (Veerman and Van Ewijk 1975); together they form the white pulp. The central artery gives off several arterial terminals. Part of these arterial terminals give rise to the meshwork of white pulp capillaries. The terminal branches of this meshwork end in the follicles in the marginal sinus surrounding the white pulp (Sasou et al. 1976) or directly in the marginal zone (Van Rooijen et al. 1972). After passage through the reticular meshwork of the marginal zone, the blood is collected in the venous sinuses (Sasou et al. 1980). Another part of the arterial branches of the central arteriole traverse the different compartments of the white pulp, including the marginal zone, toward the red pulp (Van Rooijen et al. 1986). The central artery itself leaves the white pulp and is then designated as a penicillar artery, which divides into several arterial terminals ending up in the splenic red pulp. These arterial terminals are tubular or funnel-shaped and open into the reticular meshwork of the splenic cords in the red pulp (Satodate et al. 1986). Therefore, the rat has an "open end" vascular system in the spleen. Venous blood is collected by the red pulp sinuses which are surrounded by a discontinuous layer of endothelial cells and is then transported by the trabecular veins toward the hilus. Lymphatics are recognizable after ligation of the thoracic duct and occur in the periarteriolar lymphocyte sheath (PALS) close to the larger central arteries (Koshikawa et al. 1984).

Microscopic Features

Red Pulp

The red pulp (Figs. 191, 192) consists of venous sinuses filled with blood, giving this compartment its typical deep red color, and the splenic cords. The venous sinuses are recognizable by their content, mainly red blood cells surrounded by endothelial cells. The splenic cords are conspicuous, consisting predominantly of nucleated cells between the sinuses. Among macrophages, lymphocytes, and occasionally megakaryocytes, all types of blood cells can be found in the reticular meshwork of the splenic cords. This meshwork consists of reticular cells supported by fine reticular fibers.

White Pulp

The splenic white pulp consists of three major compartments which are, especially in the rat, easily recognizable in routine stained sections:

1. The *periarteriolar lymphocyte sheath (PALS)* surrounds the central artery and consists of predominantly small lymphocytes and therefore appears somewhat darker than the two

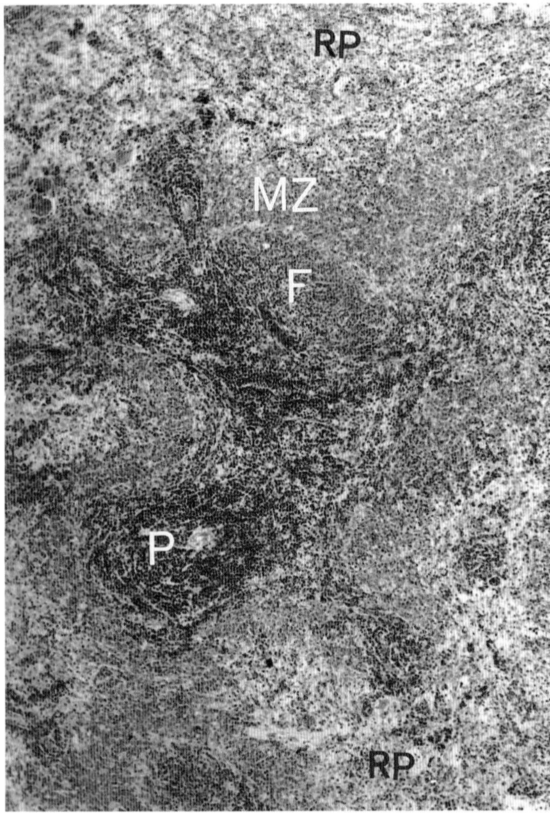

◀ **Fig. 191** *(above).* Spleen, rat, with both red pulp *(RP)* and white pulp compartments. Periarteriolar lymphocytic sheaths, PALS *(P)* is dark due to densely packed small lymphocytes. *F,* follicle; *MZ,* marginal zone. Methyl green-pyronine, × 40

Fig. 192 *(below).* Spleen, rat, detail of the white pulp with a follicle *(F)* containing pyroninophylic blast cells in the center of the follicle *(arrow).* P, periarteriolar lymphocyte sheath, PALS; *F,* follicle; *MZ,* marginal zone; *RP,* red pulp. Methyl green-pyronine, × 100

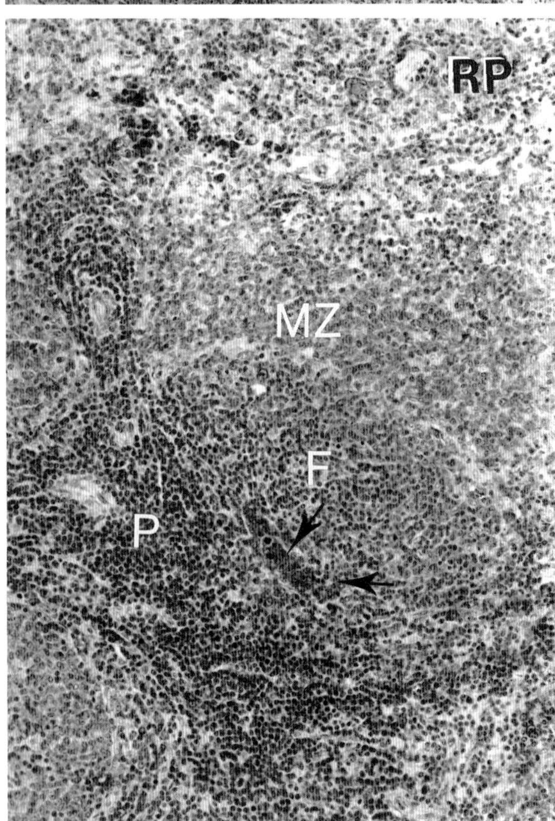

other compartments of the white pulp in routine stained sections. With silver staining, the sparse, thick reticular fibers are recognizable running parallel to the central artery. Apart from the lymphocytes, nonlymphoid cells are also present in the PALS, but they are difficult to recognize in routine stained sections. The PALS can be subdivided in an inner and an outer PALS, each differing in cellular composition. The inner PALS contains almost exclusively small lymphocytes, whereas in the outer PALS small and medium sized lymphocytes occur, and, especially after antigenic stimulation, many plasma cells are present (Sminia and Janse 1982).

2. The *follicles* are globular structures attached to the PALS, consisting of a mantle zone or corona, with densely packed small and medium sized lymphocytes, and a follicular center with larger lymphocytes. The follicular center appears in routine stained sections somewhat paler than the surrounding compartments due to its relative low number of nucleated cells. After antigenic stimulation the follicular centers contain many blast cells, large cells with a pyroninophylic cytoplasm (Sminia and Janse 1982) (Fig. 192). Apart from the lymphoid cells the follicular centers contain large macrophages, filled with condensed nuclear material with high affinity for dyes, the so-called tingible body macrophages. Other nonlymphoid cells are not recognizable at the light microscopic level.

3. The *marginal zone* of rat spleen is very prominent in comparison with other species and consists of several layers of medium sized, slightly pyroninophylic lymphocytes. It surrounds both the PALS and the follicle and is separated from the follicle by the marginal sinus. Considering its vascularization, the marginal zone compartment is distinct from the other two white pulp compartments. On the other hand its structure and function designate it as

Fig. 193 *(above).* Spleen, rat, stained by immunoperoxidase method for macrophages; monochromal antibody (moab) ED2 recognized red pulp macrophages *(RP)*. *WP,* white pulp. Cryostat section, ×400

Fig. 194 *(below).* Spleen, rat, stained by immunoperoxidase method using monoclonal antibody (moab) ED3 which recognizes marginal zone macrophages *(MZ)* and marginal metallophils *(MM)*. *RP,* red pulp; *WP,* white pulp. Cryostat section, ×400

a typical lymphoid compartment, and therefore it should be considered as belonging to the white pulp. As for the nonlymphoid cells, a rim of macrophages at the inner border of the marginal sinus is detectable by silver impregnation techniques, the so-called marginal metallophils (Snook 1964; Katsura et al. 1970; Satodate et al. 1971). The arterial terminals running through the marginal zone towards the red pulp are designated by some authors as "marginal zone bridging channels" (Mitchell 1973) and are accompanied by a few layers of predominantly small lymphocytes.

Immunohistochemistry

Application of monoclonal antibodies against the different cell types populating the reticular meshwork of red and white pulp clearly shows that each of the compartments is preferentially populated by certain cell types (Barclay 1981a, b; Eikelenboom et al. 1985).

Red Pulp

Macrophages form the most important cell population of the splenic red pulp, as is shown by the macrophage-specific monoclonals ED1 and ED2 (Dijkstra et al. 1985a) and Ki-M2R (Wacker et al. 1985) (Figs. 193, 194). Furthermore, dispersed throughout the red pulp are T and B lymphocytes and granulocytes (Barclay 1981a; Dijkstra et al. 1983). The arterial terminals appear to be surrounded by T lymphocytes and plasma cells (Van Rooijen et al. 1986; Claassen et al. 1986).

White Pulp

The lymphocytes in the inner PALS are almost exclusively T lymphocytes (W3/13) (Figs. 195,

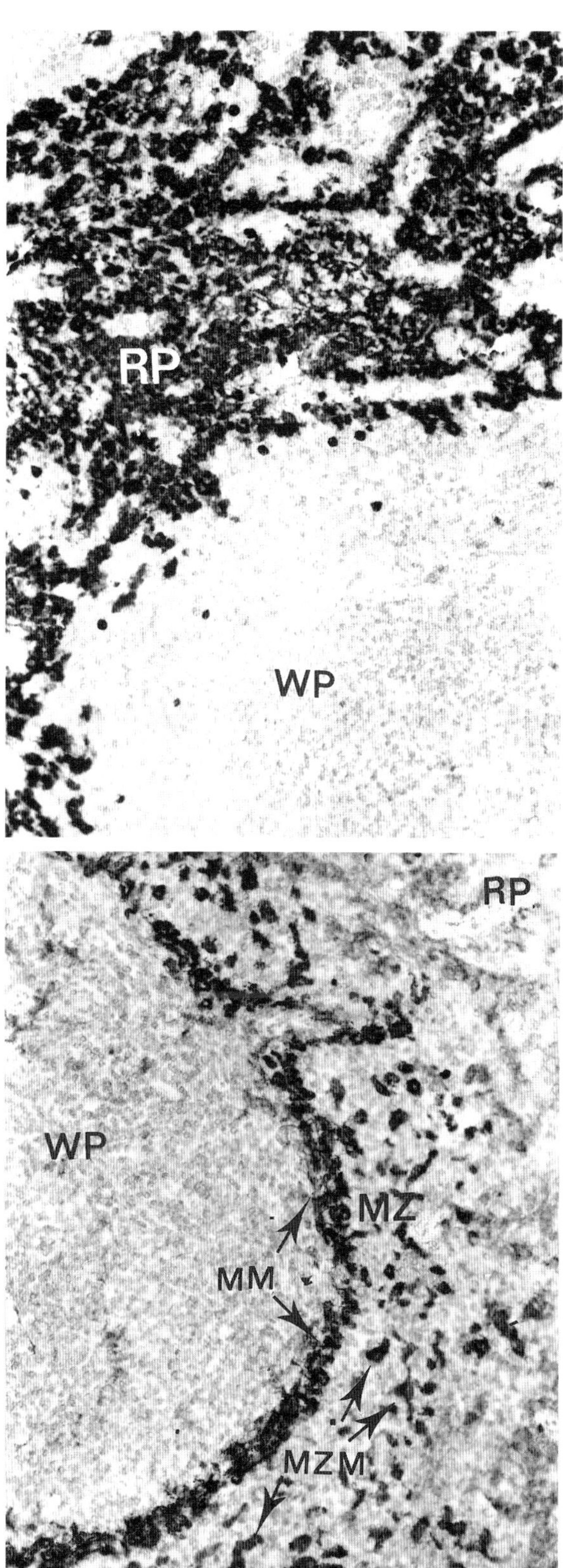

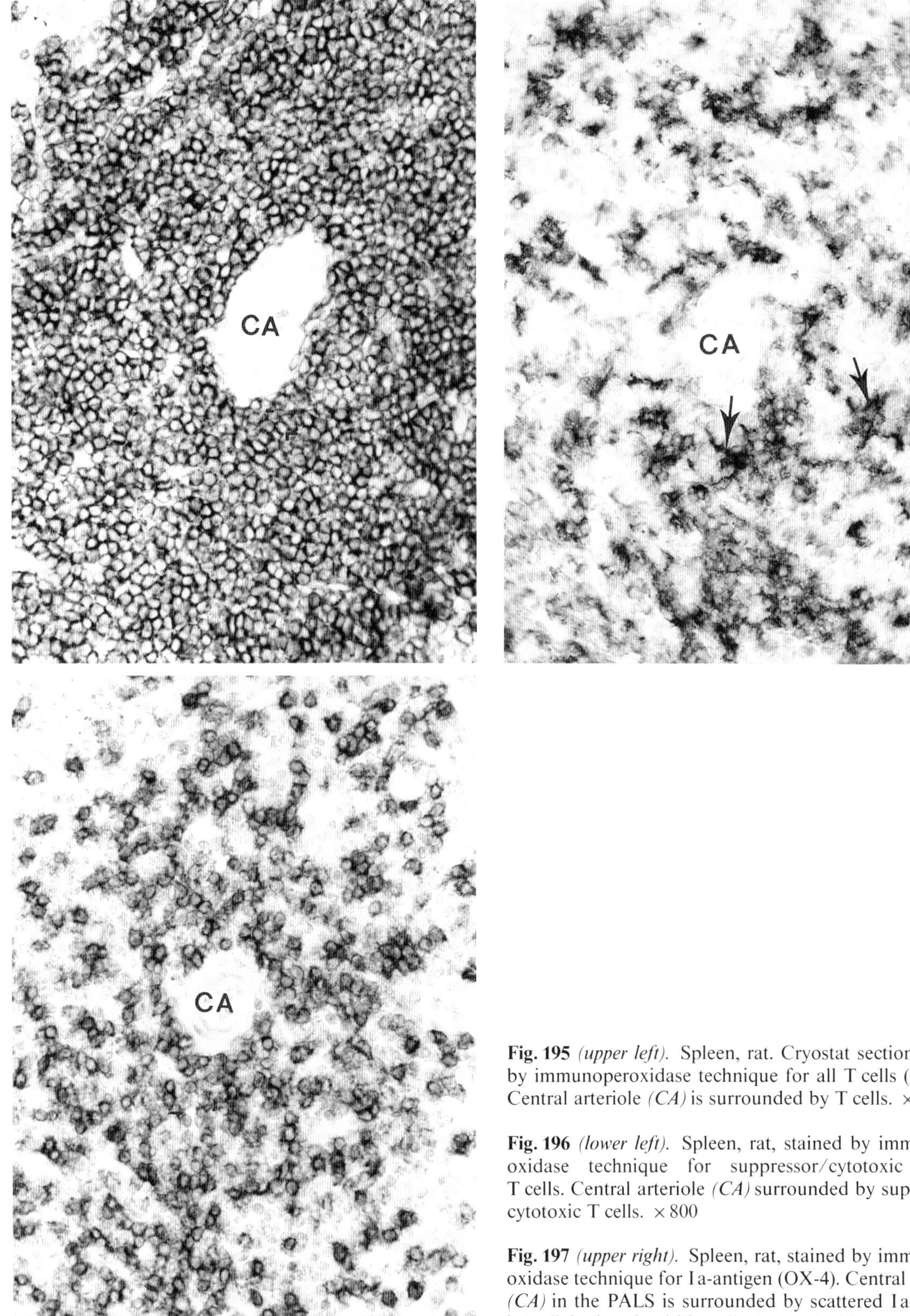

Fig. 195 *(upper left)*. Spleen, rat. Cryostat section stained by immunoperoxidase technique for all T cells (W3/13). Central arteriole *(CA)* is surrounded by T cells. × 800

Fig. 196 *(lower left)*. Spleen, rat, stained by immunoperoxidase technique for suppressor/cytotoxic (OX-8) T cells. Central arteriole *(CA)* surrounded by suppressor/cytotoxic T cells. × 800

Fig. 197 *(upper right)*. Spleen, rat, stained by immunoperoxidase technique for I a-antigen (OX-4). Central arteriole *(CA)* in the PALS is surrounded by scattered I a-positive interdigitating dendritic cells *(arrows)* with extensive cell processes among the unstained lymphocytes. × 800

Fig. 198 *(above)*. Spleen, rat. T lymphocytes are stained in ▶ periarteriolar lymphocyte sheath, PALS *(P)*, but only a few are seen in the follicle *(F)* or marginal zone *(MZ)*. Immunoperoxidase stain for T cells, × 200

Fig. 199 *(below)*. Spleen, rat. Immunoperoxidase stain technique for B cells. Lymphocyte populations in follicle *(F)* and marginal zone *(MZ)* are stained, and T cells in periarteriolar lymphocyte sheath, PALS *(P)*, are unstained. Central arteriole *(arrow)*. × 200

196) whereas in the outer PALS, T and B lymphocytes occur intermingled. The minority of the T cells is of the suppressor/cytotoxic phenotype (OX-8) (Fig. 196); most are T helper cells (W 3/25) (Barclay 1981 a). Staining for I a-antigen (OX-4) reveals large cells in the inner PALS with dendritic cell processes (Fig. 197). These are the so-called interdigitating cells (IDC) (Barclay 1981 b; Dijkstra 1982).

In the follicles the lymphocytes are almost all of the B phenotype, although a few T lymphocytes are always present in the follicular centers (Fig. 198). The T cells in the follicles are of the helper phenotype (Kroese et al. 1985). Follicular dendritic cells can be demonstrated by the appropriate monoclonal antibodies (OX-2: Barclay 1981 b; ED 5: Jeurissen and Dijkstra 1986; KiMR 4: Wacker et al. 1987). Surprisingly, no currently available macrophage-specific monoclonal antibody recognizes the tingible body macrophages.

The marginal zone forms the major B-cell compartment of the rat spleen (Kumararatne et al. 1981) (Fig. 199). The B lymphocytes of the marginal zone differ from most other B lymphocytes by their lack of IgD on the cell surface (Gray et al. 1982). Only a few T lymphocytes are present in the marginal zone. The arterial terminals running through the marginal zone are accompanied by a few layers of T lymphocytes. The nonlymphoid cells of the marginal zone are easily recognizable by the application of the macrophage-specific monoclonal antibody ED 3 (Fig. 194). ED 3 recognizes very large cells with extensive cell processes dispersed throughout the marginal zone (Dijkstra et al. 1985 b), the so-called marginal zone macrophages (Humphrey and Grennan 1981). In addition, staining with ED 3 monoclonal antibody clearly reveals the rim of marginal metallophils at the inner border of the marginal sinus (Dijkstra et al. 1985).

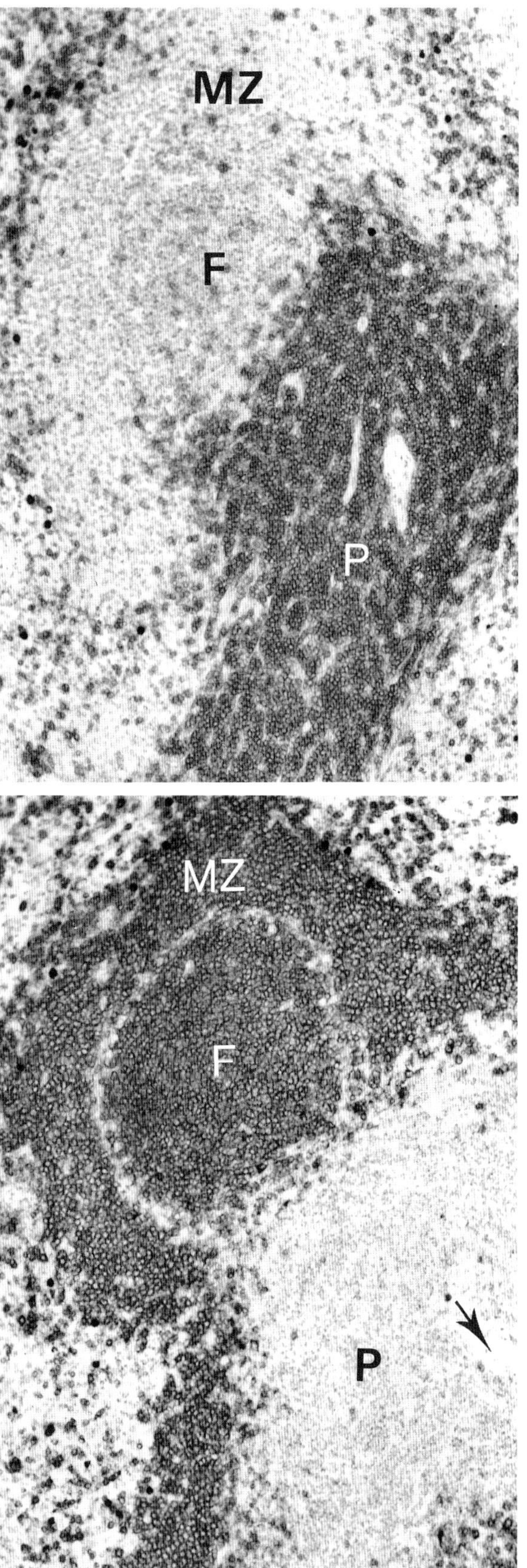

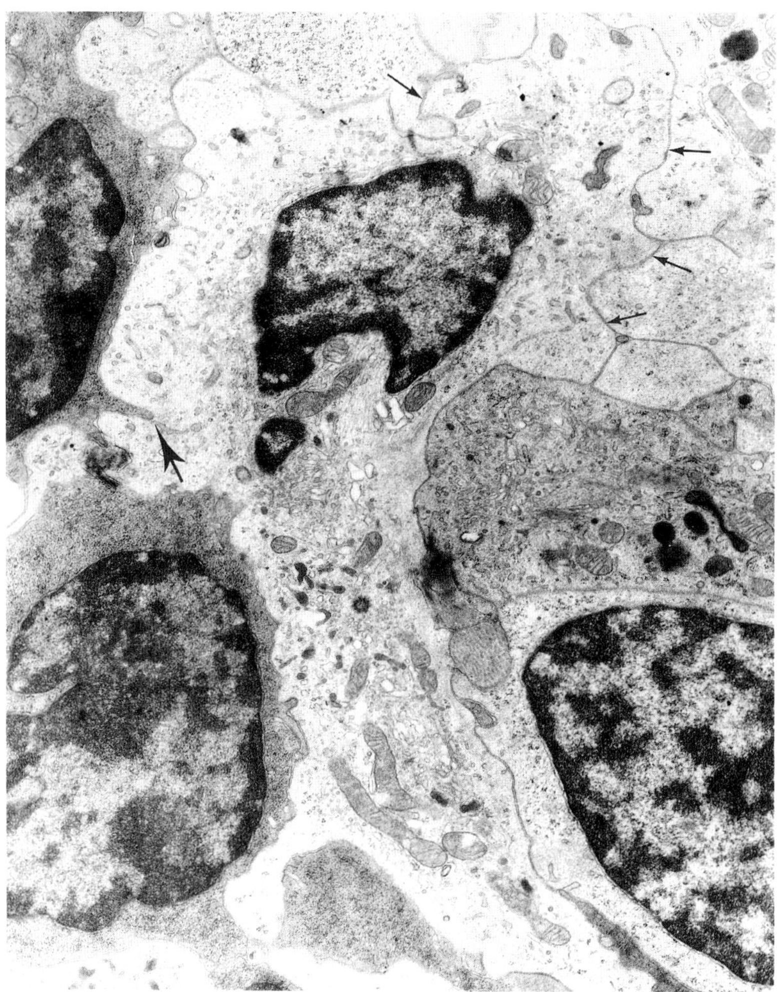

Fig. 200. Spleen, rat. Interdigitating dendritic cell (IDC) from the inner periarteriolar lymphocyte sheath (PALS). The irregularly shaped nucleus, electron-dense cytoplasm, and extensive membrane invaginations *(thin arrows)* are characteristic of IDC. Fingerlike extensions of lymphocytes *(large arrow)* indent the cytoplasm of the IDC. Glutaraldehyde fixed, contrasted with uranylacetate acid-lead citrate, TEM, × 16000

Ultrastructure

Ultrastructural studies of the red pulp are of particular importance for the evaluation of the blood supply of the spleen (as described under Gross Appearance).

The nonlymphoid cells of the white pulp are difficult to recognize at the light microscopic level in routine stained sections, but ultrastructural observations reveal that each compartment of the white pulp contains its characteristic nonlymphoid cell. For the PALS this is the IDC, occurring predominantly in the inner PALS (Fig. 200). They are recognizable as large cells with typical electron-lucent cytoplasm and an irregularly shaped nucleus. The most conspicuous feature of the IDC is formed by the well-developed cell processes with small fingerlike protrusions in close contact with the surrounding lymphocytes (Veerman 1974; Brelinska and Pilgrim 1983). IDC are considered to belong to the mononuclear phagocyte system but differ in many aspects from classical macrophages.

The follicular dendritic cell (FDC) is a cell that is able to trap and retain immune complexes, present only in lymphoid follicles. It probably originates from the reticulum network (Veerman 1975; Humphrey et al. 1984; Dijkstra et al. 1984) and has characteristic morphologic features at the ultrastructural level (Nossal et al. 1968) (Fig. 201). The nucleus is lobated or quadrangular and euchromatic. The cytoplasm is relatively devoid of organelles, virtually no phagolysosomes are present. The most striking features,

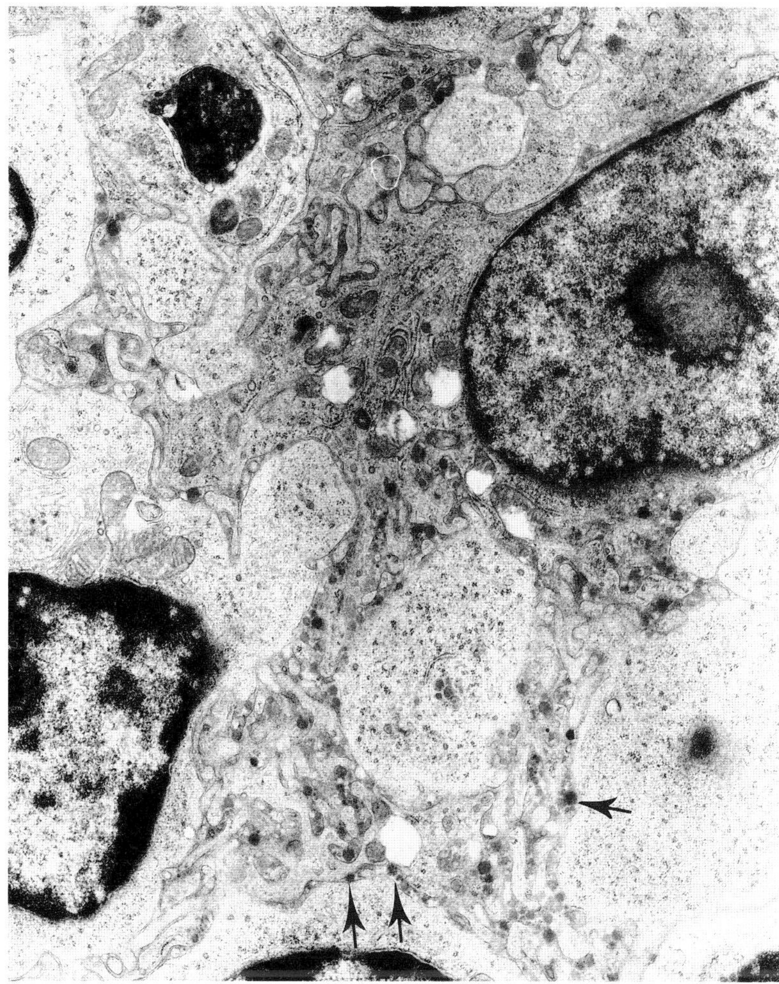

Fig. 201. Spleen, rat, follicle center. The cytoplasm of the follicular dendritic cell has many fine invaginations; between these invaginations electron-dense material is present, often in the form of small globules *(arrows)*. TEM, × 13 000

however, are the extensive cell processes, very elongated and slender, forming an intricate network between the follicular lymphocytes. These processes, especially in well-developed germinal centers after stimulation, have numerous invaginations of the cell membrane, covered with electron-dense material (immune complexes).

The third compartment of the white pulp contains the marginal zone macrophage as the typical nonlymphoid cell. The marginal zone macrophage is characterized by its phenotypical (Dijkstra et al. 1985a, b) and functional (Humphrey 1981; Matsuno et al. 1986) properties, rather than by its morphologic features at the ultrastructural level (Veerman and Van Ewijk 1975).

Comparison with Other Species

Although functional analogues are present in different species, the distinct boundaries between PALS, follicles, and marginal zone are quite characteristic of the rat spleen. In mice, rabbits, and humans the bounderies seem to be more diffuse.

The immunohistochemical detection of different cell populations in mice reveals a distribution of T and B cells (Van Ewijk and Nieuwenhuis 1985) and nonlymphoid cells (Hume et al. 1983; Witmer and Steinman 1984; Dijkstra et al. 1985b; Kraal et al. 1987) very similar to that described for the rat. In the human spleen the same compartments are found in the white pulp with the same distribution of lymphocyte subsets (Timens and Poppema 1985).

Hemopoiesis in the red pulp of the spleen is only present under pathological conditions in humans and rabbits. In adult rats it is present to a small extent, whereas in mice the spleen is a major site of hemopoiesis in both adult and neonatal animals (Seifert and Marks 1985).

References

Barclay AN (1981a) The localization of populations of lymphocytes defined by monoclonal antibodies in rat lymphoid tissues. Immunology 42: 593–600

Barclay AN (1981b) Different reticular elements in rat lymphoid tissue identified by the localization of Ia, Thy-1 and MRC OX2 antigens. Immunology 44: 727–736

Brelinska R, Pilgrim C (1983) Macrophages and interdigitating cells; their relationship to migrating lymphocytes in the white pulp of rat spleen. Cell Tissue Res 233: 671–688

Claassen E, Kors N, Dijkstra CD, Van Rooijen N (1986) Marginal zone of the spleen and the development and localization of the specific antibody-forming cells against thymus-dependent and thymus-independent type-2 antigens. Immunology 57: 399–403

Dijkstra CD (1982) Characterization of nonlymphoid cells in rat spleen, with special reference to strongly Ia-positive branched cells in the T-cell areas. J Reticuloendothel Soc 32: 167–178

Dijkstra CD, Dopp EA, Langevoort HL (1983) Regeneration of splenic tissue after autologous subcutaneous implantation: homing of T- and B- and Ia-positive cells in the white pulp of the rat spleen. Cell Tissue Res 229: 97–107

Dijkstra CD, Kamperdijk EW, Dopp EA (1984) The ontogenetic development of the follicular dendritic cell. An ultrastructural study by means of intravenously injected horseradish peroxidase (HRP)-anti-HRP complexes as marker. Cell Tissue Res 236: 203–206

Dijkstra CD, Dopp EA, Joling P, Kraal G (1985a) The heterogeneity of mononuclear phagocytes in lymphoid organs: distinct macrophage subpopulations in the rat recognized by monoclonal antibodies EDI, ED2 and ED3. Immunology 54: 589–599

Dijkstra CD, van Vliet E, Dopp EA, van der Lelij AA, Kraal G (1985b) Marginal zone macrophages identified by a monoclonal antibody: characterization of immuno- and enzyme-histochemical properties and functional capacities. Immunology 55: 23–30

Eikelenboom P, Dijkstra CD, Boorsma DM, Van Rooijen N (1985) Characterization of lymphoid and nonlymphoid cells in the white pulp of the spleen using immunohistperoxidase techniques and enzyme-histochemistry. Experientia 41: 209–215

Gray D, MacLennan IC, Bazin H, Khan M (1982) Migrant mu + delta + and static mu + delta − B lymphocyte subsets. Eur J Immunol 12: 564–569

Hume DA, Robinson AP, MacPherson GG, Gordon S (1983) The mononuclear phagocyte system of the mouse defined by immunohistochemical localization of antigen F4/80. Relationship between macrophages, Langerhans cells, reticular cells, and dendritic cells in lymphoid and hematopoietic organs. J Exp Med 158: 1522–1536

Humphrey JH, Grennan D (1981) Different macrophage populations distinguished by means of fluorescent polysaccharides. Recognition and properties of marginal zone macrophages. Eur J Immunol 11: 221–228

Humphrey JH, Grennan D, Sundaram V (1984) The origin of the follicular dendritic cells in the mouse and the mechanism of trapping immune complexes on them. Eur J Immunol 14: 859–864

Jeurissen SHM, Dijkstra CD (1986) Characteristics and functional aspects of nonlymphoid cells in rat germinal centers, recognized by two monoclonal antibodies ED5 and ED6. Eur J Immunol 16: 562–568

Katsura S, Satodate R, Makita Y (1970) Demonstration of splenic metallophilic cells in bacterial infectious disease. Acta Pathol Jpn 20: 127–139

Koshikawa T, Asai J, Iijima S (1984) Cellular and humoral dynamics in the periarterial lymphatic sheaths of rat spleens. Acta Pathol Jpn 34: 1301–1311

Kraal G, Rep M, Janse M (1987) Macrophages in T and B cell compartments and other tissue macrophages recognized by monoclonal antibody MOMA-2: an immunohistochemical study. Scand J Immunol 26: 653–661

Kroese FG, Wubbena AS, Joling P, Nieuwenhuis P (1985) T lymphocytes in rat lymphoid follicles are a subset of T helper cells. Adv Exp Med Biol 186: 443–449

Kumararatne DS, Bazin H, MacLennan IC (1981) Marginal zones: the major B cell compartment of rat spleens. Eur J Immunol 11: 858–864

Matsuno K, Fujii H, Kotani M (1986) Splenic marginal-zone macrophages and marginal metallophils in rats and mice. Cell Tissue Res 246: 263–269

Mitchell J (1973) Lymphocyte circulation in the spleen. Marginal zone bridging channels and their possible role in cell traffic. Immunology 24: 93–107

Nossal GJV, Abbot A, Mitchel J, Lummus Z (1968) Antigens in immunity XV ultrastructural features of antigen capture in primary and secondary follicles. J Exp Med 127: 277–289

Sasou S, Satodate R, Katsura S (1976) The marginal sinus in the perifollicular region of rat spleen. Cell Tissue Res 172: 195–203

Sasou S, Satodate R, Suzuki A (1980) A scanning electron microscopical study of the perifollicular region of the rat spleen. J Reticuloendothel Soc 27: 461–9

Satodate R, Ogasawara S, Sasou S, Katsura S (1971) Characteristic structure of the splenic white pulp of rats. J Reticuloendothel Soc 10: 428–433

Satodate R, Tanaka H, Sasou S, Sakuma T, Kaizuka H (1986) Scanning electron microscopical studies of the arterial terminals in the red pulp of the rat spleen. Anat Rec 215: 214–216

Seifert MF, Marks SCJr (1985) The regulation of hemopoiesis in the spleen. Experientia 41: 192–199

Sminia T, Janse EM (1982) Distribution of IgM- and IgG-containing cells during the primary immune response in the rat spleen. Cell Tissue Res 224: 25–31

Snook T (1964) Studies on the perifollicular region of the rat's spleen. Anat Res 148: 149–159

Timens W, Poppema S (1985) Lymphocyte compartments in human spleen. An immunohistologic study in normal spleens and noninvolved spleens in Hodgkin's disease. Am J Pathol 120: 443–454

Van Ewijk W, Nieuwenhuis P (1985) Compartments, domains and migration pathways of lymphoid cells in the splenic white pulp. Experientia 41: 199–208

van Rooijen N (1972) The vascular pathways in the white pulp of the rabbit spleen. Acta Morphol Neerl Scand 10: 351–357

van Rooijen N, Claassen E, Eikelenboom P (1986) Is there a single differentiation pathway for all antibody-forming cells in the spleen? Immunol Today 7: 193–196

Veerman AJ (1974) On the interdigitating cells in the thymus-dependent area of the rat spleen: a relation between the mononuclear phagocyte system and T-lymphocytes. Cell Tissue Res 148: 247–257

Veerman AJ (1975) The postnatal development of the white pulp in the rat spleen and the onset of immunocompetence against a thymus-independent and a thymus-dependent antigen. Z Immunitaetsforsch 150: 45–59

Veerman AJ, Van Ewijk W (1975) White pulp compartments in the spleen of rats and mice. A light and electron microscopic study of lymphoid and non-lymphoid cell types in T- and B-areas. Cell Tissue Res 156: 417–441

Wacker HH, Radzun HJ, Parwaresch MR (1985) Ki-M2R, a new specific monoclonal antibody, discriminates tissue macrophages from reticulum cells and monocytes in vivo and in vitro. J Leukocyte Biol 38: 509–520

Wacker HH, Radzun HJ, Mielke V, Parwaresch MR (1987) Selective recognition of rat follicular dendritic cells (dendritic reticulum cells) by a new monoclonal antibody Ki-M4R in vitro and in vivo. J Leukocyte Biol 41: 70–77

Witmer MD, Steinman RM (1984) The anatomy of peripheral lymphoid organs with emphasis on accessory cells: light-microscopic immunocytochemical studies of mouse spleen, lymph node, and Peyer's patch. Am J Anat 170: 465–481

NEOPLASMS

Large Granular Lymphocyte Leukemia, Rat

Paul C. Stromberg

Synonyms. Mononuclear cell leukemia; Fischer rat leukemia; large granular lymphocyte leukemia.

Gross Appearance

Large granular lymphocyte leukemia of Fischer 344 rats is characterized by splenomegaly (Stromberg and Vogtsberger 1983). The spleens in leukemic rats are enlarged (up to 25 times normal weight) and may be palpated as an elongated mass in the left abdomen. Grossly, these spleens are dark red, congested, pulpy, friable, and bulge on the cut surface. Rarely, poorly demarcated white masses may be seen. The clinical appearance of rats with marked splenomegaly often includes pallor of the eyes and external ears. Some rats develop icterus. Occasionally, petechiae are visible on the surface of the lungs, lymph nodes, and brain. Affected animals become depressed, are reluctant to move, and have rapid respirations.

Microscopic Features

Neoplastic large granular lymphocytes are typically pleomorphic (Stromberg and Vogtsberger 1983; Ward and Reynolds 1983). They range from 10 to 20 µm in diameter. The nucleus is round to irregular, but many are uniform; it is often eccentrically located in the cell. The abundant, pale cytoplasm may contain variable numbers of distinct, minute, azurophilic granules and vacuoles of differing sizes (Fig. 202). Erythrophagocytosis by tumor cells can often be observed in peripheral blood smears (Fig. 203). The tumor cells are strongly positive for naphthol AS-D acetate esterase. The reaction appears as minute, discrete granules scattered throughout the cytoplasm with a concentration near the nuclear indentation (Stromberg et al. 1983 c).

Peripheral blood smears have the characteristics seen in hemolytic anemia (Stromberg et al. 1983 a). The WBC count may be very high (200000–400000 cells/µl), and most of the cells are neoplastic large granular lymphocytes. Anisocytosis is marked, with polychromasia and spherocytosis. The numbers of reticulocytes are increased, nucleated red blood cells are numerous, and the mean corpuscular volume is increased.

Histologic manifestations of this leukemia are widespread in rats (Stromberg and Vogtsberger 1983). Sinusoidal leukocytosis and perivascular accumulation of neoplastic cells occur in most well-vascularized tissues. Characteristic changes occur in the spleen of rats with this type of leukemia (Losco and Ward 1984). These include diffuse infiltration of large granular lymphocytes in the splenic sinusoids and depletion of lymphocytes in the periarteriolar lymphoid sheaths (Fig. 204). Erythrophagocytosis is widespread. Sinusoidal leukocytosis is conspicuous in the liver, and multifocal necrosis of individual hepatocytes as well as centrilobular hepatocellular degeneration and necrosis may be evident (Fig. 205). Small aggregates of tumor cells are often observed in the alveolar septae of the lungs and in the renal cortical interstitium. Mesenteric lymph nodes and bone marrow are infiltrated with tumor cells late in the course of the disease. Nonneoplastic proliferation of erythroid and myeloid cells as well as megakaryocytes is a more consistent change in the bone marrow. Medullary osteosclerosis and myelofibrosis are observed more frequently in the femurs of leukemic rats than in age- and sex-matched rats without leukemia. Serum from leukemic rats stimulates marrow fibroblast proliferation in vitro (Bauldry et al. 1985) making it appear likely that some of the marrow stromal alterations are mediated by the leukemia.

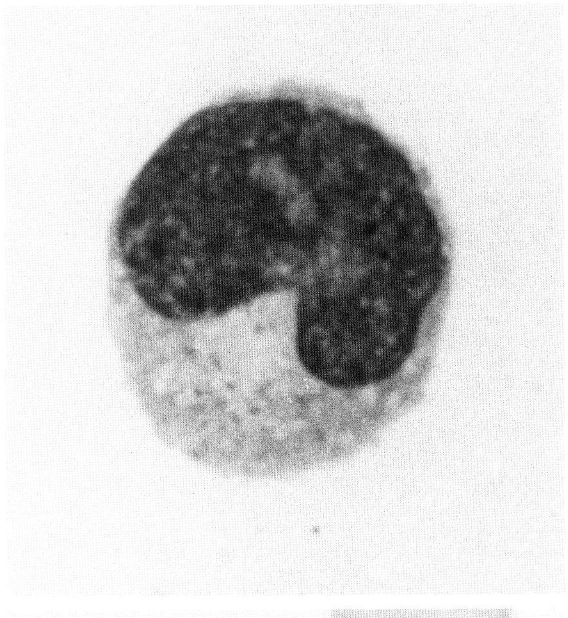

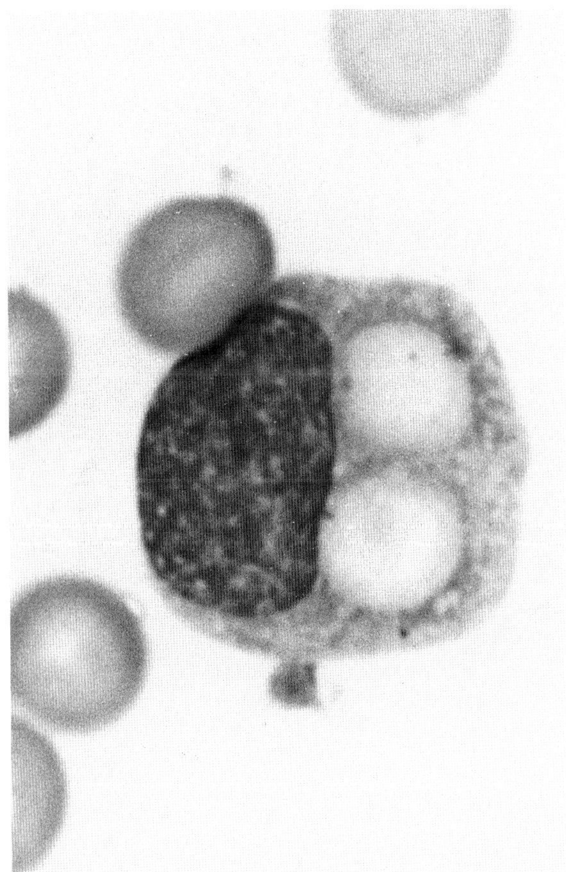

Ultrastructure

Neoplastic LGLs have round, uniform, or irregular nuclear membranes (Stromberg et al. 1983c; Ward and Reynolds 1983). The chromatin is coarsely clumped and marginated, and often there is a single nucleolus. The cytoplasm contains free ribosomes, numerous short segments of rough endoplasmic reticulum, tubular arrays of Golgi apparatus, scattered vacuoles, and few mitochondria (Fig. 206). The granules appears as densely osmiophilic, membrane-bound lysosomes. The plasma membrane is ruffled and has numerous microvilli. Tumor cell thrombophagocytosis as well as erythrophagocytosis have been observed with the electron microscope (Stromberg et al. 1983c). No virus particle has been seen.

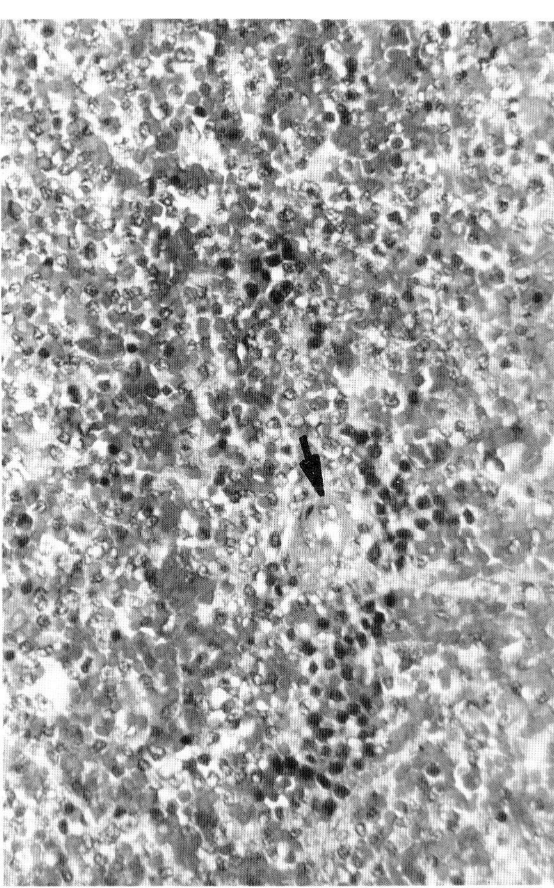

Fig. 202 *(above).* Neoplastic large granular lymphocyte with eccentric, reniform nucleus, nucleolus, and minute cytoplasmic granules concentrated in the nuclear notch. Wright-Giemsa stain, × 3060

Fig. 203 *(below).* Erythrophagocytosis by a neoplastic large granular lymphocyte in peripheral blood smear. Wright-Giemsa stain, × 2950

Fig. 204. Spleen, large granular lymphocyte leukemia. Diffuse infiltration of sinusoids by tumor cells. There is severe depletion in the lymphoid sheaths surrounding central arterioles *(arrow).* H and E, × 315

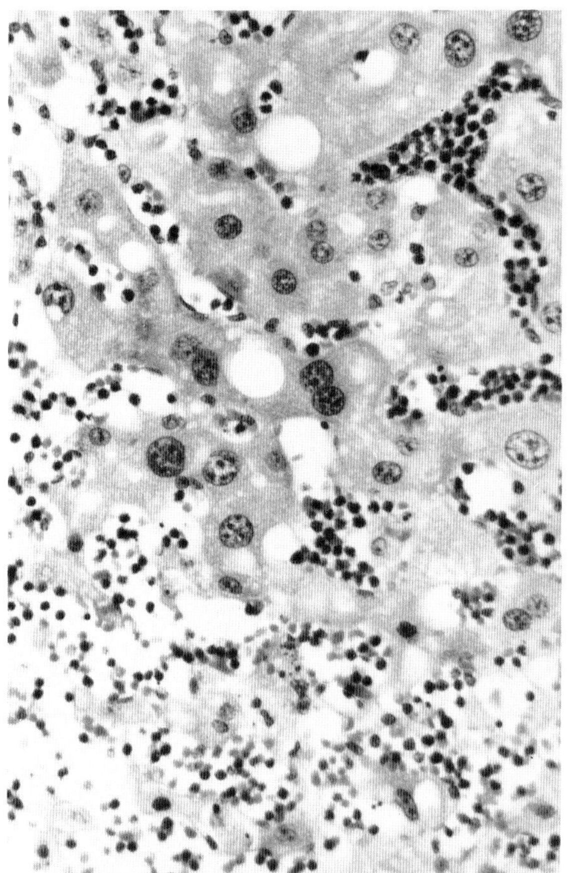

Differential Diagnosis

The occurrence of splenomegaly in rats of any strain requires a consideration of lymphoreticular neoplasia. Although lymphomas occur in many strains, the presence of leukemia, appearance of the typical characteristics of the neoplastic cell, and evidence of hemolytic anemia should aid in arriving at the diagnosis. Large granular lymphocyte leukemia is extremely common in aged F344 and Wistar/Furth rats but rare in other strains (Tarone et al. 1981; Moloney et al. 1969; Abbott et al. 1983). Although other lymphomas occur in F344 rats, they are uncommon, and LGL leukemia should be considered very carefully before diagnosing another lymphoreticular neoplasm in this strain of rat.
Extramedullary hemopoiesis (see p. 232, this volume) should be clearly differentiated.

Fig. 205 *(above).* Liver, large granular lymphocyte leukemia. Sinusoidal leukocytosis in a rat with severe leukemia. There is hepatocellular degeneration and necrosis. H and E, × 500

Fig. 206 *(below).* Neoplastic large granular lymphocyte from the spleen of a leukemic F344 rat. Lysosomal granules *(arrow)* and Golgi apparatus are prominent in the cytoplasm near the nuclear indentation. TEM, × 14030

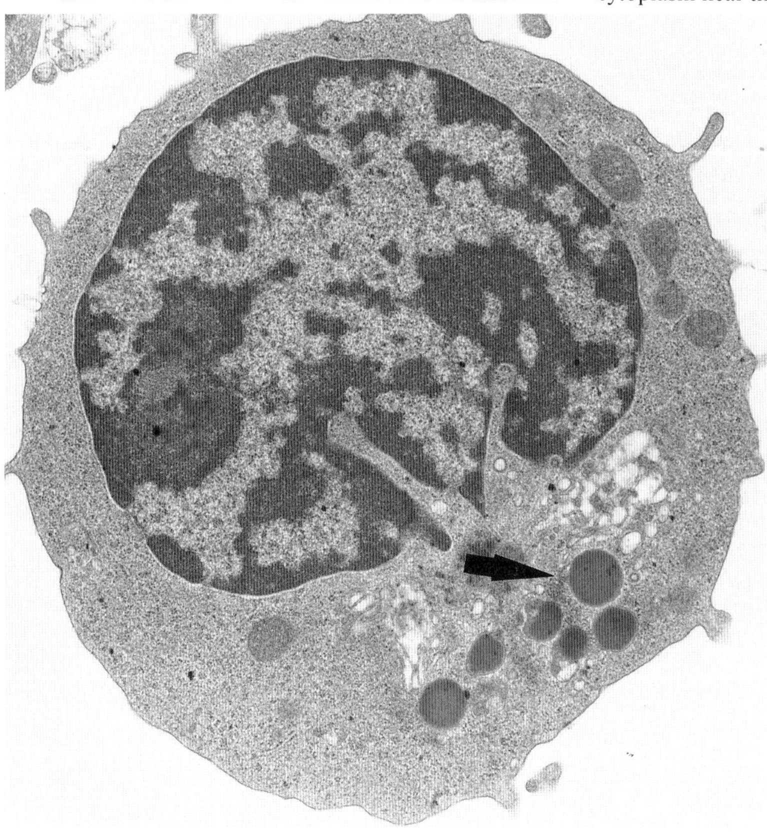

Biologic Features

Large granular lymphocytic leukemia appears to originate in the spleen, because the tumor always involves the spleen, and splenectomized rats have a markedly lower incidence of this neoplasm (Moloney et al. 1971; Moloney and King 1973).

The cells have the appearance of normal large granular lymphocytes of rat. Marked increases in glycolytic, pentose shunt, and Krebs cycle enzyme activities have been reported in the tumor cells (Dieter et al. 1985). They bear Fc receptors, are positive for esterase, have a low capacity for in vitro phagocytosis, and have some ability to adhere to plastic (Stromberg et al. 1983c). In addition, they share surface antigens in common with normal rat large granular lymphocytes (Reynolds et al. 1981, 1984; Ward and Reynolds 1983). The lysosomal granules contain potent lytic activity (Millard et al. 1984), and although variable between tumors, the cells have clear NK activity against YAC-1 targets (Ward and Reynolds 1983). There is no evidence of either cytoplasmic or surface immunoglobulin. These features strongly argue that this tumor in rats is derived from normal large granular lymphocytes (see p. 103, this volume). A consistent and important feature of this leukemia is the occurrence of hemolytic anemia and thrombocytopenia. With the progressive increase in the magnitude of leukocytosis, splenic enlargement, and severity of hemolytic anemia there are concomitant changes in other clinical parameters (Stromberg et al. 1983b). Hemostasis is affected as indicated by prolonged prothrombin times, slightly elevated partial thromboplastin times, and hypofibrinogenemia.

Increases occur in conjugated and unconjugated bilirubin, lactate dehydrogenase, alanine and aspartate aminotransferase. There are marked alterations in serum proteins and serum lipoproteins (Stromberg et al. 1988). Positive direct Coombs' tests in terminally ill rats indicate that the anemia is at least partially immune-mediated. Histologic evidence of lymphoid depletion in the splenic white pulp and immunocytochemical T suppressor cell depletion suggest that the tumor may induce immunoregulatory abnormalities (Losco and Ward 1984). All these associated features may potentially interfere with the interpretation of chronic toxicity studies.

Etiology and Frequency

The original description of large granular lymphocyte leukemia was in Wistar-Furth rats (Moloney et al. 1969). In this study, between 15% and 22% of control rats develop leukemia spontaneously. In a second study 26.8% of 298 Wistar-Furth rats spontaneously developed leukemia (Moloney et al. 1971). The incidence of leukemia in Wistar rats (2%) and Sprague-Dawley rats (0.03%) is very low (Moloney et al. 1971; Abbott et al. 1983). The first studies of this leukemia in F344 rats revealed that 24.4% of 86 female rats (Moloney et al. 1970) and 24.4% of 86 male and female rats (Davey and Moloney 1970) developed leukemia. A retrospective analysis of the incidence of leukemia in control groups from 2-year chronic studies from the National Toxicology Program Carcinogenesis Bioassay indicated that 22.2% of 573 male rats and 20.5% of 572 female F344 rats had this disease. The tumor was rare in rats less than 20 months old but rapidly increased in frequency with advancing age up to 24 months (Stromberg and Vogtsberger 1983). The incidence in small groups of rats can be quite variable and may be much higher than previously reported. There is some evidence that the incidence of large granular lymphocyte leukemia in F344 rats is increasing. It remains one of the most common neoplasms in this strain of rat and accounts for over 50% of the early death loss in 2-year studies (Solleveld et al. 1984; Tarone et al. 1981).

Large granular lymphocyte leukemia is readily transplanted to syngeneic recipients, and the resultant syndrome is identical to the spontaneous disease (Reynolds et al. 1984; Stromberg et al. 1985). Transplantation of cell-free lysates is not followed by tumor growth. Transplanted tumor cells which accumulate in the spleen do not have the host's alloantigens, indicating that transplantation results in the growth of inoculated cells, not the induction of neoplasia in a host cell population. No viruses have been observed or isolated, and no reverse transcriptase activity has been associated with this leukemia.

The occurrence of large granular lymphocyte leukemia in F344 rats is modified by several factors. Splenectomy at a young age and irradiation markedly decrease the incidence of leukemia (Moloney et al. 1971; Moloney and King 1973). Administration of the following nine chemical compounds for 2 years appears to have reduced the incidence of leukemia: 11-aminoundecanoic acid, 2-biphenylamine, CI-disperse yellow 3, CIsolvent yellow 14, CI-acid orange 10, D&C red 9, propyl gallate, monuron, and monoethylglycerol ether. The following chemicals appear to have increased the incidence of leukemia in F344 rats: 3-methylcholanthrene, 2-amino-5-nitrothiazole, arochlor 1254, allyisothiocyanate, allyisovalerate, butylbenzylphthalate, diazinon, 3,3′-dimethoxybenzidine-4,4′-diisocyanate, dimethylmorpholinophospharamidate, lasiocarpine, peperonyl butoxide, phenol, pyridine, sulfisoxazole, and 2,3,4-trichlorophenol (National Toxicology Program, personal communication).

Comparison with Other Species

Lymphoproliferative disorders of large granular lymphocytes have been recognized in cats (Franks et al. 1986) and humans (Reynolds and Foon 1984). Although there is substantial variability in the phenotypic expression of human disorders, some cases of leukemia with autoimmune disorders similar to this leukemia in rats have been reported (Loughran et al. 1985).

References

Abbott DP, Prentice DE, Cherry CP (1983) Mononuclear cell leukemia in aged Sprague-Dawley rats. Vet Pathol 20: 434–439

Bauldry SA, Wilson FD, Stromberg PC, Ackerman GA (1985) Stimulation of normal rat bone marrow fibroblast proliferation by sera from leukemic Fischer rats. Exp Hematol 13: 750–759

Davey FR, Moloney WC (1970) Postmortem observations on Fischer rats with leukemia and other disorders. Lab Invest 23: 327–334

Dieter MP, Maronpot RR, French JE (1985) Comparison of the morphology and enzyme activity of mononuclear cells from Fischer 344 rats with either spontaneous or transplanted leukemia. Cancer Res 45: 4301–4307

Franks PT, Harvey JW, Calderwood-Mays M, Senior DF, Bowen DJ, Hall BJ (1986) Feline large granular lymphoma. Vet Pathol 23: 200–202

Losco PE, Ward JM (1984) The early stage of large granular lymphocyte leukemia in the F344 rat. Vet Pathol 21: 286–291

Loughran TP, Kadin ME, Starkbaum G, Abkowitz JL, Clark EA, Disteche C, Lum LG, Slichter SJ (1985) Leukemia of large granular lymphocytes: association with chromosomal abnormalities and autoimmune neutropenia, thrombocytopenia and hemolytic anemia. Ann Intern Med 102: 169–175

Millard PJ, Henkart MP, Reynolds CW, Henkart PA (1984) Purification and properties of cytoplasmic granules from cytotoxic rat LGL tumors. J Immunol 132: 3197–3204

Moloney WC, King VP (1973) Reduction of leukemia incidence following splenectomy in the rat. Cancer Res 33: 573–574

Moloney WC, Boschetti AE, King V (1969) Observations on leukemia in Wistar Furth rats. Cancer Res 29: 938–946

Moloney WC, Boschetti AE, King VP (1970) Spontaneous leukemia in Fischer rats. Cancer Res 30: 41–43

Moloney WC, Batata M, King V (1971) Leukemogenesis in the rat: further observations. JNCI 46: 1139–1144

Reynolds CW, Foon KA (1984) T gamma-lymphoproliferative disease and related disorders in humans and experimental animals: a review of the clinical, cellular, and functional characteristics. Blood 64: 1146–1158

Reynolds CW, Sharrow SO, Ortaldo JR, Herberman RB (1981) Natural killer activity in the rat. II. Analysis of surface antigens on LGL by flow cytometry. J Immunol 127: 2204–2208

Reynolds CW, Bere EW Jr, Ward JM (1984) Natural killer activity in the rat. III. Characterization of transplantable large granular lymphocyte (LGL) leukemias in the F344 rat. J Immunol 132: 534–540

Solleveld HA, Haseman JK, McConnell EE (1984) Natural history of body weight gain, survival and neoplasia in the F344 rat. JNCI 72: 929–940

Stromberg PC, Vogtsberger LM (1983) Pathology of the mononuclear cell leukemia of Fischer rats. I. Morphologic studies. Vet Pathol 20: 698–708

Stromberg PC, Vogtsberger LM, Marsh LR, Wilson FD (1983a) Pathology of the mononuclear cell leukemia of Fischer rats. II. Hematology. Vet Pathol 20: 709–717

Stromberg PC, Vogtsberger LM, Marsh LR (1983b) Pathology of the mononuclear cell leukemia of Fischer rats. III. Clinical chemistry. Vet Pathol 20: 718–726

Stromberg PC, Rojko JL, Vogtsberger LM, Cheney C, Berman R (1983c) Immunologic, biochemical, and ultrastructural characterization of the leukemia cell in F344 rats. JNCI 71: 173–181

Stromberg PC, Vogtsberger LM, McMurray DN, Marsh LR, Kotur MS, Brown CA (1985) Behavior of transplanted large granular lymphocyte leukemia in Fischer 344 rats. Lab Invest 53: 200–208

Stromberg PC, McMurray DN, Brown CA (1988) Inhibition of in vitro mitogen-induced lymphoproliferative responses by sera from F344 rats with large granular lymphocyte leukemia. J Clin Lab Immunol 25: 89–95

Tarone RE, Chu KG, Ward JM (1981) Variability in the ratio of some naturally occurring tumors in Fischer 344 rats and (C 57 BL/6 N × C 3 H/HeN) F₁ (B6C3F1) mice. JNCI 66: 1175–1181

Ward JM, Reynolds CW (1983) Large granular lymphocyte leukemia. A heterogeneous lymphocytic leukemia in F344 rats. Am J Pathol 111: 1–10

Immunohistochemistry of Large Granular Lymphocyte Leukemia, Rat

Jerrold M. Ward

The large granular lymphocyte of the rat, the effector cell of natural killer (NK) activity, possesses specific antigenic markers which allow one to use them to identify the normal and neoplastic LGL in frozen and fixed tissue sections. Many of them represent cell surface glycoproteins with unknown cellular functions. In normal LGLs, antigens immunoreact with monoclonal antibodies OX-1 (CD45), W3/13, ASGM1, OX-34 (CD2), and OX-8 (CD8) (Reynolds, p. 103, this volume; Barclay 1981; Brideau et al. 1980). The OX-8 antibody is available from Sera Labs., Oxford, UK, or Accurate Chemical & Scientific Corp., Westbury, New York. OX-8 reactivity is also found on rat cytotoxic/suppressor T cells and parotid salivary gland epithelium. In young nude rats, OX-8 is not found on cytotoxic/suppressor T cells (Ward et al. 1983) but may be found on these cells in older nude rats. OX-8 immunoreactivity is well protected by freezing, Bouin's, Zenker's or B-5 fixatives but poorly preserved with formalin. After trypsinization, immunoreactivity may be seen in formalin-fixed tissues, but this phenomenon is not consistently found. Most other cell surface antigens of normal or neoplastic rat LGLs can be demonstrated only with frozen sections, while other antigens such as esterases and acid phosphatase can be demonstrated by the histochemistry of frozen sections as well. In normal tissues, reactivity is seen in the T-cell areas of the lymph nodes and spleen and in areas in which large granular lymphocytes are found, including the intestinal lamina propria and within the epithelial layer of the small intestine. Inflammatory lymphocytes are often reactive, especially in nude rats (Ward et al. 1983). Cell surface staining of OX-8 is evident in normal large granular lymphocytes and neoplastic large granular lymphocyte leukemia cells (Fig. 207).

In rat leukemias of large granular lymphocytes more than 85% of the animals are immunoreactive with the OX-8 monoclonal antibody (Ward and Reynolds 1983; Ward and Lynch 1984; Reynolds et al. 1984; Losco and Ward 1984). Membrane staining can be clearly seen in fixed tissue sections. In early cases of naturally occurring large granular lymphocyte leukemia in aging rats (Losco and Ward 1984) and in those with early stages of the transplantable leukemia (Reynolds et al. 1984), many neoplastic lymphocytes in the marginal zones of the spleen are reactive (Fig. 208); few are normally present. In advanced leukemia, the red pulp is diffusely infiltrated by reactive cells as well as by these leukemic cells in other tissues (Fig. 209) (Reynolds et al. 1984).

Recently, a rabbit polyclonal antibody was developed to rat LGL granule antigens. These antigens include a calcium-dependent cytolytic enzyme, β-gluronidase, acid phosphatase, and other lysosomal enzymes (Reynolds et al. 1987; Millard et al. 1984). The reactivity is specific for large granular lymphocytes in cell suspensions and not other lymphocytes. The antisera may, however, react with other types of lymphocytes in tissue sections but to a considerably lesser degree than with large granular lymphocytes. The antigens are reactive in formalin-fixed tissue sections, and abundant granules can be seen in leukemic cells (Fig. 210). If other types of lymphomas or leukemias are reactive with this antibody, they probably will not have the tissue distribution and cell morphology of this specific leukemia (see p. 194, this volume).

The antibodies described above may be valuable adjuncts for the diagnosis of LGL leukemia in rats. With the utilization of these antibodies, blood smears, and histopathology, we have seen this leukemia in F344, Wistar, Sprague-Dawley, ACI, and Wistar-Furth rats, although it is most common in the F344 rat. LGL leukemia is not reactive with antibodies to lysozyme, rat granulocyte antigens (Ward et al. 1989), or rat immunoglobulins.

References

Barclay AN (1981) The localization of populations of lymphocytes defined by monoclonal antibodies in rat lymphoid tissues. Immunology 42: 593–600

Brideau RJ, Carter PB, McMaster WR, Mason DW, Williams AF (1980) Two subsets of rat T lymphocytes defined with monoclonal antibodies. Eur J Immunol 10: 609–615

Losco PE, Ward JM (1984) The early stage of large granular lymphocyte leukemia in the F344 rat. Vet Pathol 21: 286–291

Millard PJ, Henkart MP, Reynolds CW, Henkart PA (1984) Purification and properties of cytoplasmic granules from cytotoxic rat LGL tumors. J Immunol 132: 3197–3204

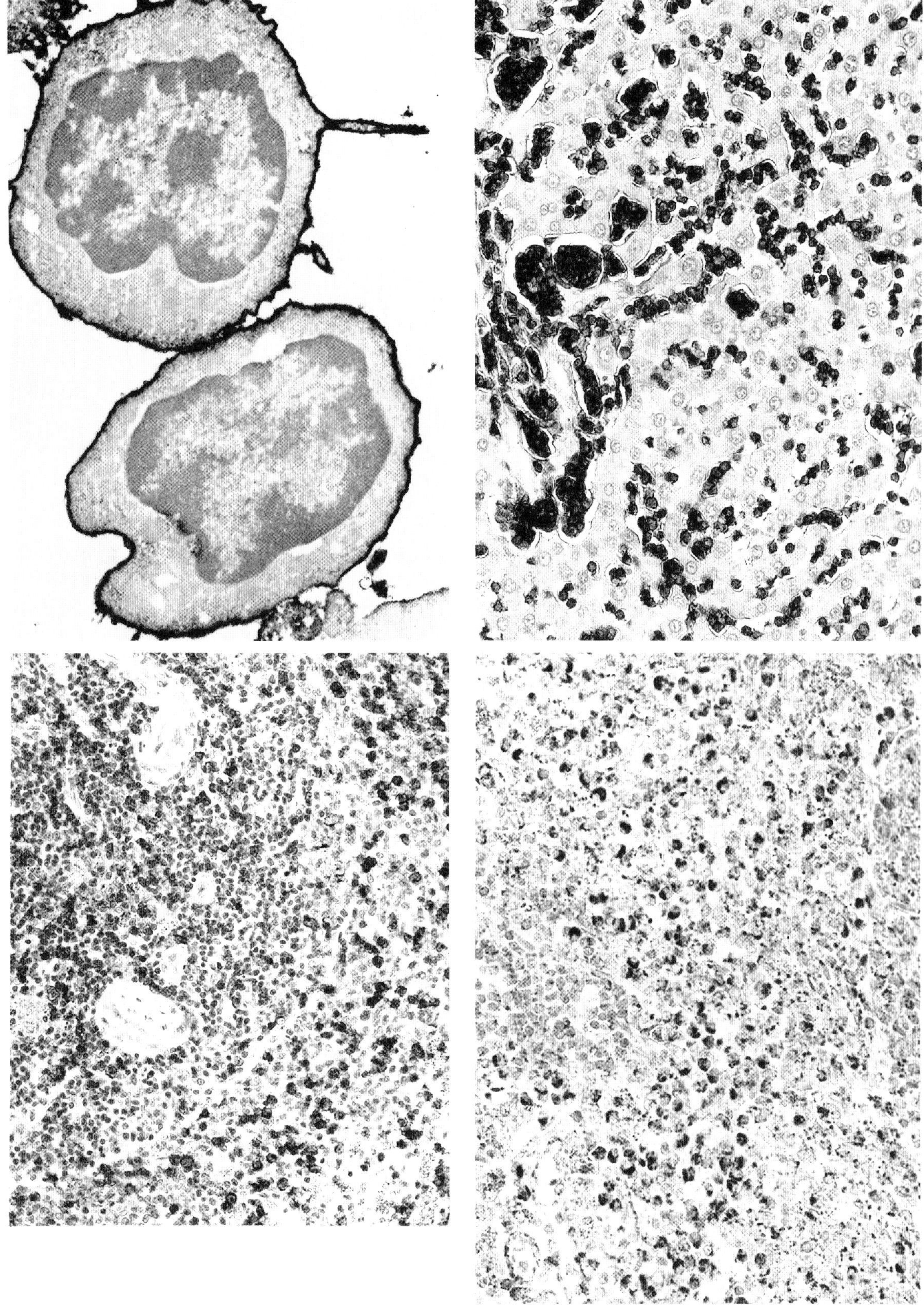

◄ **Fig. 207** *(upper left).* Cell surface reactivity of neoplastic large granular lymphocytes, F344 rat, with mouse monoclonal antibody OX-8. Immunoelectron microscopy, DAB, × 5000

Fig. 208 *(lower left).* Early large granular lymphocyte leukemia, spleen, aging F344 rat. OX-8 reactive lymphocytes are increased in number in the marginal zone. There is lymphocyte depletion of the white pulp. Avidin-biotin complex immunoperoxidase, OX-8, hematoxylin, × 250

Fig. 209 *(upper right).* OX-8 immunoreactive neoplastic large granular lymphocytes, hepatic sinusoids, aging F344/NCr rat. Avidin-biotin complex immunoperoxidase, OX-8 hematoxylin, × 250

Fig. 210 *(lower right).* Immunoreactivity of rabbit antiserum to large granular lymphocyte (LGL) granule antigens in LGL leukemia, red pulp, spleen, F344 rat. Note granular staining. Avidin-biotin complex immunoperoxidase, hematoxylin, × 250

Reynolds CW, Bere EWJr, Ward JM (1984) Natural killer activity in the rat. III. Characterization of transplantable large granular lymphocyte (LGL) leukemias in the F344 rat. J Immunol 132: 534–540

Reynolds CW, Richardt D, Henkart M, Millard P, Henkart P (1987) Inhibition of NK and ADCC activity by antibodies against purified cytoplasmic granules from rat LGL tumors. J Leukocyte Biol 42: 642–652

Ward JM, Reynolds CW (1983) Large granular lymphocyte leukemia: a heterogeneous lymphocytic leukemia in F344 rats. Am J Pathol 111: 1–10

Ward JM, Argilan F, Reynolds CW (1983) Immunoperoxidase localization of large granular lymphocytes in normal tissues and lesions of athymic nude rats. J Immunol 131: 132–139

Ward JM, Lynch PH (1984) Transplantability of naturally occurring benign and malignant neoplasms and age-associated nonneoplastic lesions of the aging F344 rat as biological evidence for the histological diagnosis of neoplasm. Cancer Res 44: 2608–2615

Ward JM, Rehm S, Reynolds CW (1990) Tumours of the haematopoietic system. In: Turusov VS (ed) Pathology of tumours in laboratory animals. I. Tumours of the rat, 2nd edn. IARC, Lyon (in press)

Mast Cell Neoplasms, Mouse

Sabine Rehm, Jerrold M. Ward, Deborah E. Devor, and Robert M. Kovatch

Synonyms. Mast cell tumor; mastocytoma; mast cell leukemia; mast cell sarcoma.

Gross Appearance

Mast cell neoplasms of the mouse appear grossly as soft, white, opaque nodules originating in the subcutis or in other organs such as the lymph nodes, omentum, spleen, and stomach where mast cells are normally found (Deringer and Dunn 1947; Furth et al. 1957). Occasionally, hemorrhagic foci or a canary-yellow margin can accompany the neoplastic growth, and the liver, spleen, or lymph nodes may be swollen. Some cases, however, are detectable only by light microscopic examination (Deringer and Dunn 1947; Dunn and Potter 1957; Frith et al. 1976).

Microscopic Appearance

Mast cell neoplasms may occur in mice as solitary processes without involvement of other tissues or develop as systemic disease with neoplastic cells growing in several organs (Figs. 211–214). Leukemic forms are extremely rare (Deringer and Dunn 1947; Frith et al. 1976). In cases of systemic spread, the tumorous mast cells may invade organs in a nodular or diffuse fashion or grow chainlike along pre-existing structures such as sinuses or trabeculae. Histologically, the tumors have an impressively uniform appearance (Figs. 211, 213). The cells are usually closely packed in clusters or rows and possess distinct cell boundaries, abundant cytoplasm, and a centrally located nucleus. In H and E stained specimens the cytoplasm appears faintly eosinophilic or amphophilic and is slightly granular. Metachromatic stains (Giemsa, toluidine blue) usually reveal an abundance of red or blue (orthochromatic) granules in many cells (Figs. 212, 213), but varying numbers of cells may be present that contain only few or no granules (Deringer and Dunn 1947; Rask-Nielsen and Christensen 1963). Round basophilic inclusions can be found in the cytoplasm of mast cells, probably resulting from the fusion of degenerative granules (Frith et al. 1976).

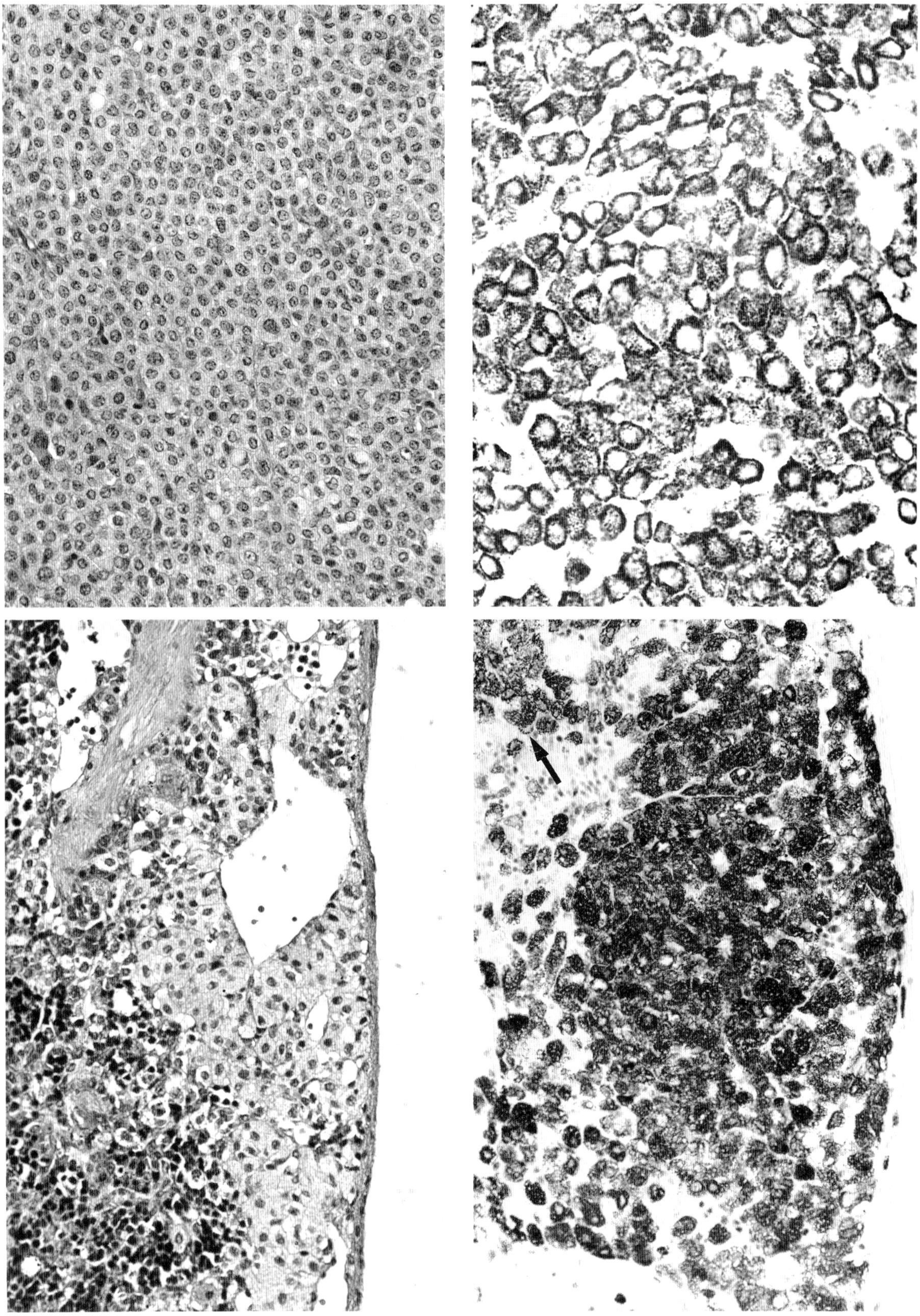

◄ **Fig. 211** *(upper left)*. Mast cell neoplasm, mouse, subcutis. Solid growth of homogenously round cells with abundant dusty cytoplasm and central, round, pale nuclei. H and E, × 250

Fig. 212 *(upper right)*. Mast cell neoplasm, mouse, same specimen as in Fig. 211, stained with Giemsa stain to demonstrate presence of metachromatic cytoplasmic granules. × 630

Fig. 213 *(lower left)*. Metastasis of mouse mast cell neoplasm to the spleen from primary tumor in the skin. Focal subcapsular proliferation of neoplastic mast cells. H and E, × 250

Fig. 214 *(lower right)*. Metastasis of mouse mast cell neoplasm to the spleen, same specimen as in Fig. 213 stained with Giemsa stain to show coarse, dense, metachromatic granules in the cytoplasm *(arrow)*. × 250

Ultrastructure

Ultrastructural studies were carried out on transplanted mast cell neoplasms from different sources and different transplantation passages, therefore descriptions may vary (Mengel and Trier 1961; Christensen et al. 1963; Bloom 1963; Murata et al. 1979). The most important ultrastructural cytoplasmic structures of neoplastic mast cells are membrane-bound granules or vesicles located preferentially towards the cell periphery (Christensen et al. 1963). In contrast to the normally homogeneous granule contents, those from neoplastic cells are heterogeneous and have the appearance of multivesicular bodies (Murata et al. 1979) or of electron-lucent empty vesicles (Mengel and Trier 1961; Christensen et al. 1963). Changes in the number and morphology of granules or vesicles are probably related to biochemical changes such as a decrease in serotonin and an increase in histamine, both consequences of tumor dedifferentiation during repeated transplantation (Mengel and Trier 1961). The nuclei of cells from mast cell tumors regularly contain nucleoli (absent in normal mast cells), and the surface is covered by numerous, irregular, short microvilli (Murata et al. 1979; Inoue and Harada 1983).

Differential Diagnosis

Mast cell neoplasms should be differentiated from mast cell hyperplasia or mastocytosis (Frith and Wiley 1981). Focal hyperplasia of mast cells is observed in the subcutis following skin pain-

ting studies with methylcholanthrene (Cramer and Simpson 1944), can be seen within or around tumors (Bali and Furth 1949), or may occur in the lymph nodes, spleen, or other organs of aging mice (Frith and Wiley 1981). Even strain-dependent variations in the normal number of mast cells in a given organ can be considerable (Deringer and Dunn 1947). Other neoplasms that may have a fairly uniform growth of round cells such as histiocytic sarcomas, granular cell tumors, or plasmacytomas can easily be distinguished from mast cell tumors with the aid of metachromatic stains.

Biologic Features

Mast cell neoplasms are rare, naturally occurring lesions in mice 20 months of age or older with an overall incidence below 1% (Ward et al. 1979; Zurcher et al. 1982; Rehm et al. 1985). In a recent study we found 9 spontaneous tumors in 1111 mice from an experiment involving different congenic NFS strains. Mast cell tumors have been induced in mice treated with pristane and infected with the Abelson murine leukemia virus (Barsumian et al. 1985). Two of the mast cell neoplasms studied most frequently and kept as transplants or cell lines are P-815, induced by methylcholanthrene (Dunn and Potter 1957), and the Furth murine mastocytoma, induced by irradiation (Furth et al. 1957). Although the neoplastic mast cells undergo morphological and functional changes during successive transplantation, they are still useful in assessing the morphological, physiological, and biochemical aspects of mast cell function (van Orden et al. 1967; Mori et al. 1979; Laeng et al. 1985; Inoue and Harada 1987). The tumor cells have been shown to produce histamine, heparin, and serotonin (Hagen et al. 1959; Green and Day 1960) and to possess antibody receptors (Ovary 1971; Minard and Levy 1972); they are used to test anticancer (Warrington et al. 1987) or antiallergic (Umezu et al. 1985) drugs.

Comparison with Other Species

The mast cell tumor in the dog is the most frequent skin tumor (13%), and it constitutes 6% of all tumors, with a predisposition in several breeds (Moulton 1978). Canine mast cell tumors can be classified according to the degree of morphologic differentiation (Hottendorf and Nielsen 1967); they are often associated with eosinophil infiltration and collagen degeneration and may well disseminate to other organs. Affected animals may develop gastrointestinal ulcers due to histamine release (Moulton 1978). Cats more commonly develop systemic mast cell leukemia involving blood, bone marrow, and spleen, although the neoplasms are rare, and localized tumors have been reported to arise in the wall of the small intestine and in the skin. Mast cell neoplasms are also found as rare tumors in horses, cattle, pigs, and sheep. These usually occur as cutaneous tumors but can also be seen in other organs (Moulton 1978). Reports on the spontaneous occurrence or induction of mast cell tumors in other experimental animals, besides the mouse, are extremely rare. In humans, mast cell tumors are referred to as mastocytomas or urticaria pigmentosa arising in the skin and sometimes systemically involving the liver, spleen, lymph nodes, and bone marrow (Rywlin 1985). The bone marrow may undergo eosinophilia or myelofibrosis.

References

Bali T, Furth J (1949) A transplantable splenic tumor rich in mast cells. Observations on mast cells in varied neoplasms. Am J Pathol 25: 605–625

Barsumian EL, McGivney A, Basciano LK, Siraganian RP (1985) Establishment of four mouse mastocytoma cell lines. Cell Immunol 90: 131–141

Bloom GD (1963) Electron microscopy of neoplastic mast cells: a study of the mouse mastocytoma mast cell. Ann NY Acad Sci 103: 53–86

Christensen HE, Iversen OH, Rask-Nielsen R (1963) Studies on a transplantable mastocytoma in mice. II. Electron microscopic observations. JNCI 30: 763–781

Cramer W, Simpson WL (1944) Mast cells in experimental skin carcinogenesis. Cancer Res 4: 601–616

Deringer MK, Dunn TB (1907) Mast-cell neoplasms in mice. JNCI 7: 289–298

Dunn TB, Potter M (1957) A transplantable mast-cell neoplasm of the mouse. JNCI 18: 587–601

Frith CH, Wiley LD (1981) Morphologic classification and correlation of incidence of hyperplastic and neoplastic hematopoietic lesions in mice with age. J Gerontol 36: 534–545

Frith CH, Sprowls RW, Breeden CR (1976) Mast cell neoplasia in mice. Lab Anim Sci 26: 478–481

Furth J, Hagen P, Hirsch EI (1957) Transplantable mastocytoma in the mouse containing histamine, heparin, 5-hydroxytryptamine. Proc Soc Exp Biol Med 95: 824–828

Green JP, Day M (1960) Heparin, 5-hydroxytryptamine, and histamine in neoplastic mast cells. Biochem Pharmacol 3: 190–205

Hagen P, Barrnett RJ, Lee F-L (1959) Biochemical and electron microscopic study of particles isolated from mastocytoma cells. J Pharmacol Exp Ther 126: 91–108

Hottendorf GH, Nielsen SW (1967) Pathologic survey of 300 extirpated canine mastocytomas. Zentralbl Veterinarmed [A] 14: 272–281

Inoue K, Harada T (1983) Electron microscopic observations of a mouse mastocytoma cell line. J Electron Microsc 32: 54–56

Inoue K, Harada T (1987) Induction of granulopoiesis of mastocytoma cells: ultrastructural and cytochemical studies on production of serotonin in a cultured mouse mastocytoma cell line. Virchows Arch [B] 53: 153–160

Laeng H, Harris DT, Schindler R (1985) Proliferative quiescence of normal mast cells resembles that of cold-sensitive mutant mastocytoma cells. Dominant expression of the quiescent state in heterokaryons. Exp Cell Res 158: 170–176

Mengel CE, Trier JS (1961) Biochemical and morphologic heterogeneity in a transplantable mast-cell neoplasm. JNCI 27: 1341–1359

Minard P, Levy DA (1972) Reaginic antibody receptors on murine mastocytoma cells. J Immunol 109: 887–890

Mori Y, Akedo H, Tanaka K, Tanigaki Y, Okada M (1979) Effect of sodium butyrate on the granulopoiesis of mastocytoma cells. Exp Cell Res 118: 15–22

Moulton JE (ed) (1978) Tumors in domestic animals. University of California Press, Berkeley, pp 26–33, 195, 268

Murata F, Ikeda S, Yoshida K, Ohno S, Nagata T (1979) Fine structure of mastocytoma cells and mast cells of mice and rats. Okajimas Folia Anat Jpn 56: 159–192

Ovary Z (1971) Immunoglobulin receptors on mouse mast cells. II. Mast cells of different strains and mastocytomas. J Immunol 107: 1795–1797

Rask-Nielsen R, Christensen HE (1963) Studies on a transplantable mastocytoma in mice. I. Origin and general morphology. JNCI 30: 743–761

Rehm S, Rapp KG, Deerberg F (1985) Influence of food restriction and body fat on life span and tumour incidence in female outbred Han: NMRI mice and two sublines. Z Versuchstierkd 27: 240–283

Rywlin AM (1985) Hematopoietic system: reticuloendothelial system, spleen, lymph nodes, bone marrow, and blood. In: Kissane JM (ed) Anderson's pathology, vol 2. Mosby, St Louis, pp 1257–1351

Umezu K, Yuasa S, Sudoh A, Kikumoto R, Ichikawa A (1985) Inhibitory effect of tritoqualine (TRQ) on histamine release from mast cells. Jpn J Pharmacol 38: 153–160

Van Orden LS 3rd, Vugman I, Bensch KG, Giarman NJ (1967) Biochemical, histochemical and electron-microscopic studies of 5-hydroxytryptamine in neoplastic mast cells. J Pharmacol Exp Ther 158: 195–205

Ward JM, Goodman DG, Squire RA, Chu KC, Linhart MS (1979) Neoplastic and nonneoplastic lesions in aging (C57BL/6N × 63H/HeN)F$_1$ (B6C3F$_1$) mice. JNCI 63: 849–854

Warrington RC, Cheng I, Fang WD (1987) Effects of L-Histidinol on the susceptibility of P815 mastocytoma cells to selected anticancer drugs in vitro and in DBA/2J mice. JNCI 78: 1177–1183

Zurcher C, van Zwieten MJ, Solleveld HA, Hollander CF (1982) Aging research. In: Foster HL, Small JD, Fox JG (eds) The mouse in biomedical research. IV. Experimental biology and oncology. Academic, New York, pp 11–35

Erythroleukemia, Mouse

Torgny N. Fredrickson

Synonyms. Erythroblastosis; Friend disease; Rauscher disease; erythroblastic leukemia; erythremic myelosis.

Gross Appearance

Erythroleukemia induced with retrovirus occurs in one of three distinct forms. Two of these are associated with rapid onset and death (<3 months) and cause either a polycythemic or anemic blood picture. There is also a chronic type of the anemic form. Viruses comprising the Friend complex are capable of inducing all forms, including FVP (polycythemic form), FVA (anemic form), and Friend murine leukemia virus (F-MuLV) (chronic form). The Rauscher virus complex also contains components which induce acute or chronic anemic forms, and viruses of both complexes will be used as models for the descriptions of gross and microscopic aspects given below.

Splenic changes are the most obvious gross lesions associated with all three forms, and the degree of splenomegaly has been used as a measurement of dose for those viruses inducing the acute forms. In advanced cases, the spleen may weigh as much as 4 g. In even moderate stages of enlargement, the spleen is easily palpable as a smooth mass lying crosswise in the abdominal cavity, so that affected mice have a "pot-bellied" appearance. The gross appearance of the spleen varies somewhat according to latent period. When splenomegaly develops slowly, i. e., over a period of 2–3 months, as with F-MuLV, the organ is symmetrically enlarged, the capsule tense but usually intact, and the color a uniform dark red; however, when splenomegaly occurs within 2–3 weeks, as with FVP or FVA, disruption of the normal architectural components usually occurs. This breakdown in structure causes localized hematomas, irregular in both size and shape, throughout the splenic parenchyma. These "blood lakes" are easily seen as purplish-red, fluid blood underneath the capsule. Partial resolution of these hemorrhages by clot formation and fibrosis produces firm, irregular, gray areas giving the spleen a mottled appearance. In cases of acute disease, especially with extensive bleeding and thrombosis, the stretched capsule may rupture, causing extravasation of blood into the abdominal cavity and rapid death. These destructive lesions are in contrast to proliferative foci of erythroblasts seen in the early stages of erythroleukemia as small gray areas underneath the capsule within 9 days after inoculation of virus. The number of these splenic foci has also been used as a measure of virus dose for the Friend and Rauscher virus complexes, hence the acronym SFFV for spleen focus-forming virus (Steeves 1975).

The liver in those cases of erythroleukemia with a more protracted course also undergoes severe enlargement and may be double normal size and have the same dark red color as that of the spleen. As in the spleen, there may be patchy gray areas of hepatic necrosis caused by thrombosis due to tumor emboli (Siegler and Rich 1964).

The gross appearance of the blood is characteristic of the inductive virus, and for Friend virus complex, the hematocrit may vary from >60% to <30% and the blood may be so thick in the polycythemic form that it is difficult to make a well-dispersed film, or it may be so thin in the anemic form that even a thick film contains relatively few cells. Extremely low hematocrits (10%–20%) are usually seen in erythroleukemia induced by helper virus alone as opposed to helper virus and SFFV. In none of these forms is there an impressive buffy coat.

The lymph nodes and thymus are generally unaffected in erythroleukemia although in the chronic form nodes may be slightly enlarged and dark tan in color because of the hemosiderin content of the macrophages.

Microscopic Features

The most obvious change in susceptible mice occurs in the spleen within hours after inoculation of the Friend virus complex, due to focal accumulations of actively proliferating, large, basophilic cells throughout the red pulp, but particularly under the capsule. These cells have been called reticulum cells (Friend 1957; Dawson et al. 1963), Friend cells (Metcalf et al. 1959), hyperbasophilic cells (Tambourin et al. 1979), basophilic erythroblasts (Russo et al. 1976), and pro-

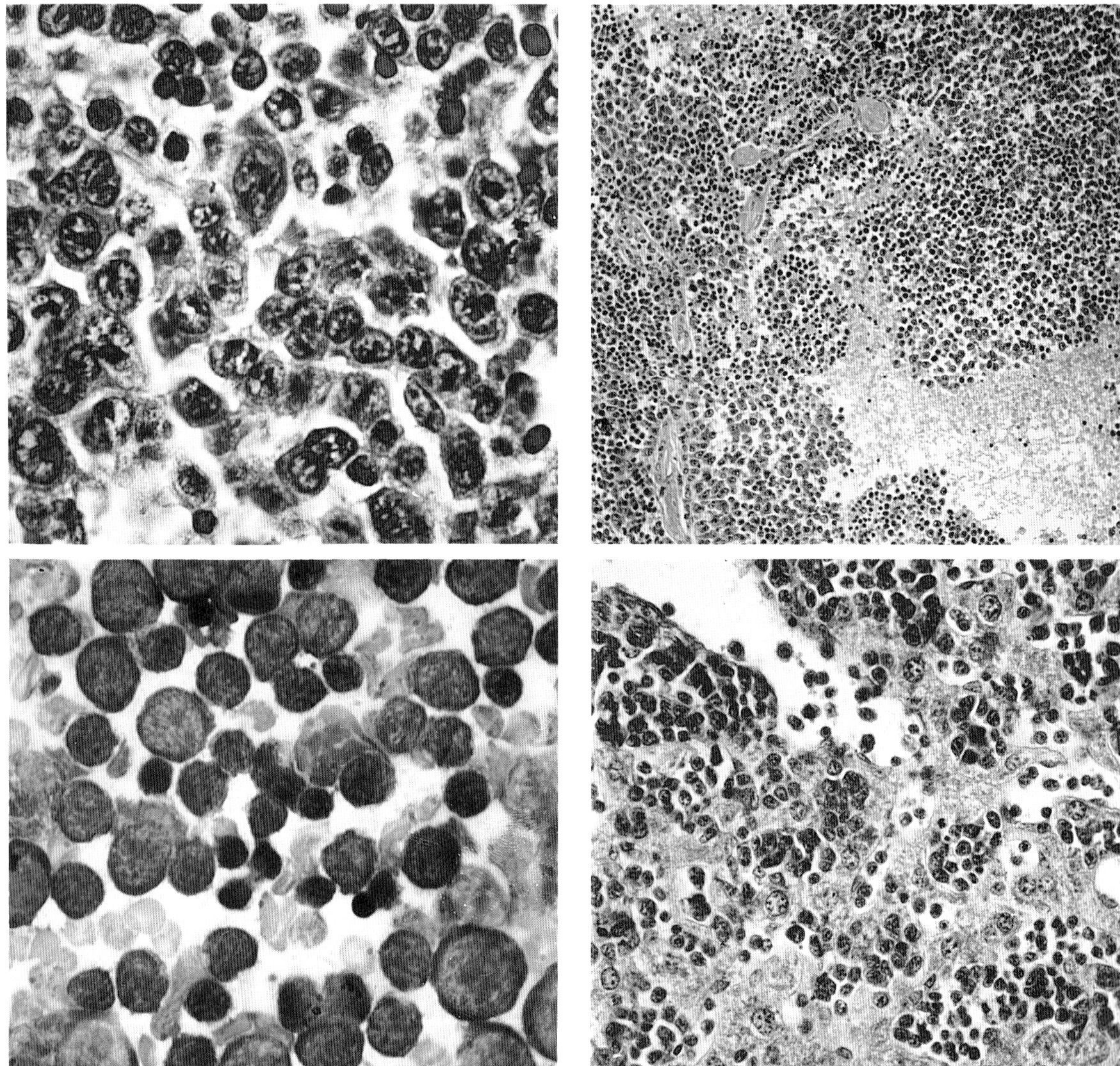

Fig. 215 *(upper left).* Typical spleen (weight 2.64 g), Swiss mouse given SFFV$_P$. Hematocrit was 64%. Extremely large proerythroblasts are intermingled with basophilic erythroblasts and normoblasts. H and E, × 1000

Fig. 216 *(lower left).* Imprint of a spleen (weight 2.00 g), Swiss mouse given SFFV$_A$. Hematocrit was 31%. The cell population is very similar to that shown in Fig. 215. Wright-Giemsa stain, × 1000

Fig. 217 *(upper right).* Spleen of mouse shown in Fig. 216. Note degenerative changes typical of advanced Friend disease. The hemorrhagic lesion *(lower right)* is similar to that seen throughout the organ. These usually cause splenic rupture but may also undergo consolidation. H and E, × 160

Fig. 218 *(lower right).* Liver, NFS/N mouse given helper MuLV. Erythroblasts fill the sinusoids. H and E, × 400

erythroblasts (DeBoth et al. 1978). This latest designation is in accordance with observations made by Zajdela (1962) who concluded that similar cells could be seen in low numbers in normal spleens and that they represented very early erythroid progenitors. Using the morphologic criteria of hyperbasophilia, a high nuclear to cytoplasmic ratio, and the presence of a round nucleus containing nucleoli, such cells have been

shown to comprise about 80% of all splenic cells within 28 days after inoculation with a large dose of virus (Smadja-Joffe et al. 1973; Russo et al. 1976).

Most of the other splenic cells in such cases were more mature erythroid progenitors. The early sites of initial proliferation within the red pulp rapidly expand to form microscopic foci. Histologically, these foci are composed largely of pro-

Fig. 219 *(above)*. Blood smear, same mouse as in Fig. 215. ▶
A normoblast *(middle right)* represents the few erythroid
precursors seen in the film. The variable chromicity and
size of the erythrocytes are evident. Wright-Giemsa stain,
× 1000

Fig. 220 *(middle)*. Blood smear, same mouse as in
Figs. 216 and 217 with a basophilic erythroblast in the
center. The number of large, basophilic erythrocytes is
negligible; various schistocytes can be seen. Wright-
Giemsa stain, × 1000

Fig. 221 *(below)*. Blood smear, NFS/N mouse given helper MuLV. The large number of erythroid precursors vary
from basophilic erythroblasts *(b)* to more mature, darkly
staining normoblasts *(n)*. The smudge cell *(s)* was possibly
a very immature cell similar to that shown *(arrow)* with an
eccentric nucleus, containing a single pale nucleolus and
pale basophilic cytoplasm. Erythrocytes are generally normal. Wright-Giemsa stain, × 1000

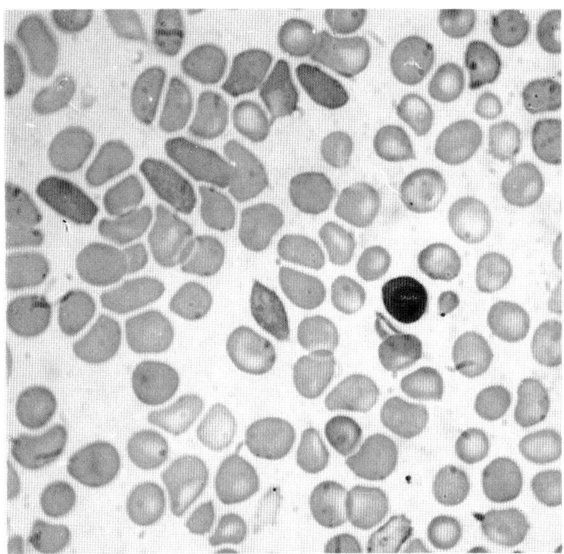

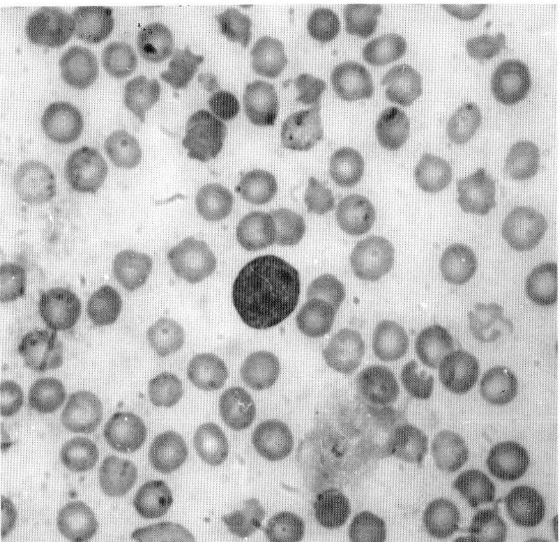

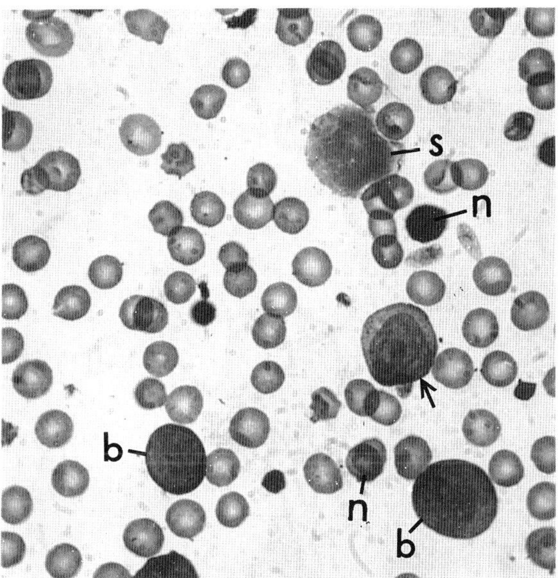

erythroblasts with an admixture of basophilic
erythroblasts and normoblasts. Foci coalesce
within as short a time as 10 days after inoculation of the virus to form solid sheets so that
erythroid precursors (Figs. 215–216) replace myeloid progenitors and megakaryocytes in the red
pulp almost entirely and cause compression of
the PALS. At this point normal structural components start to break down with the resultant
hemorrhage forming blood lakes (Fig. 217) which
undergo consolidation if rupture does not cause
death at this stage (Fredrickson et al. 1972).
In the chronic form (helper virus alone) there is
usually no destructive phase accompanying the
massive accumulation of erythroid precursors. In
the bone marrow erythroid cells also accumulate
and may comprise 20% of the total cellularity
(Ludwig et al. 1964); however, these are not
clearly seen histologically although areas of
Friend cells and erythroblasts can sometimes be
distinguished as small clusters within an otherwise normal marrow.
The liver is also affected, but to a variable degree. Acute cases with splenic rupture may have
little accompanying hepatic involvement, but in
more prolonged cases, erythroid precursors, presumably of splenic origin (Siegler and Rich
1964), lodge within hepatic sinusoids in a fairly
even distribution (Fig. 218) and generally to a
lesser extent around triads. Other organs are not
sites of significant infiltration.
The blood picture varies according to the initiat-
ing virus and stage of the disease. In both the
acute forms induced by the Friend virus complex, there is severe reticulocytosis of up to about

fourfold for the anemic and about tenfeld for the polycythemic form (Sassa et al. 1968; Tambourin et al. 1973; Steinhelder et al. 1979). However, no pronounced reticulocytosis occurs in the chronic form (Weitz-Hamburger et al. 1975). Lymphocytosis (Metcalf et al. 1959; Ludwig et al. 1964) and thrombocytopenia (Dennis and Brodsky 1965) have been associated with the Friend complex; however, they are not prominent features. Blood films reveal a surprising similarity in both acute forms; polychromasia and anisocytosis due to the presence of numerous, large, basophilic erythrocytes are the most obvious abnormalities (Figs. 219, 220). The blood picture is considerably different in the case of chronic erythroleukemia (Oliff et al. 1980): many normoblasts, some basophilic erythroblasts, and even occasional pro-erythroblasts may be seen (Fig. 221). The number of smudge cells can be reduced if the blood is allowed to run down a microslide without using a spreader slide. Thus cells which would be unrecognizable are seen to be erythroid precursors. Poikilocytosis is variably part of the picture in the chronic form. (It should be noted that the above description of the polycythemic and anemic forms of erythroleukemia were derived from studies of blood from mice which were inoculated with molecularly cloned viruses. They do not exactly match earlier descriptions of Friend disease, possibly because such clones were not then available, and the diseases described at that time were due to a mixture of viruses.)

Ultrastructure

Investigations of erythroleukemia using electron microscopy have been limited and have revealed only two features among leukemic cells that are not seen in normal erythroid progenitors. These include budding of retroviral particles from the plasma membranes of erythroblasts, normoblasts, and reticulocytes (LoBue et al. 1974) and the presence of cytoplasmic vacuoles (Orlic and Mirand 1977).

Differential Diagnosis

Splenic enlargement, subcapsular foci, hematocrit values, the presence of erythroid precursors in splenic imprints, as well as tissue sections or blood films are criteria by which the various forms of erythroleukemia can be positively identified. On a gross basis they can be differentiated from lymphomas which are characterized by the presence of enlarged lymph nodes and/or thymus. Also, in lymphomas the splenic white pulp is generally enlarged and prominent, either as a diffuse white mottling or as discrete nodular tumor masses. In contrast to the severe aberrations seen in erythroleukemia, hematocrit values are generally between 30% and 40% in lymphomas. Distinction between erythroblasts and lymphoblasts in splenic imprints may be difficult using Romanovsky stains, and use of esterase positivity of erythroblasts but not lymphoblasts (Silver 1986) can be helpful. Erythroleukemia in mice must also be differentiated from myelogenous leukemia since both are primarily diseases of the splenic red pulp. Spleno- and hepatomegaly are features of both diseases, but there is usually a distinct difference in color with these organs: in myelogenous leukemia, a dull brown to brick red, in contrast to the dark red characteristic of erythroleukemia. The hematocrit is very depressed in advanced cases of chronic myelogenous leukemia and anemic forms of erythroleukemia but usually is lower in the latter. The blood picture of myelogenous leukemia is characteristically one of a severe leukemia representing all stages of neutrophilic maturation, and myeloid cells predominate in splenic imprints. Myeloblasts have an eccentric ovoid nucleus, a much more dispersed chromatin, and less basophilic cytoplasm than erythroblasts. In the liver, myeloid leukemic cells accumulate in the triad areas rather than evenly within sinusoids as in erythroleukemia. Lymph nodes may be moderately enlarged with a greenish tinge in cases of myelogenous leukemia, due to a medullary accumulation of myeloid precursors.

In the early stages of the polycythemic form of erythroleukemia there may be some confusion with a physiologically appropriate, secondary polycythemia. However, even in such severe situations as the response to hemolysis caused by phenylhydrazine, macroscopic erythroblastic colonies are not seen in the spleen, since secondary polycythemia erythroid precursors are evenly distributed through the red pulp. Also, the number of circulating reticulocytes is less in secondary than in virus-induced polycythemia. With the anemic forms of erythroleukemia, differentiation from physiologically reduced erythropoiesis or accelerated destruction of circulating erythrocytes depends on the presence in erythroleukemia, particularly the chronic form, of large numbers of circulating normoblasts and the accumulation of erythroid precursors within the hepatic sinusoids. It generally is not appreciated that chronic inflammation can cause severe splenomegaly, and even antigenically challenged mice may have moderately enlarged spleens. Such conditions may be difficult to differentiate from early erythroleukemia induced by helper virus. Microscopically, such a differentiation is easier because reactive spleens maintain normal architectural compartmentalization of red and white pulp, and the periarteriolar sheaths are enlarged rather than compressed. It is also not usually appreciated that erythroleukemia may occur in the same animal along with lymphoma, in which case both the red and white pulp are filled with erythroblasts and lymphoblasts, respectively, although in some cases individual nodes are lymphomatous, and the splenic white pulp appears normal. Mixed erythro- and myelogenous leukemias also have been mentioned, but these appear to occur very rarely in the same mouse.

Biologic Features

Natural History

It appears that erythroid progenitors in the mouse are particularly vulnerable to transformation through retroviral infection. That this represents transformation in the sense that proliferating cells are released from normal replication controls, i. e., that they are truly "malignant", has been indicated by transplantation experiments. Although such transplantation in syngeneic mice is unsuccesful when donor cells are derived early in the course of Friend disease, several transplantable cell lines have been developed from cases of advanced erythroleukemia (Friend and Haddad 1960; Dawson et al. 1963; Mager et al. 1980; Wendling et al. 1981). This can be explained as the result of a multistep process leading to autonomy which requires time to develop and is not a component of early disease. Progression of erythroleukemia has been studied extensively by culturing in vitro progenitor cells derived from SFFV-infected mice. There is a difference in dependency on erythropoietin for colony growth, with SFFV$_P$-derived progenitors (see below) being erythropoietin-independent, whereas SFFV$_A$-derived are erythropoietin-dependent (Ruscetti and Wolff 1984). In mice this difference is reflected in the erythropoietin-diminishing effect of hypertransfusion which inhibits SFFV$_A$- but not SFFV$_P$-induced disease (Milrand 1966). Tran-

scription of gp52 glycoprotein from the env portion of the SFFV genome has been shown to be required for induction of acute erythroleukemia (Oliff et al. 1980). The replication-competent viruses inducing chronic erythroleukemia do not transcribe such a protein. These viruses appear to belong to the MCF class of murine retroviruses, which is in accordance with a requirement for infection of neonatal mice as compared with the ability of SFFV to induce erythroleukemia when given to adults. One strain of the anemic form of Friend virus (FVA) induces erythroleukemia which spontaneously regresses (Russo et al. 1976).

Etiology and Frequency

A number of murine retroviruses have been associated with erythroid neoplasia, a very rare spontaneous event in all strains of mouse. The prototype is Friend leukemia virus complex (Friend 1957), which has been the subject of extensive investigations. It was established that the complex consisted of either of two defective viral components (SFFV$_P$ or SFFV$_A$) and a replication component, helper virus (F-MuLV), which allowed the defective component to become infectious and integrate into cellular genomes (Steeves 1975). As described above, the disease differs according to which of the two types of SFFV become integrated into the genome of the target cell so that either polycythemia (SFFV$_P$) or anemia (SFFV$_A$) develops (Mirand 1966; Tambourin et al. 1973). F-MuLV, by itself, also induces the anemic form (MacDonald et al. 1980; see reviews by Tambourin et al. 1979; Ruscetti and Wolff 1984; Schiff and Oliff 1986 for the virologic aspects of erythroleukemia in mice). Another intensively studied murine retrovirus causing erythroleukemia is the Rauscher virus (Rauscher 1962), which induces a disease similar to SFFV$_A$ (Siegler and Rich 1964), and the original virus was shown to be a complex of a defective SFFV and a helper virus component (Van Griensven and Vogt 1980). The latter is probably the component of the Rauscher complex inducing a response similar to F-MuLV (LoBue et al. 1974).

The erythroid precursor appears to be the target for a number of complete murine retroviruses including several derived from California wild mice which mimic either F-MuLV or SFFV (Langdon et al. 1983; Fredrickson et al. 1984). Some murine sarcomaviruses (MSV), including

Kirsten (Kirsten and Mayer 1967), Harvey (Harvey 1964; Chesterman et al. 1966), BALB/c (Peters et al. 1974), NS-AKV-1 and NS-AKV-2 MSVs (Fredrickson et al. 1987) induce some degree of erythroid proliferation. All of these contain an activated *ras* oncogene. Genetically engineered retroviral constructs containing v-*myc* or v-*raf* oncogenes (Rapp et al. 1985) also induce erythroleukemia. Another complete murine retrovirus which induces a disease in mice with a distinct erythroid component is the recently isolated myeloproliferative sarcomavirus (Le-Bousse-Kerdiles et al. 1980).

Comparison with Other Species

Among all species, spontaneous erythroleukemia appears to be a rare occurrence; however, such cases occur in both mice and chickens (Fredrickson, personal observations). Thus, induction with retrovirus in rats, chickens, and mice cannot be regarded entirely as a laboratory artifact. In rats, Friend virus complex causes lymphomas, but Kirsten and Harvey MSVs and a variant of Moloney MuLV (Taylor et al. 1972) cause a disease which features all aspects of erythroleukemia in mice. These lesions are typical of erythroleukemia; however, they are mixed with sarcomatous lesions, and in the spleen, the formation of blood lakes or rupture of the capsule is rarely seen. In chickens, avian erythroblastosis virus, which contains within its genome the oncogenes *erb*A and *erb*B, induces a fulminating proliferation of basophilic erythroblasts, causing profound normocytic anemia. Unlike the mouse, the bone marrow is the principal source of these erythroblasts hematogeneously spread to the spleen and liver, which undergo severe enlargement due to the accumulation of erythroblasts in the splenic red pulp and hepatic sinusoids. Ascites is moderately frequent, and HCT levels may be extremely low, generally less than 20%. The polycythemic form of erythroleukemia does not occur in rats or chickens. Erythroid neoplastic disease has been reported in the domestic cat as a rare spontaneous disease which appears to be associated with feline leukemia virus (Ward et al. 1969; Hardy 1981; Grindem et al. 1985). Following the nomenclature for human myeloproliferative diseases, the pure erythroid neoplastic condition is referred to by some investigators as erythremic myelosis rather than erythroleukemia. Feline erythroid neoplastic disease originates in the bone marrow, so splenic lesions are not invariably seen as part of the disease syndrome as they are in mice. Anemia with erythroid progenitors in the peripheral blood and a marrow crammed with erythroblasts are the hallmarks of the disease. The human disease, polycythemia vera, is associated with overproduction of erythrocytes and thus has some resemblance to polycythemia induced with SFFV$_P$ in mice. There are, however, differences including the long, indolent course in polycythemia vera often with the development of terminal myeloproliferative disease involving nonerythroid hematopoietic elements.

Acknowledgment. The help of Dr. S. Ruscetti is gratefully acknowledged.

References

Chesterman FC, Harvey JJ, Dourmashkin RR, Salaman MH (1966) The pathology of tumors and other lesions induced in rodents by virus derived from a rat with Moloney leukemia. Cancer Res 26: 1759–1768

Dawson PJ, Fieldsteel AH, Bostick WL (1963) Pathologic studies of Friend virus leukemia and the development of a transplantable tumor in BALB/c mice. Cancer Res 23: 349–354

de Both NJ, Vermey M, Van Griensven LJLD (1978) The effect of Rauscher murine leukemia virus infection on the hemopoietic system of BALB/c mice. Cell proliferation and cell loss. Exp Hematol 6: 515–527

Dennis LH, Brodsky I (1965) A dose-response curve employing thrombocytopenia induced by the Friend leukemia virus. Proc Soc Exp Biol Med 120: 683–685

Fredrickson TN, LoBue J, Alexander PA Jr, Schultz EF, Gordon AS (1972) A transplantable leukemia from mice inoculated with Rauscher leukemia virus. JNCI 48: 1597–1605

Fredrickson TN, Langdon WY, Hoffman PM, Hartley JW, Morse HC III (1984) Histologic and cell surface antigen studies of hematopoietic tumors induced by Cas-Br-M murine leukemia virus. JNCI 72: 447–454

Fredrickson TN, O'Neill RR, Rutledge RA, Theodore TS, Martin MA, Ruscetti SK, Austin JB, Hartley JW (1987) Biologic and molecular characterization of two newly isolated ras-containing murine leukemia viruses. J Virol 61: 2109–2119

Friend C (1957) Cell-free transmission in adult Swiss mice of a disease having the character of a leukemia. J Exp Med 105: 307–318

Friend C, Haddad JR (1960) Tumor formation with transplants of spleen or liver from mice with virus-induced leukemia. JNCI 25: 1279–1289

Grindem CB, Perman V, Stevens JB (1985) Morphological classification and clinical and pathological characteristics of spontaneous leukemia in 10 cats. J Am Anim Hosp Assoc 21: 227–236

Hardy WD Jr (1981) Hematopoietic tumors of cats. J Am Anim Hosp Assoc 17: 921–940

Harvey JJ (1964) An unidentified virus which causes the rapid production of tumours in mice. Nature 204: 1104–1105

Kirsten WH, Mayer LA (1967) Morphologic responses to a murine erythroblastosis virus. JNCI 39: 311–335

Langdon WY, Hoffman PM, Silver JE, Buckler CE, Hartley JW, Ruscetti SK, Morse HC 3rd (1983) Identification of a spleen focus-forming virus in erythroleukemic mice infected with a wildmouse ecotropic murine leukemia virus. J Virol 46: 230–238

Le Bousse-Kerdiles MC, Smadja-Joffe F, Klein B, Caillou B, Jasmin C (1980) Study of a virus-induced myeloproliferative syndrome associated with tumor formation in mice. Eur J Cancer 16: 43–51

LoBue J, Gordon AS, Weitz-Hamburger A, Ferdinand P, Camiscoli JF, Fredrickson TN, Hardy WD Jr (1974) Erythroid differentiation in murine erythroleukemia. In: Clarkson B, Baserga R (eds) Control of proliferation in animal cells. Cold Spring Harbor Laboratory, Cold Spring Harbor, pp 863–885

Ludwig FC, Bostick WL, Epling ML (1964) Quantitative analysis of Friend's disease in two inbred strains of mice with emphasis on bone marrow response. Cancer Res 24: 1308–1317

MacDonald ME, Mak TW, Bernstein A (1980) Erythroleukemia induction by replication-competent type C viruses cloned from the anemia- and polycythemia-inducing isolates of Friend leukemia virus. J Exp Med 151: 1493–1503

Mager D, Mak TW, Bernstein A (1980) Friend leukaemia virus-transformed cells, unlike normal stem cells, form spleen colonies in S 1/S 1 d mice. Nature 288: 592–594

Metcalf D, Furth J, Buffett RF (1959) Pathogenesis of mouse leukemia caused by Friend virus. Cancer Res 19: 52–58

Mirand EA (1966) Erythropoietic response of animals infected with various strains of Friend virus. NCI Monogr 22: 483–503

Oliff A, Linemeyer D, Ruscetti S, Lowe R, Lowy DR, Scolnick E (1980) Subgenomic fragment of molecular cloned Friend murine leukemia virus DNA contains the gene(s) responsible for Friend murine leukemia virus-induced disease. J Virol 35: 924–936

Orlic D, Mirand EA (1977) An electron microscopic study of hepatic erythropoiesis in adult mice with Friend virus disease. Lab Invest 37: 579–587

Peters RL, Rabstein LS, Van Vleck R, Kelloff GJ, Huebner RJ (1974) Naturally occurring sarcoma virus of the BALB/cCr mouse. JNCI 53: 1725–1729

Rapp UR, Cleveland JL, Fredrickson TN, Holmes KL, Morse HC III, Jansen HW, Patschinsky T, Bister K (1985) Rapid induction of hemopoietic neoplasms in newborn mice by a raf(mil)/myc recombinant murine retrovirus. J Virol 55: 23–33

Rauscher FJ (1962) A virus-induced disease of mice characterized by erythrocytopoiesis and lymphoid leukemia. JNCI 29: 515–543

Ruscetti S, Wolff L (1984) Spleen focus-forming virus: relationship of an altered envelope gene to the development of a rapid erythroleukemia. Curr Top Microbiol Immunol 112: 21–44

Russo I, Russo J, Baldwin J, Rich MA (1976) Histopathology of spontaneous regression in virus-induced murine leukemia. Am J Pathol 85: 73–84

Sassa S, Takaku F, Nakao K (1968) Regulation of erythropoiesis in the Friend leukemia mouse. Blood 31: 758–765

Schiff RD, Oliff A (1986) The pathophysiology of murine retrovirus-induced leukemias. CRC Crit Rev Oncol Hematol 5: 257–323

Siegler R, Rich MA (1964) Comparative pathogenesis of murine viral lymphoma. Cancer Res 24: 1406–1417

Silver J (1986) Genetic study of lymphoma induction by Friend murine leukemia virus in crosses involving AKR mice. JNCI 77: 793–799

Smadja-Joffe F, Jasmin C, Malaise EP, Bournoutian C (1973) Study of the cellular proliferation kinetics of Friend leukemia. Int J Cancer 11: 300–313

Steeves RA (1975) Spleen focus-forming virus in Friend and Rauscher leukemia virus preparations. JNCI 54: 289–297

Steinheider G, Seidel HJ, Kreja L (1979) Comparison of the biological effects of anemia inducing and polycythemia inducing Friend virus complex. Experientia 35: 1173–1175

Tambourin PE, Gallien Lartique O, Wendling F, Huaulme D (1973) Erythrocyte production in mice infected by the polycythaemia-inducing Friend virus or by the anaemia-inducing Friend virus. Br J Haematol 24: 511–524

Tambourin PE, Wendling F, Jasmin C, Smadja-Joffe F (1979) Review: the physiopathology of Friend leukemia. Leuk Res 3: 117–129

Taylor DON, Cremer NE, Oshiro LS, Lennette EH (1972) An anemia-inducing virus derived from tumors caused by murine sarcoma virus-Moloney. JNCI 49: 829–845

Van Griensven LJLD, Vogt M (1980) Rauscher 'mink cell focus-inducing' (MCF) virus causes erythroleukemia in mice: its isolation and properties. Virology 101: 376–388

Ward JM, Sodikoff CH, Schalm OW (1969) Myeloproliferative disease and abnormal erythrogenesis in the cat. J Am Vet Med Assoc 155: 879–888

Weitz-Hamburger A, Fredrickson TN, LoBue J, Hardy WD Jr, Camiscoli JF, Ferdinand P, Gallicchio V, Gordon AS (1975) Stimulation of erythropoietic differentiation in BALB/c mice infected with Rauscher leukemia virus. JNCI 55: 1171–1175

Wendling F, Moreau-Gachelin F, Tambourin P (1981) Emergence of tumorigenic cells during the course of Friend virus leukemias. Proc Natl Acad Sci USA 78: 3614–3618

Zajdela F (1962) Contribution a l'étude de la cellule de Friend. Assoc Fr Etude Cancer Bull 49: 351–373

Early Follicular Center Cell Lymphoma, Mouse

Jerrold M. Ward

Synonyms. Follicular center cell lymphoma; B cell lymphoma of splenic follicles; reticulum cell sarcoma, type B; lymphoma, pleomorphic or mixed; prelymphomatous changes; progressively transformed follicular centers.

Gross Appearance

The early stage of follicular center cell lymphoma in mice usually occurs in a spleen of normal size and weight. Occasionally, the spleen is also slightly enlarged (Yumoto et al. 1980).

Microscopic Features

Follicular center cell lymphoma, a common lymphoma of certain mouse strains, frequently arises in the white pulp of the spleen of an aging mouse. It is especially observed in aging female BALB/c mice (Pattengale and Frith 1983; Frith et al. 1985; Pattengale and Frith 1986). One or more white pulp areas may be involved in the early lesions in an individual section. The early lesion often stands out as a pale zone in the white pulp (Figs. 222-224). More severe involvement includes all follicles in the section. The earliest neoplastic lesions are seen in the B- or T-cell zones (PALS) of the white pulp. Several forms of prelymphomatous and lymphomatous lesions were described by Japanese pathologists in NZB mice including those predominant in follicles, PALS, red pulp, or marginal zone (Yumoto et al. 1980). In the T-cell area, the early lesion may be adjacent to the PALS, the potential location of Lyt-1 positive B cells (Davidson et al. 1984), the possible cell of origin of FCC lymphomas. There is depletion of the normal small follicular lymphocytes and of the normal follicular architecture. Normal lymphocytes are usually replaced by pleomorphic, cleaved or noncleaved cells with a reticular cell appearance, hence the earlier descriptions as reticulum cell sarcoma (Figs. 223-225). The cell population may be uniform or pleomorphic. Cytoplasm may be abundant or sparse, and mitotic figures are not usually prominent.
If the spleen is fixed in Bouin's B-5, or Zenker's fixatives or frozen sections are used, immuno-

globulins can usually be demonstrated by immunoperoxidase techniques. Although formalin-fixed tissues can be trypsinized, the immunoreactivity of immunoglobulins is not always enhanced. If the early lesion is a neoplastic proliferation of B-lymphocyte precursors, immunoglobulins can usually be demonstrated in a portion of the tumor cells (Figs. 225, 226). Specific immunoglobulins can be seen or antisera against heavy or light chains or against several immunoglobulins can be used as screening reagents. I use a commercially prepared goat polyclonal antiserum to mouse immunoglobulins (IgA, IgG, IgM) for the detection of immunoglobulin-containing cells. Theoretically, if the proliferation is monoclonal, either κ or λ immunoglobulin light chains are seen, although κ immunoreactivity is more common in advanced lymphomas (Pattengale and Frith 1983; Fredrickson et al. 1985; Picker et al. 1987). If the proliferation is polyclonal and not neoplastic, cells containing either type of light chains can be found in the lesion. Unfortunately, normal nonneoplastic B cells can be found throughout the spleen and may intermingle with neoplastic B cells of one light chain type. Frequently, normal plasma cells may be seen around the PALS (Fig. 225) and in some areas of normal and neoplastic follicles. Thus, one must be cautious in interpretation. In normal follicles, T cells may also be found whereas fewer are seen in neoplastic B-cell proliferations. As the FCC lymphoma progresses, additional follicles become involved, and the spleen becomes enlarged. The spleen appears nodular, and neoplastic follicles may coalesce. The morphology and immunocytochemistry of the earliest lesion in individual follicles frequently is identical to the diffuse process (see p. 147, this volume).
More recently, we have found that some of the early follicular center cell tumor cells and many tumor cells in advanced lymphoma bind to peanut lectin (agglutinin) (Fig. 227). Such prominent binding is not found in nonneoplastic reactive B-cell hyperplasia nor in normal tissues. The pattern of binding can serve as a marker for early neoplastic lesions and differentiation from reactive lesions. Similar findings have been reported in humans (Hsu and Ree 1983; Ree and Hsu 1983).

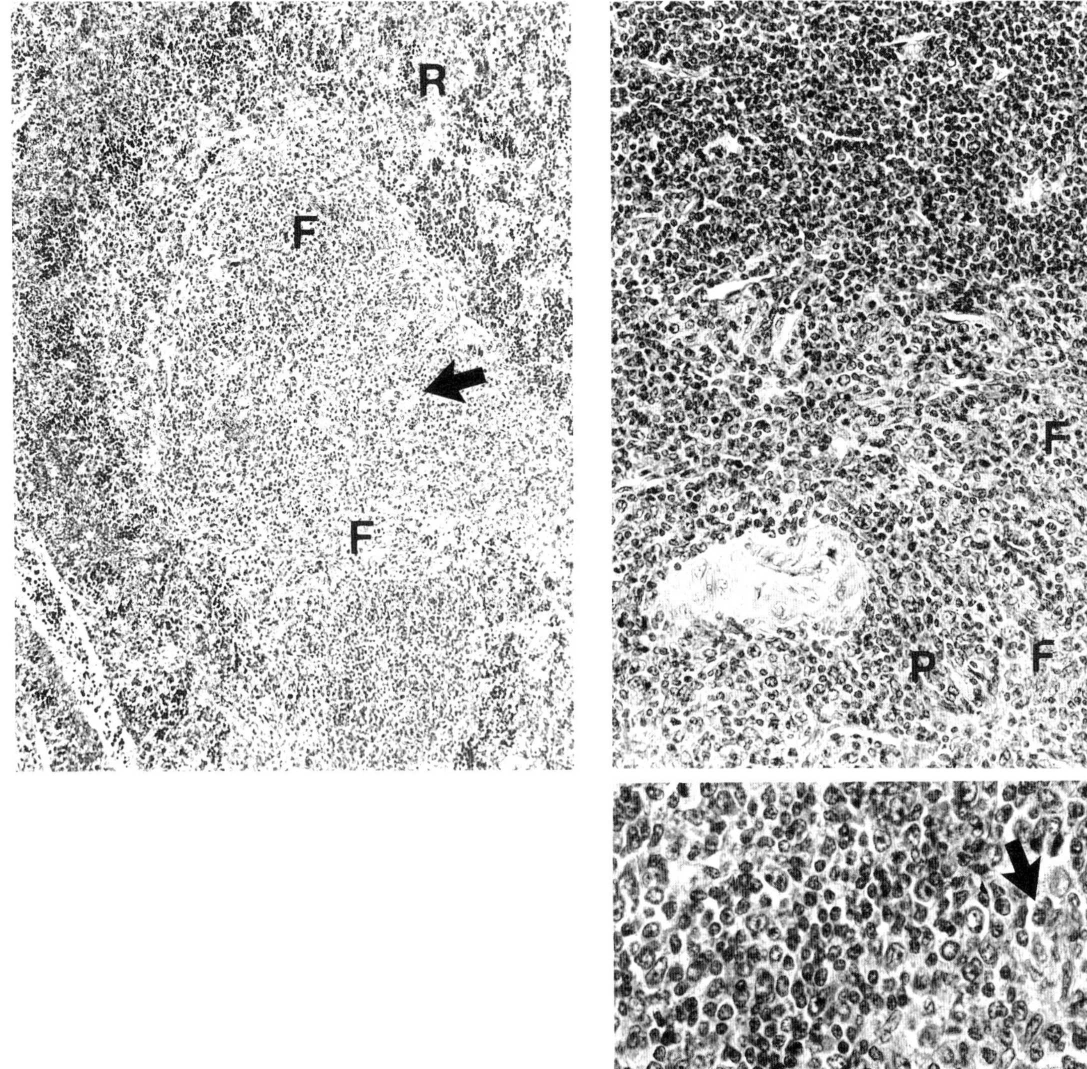

Fig. 222 *(upper left).* Spleen, aging BALB/c mouse. Pale white pulp zone of early follicular center cell lymphoma *(F).* In this spleen, only a few white pulp areas were involved. *Arrow,* periarteriolar lymphoid sheath; *R,* red pulp. H and E, × 100

Fig. 223 *(upper right).* Spleen, mouse, Portion of white pulp area showing early follicular center cell lymphoma with pale pleomorphic cells *(F).* Normal small lymphocytes at *top* of figure. *P,* periarteriolar lymphoid sheath. H and E, × 250

Fig. 224 *(lower right).* Spleen, mouse. Early follicular center cell lymphoma with pale pleomorphic cells *(arrows).* Note normal small lymphocytes at *top* of figure. H and E, × 400

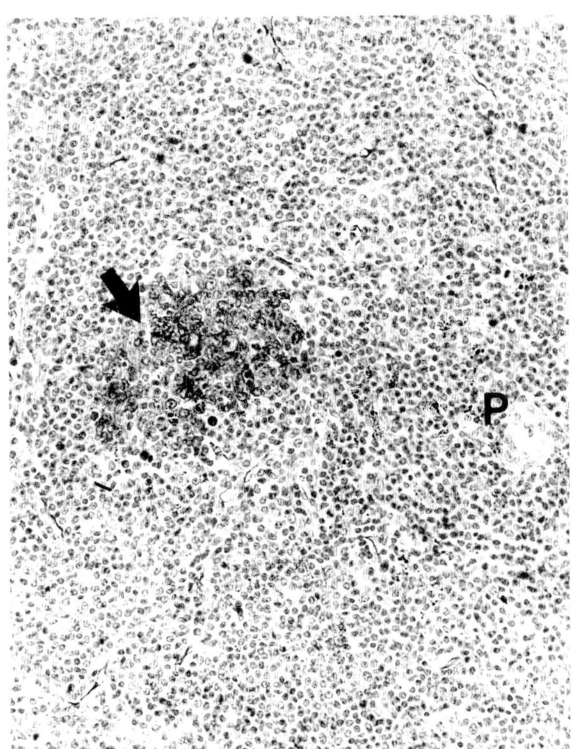

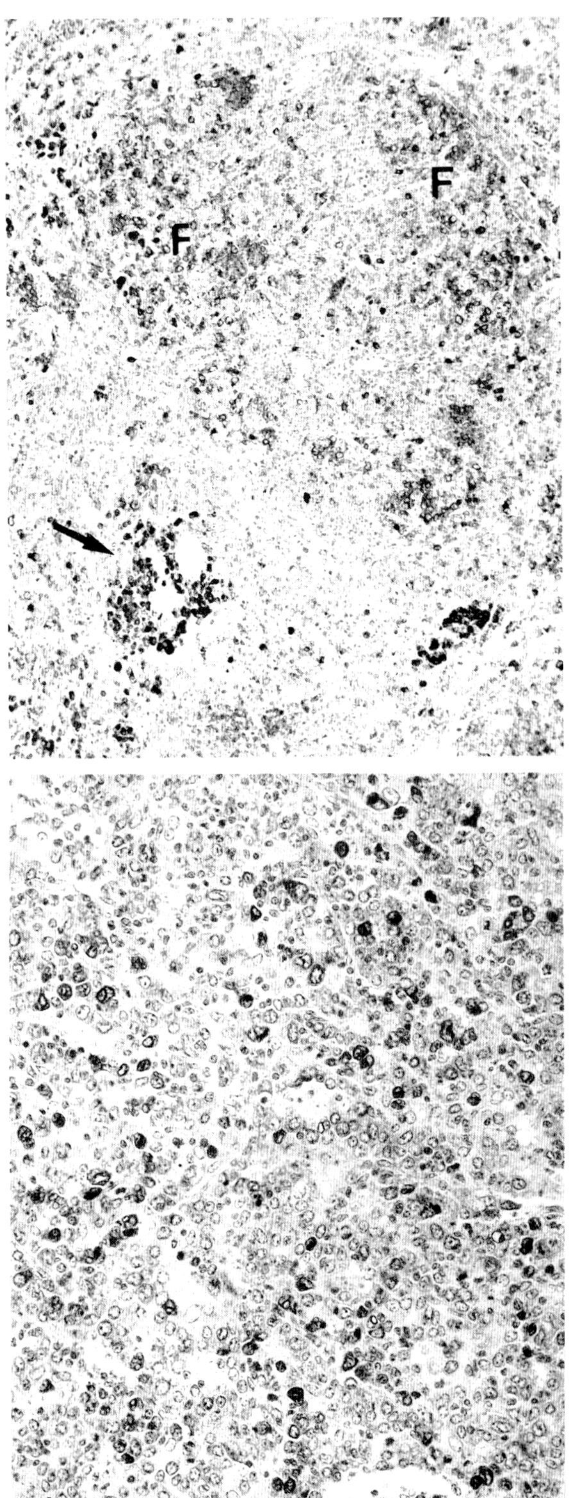

Fig. 225 *(upper left).* Spleen, BALB/c mouse. Immunoglobulin immunoreactive neoplastic cells in white pulp with early follicular center cell lymphoma *(F).* Note mature plasma cells with intense immunoreactivity in the periarteriolar lymphoid sheath *(arrow).* Avidin-biotin complex immunoperoxidase for mouse immunoglobulins, Bouin's fixative, hematoxylin, × 100

Fig. 226 *(lower left).* Spleen, mouse. Immunoglobulins in follicular center cell lymphoma in white pulp. Note the cytoplasms of a proportion of tumor cells are immunoreactive *(dark).* Avidin-biotin complex immunoperoxidase for mouse immunoglobulins, Bouin's fixative, hematoxylin, × 250

Fig. 227 *(upper right).* Spleen, mouse. Peanut lectin binding to small focus of neoplastic B cells *(arrow)* in early stage of follicular center cell lymphoma arising in B-cell zone of white pulp. Avidin-biotin complex immunoperoxidase with biotinylated peanut lectin. *P,* periarteriolar lymphoid sheath. Hematoxylin, × 250

Ultrastructure

Not reported.

Differential Diagnosis

The early lesions must be differentiated from reactive lesions due to the immune response to antigens or aging processes. The pleomorphism of the infiltrated cells and paleness of the affected area are usually very different from those seen in reactive or aging lesions. Chronic infectious or degenerative processes in other tissues which stimulate the splenic B-cell response may make the reactive lesion more complex. A single or a few potentially neoplastic follicles should be interpreted with caution since one may be uncertain of their outcome. Several or many affected follicles may strengthen the diagnosis of neoplasia. Although reactive lesions are frequently diffuse, they may be focal as well. Although immunocytochemistry is conclusive to some, it may also add additional problems in interpretation. Monoclonality can be shown although only a small percentage of the neoplastic population in the small early lesion may contain monoclonal immunoglobulins. If the population of cells contains only κ or λ light chains, the population is probably monoclonal, while if it contains cells with either light chain, it is probably polyclonal. Normal nonneoplastic cells containing either light chain can be found in areas of neoplastic cells also. We use polyclonal antisera to mouse immunoglobulins to demonstrate cells containing immunoglobulins of any type and then show cells containing κ or λ light chains in the lesion.

Biological Features

Although not documented in the literature, the early follicular lesions are progressive in nature. They may also occur in Peyer's patches of the small intestine, follicles of mesenteric lymph nodes, or in any lymphoid tissue. From serial sacrifice studies, the progression of these lesions to advanced PCC lymphomas may be followed. They are slow growing lesions at least during the early stages and resemble lesions of progressively transformed germinal centers seen in human lymph nodes (van den Oord et al. 1985). The cause of follicular center cell lymphoma in mice is not known, although some evidence for a retroviral etiology has been presented but not proved (Fredrickson et al. 1985). B-cell lymphomas of B-cell and follicular cell origin have been induced by retroviruses (Pattengale et al. 1982). Retroviral antigens can be demonstrated in a few megakaryocytes and rare nonneoplastic and neoplastic lymphocytes in the spleen of these mice by immunocytochemistry (J. Ward, unpublished observations), but retroviruses have not been shown to cause the naturally occurring disease.

Comparison with Other Species

Follicular center cell lymphomas have been described in humans (Taylor 1986) and compared with those of the mouse. Many similarities exist, and the mouse has been proposed as a model for the human counterparts (Pattengale and Taylor 1983).

References

Davidson WP, Fredrickson TN, Rudikoff EK, Coffman RL, Hartley JW, Morse HC III (1984) A unique series of lymphomas related to the Ly-1+ lineage of B lymphocyte differentiation. J Immunol 133: 744–753

Fredrickson TN, Morse HC III, Yetter RA, Rowe WP, Hartley JW, Pattengale PK (1985) Multiparameter analyses of spontaneous nonthymic lymphomas occurring in NFS/N mice congenic for esotropic murine leukemia viruses. Am J Pathol 121: 349–360

Frith CH, Pattengale PK, Ward JM (1985) A color atlas of hematopoietic pathology of mice. Toxicology Pathology Associates, Little Rock, Abst 8326

Hsu SM, Ree HJ (1983) Histochemical studies on lectin binding in reactive lymphoid tissues. J Histochem Cytochem 31: 538–546

Pattengale PK, Frith CH (1983) Immunomorphologic classification of spontaneous lymphoid cell neoplasms occurring in female BALB/c mice. JNCI 70: 169–179

Pattengale PK, Frith CH (1986) Contributions of recent research to the classification of spontaneous lymphoid cell neoplasms in mice. CRC Crit Rev Toxicol 16: 185–212

Pattengale PK, Taylor CR (1983) Experimental models of lymphoproliferative disease: the mouse as a model for human non-Hodgkins lymphomas and related leukemias. Am J Pathol 113: 237–265

Pattengale PK, Taylor CR, Twomey P, Hill S, Jonasson J, Beardsley T, Haas M (1982) Immunopathology of B-cell lymphomas induced in C57BL/6 mice by dualtropic murine leukemia virus (MuLV). Am J Pathol 107: 362–377

Picker LJ, Weiss LM, Medeiros LJ, Wood GS, Warnke RA (1987) Immunophenotypic criteria for the diagnosis of non-Hodgkin's lymphoma. Am J Pathol 128: 181–201

Ree HJ, Hsu SM (1983) Lectin histochemistry of malignant tumors. I. Peanut agglutinin (PNA) receptors in

follicular lymphoma and follicular hyperplasia: an immunohistochemical study. Cancer 51: 1631–1638
Taylor CR (1986) Immunomicroscopy: a diagnostic tool for the surgical pathologist. Saunders, Philadelphia
van den Oord JJ, de Wolf-Peeters C, Desmet VJ (1985) Immunohistochemical analysis of progressively transformed follicular centers. Am J Clin Pathol 83: 560–564

Yumoto T, Yoshida Y, Yoshida H, Ando K, Matsui K (1980) Prelymphomatous and lymphomatous changes in splenomegaly of New Zealand black mice. Acta Pathol Jpn 30: 171–186

Fibrosarcoma, Spleen, Rat

James A. Popp

Synonyms. Stromal sarcoma; capsular sarcoma.

Gross Appearance

Fibrosarcoma of the spleen are generally single lesions and vary in size from a few millimeters up to several centimeters in diameter. Most lesions cause the splenic capsule to bulge, but smaller lesions may occasionally be embedded in the splenic parenchyma and cause little or no external distortion. Rarely, these neoplasms appear to be associated only with the deep surface of the capsule with little evidence of extension into the parenchyma. Such lesions have been designated capsular sarcomas.

These neoplasms are generally firm with a slightly irregular and occasionally multinodular surface. Most are pale gray, similar to sarcomas which occur in other organs. On cut surfaces, areas of hemorrhage, necrosis, or fatty metamorphosis may cause an irregular color pattern. The neoplastic tissue merges with the surrounding splenic tissue with no sharp line of demarcation.

Microscopic Features

Fibrosarcomas are usually well-differentiated and composed of large sheets of irregular, spindle-shaped fibroblasts with ovoid nuclei (Ward et al. 1980). These neoplastic cells form parallel arrays and lack any orientation around vessels or other splenic structures. The cytologic characteristics of typical fibrosarcoma are similar to those found in other organs (Fig. 228). In the less well-differentiated neoplasms, the nuclei are relatively uniform, large, oval to elongated, vesicular and lack nucleoli. In contrast the nuclei in less well-differentiated neoplasms may vary in size and may contain large nucleoli. Cell boundaries are indistinct as the cytoplasm is difficult to distinguish from the adjacent collagen. Mitotic figures are infrequently observed except in the most poorly differentiated neoplasms.

Although variable in amount, collagen is a common feature in splenic fibrosarcomas. Many neoplasms, particularly the more well-differentiated, have extensive collagen deposition throughout the lesion (Fig. 229). Masson trichrome stain can be used to identify the collagen if necessary. Areas of osteoid metaplasia may occasionally be found, although the percentage of the lesion composed of osteoid is always minimal. Individual and/or clusters of mature adipocytes are common features of splenic fibrosarcomas (Goodman et al. 1984). Hemorrhage and necrosis are often observed in the larger neoplasms.

Fibrosarcomas interdigitate with the surrounding splenic tissue, forming no distinct line of demarcation. Local invasion of the adjacent tissue is readily apparent. Invasion generally affects all internal structures of the spleen, but the neoplasm rarely extends through the capsule or into large vessels.

Ultrastructure

TEM supports the fibroblastic characteristics of these neoplasms (Fig. 230). The cells are generally elongated with a moderate amount of cytoplasm containing few organelles. The nuclei conform to the architecture of the cells and characteristically have marginated chromatin and indistinct nucleoli. The extracellular stroma of the

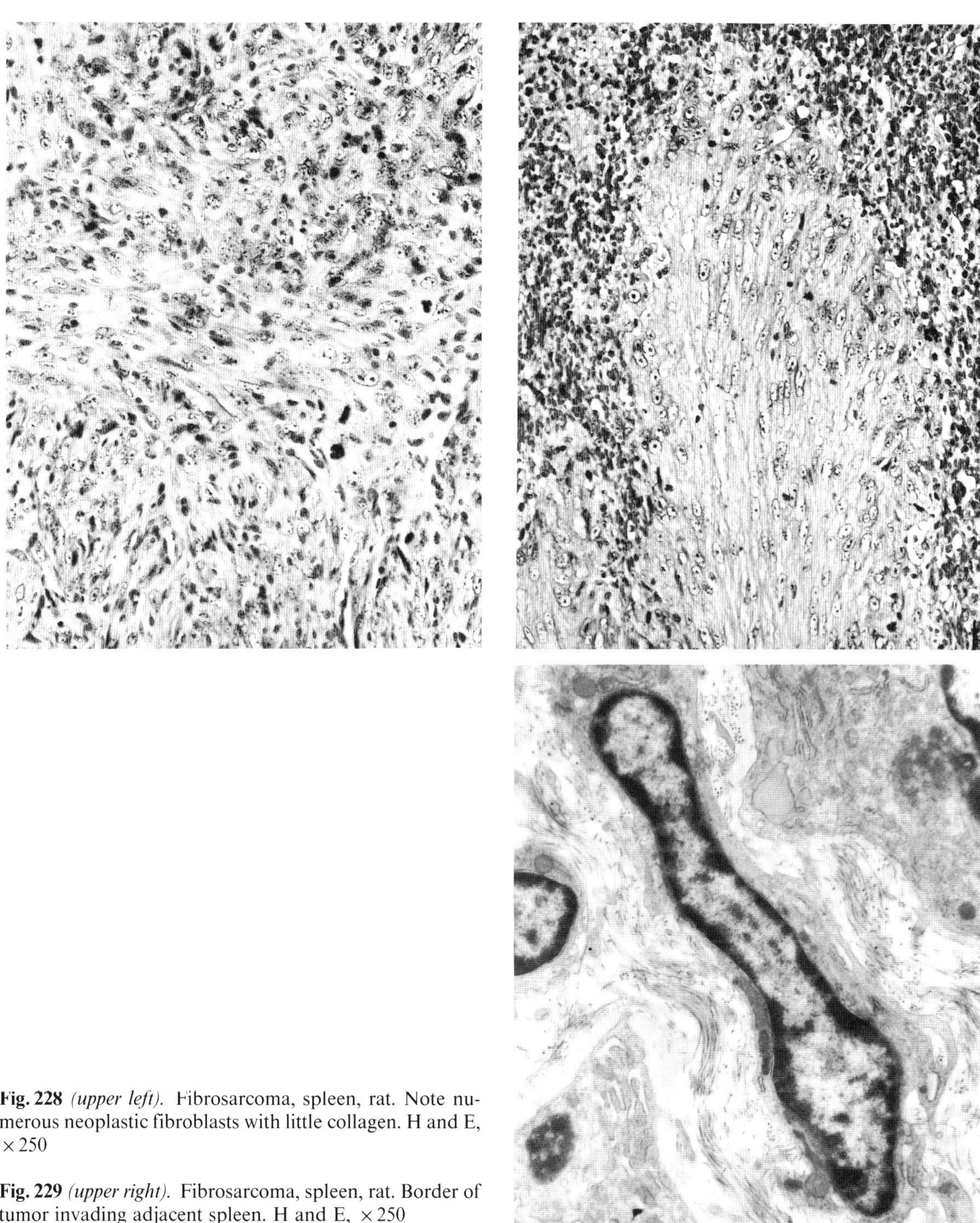

Fig. 228 *(upper left).* Fibrosarcoma, spleen, rat. Note numerous neoplastic fibroblasts with little collagen. H and E, ×250

Fig. 229 *(upper right).* Fibrosarcoma, spleen, rat. Border of tumor invading adjacent spleen. H and E, ×250

Fig. 230 *(lower right).* Neoplastic fibroblast in a fibrosarcoma of the spleen of a rat. TEM, ×6600 neoplasm is frequently made up of extensive collagen.

Fibrosarcomas usually have a well-developed Golgi complex and characteristically lack a basal lamina and cell junctions. These ultrastructural features may help differentiate fibroblastic tumors from other primitive mesenchymal tumors.

Differential Diagnosis

Fibrosarcomas must be distinguished from splenic fibrosis, the precursor lesion from which the neoplasm appears to arise (Ward et al. 1980). While poorly differentiated neoplasms are readily distinguished from fibrosis, well-differentiated fibrosarcomas with extensive collagen must be distinguished from fibrosis based on the cytologic characteristics of the cells. That fibrosarcomas are infrequently observed within areas of well-differentiated fibrosis supports the supposition that the neoplasms arise from areas of preexisting fibrosis (Goodman et al. 1984; Weinberger et al. 1985). While fibrosarcomas are frequently associated with fibrosis, benign fibroblastic neoplasma, i. e., fibromas, have rarely been observed in the rat spleen (Goodman et al. 1984).

Fibrosarcomas of the spleen must also be differentiated from other mesenchymal neoplasms particularly hemangiopericytomas, osteosarcomas, angiosarcomas, and hemangiosarcomas (Goodman et al. 1984). By light microscopy hemangiopericytomas are distinguished by the "strap" shape of the elongated cells and their frequent concentric arrangement around blood vessels. Osteosarcomas are distinguished by the presence of neoplastic osteocytes producing osteoid. Osteosarcomas must be distinguished from poorly differentiated fibrosarcomas which may contain multiple areas of osseous metaplasia. Osseous metaplasia is relatively common within both poorly and well-differentiated splenic fibrosarcomas. Splenic fibrosarcomas must also be differentiated from hemangiosarcomas (angiosarcomas) which may be present in the same spleen. Hemangiosarcomas consist of endothelial cells in solid masses and often form poorly organized vascular channels. True vascular channels lined by neoplastic endothelial cells should be distinguished from areas of necrosis and hemorrhage that may be observed in splenic fibrosarcomas.

Although splenic fibrosarcomas must be distinguished from the several mesenchymal neoplasms mentioned above, it should be remembered that these various neoplasms can and do occur in the same groups of animals when splenic neoplasms are induced by chemicals (Goodman et al. 1984; Weinberger et al. 1985). Fibrosarcomas are generally the most common histologic type of neoplasms, but they may be associated with a smaller number of other neoplasms, particularly osteosarcomas and hemangiosarcomas.

Biological Features

Most splenic fibrosarcomas of the rat are localized lesions with obvious local invasion. The metastatic rate of splenic fibrosarcomas appears to be variable from study to study. When they metastasize, they tend to involve the abdominal viscera most severely (Goodman et al. 1984). The liver is one of the most frequent sites of metastasis since this organ is secondarily involved by both direct invasion as well as hematogenous spread. Direct extension may occur to the pancreas, stomach, diaphragm, mesentery, kidney, and regional lymph nodes (Weinberger et al. 1985). Hematogenous metastasis to distant sites is occasionally observed.

Splenic fibrosarcomas are relatively uncommon in the rat as a result of chemical treatment (Bus and Popp 1987) and are rarely found as spontaneous lesions (Goodman et al. 1979). Chemical induction of these neoplasms has been reported following the administration of six different aromatic amines or their derivatives (Bus and Popp 1987; Goodman et al. 1984). They have been associated with a variety of other morphologic changes that are primarily characterized by nonneoplastic proliferation of splenic stromal cells and/or fibroblasts (Goodman et al. 1984). The neoplasms are associated with or preceded by the appearance of stromal fibrosis, stromal hyperplasia, and capsular fibrosis. Neoplastic lesions appear to arise from these preexisting nonneoplastic lesions. In addition, hemosiderosis is usually present, indicating substantial red cell destruction. Proposed steps in the formation of splenic sarcomas have been published (Goodman et al. 1984; Weinberger et al. 1985), and the proposed mechanism of splenic injury and tumor formation has been reviewed (Bus and Popp 1987).

Chemical-induced splenic fibrosarcomas occur more frequently in male than in female rats (Bus and Popp 1987). Mice rarely develop sarcomas of the spleen in response to chronic administration of aromatic amines (Bus and Popp 1987).

Comparison with Other Species

Splenic fibrosarcomas are uncommon in all species, limiting detailed species comparisons.

References

Bus JS, Popp JA (1987) Perspectives on the mechanism of action of the splenic toxicity of aniline and structurally-related compounds. Food Chem Toxicol 25 (8): 619–626

Goodman DB, Ward JM, Squire RA, Chu KC, Linhart MS (1979) Neoplastic and nonneoplastic lesions in aging F344 rats. Toxicol Appl Pharmacol 48: 237–248

Goodman DB, Ward JM, Reichardt WD (1984) Splenic fibrosis and sarcomas in F344 rats fed diets containing aniline hydrochloride, p-chloroaniline, azobenzene, o-toluidine hydrochloride, 4,4'-sulfonyldianiline, or D&C red no. 9. JNCI 73 (1): 265–273

Ward JM, Reznik G, Garner FM (1980) Proliferative lesions of the spleen in male F344 rats fed diets containing p-chloroaniline. Vet Pathol 17: 200–205

Weinberger MA, Albert RH, Montgomery SB (1985) Splenotoxicity associated with splenic sarcomas in rats fed high doses of D&C red no. 9 or aniline hydrochloride. JNCI 75: 681–690

Classification of Reactive Lesions, Spleen

Jerrold M. Ward

The reactive and functional anatomic areas of the spleen include the capsule, vascular red pulp, and cellular white pulp (Table 41). Each region contains cells or anatomical units which may react to endogenous and exogenous insults. Reactive lesions of the human spleen have been described (Burke 1981 a, b).

Splenic Capsule

The splenic capsule contains fibroblasts which may proliferate in response to chronic insults. Focal or diffuse fibrosis can be seen in peritonitis or in response to peritoneal tumors and can be induced by specific chemicals including aniline and Red 9 (Goodman et al. 1984; see p. 216, this volume).

Red Pulp

The vascular red pulp contains sinuses lined by endothelial cells in close apposition with reticular cells and macrophages. *Congestion* and *hemorrhage* are often seen in a variety of processes in the red pulp. The reticular cells and macrophages may phagocytize erythrocytes, foreign materials, microorganisms, and other substances, giving the appearance of a reactive reticuloendothelial red pulp reaction. Focal or diffuse *necrosis* may also be found, sometimes associated with vascular lesions including infarcts. Various types of *pigments* and associated *histiocytosis* are seen in the spleen of aging rodents including hemosiderin and lipofuscin (Ward and Reznik-Schuller 1980; Crichton et al. 1980) and after exposure to certain chemicals which induce *hemosiderosis* or other pigmented lesions. Focal *fibrosis* of the splenic red pulp has been reported for aniline and related aromatic amines in rats (Goodman et al. 1984), perhaps as a sequel to marked methemoglobinemia and splenic pigmentation or necro-

Table 41. Classification of reactive splenic lesions of rodents

Capsule
Inflammation
Fibrosis

Red pulp
Congestion
Hemorrhage
Necrosis
Fibrosis (focal)
Hematopoiesis
   Erythroblastosis (erythropoiesis)
   Myeloid hyperplasia
Plasmacytosis
Amyloidosis
Pigmentation
Histiocytosis
Angiectasis

White pulp
Lymphoid
   Necrosis
   Atrophy (lymphocyte depletion)
   Hyperplasia
      B-cell zone (follicular)
         Immunoblastic
         Lymphocytic
      T-cell zone (periarteriolar lymphoid sheath)
         Lymphoblastic
         Lymphocytic

Marginal zone
Atrophy
Hyperplasia

sis but rarely occurs spontaneously. Focal *angiectasis* in mice and rats is often the early stage of hemangioma or hemangiosarcoma and may be associated with trabecular fibrosis.

The splenic cords contain blood vessels, macrophages, and hemopoietic elements. *Hemopoiesis* is normal in the spleens of young rats and mice, and an increase in the degree of this response occurs readily after inflammatory, neoplastic, or hemopoietic insults. The spleen may enlarge several times during reactive hemopoiesis (mye-

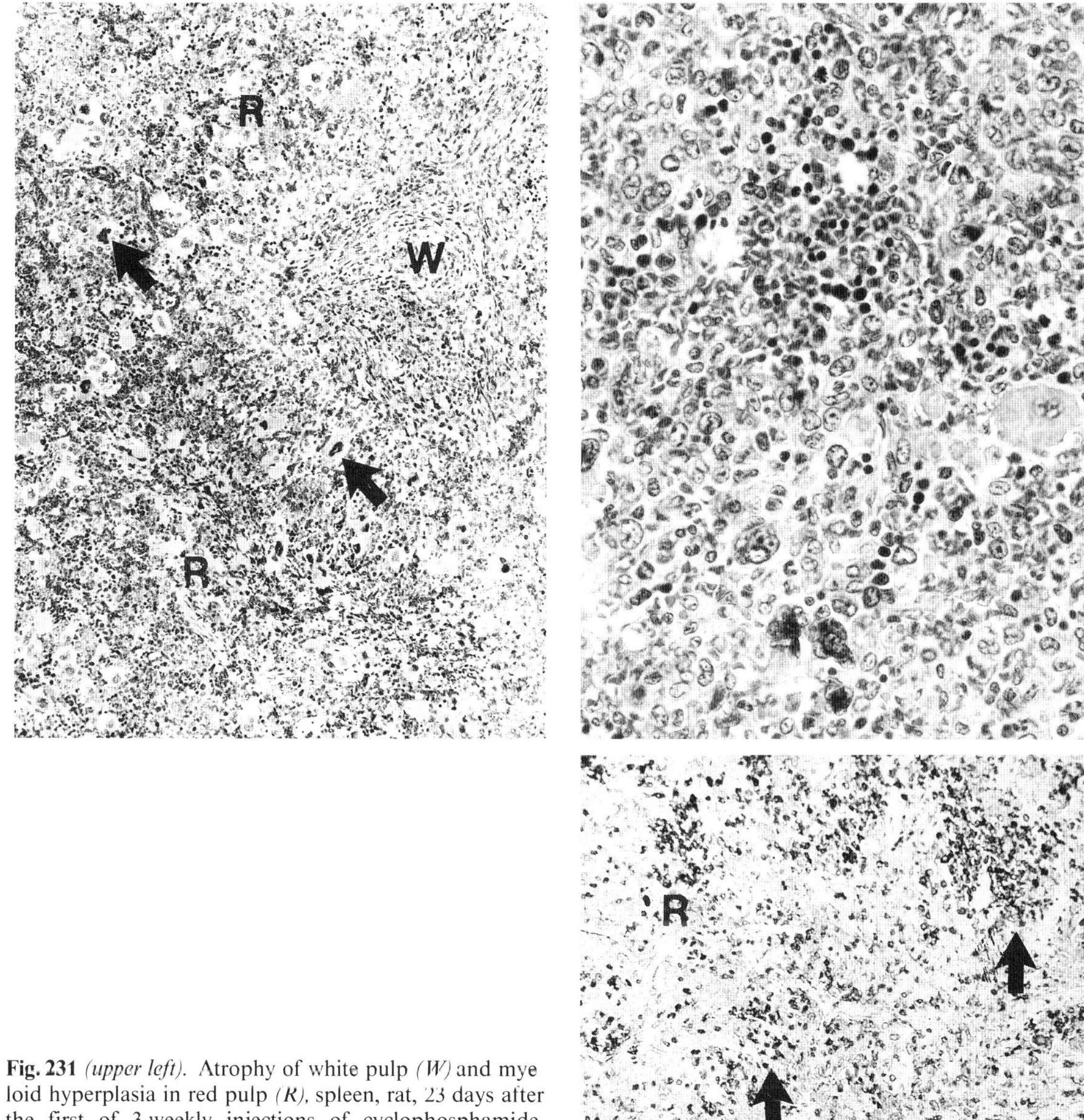

Fig. 231 *(upper left).* Atrophy of white pulp *(W)* and mye loid hyperplasia in red pulp *(R)*, spleen, rat, 23 days after the first of 3 weekly injections of cyclophosphamide. Large nuclei belong to megakaryocytes *(arrows)*. H and E, × 100

Fig. 232 *(upper right).* Myeloid hyperplasia, splenic red pulp, aging Sprague-Dawley derived rat. Immature mye loid elements and megakaryocytes are observed. H and E, × 400

Fig. 233 *(lower right).* Aging Sprague-Dawley rat, spleen, with numerous immunoglobulin-containing plasma cells *(arrows)* in red pulp *(R)* and white pulp *(W)* associated with myeloid metaplasia and atrophy of white pulp. Avid-in-biotin complex immunohistochemistry for rat immuno-globulins, Bouin's fixative, hematoxylin, × 100

222   Jerrold M. Ward

loid hyperplasia), which may involve erythropoiesis, myelopoiesis, and/or megakaryocyte hyperplasia to varying degrees (Long et al. 1986). It
must be differentiated from granulocytic leukemia. The cords are usually filled with hemopoietic elements in varying degrees of differentiation,
and there is frequently atrophy of the white pulp
(Figs. 231, 232). In some areas of the spleen, immature cells may predominate, while in others,
more mature forms are evident. In aging rats, especially of the Sprague-Dawley stock, enlarged
spleens may be common without evidence of
etiology. These spleens can mimic neoplasia, in
part, because the white pulp is depleted of lymphocytes, and the entire spleen may be filled
with immature and mature myeloid elements
(Fig. 232). Often, marked *plasmacytosis* is evident, which contributes to the degree of cellularity. Plasmacytosis may be associated with inflammatory, infectious, or neoplastic lesions in other
organs. Plasma cells and their precursors, the
immunoblasts, may be difficult to visualize in a
cellular spleen but are readily evident after immunoperoxidase staining for immunoglobulins
(Fig. 233). Bouin's, B-5, or Zenker's fixatives
must be used, however, to demonstrate readily
the presence of immunoglobulins.

Amyloidosis in mice usually arises in the red pulp
and may spread to the white pulp. Characteristics of this lesion are described by Sass, p. 235,
this volume.

Erythroblastosis, especially in mouse spleen, occurs after severe insults to erythrocytes or infection by specific retroviruses. Immature erythroblasts proliferate and may eventually fill the
entire red pulp and also result in depletion of
lymphocytes in the white pulp (Figs. 234, 235).
Drug-induced methemoglobinemia may induce
splenic enlargement and a marked degree of
erythropoiesis (erythroid hyperplasia) which can
be seen after injection of 5-bromo-2'-deoxyuri-
dine (BrdU) and BrdU immunohistochemistry
(deFazio et al. 1987) as an increase in the labelling index compared with that of normal red
pulp cells (Figs. 236, 237). Immunoreactive cells
are in active DNA synthesis.

White Pulp

The white pulp of the spleen is composed of a
T-cell zone, the periarteriolar lymphoid sheath
(PALS), follicular B-cell zone, and marginal
zone. Each zone may have lesions of lymphoid
atrophy or hyperplasia or other lesions, including

Fig. 234 *(upper left).* Marked erythroblastosis in red pulp ▶
(arrows) and atrophy of white pulp *(W)* of mouse spleen,
induced by Harvey sarcomavirus/Moloney leukemia virus. H and E, × 100

Fig. 235 *(lower left).* High magnification of splenic erythroblastosis from Fig. 234. Large erythroblasts *(arrows)*
along trabeculae are associated with small nucleated
erythrocytes *(N).* H and E, × 400

Fig. 236 *(upper right).* 5-Bromo-2'-deoxyuridine immunohistochemistry of mouse spleen in phenacetin-induced
erythroblastosis after 10 days of exposure. Erythroblasts
in the red pulp have a high immunoreactive nuclear labeling index *(arrows)* as compared with normal spleen
(Fig. 237). Note relatively fewer labeled cells in white
pulp *(W).* Avidin-biotin complex immunohistochemistry
for BrdU, after BrdU injection, Bouin's fixative, hematoxylin, × 100

Fig. 237 *(lower right).* Normal young adult mouse spleen
after BrdU injection. Immunoreactive cells in red *(R)* and
white *(W)* pulp are much less numerous than in Fig. 236.
Bouin's fixative, hematoxylin, × 100

the presence of pigmented macrophages, dendritic cell hyperplasia, and plasmacytosis.

The T-cell zone develops *atrophy* after exposure
to irradiation, viruses (Mims and Gould 1978), or
drugs which cause *necrosis* of lymphocytes.
Athymic animals also have atrophic T-cell zones.
Depletion of lymphocytes in the PALS often accompanies atrophy of lymphocytes in the B-cell
zone, especially after drugs (Fig. 231). T-cell zone
hyperplasia may be seen in early metastasis of
thymic T-cell lymphomas (lymphoblastic) and
other lymphomas or leukemias (lymphoblastic or
lymphocytic). Pigmented macrophages or reticular cells can be seen in aging rats in this zone.

Hyperplasia of B cells (follicular hyperplasia) in
the B-cell area of the white pulp occurs in acute
immune responses to antigens. For example, after intraperitoneal injection of *Escherichia coli*
endotoxin (McMaster and Franzl 1968; Dardick
et al. 1983), immature B cells (immunoblasts)
proliferate within hours (Fig. 238-240) in this
zone. These immunoblasts have roundish, regular nuclear membranes and do not resemble
those pleomorphic cleaved cells seen in mouse
follicular center cell lymphomas. They mature to
plasma cells which migrate into the red pulp
(Fig. 241). The numbers of immunoglobulin-containing cells in the spleen, especially the red
pulp, increases greatly for several days after exposure to endotoxin. Large B-cell zones (follicular hyperplasia) and/or a cellular marginal zone
may be seen in aging rat or mouse spleens with-

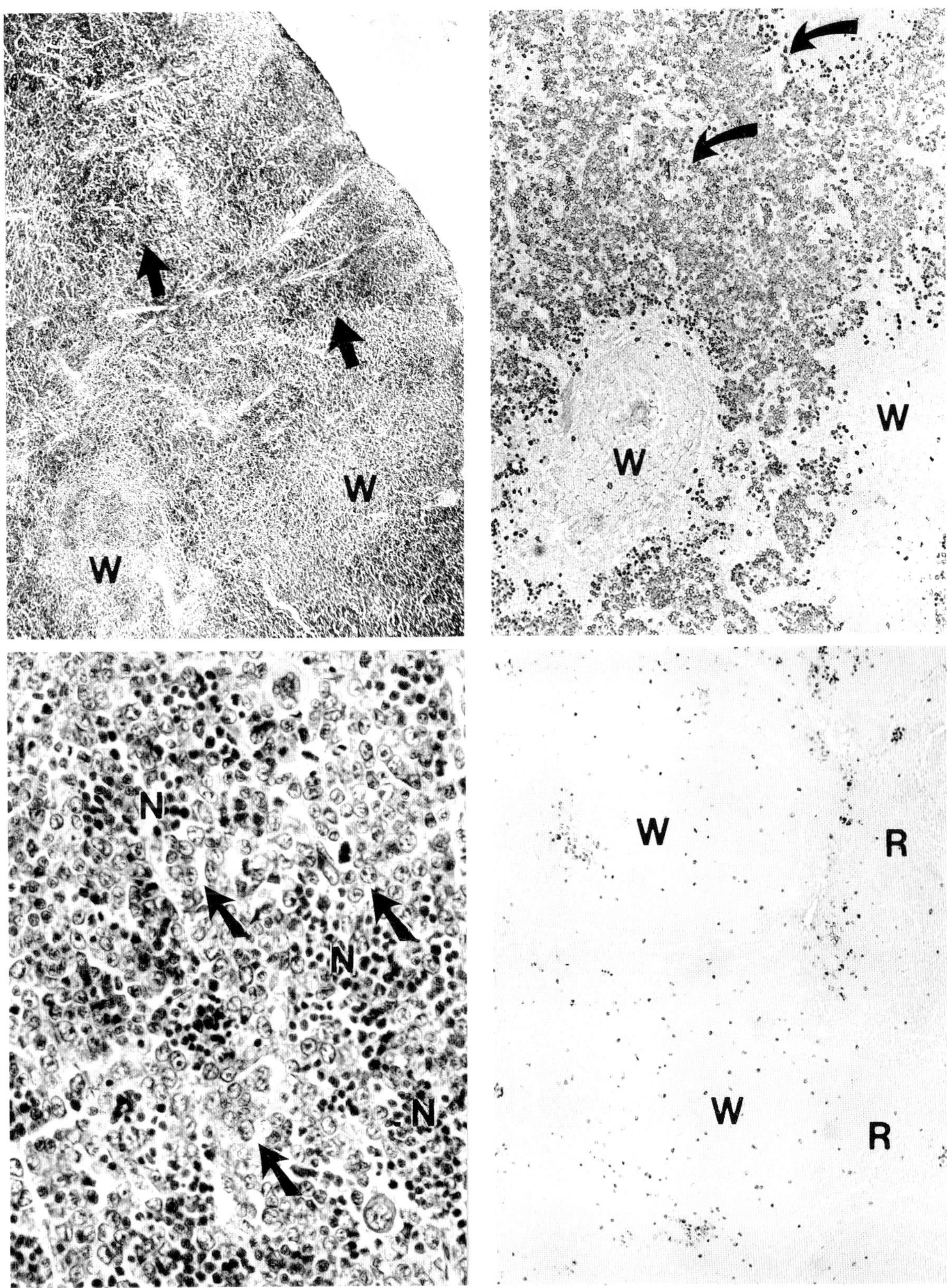

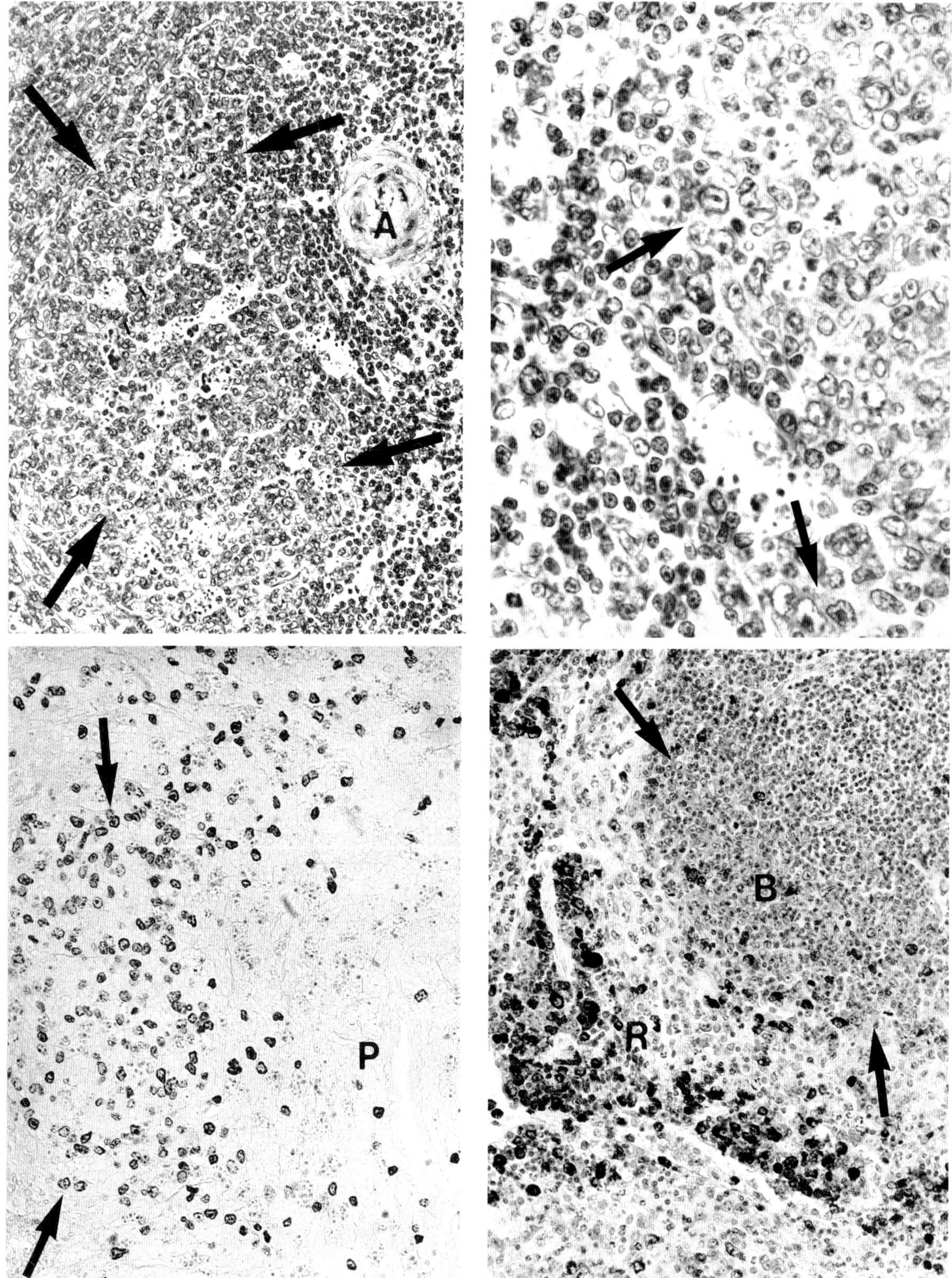

◄ **Fig. 238** *(upper left).* Hyperplasia of immunoblasts in follicular B-cell zone *(arrows)* in white pulp, F344 rat, spleen, 24 h after injection of *Escherichia coli* endotoxin. *A*, central arteriole. H and E, ×250

Fig. 239 *(lower left).* Mouse, spleen, 24 h after injection of *Escherichia coli* endotoxin showing high labeling index of immunoblasts in B-cell zone *(arrows)* compared with normal (Fig. 237). *P*, periarteriolar lymphoid sheath. Avidin-biotin complex immunohistochemistry for BrdU after BrdU injection, Bouin's fixative, hematoxylin, ×250

Fig. 240 *(upper right).* Immunoblasts *(arrows)* in hyperplastic B-cell zone, spleen, F344 rat, 24 h after *Escherichia coli* endotoxin. H and E, ×630

Fig. 241 *(lower right).* Mouse, spleen, 48 h after injection of *Escherichia coli* endotoxin. Many immunoglobulin-containing plasma cells in red pulp *(R)* adjacent to reactive follicular B-cell zone *(B)* containing some reactive immunoblasts *(arrows).* Avidin-biotin complex immunohistochemistry for mouse immunoglobulins. Hematoxylin, ×250

Fig. 242. Spleen, aged Sprague-Dawley rat with marginal ► zone *(M)* hyperplasia. *B*, follicle; *arrow*, central arteriole in white pulp; *R*, red pulp. H and E, ×100

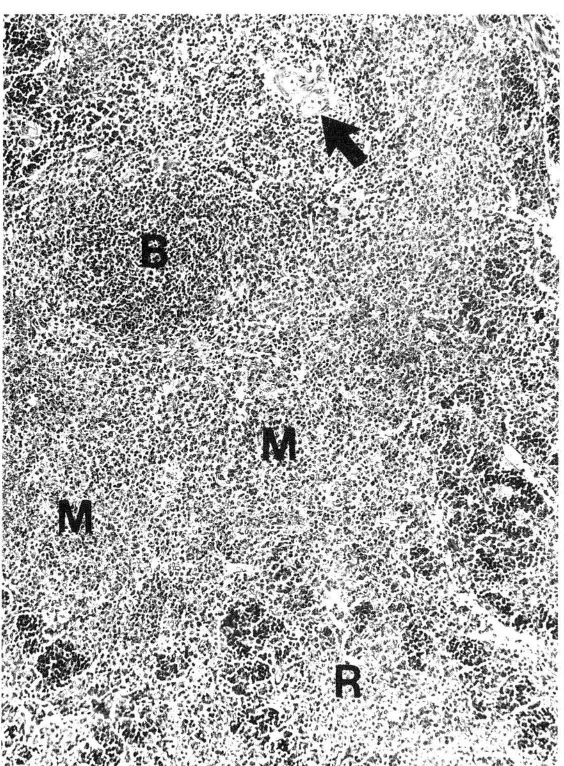

out obvious morphologic evidence of plasmacytosis. Sometimes, however, immunoperoxidase staining will reveal the presence of many immunoglobulin-containing cells in the B- or T-cell zones or marginal zone when plasmacytosis is not readily apparent in H and E sections. In aging mouse spleens, cellular white pulp areas may represent early follicular center cell lymphoma. This lesion is discussed beginning on p. 212, this volume. Rodents exposed to chronic conditions which induce splenic lymphoid and myeloid hyperplasia may develop spleens with more complex patterns of cellularity of the hyperplasia. Some of these lesions may be difficult to distinguish from early follicular center cell lymphoma.

Marginal Zone Hyperplasia

Prominent marginal zones are often seen in the spleens of aging rats. The apparently large marginal zones may occur because of the depletion of white pulp lymphocytes or from marginal zone hyperplasia (Fig. 242). In aging F344 rats, apparent marginal zone hyperplasia occurs from early infiltration or sequestration of large granular lymphocyte leukemic cells within the marginal zone meshwork (see p. 194, this volume). Marginal zones may also be altered in immune-deficient mice (Kraal et al. 1988).

References

Burke JS (1981 a) Surgical pathology of the spleen: an approach to the differential diagnosis of splenic lymphomas and leukemias. I. Diseases of the white pulp. Am J Surg Pathol 5: 551–563

Burke JS (1981 b) Surgical pathology of the spleen: an approach to the differential diagnosis of splenic lymphomas and leukemias. II. Diseases of the red pulp. Am J Surg Pathol 5: 681–694

Crichton DN, Busuttil A, Ross A (1980) An ultrastructural study of murine splenic lipofuscinosis. J Ultrastruct Res 72: 130–140

Dardick I, Sinnott NM, Hall R, Bajenko-Carr TA, Setterfield G (1983) Nuclear morphology and morphometry of B-lymphocyte transformation: implications for follicular center cell lymphomas. Am J Pathol 111: 35–49

deFazio A, Leary JA, Hedley DW, Tattersall MHN (1987) Immunohistochemical detection of proliferating cells in vivo. J Histochem Cytochem 35: 571–577

Goodman DG, Ward JM, Reichardt WD (1984) Splenic fibrosis and sarcomas in F344 rats fed diets containing aniline hydrochloride, *p*-chloroaniline, azobenzene, *o*-toluidine hydrochloride, 4,4′-sulfonyl-dianiline or D & C Red No. 9. JNCI 73: 265–273

Kraal G, Hoeben K, Janse M (1988) Splenic microenvironment of the CBA/N mouse: immunohistochemical analysis using monoclonal antibodies against lymphocytes and nonlymphoid cells. Am J Anat 182: 148–154

Long RE, Knutsen G, Robinson M (1986) Myeloid hyperplasia in the SENCAR mouse: differentiation from granulocytic leukemia. Environ Health Perspect 68: 117–123

McMaster PD, Franzl RE (1968) The primary immune response in mice. II. Cellular responses of lymphoid tissue accompanying the enhancement of complete suppression of antibody formation by a bacterial endotoxin. J Exp Med 127: 1109–1126

Mims CA, Gould J (1978) Splenic necrosis in mice infected with cytomegalovirus. J Infect Dis 137: 587–591

Ward JM, Reznik-Schuller HM (1980) Morphological and histochemical characteristics of pigments in aging F344 rats. Vet Pathol 17: 678–685

Pigment Deposition, Rat, Mouse

L. H. J. C. Danse and David N. Crichton

Synonyms. Splenic hemosiderosis; splenic lipofuscinosis; splenic ceroidosis; splenic melanosis.

Gross Appearance

Pigment deposition in the spleen leads, in most cases, to a diffuse light brown to dark brown discoloration. In splenic lipofuscinosis in C57BL mice (Crichton et al. 1978 a), the pigment distribution may vary from small foci surrounding the blood vessels at the hilus of the spleen to larger areas occupying most of the spleen and causing gross black discoloration of the organ (Fig. 243).

Microscopic Features

Hemosiderin is usually seen as intracellular golden-colored granules, 2 or 3 μm in diameter, which may become fused to form larger yellow-brown amorphous masses. The pigment is insoluble in water and most organic solvents but soluble in strong acid solutions. It occurs diffusely throughout the red pulp of the spleen, occasionally in tingible body macrophages of the white pulp (see p. 309, this volume), and in large dense, probably extracellular, clumps situated in periarteriolar lymphocyte sheaths.

Lipofuscin and ceroid should be regarded as synonymous with only their historical connotation retained (Porta and Hartroft 1969; Pearse 1985). The pigment is insoluble in fat solvents although it originates from cellular lipids and retains significant lipid characteristics during pigmentogen-

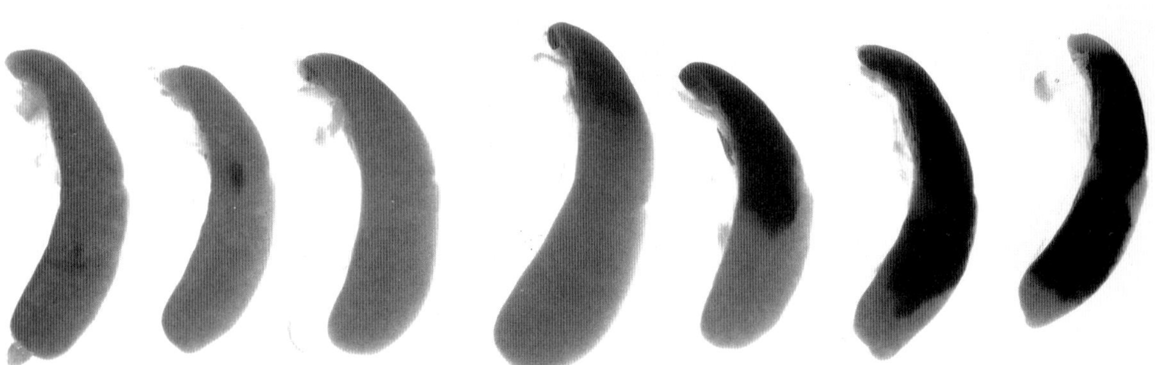

Fig. 243. Splenic lipofuscinosis, mouse. Spleens from C57BL/10 ScSn mice. Note the range of pigmentation from small focal deposits *(left)* to gross discoloration of most of the organ. Unfixed, ×2. (Reproduced from Crichton et al. 1978b)

esis. Lipofuscin is seen as an intracellular pigment varying in color from faint yellow globules to yellow brown or dark brown, more granular material. Occasionally, ceroid is colorless, causing only foaminess or vacuolation of spleen macrophages. In these cases, only special staining reactions can distinguish the pigment from intracellular fat vacuoles. Lipofuscin occurs in macrophages throughout the red pulp of the spleen in mice (Crichton et al. 1978 b) and rats. In vitamin E-deficient rats pigment also accumulates in activated macrophages of the marginal zone (Danse and Verschuren 1978).

Acid formalin pigment is a dark brown or black substance occurring in minute rhomboidal crystals and granules. It is an artifact in tissues rich in blood, when these are fixed in improperly buffered formalin at an acid pH, and is regarded as a haematin derivative (Pearse 1985).

Melanin deposition is observed in the spleens of black mice. This pigment is dark brown and is deposited in characteristic elongated strings (Frith et al. 1985). It is completely insoluble in most organic solvents or in any solution which is not markedly destructive towards the tissue preparations which contain it (Pearse 1985). Melanin has no special distribution pattern in the spleen, and it is not clear in which type of cell the pigment accumulates (Hill et al. 1977).

Ultrastructure

Hemosiderin in splenic macrophages and endothelial cells is seen as membrane-bound lysosomal structures, so-called siderosomes, of various shapes, mostly with a heterogeneous content of smaller particles (Fig. 244) (degraded ferritin). These ferritin particles may be dispersed or arranged in paracrystalline clusters (Iancu et al. 1987).

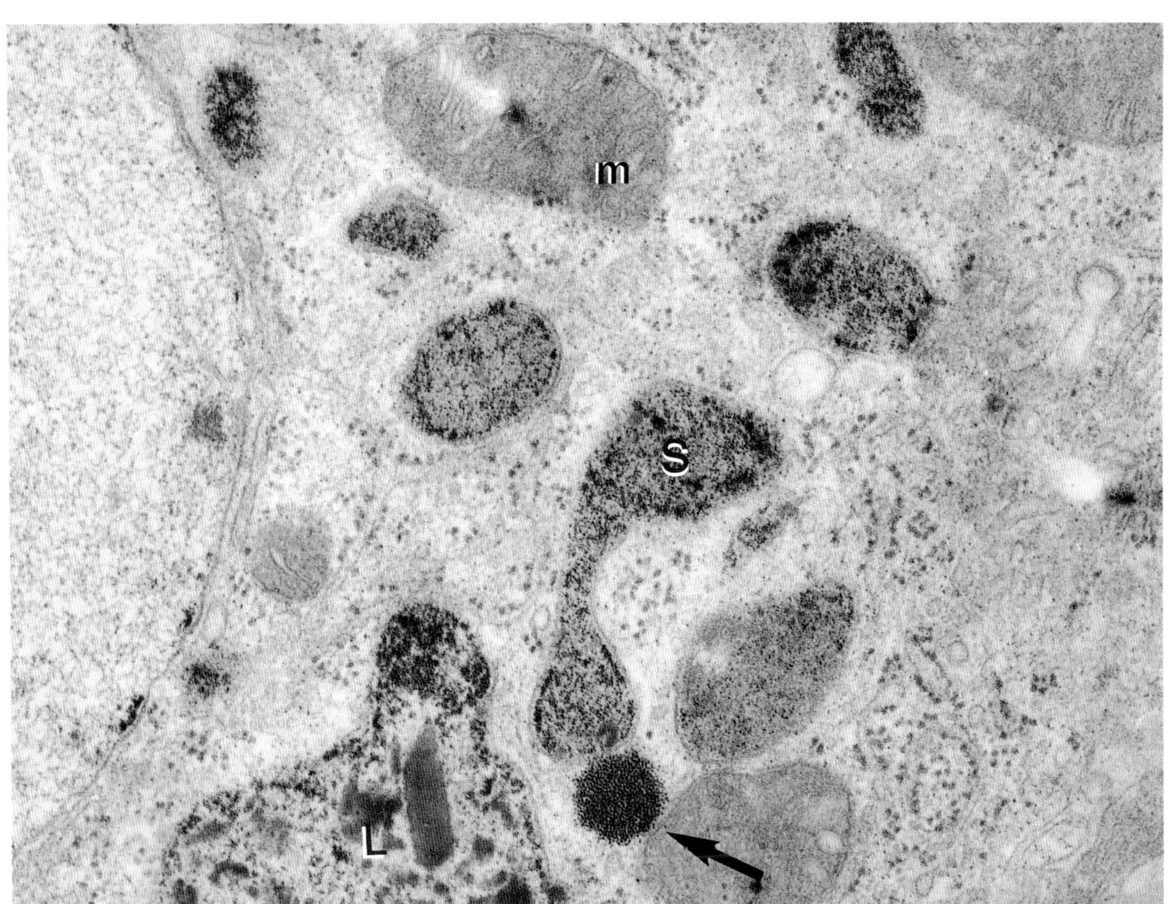

Fig. 244. Hemosiderosis, spleen, rat. Large amounts of electron-dense hemosiderin particles are seen within membrane-bound siderosomes *(S)* of various shapes; also a cluster of iron-rich particles in the cytosol *(arrow)*. *m*, mitochondrion; *L*, lipofuscin. TEM, × 44000

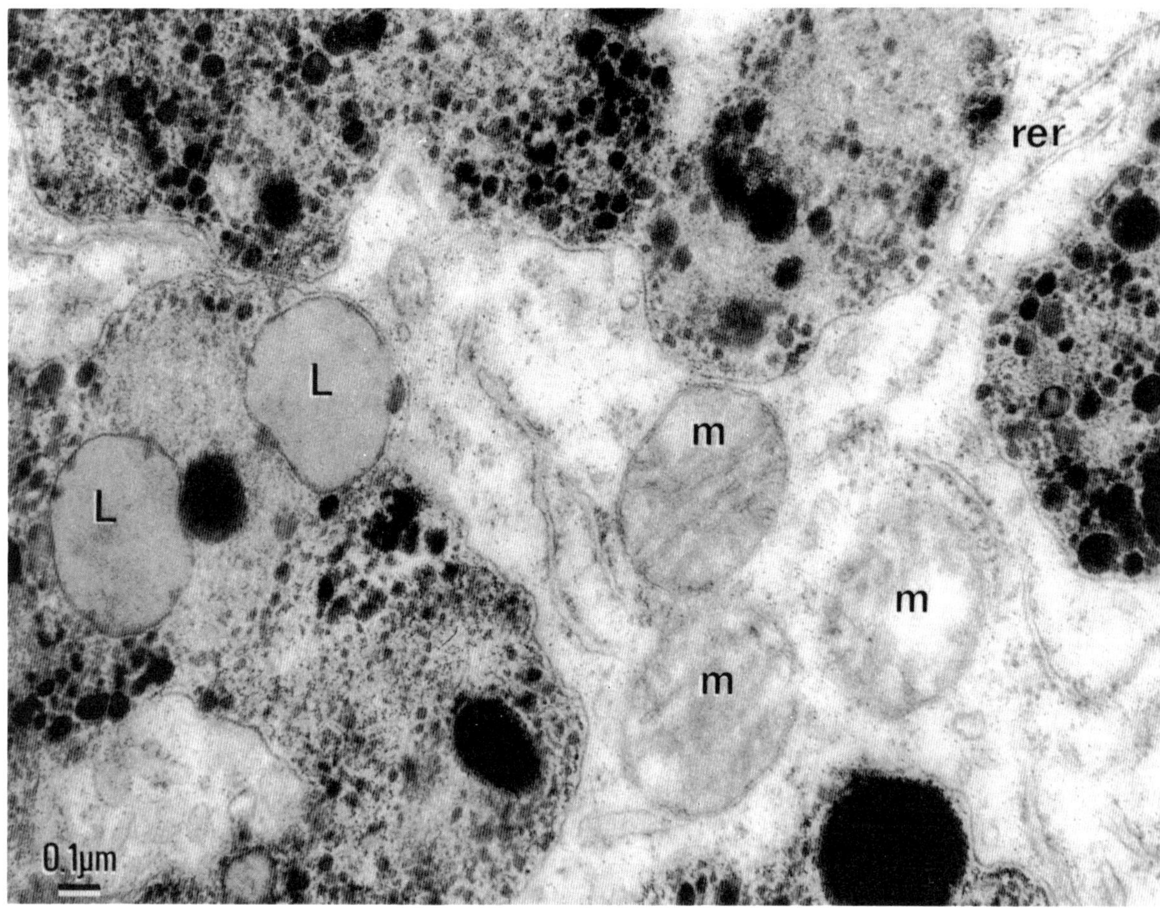

Fig. 245. Splenic lipofuscinosis, mouse. The composite arrangement of the pigment is shown. Lipid globules *(L)* are prominent within the pigment conglomerate which is composed of both electron-dense and electron-lucent material. *m*, mitochondria; *rer*, rough endoplasmic reticulum. TEM, × 44000. (Reproduced from Crichton et al. 1980)

Lipofuscin and ceroid are also derived from lysosomal structures as may be concluded from their single limiting membrane. The polymorphic internal configuration and the great variability in size are characteristic features of this pigment (Porta and Hartroft 1969). The complex internal structure of the pigment consists of droplets of modified lipid with variably sized, compact bodies of differing electron density (Fig. 245) and laminated bodies of variable shape often resembling fingerprints. Remnants of degenerated organelles and crystalloid structures are often found within the pigment conglomerate. These crystalloids are thought to be derived from red cell destruction (Crichton et al. 1980). Lipofuscin conglomerates are also called residual bodies, which refers to their content of undigested residues of lysosomal hydrolysis.

Melanin's ultrastructure in splenic cells has, to our knowledge, never been described. However, there is no reason to expect its morphology to be differ from that in other melanin-containing macrophages or melanocytes. In melanocytes, melanin is localized in melanosomes, small, membrane-limited vesicles with a very electron-dense content arranged in concentric sheets. In melanin-containing macrophages several of these melanosomes are grouped together within one lysosomal membrane (Breathnach 1969).

Differential Diagnosis

For the differentiation of pigments in paraplast sections of the spleen, in our experience, the staining techniques summarized in Table 42 are sufficient. Hemosiderin is positive with Perls' Prussian blue staining (Fig. 246). Lipofuscin and ceroid are acid-fast after Ziehl-Neelsen staining and have a bright yellow to orange autofluores-

Fig. 246 *(above).* Splenic hemosiderosis, rat. Animal sub- ▶
chronically exposed to β-hexachlorocyclohexane: note
strong Perls' positive hemosiderin deposition in the red
pulp *(R). W,* white pulp. Perls' Prussian blue staining,
×32

Fig. 247 *(below).* Splenic lipofuscinosis, rat. Animal with
vitamin E deficiency; note autofluorescent pigment in
macrophages of the red pulp *(R)* and white pulp *(W).*
M, marginal zone. Unstained section, ×80

Table 42. Staining reactions to differentiate splenic pigments in paraplast sections

Staining technique	Hemo-siderin	Lipofuscin (ceroid)	Melanin
Long Ziehl-Neelsen	−	+	−
Autofluorescence	−	+	−
Periodic acid-Schiff	−	+	−
Bleaching (KMnO₄)	−	+	+
Perls' Prussian blue	+	−	−
Schmorl's reaction	−	+	+

cence when unstained sections are studied with a
fluorescence microscope (Fig. 247) using an ex-
citing filter BG12 (wavelength 325–500 nm). This
autofluorescence is not changed after bleaching
the sections with $KMnO_4$, which enables the distinction of lipofuscin from melanin. Although
lipofuscin is also positive with the periodic acid-
Schiff reaction, this method, in general, is not
very discriminative, since it reacts with tissue mu-
copolysaccharides. Exceptionally, the lipofuscin
in murine splenic lipofuscinosis is not autofluorescent, but from the ultrastructural study of this
pigment its identity as lipofuscin may be assumed (Crichton et al. 1980). Melanin is
bleached after oxidation with $KMnO_4$. The
Schmorl's reaction, often proposed to detect melanin, is not specific since lipofuscins react positively also. Acid formalin pigment is negative in
all staining reactions listed in Table 42 and can
be recognized by its birefringence and fast
bleaching in 99% formic acid. For a more detailed account of the composition and genesis of
a great variety of organic pigments together with
extensive diagnostic schedules, we refer to the
excellent review of Pearse (1985).

A common problem in splenic pigmentation is
the simultaneous occurrence of several pigments
in the same spleen. For example, excessive erythrophagocytosis both hemosiderin and lipofuscin are generated from iron and membrane lipids
present in the cell debris. Moreover, iron is a

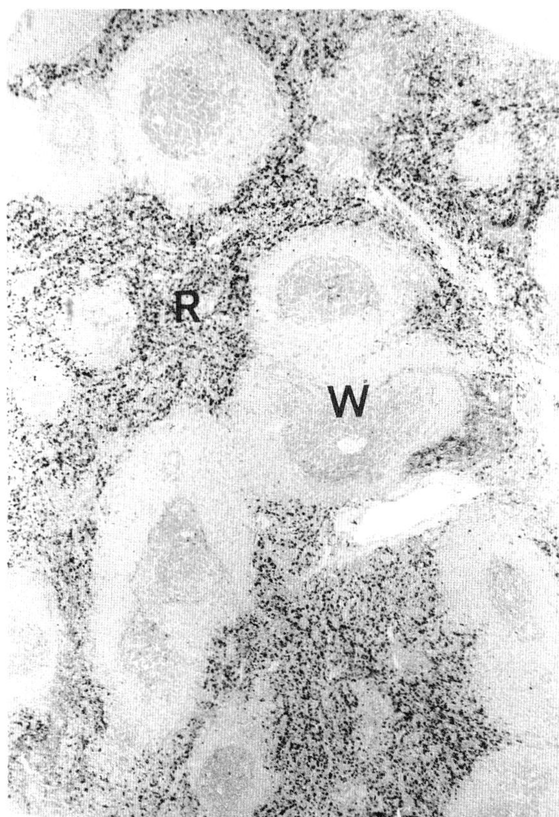

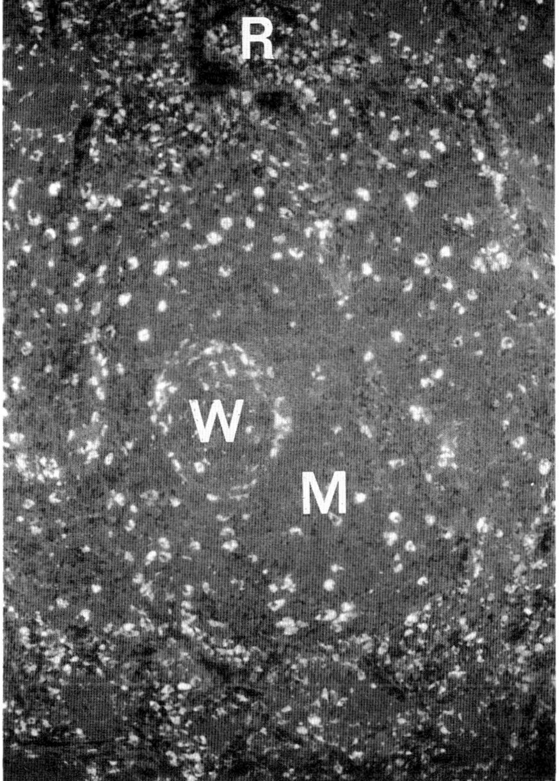

strong catalyst in lipid oxidation, which may result in the formation of lipofuscin. In these cases, careful cellular and tissue localization of the pigments and confirmation of their identity is necessary, since each pigment may indicate a specific pathogenesis.

Biological Features

Hemosiderin. Hemosiderin is a lysosomal, iron-containing, protein-polysaccharide complex (Pearse 1985), which is derived from digestion of ferritin molecules or other ferric hydroxide complexes. Ferritin is regarded as the major regular storage form of iron, while hemosiderin is considered as the storage of iron in excess. Hemosiderin accumulates in the spleens of rats and mice, following excessive erythrophagocytosis in toxic-induced (MacDonald 1969) or immune-mediated hemolytic anemia (Meryhew et al. 1984) and in iron overload resulting from nutritional iron imbalance or certain specific deficiencies such as vitamin A and zinc (Wixom et al. 1980). In nutritional iron overload in the rat, a 10-fold increase of splenic iron content was reached after 10 months loading (Iancu et al. 1987). After parenteral iron overload in rats the spleen underwent a 9-fold increase in iron content immediately after a loading period of 3 weeks, and a 20-fold increase of iron content was observed 2 months after this loading period. In the same period rats unloaded by daily phlebotomy had a spleen iron content down to control levels (Hultcrantz and Glaumann 1982), indicating that the reticuloendothelial system in the spleen is one of the primary compartments for utilization of iron during the induced synthesis of hemoglobin.

Although iron is known as a potent accelerator of lipid peroxidation and the formation of highly reactive radicals, and hemosiderin could provoke lysosomal fragility by increasing lipid peroxidation, it was found that under physiological conditions iron in the form of hemosiderin is far less active in promoting lipid peroxidation than is ferritin-bound iron (O'Connell et al. 1986). Therefore, it was concluded that hemosiderin formation in iron overload must be considered a cytoprotective mechanism.

Lipofuscin and Ceroid. Splenic lipofuscinosis is seen in aging rats and mice (Ward and Reznik-Schüller 1980), in vitamin E-deficient rats (Danse and Verschuren 1978) and mice (Csallany et al. 1977), and in mice of many C57BL sublines

(Crichton and Shire 1982). Lipofuscin is an indigestible lysosomal product of oxidized unsaturated fatty acids. These may be derived from membrane lipids, as in murine splenic lipofuscinosis. Here it is suggested that a lysosomal defect within the macrophage is the cause of decomposition of membrane lipids leading to lipofuscin accumulation (Crichton et al. 1980). On the other hand, in vitamin E-deficient rats, the lipofuscin storage in splenic macrophages has been reported to result from phagocytosis of blood-borne oxidized lipid species (Danse et al. 1979). As lipofuscin accumulation in macrophages is associated with impaired phagocytosis or overloading of the lysosomal compartment, it may have functional consequences. In this respect it is interesting that CXBH mice, a subline of C57BL with a high incidence of splenic lipofuscinosis, stand out as being highly susceptible to *Leishmania* infection, in which phagocytosis by macrophages and lysosomal fusion are essential in combatting the disease (Crichton and Shire 1982). However, in vitamin E-deficient rats with splenic lipofuscinosis, reticuloendothelial carbon clearance, phagocytosis, and digestion of *Listeria monocytogenes* in the spleen, and the immunological resistance to *L. monocytogenes* were not affected (Danse et al. 1979).

Melanin. Melanin is regarded as an oxidative derivative of tyrosine. The initial steps of oxidation to dihydroxyphenylalanine (DOPA) and dopaquinone are catalyzed by tyrosinase. The subsequent steps of oxidative polymerization and cyclization follow spontaneously. Splenic melanosis was reported to occur in black mice exclusively (Frith et al. 1985; Hill et al. 1977), and the pathogenesis of this pigmentation is not clear. However, there might be a relationship with murine splenic lipofuscinosis, since in cross-breeding experiments it appeared that this lipofuscinosis was prevented by a genetic deficiency of melanin (Crichton and Shire 1982). As there appears to be a close relationship between the production of both lipofuscin and melanin within lysosomes (Goldfischer et al. 1966), a lysosomal defect could be a logical explanation for the absence of both splenic lipofuscinosis and of melanin pigmentation. However, in another mutation of C57BL with reduced melanin pigmentation, melanosomes were severely affected, while lysosomes were normal, and a high incidence of splenic lipofuscinosis was observed (Ahmed and Shire 1985).

Comparison with Other Species

Reticuloendothelial cells of the spleen must be considered the usual overload sites for iron, and therefore hemosiderin in this organ is frequently seen in other laboratory animals, in domestic animals, e. g., in copper- and cobalt-dependent anemia (Jones and Hunt 1983), and in human hemochromatosis and some chronic anemias (MacDonald 1969; Wixom et al. 1980).

Splenic lipofuscinosis is also observed in many species such as the dog (Jones and Hunt 1983), pig, monkey (Danse et al. 1979), and mink (Danse and Steenbergen-Botterweg 1976), generally in aging or vitamin E-deficient animals. Vitamin E deficiency may often occur as a result of excessive feeding of highly unsaturated plant or fish oils. Since splenic lipofuscinosis appears at an early stage of vitamin E deficiency, its detection is important to monitor this aspect of nutritional status in individual animals or groups. In humans splenic lipofuscinosis is described as a typical morphological feature in disorders such as chronic granulomatous disease, Batten disease, and idiopathic thrombocytopenic purpura (Bianco 1983). Some of these conditions are contained in the so-called sea-blue histiocyte syndrome, referring to the lipofuscin-laden macrophages (Vacher-Lavenue et al. 1983). One of the hypotheses for the underlying pathogenetic mechanism is an inborn failure of macrophage digestion. Splenic lipofuscinosis in humans is also reported as a symptom of secondary vitamin E deficiency such as in fatal familial intrahepatic cholestasis (Byler disease) (Saito et al. 1982).

References

Ahmed F, Shire JGM (1985) Lysosomal mutations inhibit lipofuscinosis of the spleen in C57BL mice. J Hered 76: 311–312

Bianco P (1983) A histochemical study of lipoid pigment storage in chronic granulomatous disease (CGD). Basic Appl Histochem 27: 35–43

Breathnach AS (1969) Normal and abnormal melanin pigmentation of the skin. In: Wolman M (ed) Pigments in pathology. Academic, New York, pp 353–394

Crichton DN, Shire JGM (1982) Genetic basis of susceptibility to splenic lipofuscinosis in mice. Genet Res 39: 275–285

Crichton DN, Busuttil A, Price WH (1978 a) Splenic lipofuscinosis in mice. J Pathol 126: 113-120

Crichton DN, Busuttil A, Price WHL, Robertson J, Swinton J (1978 b) Lipofuscin deposition in the spleens of mice. J Inst Anim Tech 29: 31–36

Crichton DN, Busuttil A, Ross A (1980) An ultrastructural study of murine splenic lipofuscinosis. J Ultrastruct Res 72: 130-140

Csallany AS, Ayaz KL, Su LC (1977) Effect of dietary vitamin E and aging on tissue lipofuscin pigment concentration in mice. J Nutr 107: 1792–1799

Danse LHJC, Steenbergen-Botterweg WA (1976) Early changes of yellow fat disease in mink fed a vitamin-E deficient diet supplemented with fresh or oxidised fish oil. Zentralbl Veterinarmed [A] 23: 645–660

Danse LHJC, Verschuren PM (1978) Fish oil-induced yellow fat disease in rats. I. Histological changes. Vet Pathol 15: 114–124

Danse LHJC, Stolwijk J, Verschuren PM (1979) Fish oil-induced yellow fat disease in rats. IV. Functional studies of the reticuloendothelial system. Vet Pathol 16: 593–603

Frith CH, Pattengale DK, Ward JM (1985) A color atlas of hematopoietic pathology of mice. Toxicology Associates, Little Rock

Goldfischer S, Villaverde H, Forschirm R (1966) The demonstration of acid hydrolase, thermostable reduced diphosphopyridine nucleotide tetrazolium reductase and peroxidase activities in human lipofuscin pigment granules. J Histochem Cytochem 14: 641–652

Hill AC, Georgis H, Breaden J (1977) Pigment in the spleen of C57BL/10ScSn and related mice. Experientia 33: 954–955

Hultcrantz R, Glaumann H (1982) Studies on the rat liver following iron overload. Biochemical studies after iron mobilization. Lab Invest 46: 383–392

Iancu TC, Ward RJ, Peters TJ (1987) Ultrastructural observations in the carbonyl iron-fed rat, an animal model for hemochromatosis. Virchows Arch [B] 53: 208–217

Jones TC, Hunt RD (1983) Veterinary pathology. Lea and Febiger, Philadelphia

MacDonald RA (1969) Human and experimental hemochromatosis and hemosiderosis. In: Wolman M (ed) Pigments in pathology. Academic, New York, pp 115–149

Meryhew NL, Handwerger BS, Messner RP (1984) Monoclonal antibody-induced murine hemolytic anemia. J Lab Clin Med 104: 591–601

O'Connell M, Halliwell B, Moorhouse CP, Aruoma OI, Baum H, Peters TJ (1986) Formation of hydroxyl radicals in the presence of ferritin and hemosiderin. Is hemosiderin formation a biological protective mechanism? Biochem J 234: 727–731

Pearse AGE (1985) Histochemistry, theoretical and applied, vol 2. 4th edn. Churchill Livingstone, Edinburgh

Porta EA, Hartroft WS (1969) Lipid pigments in relation to aging and dietary factors (lipofuscins). In: Wolman M (ed) Pigments in pathology. Academic, New York, pp 192–235

Saito K, Matsumoto S, Yokoyama T, Okaniwa M, Kamoshita S (1982) Pathology of chronic vitamin E deficiency in fatal familial intrahepatic cholestasis (Byler disease). Virchows Arch [A] 396: 319–330

Vacher-Lavenu MC, Baron-Selme V, Abelanet R, Boissonnas A, Laroche C (1983) Le syndrome des histiocytes bleus. Revue de la literature à propos d'une observation de splenomegalie idiopathique chez l'adulte. Arch Anat Cytol Pathol 31: 342–350

Ward JM, Reznik-Schuller H (1980) Morphological and histochemical characteristics of pigments in aging F344 rats. Vet Pathol 17: 678–685

Wixom RL, Prutkin L, Munro HN (1980) Hemosiderin: nature, formation and significance. In: Richter GW, Epstein MA (eds) International review of experimental pathology, vol 22. Academic, New York, pp 193–225

Extramedullary Hemopoiesis, Spleen, Rat

Larry G. Lomax, David G. Keyes, and Richard J. Kociba

Synonyms. Extramedullary hemopoiesis myeloid metaplasia.

Gross Appearance

The normal spleen is usually a tongue-shaped organ with well-defined edges. When extramedullary hemopoiesis is present, the spleen is enlarged two or more times, but still in its normal anatomic position, and darker than normal. The splenic margins are rounded, and the surface is smooth and regular. Seen from the cut surface, the firm red pulp is prominent in comparison with the inconspicuous white pulp (Fig. 248).

Microscopic Features

The red pulp reticular meshwork of splenic cords and the venous sinuses which anastomose within the meshwork are filled with hemopoietic cells. These cells have the morphologic characteristics of immature myelocytic, erythrocytic, and megakaryocytic cells (Fig. 249). The hemopoiesis occurs within the splenic cords (Weiss 1977). The amount of white pulp present is variable; however, periarterial lymphatic sheaths and lymphatic nodules containing germinal centers are usually recognizable. MZs lying between the white and red pulp are also usually demonstrable, although distended red pulp venous sinuses contiguous to the red pulp may appear within the zone.

Ultrastructure

Electron microscopic examination is not routinely required for diagnosis. However, it is useful to differentiate splenic extramedullary hemopoiesis from early stages of large granular lymphocyte leukemia in Fischer 344 rats or other leukemic conditions. Ultrastructural examination of spleens with extramedullary hemopoiesis reveals erythrocytic, myelocytic, or megakaryocytic cells in various stages of maturation within the splenic cords.

Differential Diagnosis

Splenic extramedullary hemopoiesis in the rat should be distinguished from other conditions which result in enlargement of the organ, including leukemia/lymphoma, acute congestion, and chronic passive congestion. Leukemia/lymphoma, especially the large granular lymphocyte leukemia of Fischer 344 rats is often associated with massive splenic enlargement (see p. 194, this volume) (Ward and Reynolds 1982). Microscopic examination of tissues from affected Fischer rats reveals leukemic cells in a variety of organs but primarily in the spleen, liver, and lungs.

Acute splenic congestion due to blood stasis, which fills venous sinuses with erythrocytes, also results in enlargement of the spleen. This is a nonspecific condition that commonly occurs as an agonal event following acute overdosage with a variety of materials such as barbiturate anes-

Fig. 248 *(above).* Cut surface of *(A)* spleen from unaffect-▶ ed aged Sprague-Dawley rat and *(B)* spleen from aged Sprague-Dawley rat with extramedullary hemopoiesis. The spleen is enlarged to twice its usual size and has rounded edges; the red pulp is diffusely dark while the white pulp is inconspicuous. H and E, ×6

Fig. 249 *(below).* Spleen, aged Sprague-Dawley rat with extramedullary hemopoiesis. Splenic cords and venous sinuses are distended with erythrocytic *(e)*, myelocytic *(m)*, and megakaryocytic *(mk)* cells. A trabecula *(t)* is located at the *top*. H and E, ×560

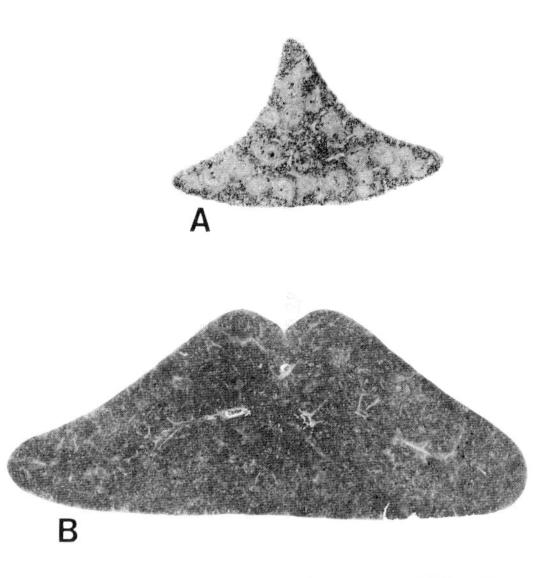

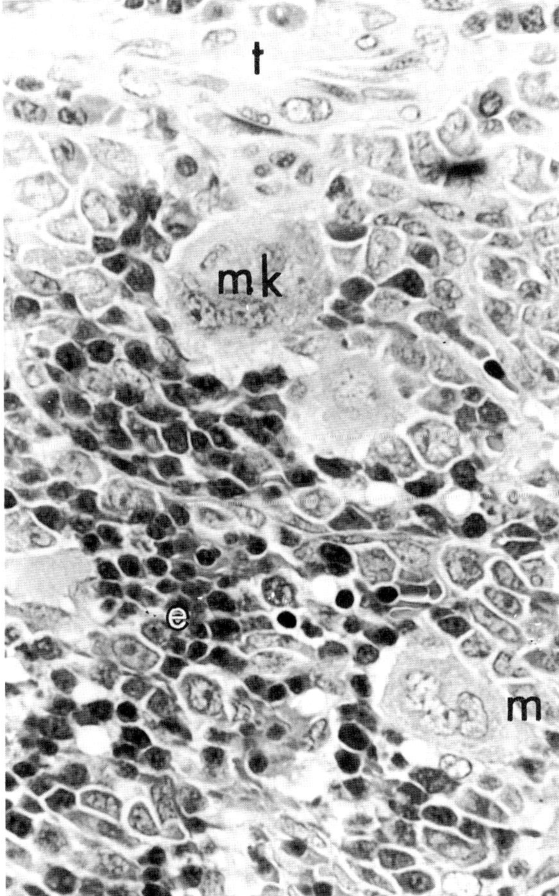

thetics. The spleen is slightly enlarged and soft. Other organs, most noticeably the liver and kidneys, are also congested due presumably to generalized circulatory stasis. Chronic passive congestive changes in the rat spleen occur infrequently and are usually caused by localized increased venous pressure of long-standing duration such as could occur with splenic venous thrombosis, periarteritis, or hepatic cirrhosis. Microscopic characteristics include distention of the red pulp venous sinuses with blood, endothelial hyperplasia, and fibrosis of the splenic cords (Jones and Hunt 1983).

Biologic Features

Splenic extramedullary hemopoiesis is the presence in the spleen of cells normally found in the bone marrow. The spleen of the rat functions as an additional hemopoietic organ during stress periods in otherwise normal animals (Loeb et al. 1978). Occasional foci of extramedullary hemopoiesis are common in young and old rats without any detectable intercurrent disease. We have not attempted to ascertain whether or not subtle stressors can influence the magnitude of this response. In addition, "clearly detectable" extramedullary hemopoiesis in rats by subjective light microscopic evaluation is a secondary phenomenon typically associated with red blood cell destruction or chronic blood loss caused by a primary condition. We are unaware of documented primary polycythemia in the rat. The distinction between low level background extramedullary hemopoiesis (to which no diagnosis of extramedullary hemopoiesis is applied) and clearly detectable changes may be somewhat arbitrary but usually is not difficult for experienced rodent pathologists, especially after consideration of other clinicopathologic findings. Furthermore, the background level of extramedullary hemopoiesis in control animals may vary slightly from study to study.

Young rats (typically 2–5 months of age) used in short-term or subchronic toxicity studies routinely have minimal extramedullary hemopoiesis naturally in the spleen without splenic enlargement or bone marrow alteration. However, increased spleen size and extramedullary hemopoiesis resulting from chemically induced hemolytic anemia has been reported (Grant et al. 1985; O'Donoghue 1986). Under these circumstances, the splenic change was a secondary manifestation of regenerative anemia.

Aging rats in long-term studies occasionally have splenic enlargement and hemopoiesis secondary to neoplastic or chronic inflammatory conditions. Animals with these conditions also usually have anemia, leukocytosis, and thrombocytosis. The anemia is characterized by decreases in red blood cell count, hemoglobin concentration, and HCT, often with accompanying reticulocytosis and polychromasia. Microscopic examination of bone marrow reveals normal or hypercellular marrow. Proliferation of white pulp lymphoid tissue may also be observed with chronic systemic inflammatory conditions in which antigenic stimulation has occurred.

Incidence

Review of control data from selected 2-year studies conducted in our laboratory using Fischer 344 rats indicated a mean incidence for splenic extramedullary hemopoiesis of 14% (55/396) in males and 16% (63/396) in females. Mesotheliomas of the abdominal cavity and ulcerated subcutaneous tumors presumably resulting in protracted intra-abdominal hemorrhage or chronic blood loss, respectively, were the most common primary conditions responsible for splenic hemopoiesis in males. In female rats a splenic lesion occurred most commonly in association with hemorrhagic intra-abdominal tumors (i. e., uterine, ovarian, and renal). Chronic gastric ulceration with intragastric hemorrhage was also an infrequent cause in both males and females. Examination of available hematologic data usually indicates normocytic normochromic anemia with polychromasia and reticulocytosis accompanied by leukocytosis and thrombocytosis. However, microcytosis and hypochromia may develop and, although unconfirmed, may indicate depletion of body stores of iron. Microscopically, the bone marrow is typically normal or hypercellular.

Aged Sprague-Dawley rats have a higher incidence of splenic extramedullary hemopoiesis than Fischer 344 rats. The mean incidence in our laboratory for control males is 32% (157/492) and 63% (314/495) for females. The high incidence in females generally parallels the high number of female rats bearing mammary tumors, many of which were ulcerated and hemorrhagic. Other associated factors in both male and females include chronic renal disease with secondary hyperparathyroidism and fibrous osteodystrophy, intra-abdominal and subcutaneous neoplasms, and chronic gastric ulceration with hemorrhage. Evaluation of pertinent hematology data indicates that affected animals often have anemia and leukocytosis.

Comparison with Other Species

The spleen of the normal adult mouse varies considerably in size and continues at all ages to play an important role in normal hemopoiesis and lymphogenesis (Hardy 1967). Most hemopoietic foci are located in the subcapsular region and adjacent to trabeculae. Erythrocytes, granulocytes, and megakaryocytes are within these foci, and dramatic increases in cell numbers can be observed following an appropriate stimulus. Extramedullary hemopoiesis of the spleen occurs in laboratory animals, domestic animals (Jubb et al. 1985), and humans. The condition occurs as a secondary process, in response to the bone marrow's inability to keep pace with production demands, in some myeloproliferative disorders, or coincident with splenic red blood cell destruction. New Zealand White rabbits orally administered a hemolytic agent develop regenerative anemia and, secondarily, splenomegaly with extramedullary hemopoiesis (Breslin et al. 1987). In humans, the manifestation is more common in the spleen than in any other organ (Richter 1966) but occurs only under pathologic conditions. A prominent example of this situation in humans is polycythemia vera, a myeloproliferative disorder characterized by erythrocytosis, leukocytosis, thrombocytosis, and splenomegaly (Glass and Wasserman 1977). In utero, the human spleen functions as a hemopoietic organ until the 5th month of gestation after which time it does not appear to provide an adequate hemopoietic microenvironment (Crosby 1977). Hemopoiesis may occur in the spleen of the dog and cat under abnormal conditions such as hemolytic anemias, myelophthisis disorders, and myeloproliferative disease of cats (Chapman 1975).

Acknowledgements. The photographic assistance of D. M. Williams and the time allowed by the Dow Chemical Co. to prepare this manuscript are greatly appreciated.

References

Breslin WJ, Phillips JE, Lomax LG, Calhoun LL, Dittenber DA, Bartels MJ, Miller RR (1987) Ethylene glycol phenyl ether (EGPE): toxicological effects in rabbits and rats. Toxicologist 7: 246

Chapman WL Jr (1975) Diseases of the lymph nodes and spleen. In: Ettinger SJ (ed) Textbook of veterinary internal medicine. Saunders, Philadelphia, pp 1664–1678

Crosby WH (1977) Structure and functions of the spleen. In: Williams WJ, Beutler E, Erslev AJ, Rundles RW (eds) Hematology. McGraw-Hill, New York, pp 74–81

Glass JL, Wasserman LR (1977) Erythrocyte disorders-polycythemia. In: Williams WJ, Beutler E, Erslev AJ, Rundles RW (eds) Hematology. McGraw-Hill, New York, pp 624–641

Grant D, Sulsh S, Jones HB, Gangolli SD, Butler WH (1985) Acute toxicity and recovery in the hemopoietic system of rats after treatment with ethylene glycol monomethyl and monobutyl ethers. Toxicol Appl Pharmacol 77: 187–200

Hardy J (1967) Haematology of rats and mice. In: Cotchin E, Roe JC (eds) Pathology of laboratory rats and mice. Blackwell Scientific, Oxford, pp 501–536

Jones TC, Hunt RD (1983) Veterinary pathology. Lea and Febiger, Philadelphia, pp 1338–1343

Jubb KVF, Kennedy PC, Palmer N (1985) Pathology of domestic animals, vol 2, 3rd edn. Academic, Orlando, pp 84–216

Loeb WF, Bannerman RM, Rininger BF, Johnson AJ (1978) Haematologic disorders. In: Benirschke K, Garner FM, Jones TC (eds) Pathology of laboratory animals, vol 1. Springer, Berlin Heidelberg New York, pp 889–1050

O'Donoghue JL (1986) Subchronic oral toxicology of 4-chloro-3-nitroaniline in the rat. Fundam Appl Toxicol 6: 551–558

Richter MN (1966) Spleen, lymph nodes and reticulo-endothelial system. In: Anderson WAD (ed) Pathology. Mosby, St Louis, pp 1009–1043

Ward JM, Reynolds CW (1982) Large granular lymphocyte leukemia: a heterogenous lymphocytic leukemia in Fischer 344 rats. Am J Pathol 111: 1–10

Weiss L (1977) The spleen. In: Weiss L, Greep RO (eds) Histology, 4th edn. McGraw-Hill, New York, pp 510–567

Amyloidosis, Spleen, Mouse

Bernard Sass

Gross Appearance

Affected spleens are sometimes enlarged. Grayish, rubbery, glassy masses are found throughout the splenic pulp.

Microscopic Appearance

Histologically, amyloid is a homogeneous, amorphous, slightly acidophilic, hyaline substance (Fig. 250). Sections of spleen containing amyloid are colored pink to red with the Congo Red coloring method, using transmitted light. Using crossed Nichol prisms, spleen sections containing amyloid exhibit red-green birefringence. The earliest lesions appear as patches of extracellular amyloid located in the red pulp in close proximity to the periphery of the follicles; more advanced lesions consist of deposits surrounding the follicles, while in extreme cases the red pulp is entirely replaced by amyloid (Figs. 251, 252). In extreme cases, the follicles are compressed (Figs. 253, 254). In such cases, fragments of red cells and hemosiderin are often present.

The spleens of affected strain A/SN mice, aged 11–17 months, contain perifollicular deposits and occasional isolated foci in the red pulp (West and Murphy 1965). Dunn (1967) found perifollicular areas of amyloid in an old, wild mouse and in the red pulp of another mouse. Chai (1976) demonstrated perifollicular deposition in mice of the low leukocyte count (LLC) strain. Schultz and Pitha (1985) studied the role of microcirculation in the development of casein-induced splenic amyloidosis in male CBA/J mice. Evans Blue dye and bovine serum albumin were injected into the thoracic aorta to demonstrate vascular changes. Autoradiography was performed in conjunction with H and E and Congo Red staining. The earliest lesions were found in the marginal zones immediately adjacent to the follicles and then spread to involve the entire marginal zone, followed by extension into the red pulp. Demonstrable by autoradiography was an absence of small vessels in areas affected by deposition of amyloid. This was interpreted by the authors as evidence of capillary injury.

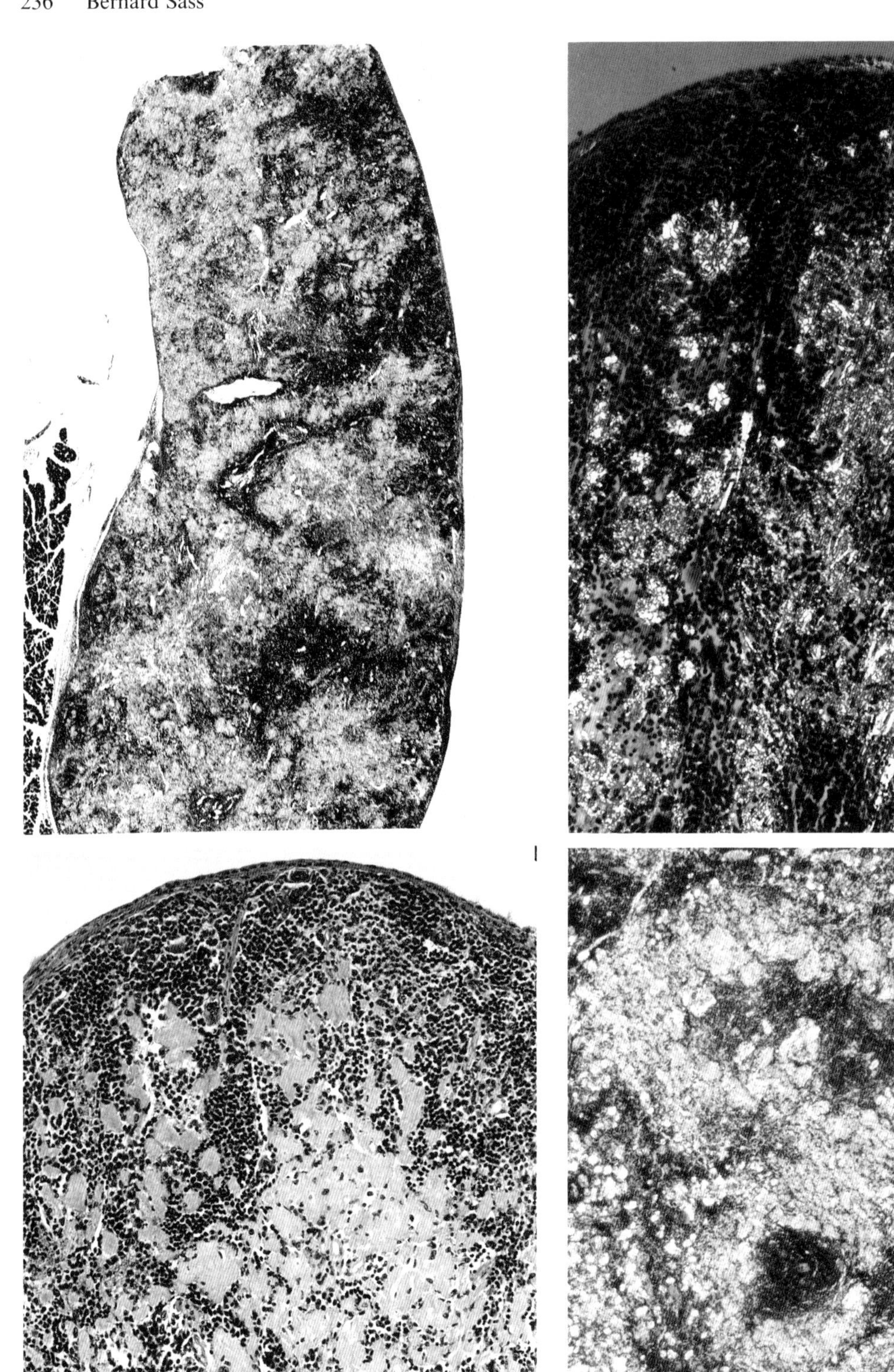

◄**Fig. 250** *(upper left).* Amyloidosis, spleen, mouse. Most of the normal architecture is replaced by amorphous, acidophilic, pale-staining hyaline material. H and E, ×20

Fig. 251 *(lower left).* Amyloidosis, spleen, mouse. The pulp is largely replaced by amyloid which occupies large confluent areas *(center)* and multiple small focal areas *(right* and *left).* H and E, ×130

Fig. 252 *(upper right).* Same spleen as in Fig. 251, sectioned at a slightly different level to demonstrate the birefringence of amyloid. Congo Red coloring method, crossed Nichol prisms, ×130

Fig. 253 *(lower right).* Amyloidosis, spleen of another mouse. Follicles *(upper center* and *center)* are compressed by surrounding amyloid material. Congo Red coloring method, crossed Nichol prisms, ×65

Fig. 254 *(above).* Spleen, higher magnification of follicle ► at center of Fig. 253 demonstrating birefringence of amyloid. Congo Red coloring method, crossed Nichol prisms, ×250

Fig. 255 *(below).* Amyloid fibrils and filaments, red pulp, mouse, spleen. Arrangement is random, but in one area *(upper left, center)* the fibrils are parallel. Uranyl acetate and lead citrate, TEM, ×34000. (Courtesy of C. K. Chai, C. Lerner, and S. Taylor, Jackson Memorial Laboratory, Bar Harbor, Maine)

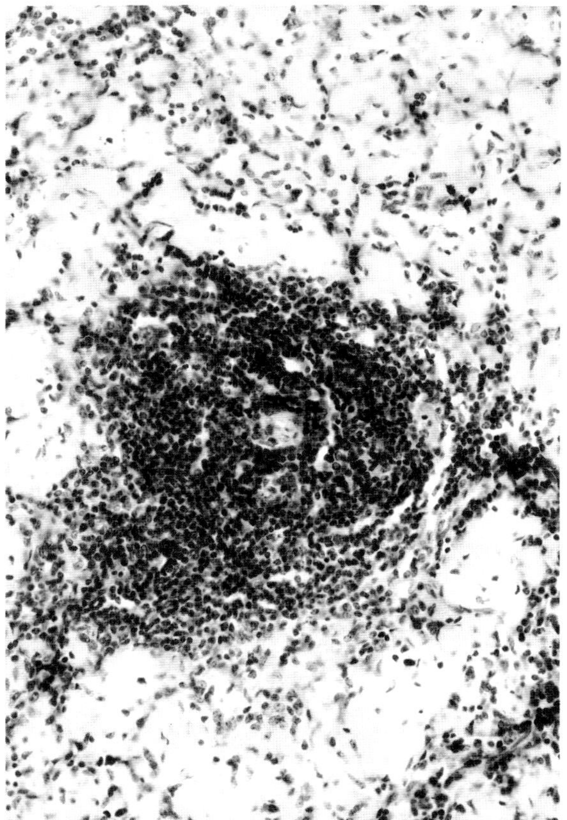

Ultrastructure

Amyloid is a collection of threadlike, unbranched, straight or slightly bent, 10-nm diameter fibrils; they may measure up to 40 nm in diameter and are then referred to as filaments. In addition to the slender, nonbranching fibrils, there is a minor component, known as the P component (see also under Natural History), which is pentagonal and doughnut-shaped and has an external diameter of 9 nm. The fibrils and filaments are often randomly arranged, resulting in a meshwork appearance (Fig. 255), but near cell borders parallel alignment is also evident (Ghadially 1982). There are two difficulties in the ultrastructural localization and identification of intracellular amyloid: the first is related to sectioning geometry which may produce the appearance of amyloid; the second involves intermediate filaments, which are of the same size as amyloid fibrils and have been at times mistaken for amyloid fibrils synthesized within the cell and discharged into the extracellular matrix (Ghadially 1982).

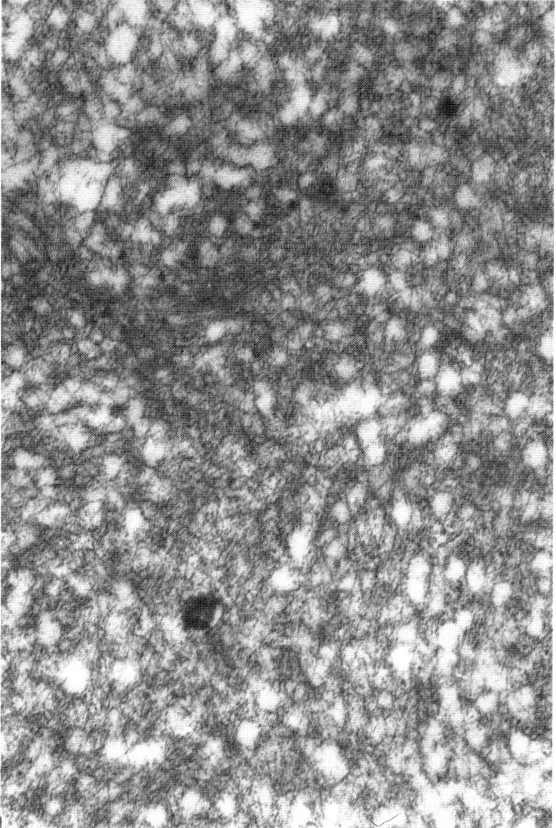

Differential Diagnosis

Amyloid must be differentiated from other hyalins which can be found in the spleen. Hyalins, including amyloid, are intracellular and extracellular substances that are translucent, homogeneous, and structureless and are colored by eosin (Robbins et al. 1984). Extracellular hyalins found in the spleens of mice include connective tissue hyalin, fibrinoid, and amyloid. Special stains such as phosphotungstic acid hemotoxylin and Masson trichrome may be used to differentiate connective tissue hyalin and fibrinoid from amyloid.

Biologic Features

Chai and Lerner (1984) demonstrated the deposition of amyloid in the cytoplasm of reticular cells of the red pulp, followed by the extracellular formation and accumulation of amyloid in LLC mice, using protein A-gold staining. In the later stages of deposition, amyloid was found in the extracellular matrix. The authors postulated that amyloid protein, as with other proteins destined for transport, is sequestered in the cisternae of the rough endoplasmic reticulum, carried by the vesicles to the Golgi complex, and then discharged by the fusion of the secretory vesicles with the plasma membrane. They also postulate that some of the amyloid protein or its precursor is then unable to be transported away and stays close to the cell border.

Natural History

The major precursor in most types of amyloidosis is the protein serum amyloid A (SAA), an α-globulin which is produced by the liver in chronic inflammation and in ageing and has a molecular weight of 12500. In serum, amyloid A is associated with a high-density lipoprotein (Robbins et al. 1984). Amyloid is found in tissues in a β-pleated sheet arrangement in which it assumes a fibrillar form, termed protein AA, which has a molecular weight of 8000 (Glenner 1980b; Kisilevsky 1983; Cohen et al. 1983). Studies in various species on the amino acid homology of protein AA demonstrated that amino residues 35–45 are identical in human and animal protein AA (Kisilevsky 1983; Westermark et al. 1985). Serum amyloid A, when denatured, releases a 12000–14000 molecular weight subunit designated SAAL. This subunit is polymorphic in mice and contains all of the immunologic cross-reactivity that exists between SAA and the AA proteins. The pathogenesis of amyloid fibril deposition is not completely elucidated (some of the postulated key events are depicted in Fig. 256). However, based upon studies in humans, there are three classes of plasma proteins from which fibrils may be formed, namely immunoglobulin, serum amyloid A, and prealbumin (Glenner 1980a). The immunoglobulin-derived amyloid is now known as the AL (amyloid light chain) type. Only the AA (SAA) type is important in mice, and it can be induced experimentally (Kisilevsky 1983; Husebekk et al. 1985). Enzymatic cleavage of circulating SAA gives rise to repetitive amyloid protein segments. Several mechanisms for the deposition of amyloid fibrils have been proposed:

1. In vitro proteolytic cleavage of some but not all Bence Jones proteins gives rise to amyloid fibrils; this is possible because of the primary structure of such proteins. Such a mechanism could operate in strain SJL/J (Scheinberg et al. 1976).
2. A second mechanism in fibrillogenesis and amyloidosis is defective enzymatic processing of plasma proteins. This mechanism is postulated on the basis that incubation of SAA with peripheral blood monocytes from human patients with amyloidosis yielded an intermediate product having amino acid sequence identity with protein AA. Monocytes from healthy individuals completely degraded SAA (Westermark et al. 1985).

Recently, Fuks and Zucker-Franklin (1985) demonstrated faulty in vitro processing of serum amyloid A by the Kupffer's cells of male C57BL/6J mice, which received from 8 to more than 30 0.5-cc injections of 10% casein. The cultures of Kupffer's cells from animals with amyloidosis contained both residual SAA and an intermediate product indistinguishable from AA. This AA product was also found in Kupffer's cell cultures prepared from animals which received only a few injections of casein and did not have amyloid deposition as determined by Congo Red stains and electron microscopy. Complete degradation of AA intermediate product occurred when Kupffer's cells from normal animals were added. Thus, the appearance of the AA peptide may be due to the inability of macrophage-type cells to degrade SAA to completion. In the CBA/J mouse (Axelrad et al. 1975), in which

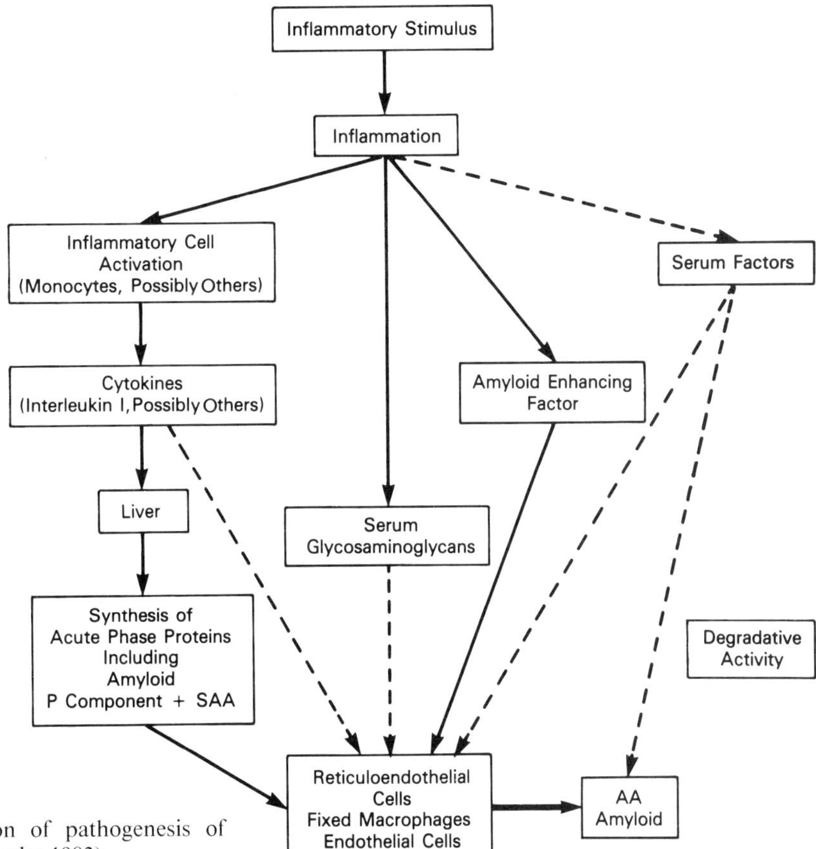

Fig. 256. Schematic representation of pathogenesis of amyloidosis. (Adapted from Kisilevsky 1983)

amyloid is rapidly deposited following an inflammatory stimulus, a protein termed amyloid enhancing factor appears within a few days and shortens the time for experimental induction of AA and precedes the formation of fibrils. Amyloid enhancing factor is a naturally occurring tissue component produced in the liver and spleen, but the exact cell of origin is not known. When CBA mice are treated with extracts of human spleens containing amyloid enhancing factor or AA and AL in addition to subcutaneous injections of casein, amyloidosis is induced in an accelerated fashion (Varga et al. 1986). The AA protein deposited in the mice is believed to be of murine origin, and the enhanced deposition is due to amyloid enhancing factor.

Glycosaminogylcans (GAGs) are carbohydrate moieties in tissue amyloid which give alcian blue positivity to amyloid deposits in tissues. Although amyloid fibrils can influence the rate of hyaluronic acid synthesis by cultured fibroblasts, this event has not been substantiated in vivo. Levels of GAG in the serum increase during inflammation and might influence the clearance and degradation of serum amyloid A. The exact function of GAGs is not known (Snow and Kisilevsky 1985).

Serum amyloid P component constitutes 10% of deposited amyloid, is a glycoprotein with a pentagonal ringlike structure composed of a protein subunit, and has a molecular weight of 25000 (Pepys et al. 1982). It is synthesized by the liver, has homology with c-reactive protein, and is an acute phase reactant to inflammation in humans. Other factors must be required for amyloid to be deposited, since interleukin I was shown to increase serum amyloid A levels in the serum experimentally, but tissue amyloid deposition did not increase (Kisilevsky 1983; Shirahama et al. 1985).

Macrophages or monocytes, when stimulated by an inflammatory reaction, release interleukin I (an inducer of acute phase protein synthesis), which causes the liver to synthesize serum amyloid A (Sztein et al. 1981). Using an in vitro macrophage model and the drug colchicine, an inhibitor of the acute SAA response to inflammatory stimulation, interleukin-1 production was induced (Brandwein et al. 1984). The authors interpreted these findings to mean that colchicine does not act to inhibit amyloidosis at the early acute phase serum amyloid A response.

Although production of the AA protein and fibrillogenesis are cellular functions, the exact sequence of events leading to the deposition of amyloid in tissues is not clear (Kisilevsky 1983) (Fig. 256). Several authors (Shirahama and Cohen 1975; Chai 1976; Chai and Lerner 1984) observed what they believed to be the initial appearance of amyloid in splenic macrophages. Since AA protein is not found in the circulating blood, it is postulated that the cells involved in its production are fixed macrophages or other fixed cells of the reticuloendothelial system.

Etiology

The exact cause of amyloidosis is unknown. Among the common triggering agents is chronic infestation with the mite *Myobia musculi* (Dunn 1967). Genetics plays an important role in the etiology of spontaneously occurring amyloidosis (Heston and Deringer 1948; Thung 1957 a). The strains 020, DBAf, C57BL, and the hybrids (020 × DBA)F1 and (C57BL × DBA)F1 develop fatal amyloidosis in old age (Thung 1957 b). Strain A similarly develops amyloidosis in old age (Heston and Deringer 1948). Wild house mice, when inbred, developed amyloidosis, although prior to inbreeding they rarely had the condition (Dunn and Andervont 1963).

The low leukocyte mouse strain (Chai 1976; Chai and Lerner 1984) and SJL/J mouse (Scheinberg et al. 1976) develop reticulum cell hyperplasia which may be related to the etiology of amyloidosis. Strain SJL/J mice develop hypergammaglobulinemia, B-cell dyscrasias, and reticulum cell tumors, all of which could be related to amyloidosis and are a model for similar diseases in humans associated with amyloidosis (Scheinberg et al. 1976).

Frequency

The frequency of spontaneous and induced amyloidosis of the spleen is shown in Tables 43 and 44. In strain C57BL, the spleen is often not the most frequent site of deposition of amyloid (Zurcher et al. 1982). In strain A/Sn, a high incidence amyloid strain, the spleen becomes involved beginning at 13 months of age, up to and including 17 months of age (West and Murphy 1965). Neither Zurcher et al. or West and Mur-

phy give actual frequencies for the incidence of splenic amyloidosis.

Splenic amyloidosis is used to monitor induction of the effects of various chemicals. The most common agents for induction are casein, azocasein, and silver nitrate (Table 44). Normal syngeneic spleen cells and amyloidotic spleen cells when administered to strain CBA mice pretreated with casein hastened the onset of amyloidosis (Axelrad et al. 1975). Recently, Varga et al. (1986) used amyloidotic human spleen cells and homogenates of amyloidotic human spleen cells containing amyloid enhancing factor to accelerate the onset of amyloidosis in strain CBA mice.

Comparison with Other Species

In humans, splenic amyloid deposition occurs not only in ageing and in chronic inflammation, but also with multiple myeloma, Alzheimer's disease (Glenner 1988), lymphoma, and some endocrine tumors. Amyloidosis occurring with myeloma, lymphoma, and certain endocrine tumors is known as the primary type and is characterized by deposition of protein AL; amyloidosis occurring with chronic inflammation and ageing is known as the secondary type and is characterized by the deposition of protein AA (Westermark et al. 1985).

McClure (1984) reviewed the literature on the occurrence of amyloidosis in monkeys. The following species are affected: baboons, pigtail macaques, squirrel, rhesus, vervet, and celebes monkeys. Concurrent diseases include granulomatous enteritis, chronic arthritis, and acquired immunodeficiency disease. Serum amyloid A protein was isolated from a single vervet monkey with amyloidosis (McClure 1984). Blanchard et al. (1986) examined 57 rhesus monkeys at necropsy; 93% or 53 animals had splenic amyloidosis. All 57 animals had lung mites, and 84% had histologic evidence of colitis.

Amyloidosis is uncommon in cats. Only 20 cases have been described in the past 20 years (DiBartola et al. 1986). In this report the authors described generalized amyloidosis in 15 Abyssinian cats. Fourteen had deposits localized in the capsule, smooth muscle trabeculae, and arteriolar walls of the spleen.

In the dog, in which amyloidosis is more frequent than in cats and other domestic animals (Maxie 1985), the disease is systemic and sometimes related to chronic inflammation, but usually it is idiopathic. The amyloid deposits are

Table 43. Frequency of spontaneous splenic amyloidosis in mice

Strain	Age (months)	No. affected/total		Reference
		M (%)	F (%)	
BL/LYDe		21/28 (75)	44/69 (64)	Deringer 1965
LLC			8/10 (80)	Eisenbud et al. 1981
LLC			(100)	Chai 1976 Chai and Lerner 1984
SJL/J	7.5–12.5		29/58 (50)	Scheinberg et al. 1976
	12.5–15.0		30/40 (75)	
	> 15.0		13/14 (95)	

Table 44. Frequency of induced splenic amyloidosis in mice

Strain	Agent	Dose	Incidence	Reference
Swiss	Casein (12%) + cyclosporin 6 × weekly	0.5 ml 2.5 mg in 5% dextrose; after 1 week 1.25 mg	100%	Shtrasburg et al. 1986
	Casein (12%)	0.5 ml subcutaneously	100%	
	Casein (10%)	0.5 cc	15/15[b] at 25 days 14/15[b] at 32 days 12/15[b] at 35 days	Ravid et al. 1985
CBA	Azocasein	50 mg	4/6	Axelrad et al. 1975
	Azocasein + syngeneic spleen cells	50 mg 10^8	4/4[a] 5/5[a]	
CBA/J	Casein (10%)	0.5 cc	0/3	Varga et al. 1986
	Casein (10%) + amyloidotic spleen tissue	1.0 cc	11/15	
	Casein (10%) + amyloid enhancing factor	1.0 cc 0.5 cc	17/24	

[a] Fourteen consecutive daily injections.

[b] Single intravenous injection of 10^8 spleen cells.

found in many organs, although several sites are preferred, such as the liver and spleen, but the kidney is most commonly involved (Maxie 1985).

A 5-year-old female mountain gazelle with anorexia, subcutaneous edema, uremia, and cachexia was euthanized (Linke et al. 1986). At autopsy, the spleen was enlarged, firm, and glassy; the cut surface contained masses of amyloid, imparting to the organ the appearance of the so-called sago spleen. In histologic sections, amyloid deposits were seen to be localized in the trabeculae, capsule, and follicles. The deposits were identified as amyloid protein type AA1.

References

Axelrad M, Kisilevsky R, Beswetherick S (1975) Acceleration of amyloidosis by syngeneic spleen cells from normal donors. Am J Pathol 78: 277–284

Blanchard JL, Baskin GB, Watson EA (1986) Generalized amyloidosis in Rhesus monkeys. Vet Pathol 23: 425–430

Brandwein SR, Sipe JD, Tatsuta E, Skinner M, Cohen AS (1984) Colchicine in acute inflammation: stimulation of production of interleukin-1 and modulation of the acute phase serum amyloid A protein response. J Rheumatol 11: 597–601

Chai CK (1976) Reticular cell hyperplasia and amyloidosis in a line of mice with low leukocyte counts. Am J Pathol 85: 49–72

Chai CK, Lerner C (1984) Amyloidosis development in LCC mice. Exp Cell Biol 52: 339–346

Cohen AS, Shirahama T, Sipe JD, Skinner M (1983) Amyloid proteins, precursors, mediator, and enhancer. Lab Invest 48: 1–4

Deringer MK (1965) Amyloidosis in strain BL/LYDe mice. Proc Soc Exp Biol Med 119: 94–96

DiBartola SP, Tarr MJ, Benson MD (1986) Tissue distribution of amyloid deposits in Abyssinian cats with familial amyloidosis. J Comp Pathol 96: 387–398

Dunn TB (1967) Amyloidosis in mice. In: Cotchin E, Roe FJC (eds) Pathology of laboratory rats and mice. Blackwell Scientific, Oxford, pp 181–212

Dunn TB, Andervont HB (1963) Histology of some neoplasms and nonneoplastic lesions found in wild mice maintained under laboratory conditions. JNCI 31: 873–901

Eisenbud LE, Lerner CP, Chai CK (1981) The effect of dimethyl sulfoxide (DMSO) upon spontaneous amyloidosis in mice. Proc Exp Biol Med 168: 172–174

Fuks A, Zucker-Franklin D (1985) Impaired Kupffer cell function precedes development of secondary amyloidosis. J Exp Med 161: 1013–1028

Ghadially FN (1982) Extracellular matrix. In: Ultrastructural pathology of the cell and matrix. A text and atlas of physiological alterations in the fine structure of cellular and extra-cellular components, 2nd edn. Butterworths, London, pp 918–921

Glenner GG (1980 a) Amyloid deposits and amyloidosis. Part I. N Engl J Med 302: 1283–1292

Glenner GG (1980 b) Amyloid deposits and amyloidosis. Part II. N Engl J Med 302: 1333–1343

Glenner GG (1988) Alzheimer's disease, its proteins and genes. Cell 52: 307–308

Heston WE, Deringer MK (1948) Hereditary renal disease and amyloidosis in mice. Arch Pathol 46: 49–58

Husebekk A, Skogen B, Husby G, Marhaug G (1985) Transformation of amyloid precursor SAA to protein AA and incorporation in amyloid fibrils in vivo. Scand J Immunol 21: 283–287

Kisilevsky R (1983) Biology of disease. Amyloidosis: a familiar problem in the light of current pathogenetic developments. Lab Invest 49: 381–390

Linke RP, Hol PR, Geisel O (1986) Immunohistochemical identification of generalized AA-amyloidosis in a mountain gazelle (Gazella gazella). Vet Pathol 23: 63–67

Maxie MG (1985) The urinary system. In: Jubb KVF, Kennedy PC, Palmer N (eds) Pathology of domestic animals, vol 2. Academic, New York, pp 343–411

McClure HM (1984) Non-human primate models for human disease. Amyloidosis. Adv Vet Sci Comp Med 28: 267–304

Pepys MB, Baltz ML, deBeer FC, Dyck RF, Holford S, Breathnach SM, Black MM, Tribe CR, Evans DJ, Feinstein A (1982) Biology of serum amyloid P component. Ann NY Acad Sci 389: 286–298

Ravid M, Chen B, Bernheim J, Kedar I (1985) Ascorbic acid induced regression of amyloidosis in experimental animals. Br J Exp Pathol 66: 137–141

Robbins SL, Cotran RS, Kumar V (1984) Diseases of immunity. Amyloidosis. In: Pathologic basis of disease, 3rd edn. Saunders, Philadelphia, pp 195–205

Scheinberg MA, Cathcart ES, Eastcott JW, Skinner M, Benson M, Shirahama T, Bennett M (1976) The SJL/J mouse: a new model for spontaneous age-associated amyloidosis. I. Morphologic and immunochemical aspects. Lab Invest 35: 47–54

Schultz RT, Pitha J (1985) Relation of the hepatic and splenic microcirculations to the development of lesions in experimental amyloidosis. Am J Pathol 119: 127–137

Shirahama T, Cohen AS (1975) Intralysozomal formation of amyloid fibrils. Am J Pathol 81: 101–116

Shirahama T, Skinner M, Sipe JD, Cohen AS (1985) Widespread occurrence of AP in amyloidotic tissues. An immunohistochemical observation. Virchows Arch [B] 48: 197–206

Shtrasburg S, Siegal B, Zemer D (1986) Repeated casein injections induce experimental amyloidosis in mice (letter to editor). Transplantation 41: 800

Snow AD, Kisilevsky R (1985) Temporal relationship between glycosaminoglycan accumulation and amyloid deposition during experimental amyloidosis. A histochemical study. Lab Invest 53: 37–44

Sztein MB, Vogel SN, Sipe JP, Murphy PA, Mizel SB, Oppenheim J, Rosenstreich DL (1981) The role of macrophages in the acute phase response: SAA inducer is closely related to lymphocyte activating factor and endogenous pyrogen. Cell Immunol 63: 164–176

Thung PJ (1957 a) The relation between amyloid and ageing in comparative pathology. Gerontologia 1: 234–254

Thung PJ (1957 b) Senile amyloidosis in mice. Gerontologia 1: 259–279

Varga J, Flinn MS, Shirahama T, Rodgers OG, Cohen AS (1986) The induction of accelerated murine amyloid with human splenic extract. Probable role amyloid enhancing factor. Virchows Arch [B] 51: 177–185

West WT, Murphy ED (1965) Sequence of deposition of amyloid in strain A mice and relationship to renal disease. JNCI 35: 167–174

Westermark P, Johnson KH, Pitkanen P (1985) Systemic amyloidosis: a review with emphasis on pathogenesis. Appl Pathol 3: 55–68

Zurcher C, van Zwieten MJ, Solleveld HA, Hollander CF (1982) Aging research. In: Foster HL, Small JD, Fox JG (eds) The mouse in biomedical research. IV. Experimental biology and oncology. Academic, New York, chap 2

Fibrosis, Spleen, Rat

James A. Popp

Synonyms. Stromal fibrosis; parenchymal fibrosis; capsular fibrosis; capsular hyperplasia; splenic fibroplasia.

Gross Appearance

Fibrosis in the rat spleen is observed in both the parenchyma and the capsule (Goodman et al. 1984). In the red pulp, fibrosis may only be recognized on cross section as areas that are from 1 mm to 1 cm in greatest dimension. Although the fibrosis is irregular in pattern, it conforms to the shape and architecture of the spleen. The white to gray fibrotic lesion, which may appear grossly as a scar or healed infarct, is firm in texture and easily distinguished from the dark red of the red pulp.

Fibrosis of the splenic capsule is characterized by capsular thickening, causing the surface of the spleen to appear white to gray in color rather than the normal dark red color. The surface of a spleen with capsular fibrosis has a rough or irregular appearance in contrast to the smooth, uniform, glistening surface of the normal spleen. Capsular fibrosis is frequently irregular, affecting some but not all areas of the surface. The edges of the spleen are preferentially affected when the distribution of the lesion is irregular. Small capsular cysts up to 2 mm in diameter and containing a slightly viscous clear fluid may be observed protruding from the surface of the capsule. Fibrosis of the capsule may be observed either alone or in conjunction with fibrosis of the red pulp of the spleen. When the two lesions occur in response to chemical treatment, fibrosis of the splenic capsule occors before fibrosis of the red pulp.

Microscopic Features

Parenchymal fibrosis of the rat spleen is characterized by numerous fibroblasts and variable amounts of collagen that have replaced the normal architecture (Goodman et al. 1984) (Fig. 257). Sinusoids are obliterated, and red blood cells are rarely found in the areas of fibrosis. The white pulp areas of the spleen are more resistant to the encroachment of the fibrosis, leaving either well-developed or remnants of lymphoid follicles trapped within the fibrosis. However, in the larger lesions and in lesions with extensive collagen deposition, remnants of lymphoid follicles are rare. Areas of fibrosis may contain small or large nests of mature fat cells (Goodman et al. 1984; Ward et al. 1980) (Fig. 258).

In addition to the focal areas of parenchymal fibrosis, focal areas of stromal hyperplasia are frequently present and characterized by hypercellularity of stromal cells; they lack collagen, however (Fig. 259).

Fibrosis of the capsule appears as a thickening of the normal capsule with increased amounts of collagen and fibroblasts (Fig. 257). The irregular distribution of the lesion is readily apparent by light microscopy. An area of normal-appearing splenic capsule can be observed adjacent to an area that is 3 or more times the normal thickness. While the increased thickness of the capsule is primarily due to fibroblasts and collagen, mononuclear cells are frequently found randomly throughout the capsule or in distinct aggregates. Cysts are occasionally found within the thickened areas of the splenic capsule (Fig. 260) and are sometimes lined by cuboidal mesothelial cells. The surface of the thickened splenic capsule is usually covered by numerous cuboidal mesothelial cells that may form papillary projections (Goodman et al. 1984; Ward et al. 1980).

Fibrotic lesions usually contain numerous typical active fibroblasts with elongated nuclei containing dense or marginated chromatin. Nucleoli are generally small, if observed. The cytoplasmic borders of the fibroblasts are usually indistinguishable from adjacent cells and collagen. Most areas of fibrosis have a moderate amount of collagen that appears to separate the fibroblasts. Lesions with extensive collagen accumulation or dense collagen are less common.

Ultrastructure

Ultrastructural studies of splenic fibrosis in the rat have not been reported.

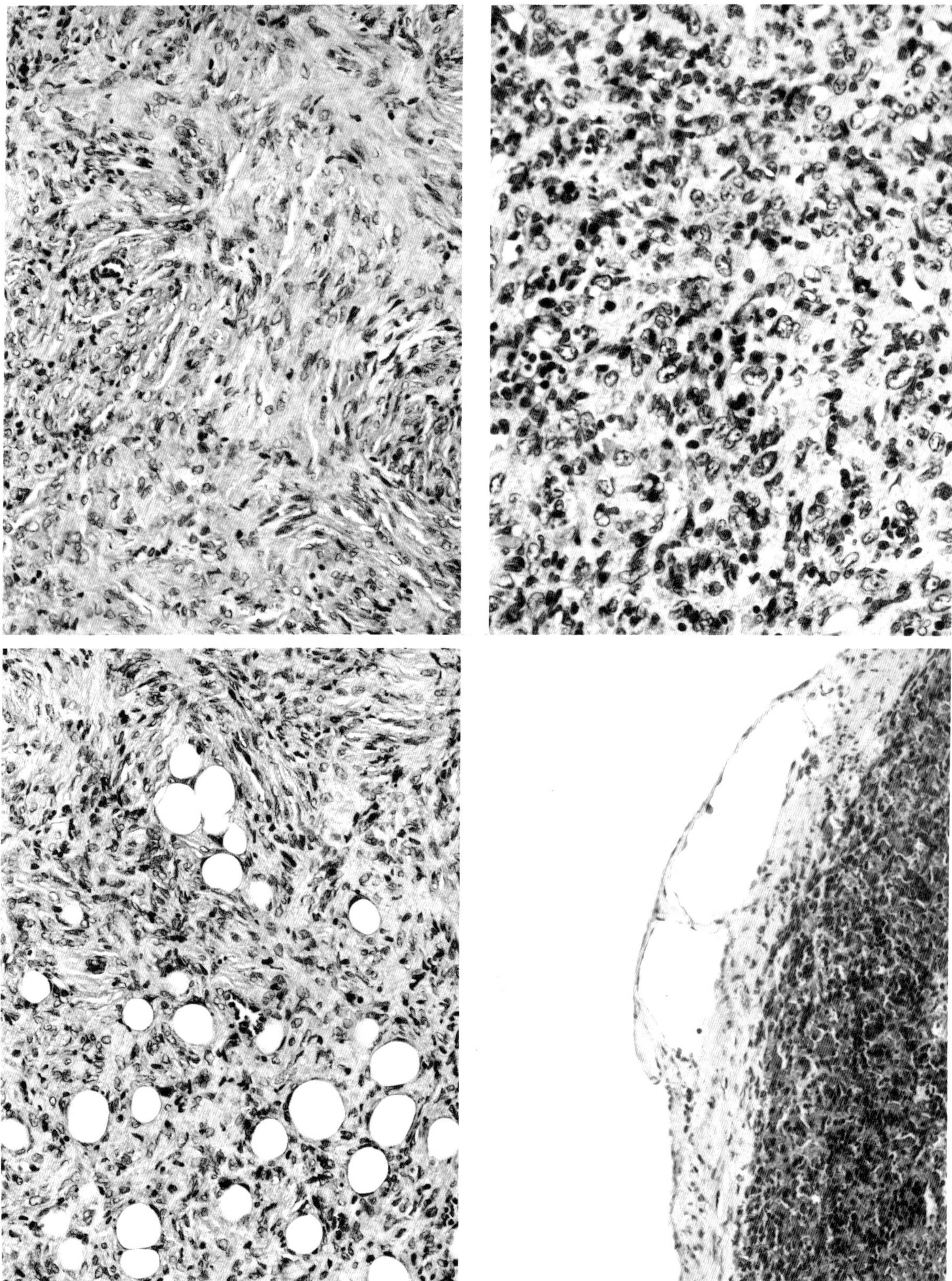

Fig. 257 *(upper left).* Fibrosis, spleen, rat. Note numerous fibroblasts and collagen deposition. Hematoxylin and phloxine, × 200

Fig. 258 *(lower left).* Fibrosis, spleen, rat. Note mature fat cells (in an area of fibrosis). Hematoxylin and phloxine, × 200

Fig. 259 *(upper right).* Stromal hyperplasia, spleen, rat. Note hypercellularity of the parenchyma of the spleen with little or no collagen. Hematoxylin and phloxine, × 400

Fig. 260 *(lower right).* Cyst of splenic capsule, rat. These cysts develop on the surface or within the capsule of the spleen. Hematoxylin and phloxine, × 200

Differential Diagnosis

Splenic fibrosis of the red pulp and capsule rarely results in a diagnostic problem due to the differentiation of the tissue and the cells within the lesion. In rare instances, splenic fibrosis must be distinguished from primary mesenchymal neoplasms of the spleen, particularly fibrosarcomas. The diagnostic distinction between these lesions is primarily made on the basis of traditional diagnostic differences between fibrosis and neoplasms of fibroblastic origin in other tissues. Cells within areas of fibrosis are better differentiated than neoplastic cells, mitotic figures are rarer, and the cells are more uniform in shape and size.

Splenic fibrosis occurs as a rare event spontaneously in F344 rats with or without LGL leukemia. Associated with this LGL leukemia (see p. 194, this volume), focal parenchymal fibrosis with gross scar formation or infarction is occasionally seen.

Biologic Features

Splenic fibrosis appears to arise through the proliferation of fibroblasts or reticuloendothelial cells within the red pulp or of fibroblasts within the capsule of the spleen. While it is a relatively uncommon lesion in the rat following chemical exposure, it has been consistently observed in the spleens of rodents chronically fed eight different aromatic amines or their derivatives (Bus and Popp 1987; Goodman et al. 1984; Weinberger et al. 1985). The earliest proliferative lesions are found in the splenic capsule, while areas of parenchymal fibrosis occur only after prolonged treatment of rats with aromatic amines. The exact mechanism of splenic fibrosis induction is unclear, although available information has been reviewed in detail (Bus and Popp 1987). It is known that methemoglobinemia, red cell destruction, and resultant splenic hemosiderosis are found following the feeding of the aromatic amines that result in splenic fibrosis. Indeed, a dose response was noted for the severity of hemosiderosis in aniline studies (Bus and Popp 1987).

Evaluation of the hematologic response, pathogenesis of the splenic lesions, and chemical disposition studies have led to the proposal that compound-derived toxicity to red blood cells is the primary lesion that results in the removal of damaged erythrocytes in the spleen, which in turn initiates splenic fibrosis (Bus and Popp 1987).

Splenic fibrosis appears to have the potential to become neoplastic, resulting in the formation of fibrosarcomas (Bus and Popp 1987; Goodman et al. 1984; Weinberger et al. 1985). This conclusion is based on (a) the presence of fibrosarcomas in the spleens of animals that develop fibrosis, (b) the time sequence of fibrosis and neoplasia, and (c) the histology of developing lesions. In rats developing fibrosarcomas associated with the chronic administration of aromatic amines, fibrosis has been a constant feature in the spleens. When sequential killings of animals during a chronic study with aniline were performed, fibrosis was found at time points preceding the appearance of neoplasms (Bus and Popp 1987). While the conversion of splenic fibrosis to fibrosarcoma is rare (based on the high incidence of animals with fibrosis and the low incidence of animals with fibrosarcomas), histological examination supports the concept that fibrosis is the precursor of fibrosarcomas. In rare fibrotic lesions in the splenic capsule or parenchyma, small areas of developing fibrosarcomas have been identified, based on the cytologic characteristics of the fibroblastic lesions.

Comparison with Other Species

Splenic fibrosis is uncommon in all species, thus preventing detailed species comparisons. Mice do not develop splenic fibrosis when exposed to the aromatic amines that cause splenic fibrosis in the rat (Bus and Popp 1987).

References

Bus JS, Popp JA (1987) Perspectives on the mechanism of action of the splenic toxicity of aniline and structurally-related compounds. Food Chem Toxicol 25(8): 619–626

Goodman DG, Ward JM, Reichardt WD (1984) Splenic fibrosis and sarcomas in F344 rats fed diets containing aniline hydrochloride, p-chloroaniline, azobenzene, o-toluidine hydrochloride, 4,4'-sulfonyldianiline, or D & C red no. 9. JNCI 73: 265–273

Ward JM, Reznik G, Garner FM (1980) Proliferative lesions of the spleen in male F344 rats feed diets containing p-chloroaniline. Vet Pathol 17: 200–205

Weinberger MA, Albert RH, Montgomery SB (1985) Splenotoxicity associated with splenic sarcomas in rats fed high doses of D & C red no. 9 or aniline hydrochloride. JNCI 75: 681–690

Thymus

Normal Anatomy, Histology, Immunohistology, Ultrastructure, Rat

Christine D. Dijkstra and Taede Sminia

Gross Appearance

The thymus is located dorsal to the cranial part of the sternum in the thorax. It is a primary or central lymphoid organ in which T lymphocytes are produced autonomously, without antigenic stimulation. The development of the fetal thymus is marked by an invagination of epithelial cells of the endodermal and ectodermal lining of the third and fourth pharyngeal pouch into the underlying mesenchyme (Owen and Jenkinson 1984).

The thymus appears as a white organ surrounded by a capsule and consists in rats and other laboratory animals of two lobi, each formed by several lobuli. At the dorsolateral border of each lobe a major septum (Sainte-Marie 1974) is found containing the hilus, the site where the blood vessels enter and leave the organ. The hilar artery bifurcates within this major septum to give rise to a cranial and a caudal branch. From the major septum arise less-developed septa that form an irregular network supporting the larger blood vessels. The lobuli vary in shape, size, and orientation. The septa often run between two adjacent lobuli but do not completely separate them (Sainte-Marie 1974). The size of the thymus relative to the rest of the body is greatest at birth. With age the thymus begins to involute, gradually diminishing in size (Hwang et al. 1974). The process of involution is accelerated by corticosteroids and sex hormones.

The thymus has no defined afferent lymphatics, but efferent lymphatics do occur. A pair of lymph nodes always accompanies the thymus at both sides of the distal part.

Microscopic Features

The connective tissue capsule consists of an outer and an inner layer; the septa are folds of the inner layer (Sainte-Marie et al. 1986). Scattered or clustered lymphocytes are present between the collagen and reticular fibers in the capsule and septa. From the capsule and the septa, trabeculae extend to the central parts of the lobuli. The course of the capsule, septa, and trabeculae is clearly visible after collagen staining or silver impregnation of the reticular fibers.

In contrast to other lymphoid organs, only the capsule, septa, trabeculae, and a thin layer of connective tissue around the blood vessels are of mesenchymal origin. The rest of the framework of the thymus is formed by an extensive network of epithelial reticular cells which, during development of the thymus, invaginate the mesenchyme. Within this epithelial network the bone marrow-derived lymphocytes (thymocytes) and nonlymphoid cells (macrophages and dendritic cells) are present (Van Haelst 1967; Duijvestijn and Hoefsmit 1981; Brelinska et al. 1985). (Fig. 263) Two compartments, cortex and medulla, can be distinguished in each lobule. The peripherally located cortex is darkly stained because of the densely packed thymocytes in the epithelial reticulum, the medulla is lighter because of the lower density of thymocytes (Figs. 261, 262). In addition to thymocytes, blood-borne macrophages and dendritic cells are present (Barclay and Mayrhofer 1981; Duijvestijn et al. 1983). In the medulla, groups of epithelial reticular cells characteristically arranged in concentric layers form Hassall's bodies (Van Haelst 1967). Between the cortex and the medulla a transitional zone can be discriminated, the corticomedullary region (Duijvestijn and Hoefsmit 1981). In this region, many blood vessels, the majority of which are arterioles, are surrounded by perivascular connective tissue (Sainte-Marie et al. 1986). Usually B lymphocytes and plasma cells can be seen in the corticomedullary region. The arterioles ramify into capillaries which extend into the cortex and medulla. In the cortex they form a special complex of capillary arcades, which empty into the medullary venules.

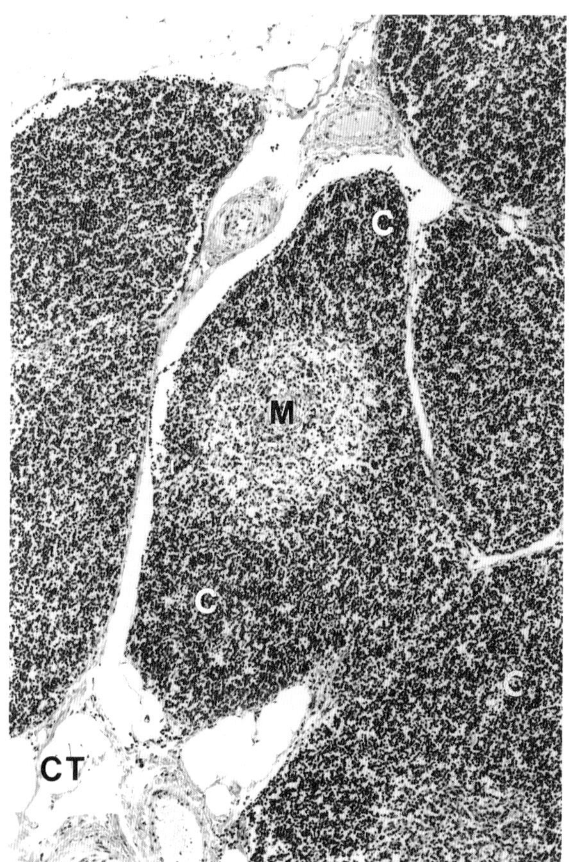
C
M
C
CT

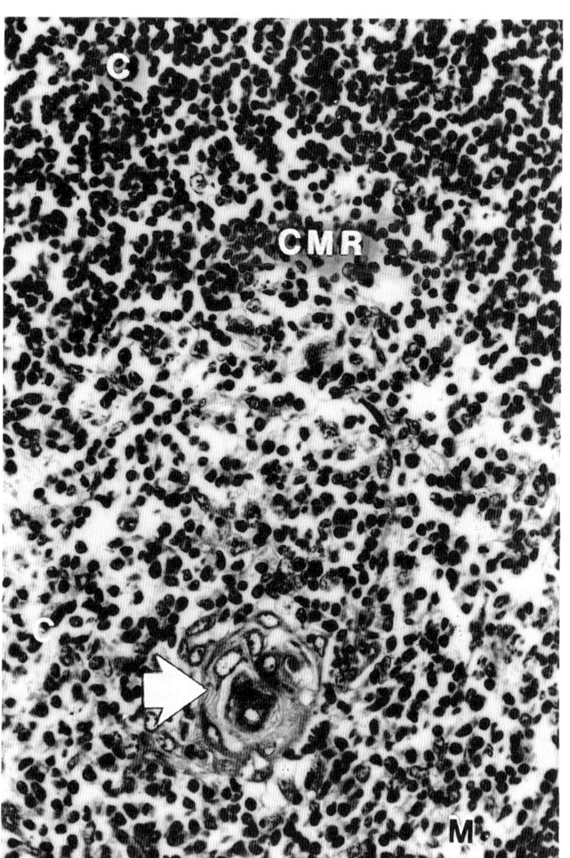
C
CMR
M

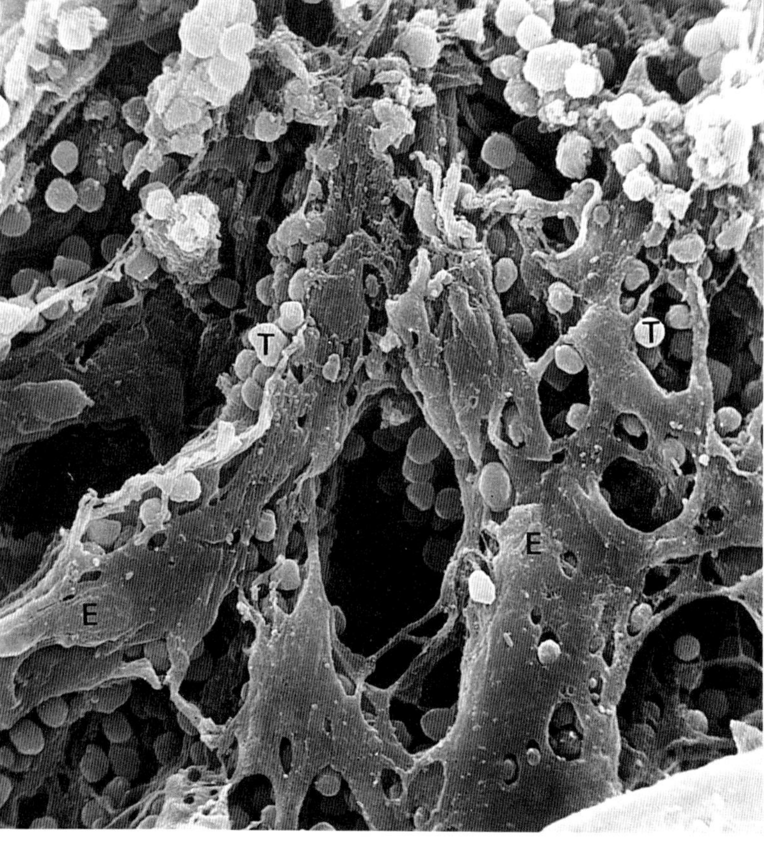
T
T
E
E

◄ **Fig. 261** *(upper left).* Rat, thymus, paraffin section. *C,* cortex; *M,* medulla; *CT,* connective tissue with fat cells. Survey showing thymic lobules separated by connective tissue and fat cells. Masson stain, × 100

Fig. 262 *(upper right).* Rat, thymus. *C,* cortex; *CMR,* corticomedullary region. Detail of Fig. 261, showing the densely packed lymphocytes in the cortex and the lighter medulla *(M)* with a typical Hassall's body *(arrow).* Masson stain, × 400

Fig. 263 *(below).* Thymic cortex thymocytes *(T)* in a network of epithelial reticular cells *(E).* SEM, × 10000. (Courtesy of W. van Ewijk)

The perivascular tissue, often containing macrophages and lymphocytes, constitutes, together with the endothelial cells and the reticular epithelial cells, the blood-thymus barrier. This barrier restricts the access of antigens to the developing T lymphocytes in the cortex; the medulla is permeable to free circulating molecules (Raviola and Karnovsky 1972).

Immunhistochemistry

Immunohistochemical analysis of the thymic cell population indicates that the diverse compartments of the thymus contain phenotypically different types of lymphoid and nonlymphoid cells. As for the nonlymphoid cells, staining for Ia-antigen reveals a typical localization of this major histocompatibility complex (MHC) class II encoded antigen (Fig. 264). In the cortex a lattice-like pattern of the Ia-positive epithelial reticular cells is obvious except for a few areas that are devoid of stromal cells (Duijvestijn et al. 1982) (Figs. 265, 266). In the medulla, a more confluent staining pattern occurs, caused by numerous bone marrow-derived cells with dendritic cell processes (Barclay and Mayrhofer 1981; Duijvestijn et al. 1983). These cells have the morphological and histochemical characteristics of interdigitating cells (Duijvestijn et al. 1983; Higley and Rowden 1984).
Use of monoclonal antibodies against rat macrophages (ED₁ and ED₂; Dijkstra et al. 1985) indicates that each compartment of the thymus contains different types of macrophages. The medulla contains predominantly dendritic cells which are positive for ED1 and Ia and negative for ED2, the corticomedullary region contains many ED1-positive monocytes, whereas in the cortex a characteristic subpopulation of ED2- and Ia-pos-

itive macrophages with large cytoplasmic processes is present (Figs. 267, 268) (Sminia et al. 1986).
As for the lymphoid cells, in this organ in which T-cell proliferation and differentiation take place almost all lymphoid cells are of the T-cell phenotype (W3/13-positive; Williams et al. 1977). In the cortex these lymphocytes are positive for both OX-8 (T suppressor/cytotoxic: Brideau et al. 1980) and W3/25 (T helper; Williams et al. 1977b), whereas in peripheral lymphoid organs T cells are either OX-8 or W3/25 positive. This implies that cortical lymphocytes are unique in phenotype; they display several surface differentiation markers that are absent on mature T cells. In the medulla, the thymocytes are either OX-8 or W3/25 positive and thus are identical to mature peripheral T lymphocytes. A minority of the cells is OX-8 positive, the majority of the medullary lymphocytes bears the W3/25 surface marker. The difference between cortical and medullary thymocytes is further stressed by observations on the presence of the differentiation marker Thy-1 (Williams et al. 1977a; Ritter and Morris 1980). This marker is strongly expressed on cortical thymocytes but only weakly on medullary thymocytes.

Ultrastructure

Epithelial Cells

The framework of the thymus in which the lymphocytes and other bone marrow-derived cells occur is formed by epithelial cells. These cells are interconnected by desmosomes (Fig. 269), contain tonofilaments, and are separated from the mesenchymal elements by a basement membrane (Van Haelst 1967; Duijvestijn and Hoefsmit 1981). The epithelial cells in the cortex differ morphologically and functionally from the medullary epithelial cells (Duijvestijn and Hoefsmit 1981). The cortical epithelial cells constitute a fine meshwork; they are interconnected by slender cytoplasmic processes and have a reticular shape. The cytoplasm is confined to a thin perinuclear layer. The most conspicuous cell organelles are vacuoles partly filled with dense and/or membranous material. Short cisternae of the rough endoplasmic reticulum, some Golgi bodies, and free polyribosomes are present (Van Haelst 1967; Duijvestijn and Hoefsmit 1981). The epithelial reticulum of the medulla is widely meshed as compared with that of the cortex. Two

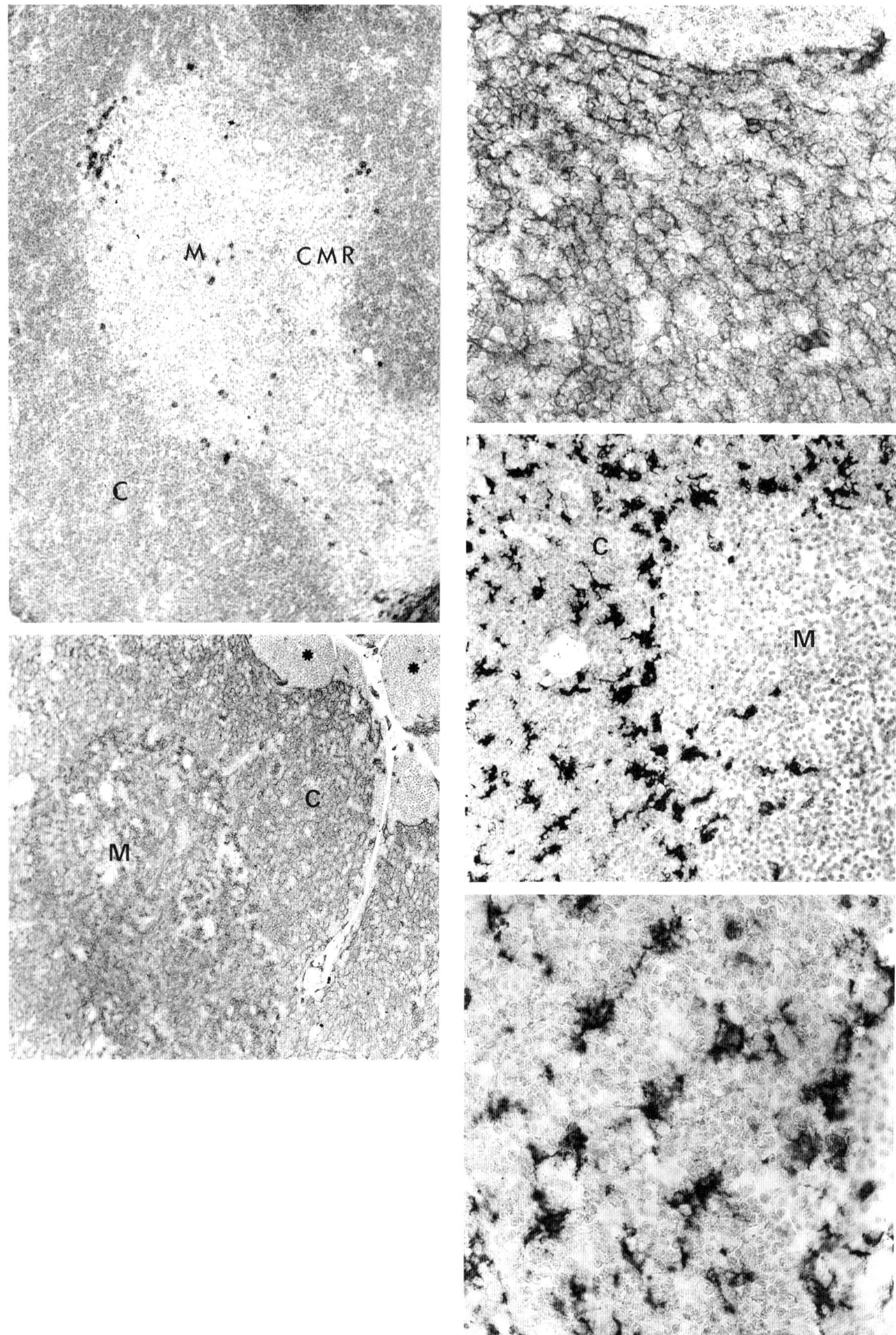

◄ **Fig. 264** *(upper left).* Rat, thymus. Ig-positive B lymphocytes and plasma cells *(dark cells)* are present in the corticomedullary region *(CMR). C,* cortex; *M,* medulla. × 80

Fig. 265 *(lower left).* Rat, thymus, immunoperoxidase localization of I a determinants. In the cortex *(C)* a reticular staining pattern is present, whereas the medulla *(M)* has a confluent I a pattern. In the cortex I a-negative areas are present *(asterisks).* × 200

Fig. 266 *(upper right).* Rat, thymus, immunoperoxidase localization of I a determinants. Higher magnification of reticular staining pattern in the cortex. × 600

Fig. 267 *(middle right).* Rat, thymus. ED$_2$-positive macrophages with cytoplasmic processes *(black cells)* among the thymocytes. *C,* cortex; *M,* medulla. × 200

Fig. 268 *(lower right).* Higher magnification of the branched ED$_2$-positive cortical macrophages in Fig. 267. × 400

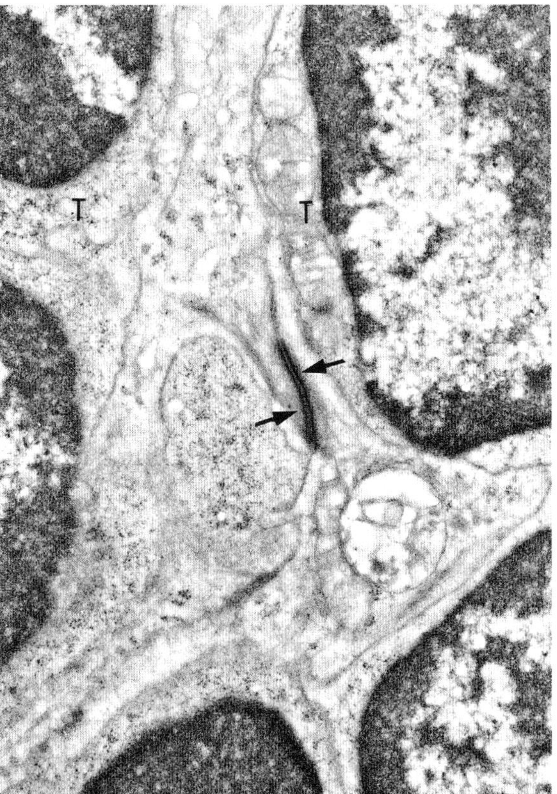

types of epithelial cells are present in the medulla. The reticular type resembles the epithelial cells of the cortex but with fewer cell processes and a more elongated shape. The other type has an eccentrically located nucleus, and the cytoplasm is marked by an abundance of vesicles, Golgi complexes, and vacuoles (Van Haelst 1967). The vacuoles often contain fingerlike membrane protrusions and sometimes clumps of fluffy dense material (Duijvestijn and Hoefsmit 1981). The epithelial cells contribute a large part to the thymic stroma, which is involved in intrathymic T-cell proliferation and differentiation. The thymic stroma exerts its effects on T-cell differentiation by secretion of various thymic hormones. Some developmental stages require direct receptor-mediated cell to cell contact of maturing T cells with stromal cells (see Van Vliet 1985). These contacts are usually firm because lymphostromal complexes can be found in thymus cell suspensions in vitro. These complexes, termed thymic nurse cells (TNC, Fig. 270), consist of a single epithelial cell filled with high numbers of fully intact thymocytes (Wekerle and Ketelsen 1980; Van Vliet et al. 1984; De Waal Malefijt et al. 1986). Thymic nurse cell formation is ascribed to the outer part of the thymus cortex, the cortical region in which numerous thymoblasts and mitotic figures are observed. The inner cortex contains mainly small thymocytes (Hwang et al. 1974; Duijvestijn and Hoefsmit 1981). Based on these observations, it has been suggested that epithelial cells of the outer cortex, and the thymic nurse cells as an in vitro equivalent of

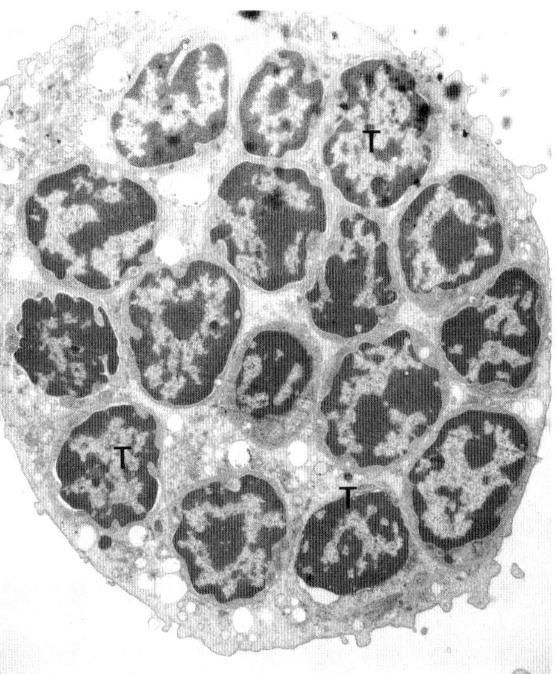

Fig. 269 *(above).* Rat, thymus. Cortical reticular epithelial cells with cytoplasmic tonifilaments near a desmosome *(arrows). T,* thymocytes. TEM, × 12000. (Courtesy of E. C. M. Hoefsmit)

Fig. 270 *(below).* Isolated thymic nurse cells with vacuoles and thymocytes *(T).* TEM, × 25000. (Courtesy of W. Leene)

them, provide a microenvironment guiding early stages of intrathymic T-cell differentiation.

Bone Marrow-Derived Stromal Cells

It is thought that in addition to the epithelial cells cortical macrophages play a part in T-cell differentiation. The most conspicuous macrophages in the cortex are the branched ED2-positive cells, and we have previously suggested that these cells do have a function in thymocyte maturation and proliferation (Sminia et al. 1986). In addition, cortical macrophages laden with numerous thymocytes in different phases of lysosomal digestion occur. They are most likely involved in the control of the number and kind of thymocytes released by the thymus. The most characteristic bone marrow-derived cell type in the medulla is the interdigitating cell (Fig. 271). These are large, nonlymphoid, bone marrow-derived cells (Barclay and Mayrhofer 1981) with characteristic morphological features. They have an irregularly shaped, excentrically located nucleus. Most cell organelles accumulate in the cytocenter. The cytoplasm is electron-lucent and has numerous processes that interdigitate with surrounding thymocytes. Occasionally, phagolysosomes with pyknotic nuclei of lymphocytes are encountered. Frequently, Birbeck granules are present in the cytoplasm of these cells (Duijvestijn and Hoefsmit 1981; Higley and Rowden 1984). These rodlike membrane structures are characteristic of interdigitating cells and related cells (such as Langerhans' cells; Birbeck et al. 1961). Their function may either involve the presentation of antigen to mature immunocompetent T cells in the medulla or the presentation of "self" antigens and hence play a part in the generation of tolerance (Barclay and Mayrhofer 1981) (Fig. 272).

Other Cell Types

In addition to epithelial cells, thymocytes, cortical macrophages, and medullary interdigitating cells, the thymus may contain B lymphocytes and plasma cells (Hwang et al. 1974). These latter cell types are in particular found in the corticomedullary area (Figs. 263, 271).
From the foregoing it is clear that the thymus in fact consists of a true primary lymphoid part, viz. the thymic cortex, and a peripheral lymphoid structure, the medulla. The thymic medulla comprises both antigen-presenting cells (interdigitating cells) and mature T lymphocytes, indicating that cellular interactions leading to an immune response may occur in this thymic compartment. During a systemic immune response and under pathological conditions, numerous plasma cells and B lymphocytes can be found in the medulla, sometimes even B-cell follicles. The thymic cortex is protected against "external" influences (antigens) by the blood-thymus barrier (Raviola and Karnovsky 1972). However, stress factors and hormones can pass this barrier and have important effects on this thymic compartment.

Comparison with Other Species

Based on studies on both invertebrates and vertebrates, T cells are considered to be phylogenetically the oldest immune cells; they execute cell-mediated immunity including the riddance of foreign tissue graft antigens and potential or outright cancerous cells. The first signs of thymic tissue have been found in the Agnata, the most primitive living vertebrates. Fishes are the first class of vertebrates in which a discrete thymus (an encapsulated lymphoid organ that produces T lymphocytes) has been reported; it consists of a cortex and a medulla. Also in other classes of vertebrates, the amphibians, reptiles, and aves, the thymus is a conspicuous lymphoid organ with several types of lymphoid and nonlymphoid cells (Van Loon et al. 1982; see Cooper 1982; Boyd et al. 1984; Holtfreter and Cohen 1987). Among the mammals, the thymus of rodents (in particular mice) and humans has been studied most extensively. Due to the development of monoclonal antibodies, cell isolation and labelling techniques, and other in vitro methods, data are available on T-cell differentiation. In mice and humans the subpopulations of thymocytes and stromal cells are well characterized (see Van Ewijk 1984; Van Vliet 1985; Van de Wijngaert et al. 1984; Nabarra and Andrianasiron 1987). However, numerous questions such as the precise cellular interactions and intrathymic migration routes of thymocytes remain unresolved, and the thymus is still a "black box" (Scollay and Shortman 1984).

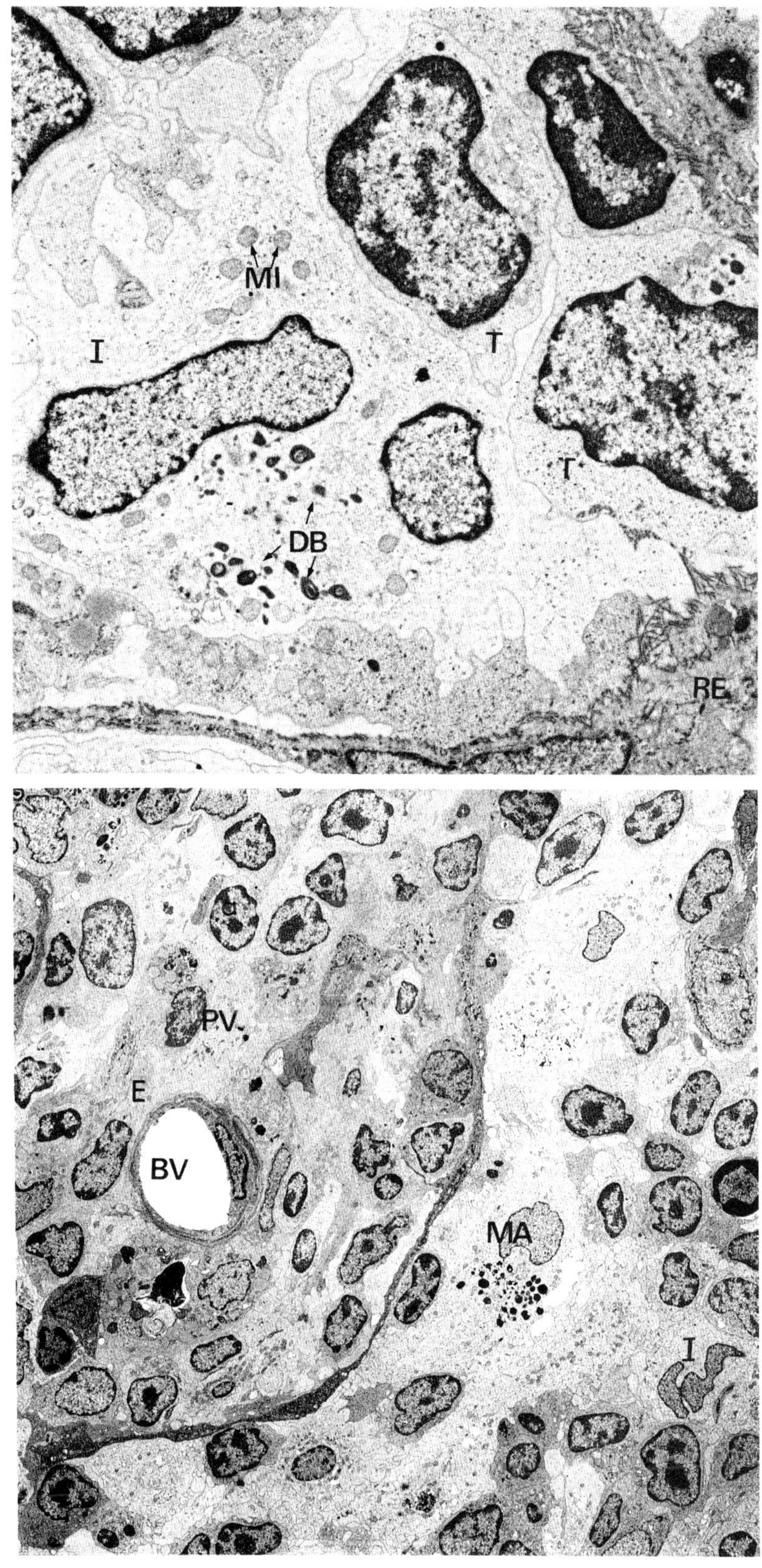

Fig. 271 *(above).* Rat thymic cortex with electron-lucent interdigitating cell *(I),* thymocytes *(T),* and reticular epithelial cell *(RE). DB,* electron-dense bodies (lysosomes); *MI,* mitochondria. TEM, × 5000. (Courtesy of E. C. M. Hoefsmit)

Fig. 272 *(below).* Thymus, rat, corticomedullary region. *BV,* blood vessel; *E,* epithelial cell; *I,* interdigitating cell; *MA,* macrophage; *PV,* perivascular space. TEM, × 1600. (Courtesy of E. C. M. Hoefsmit)

References

Barclay AN, Mayrhofer G (1981) Bone marrow origin of Ia-positive cells in the medulla of rat thymus. J Exp Med 153: 1666–1671

Brélinska R, Kaczmarek E, Warchol JB, Jaroszewski J (1985) Distribution of different cell types within the rat thymus in the neonatal period of life. Cell Tissue Res 240: 473–478

Birbeck MS, Breathnach AS, Everall JD (1961) An electronmicroscope study of basal melanocytes and high-level clear cells (Langerhans cells) in vitiligo. J Invest Dermatol 37: 51–64

Brideau RJ, Carter PB, McMaster WR, Mason DW, Williams AF (1980) Two subsets of rat T lymphocytes defined with monoclonal antibodies. Eur J Immunol 10: 609–615

Boyd RL, Oberhuber G, Hála K, Wick G (1984) Obese strain (OS) chickens with spontaneous autoimmune thyroiditis have a deficiency in thymic nurse cells. J Immunol 132: 718–724

Cooper EL (1982) General immunology. Pergamon, New York

De Waal Malefijt R, Leene W, Roholl PJM, Wormmeester J, Hoeben KA (1986) T cell differentiation within the thymic nurse cells. Lab Invest 55: 25–34

Dijkstra CD, Döpp EA, Joling P, Kraal G (1985) The heterogeneity of mononuclear phagocytes in lymphoid organs: distinct macrophage subpopulations in the rat recognized by monoclonal antibodies ED1, ED2 and ED3. Immunology 54: 589–599

Duijvestijn AM, Hoefsmit EC (1981) Ultrastructure of the rat thymus: the micro-environment of T-lymphocyte maturation. Cell Tissue Res 218: 279–292

Duijvestijn AM, Sminia T, Kohler YG, Janse EM, Hoefsmit ECM (1982) Rat thymus micro-environment: an ultrastructural and functional characterization. In: Nieuwenhuis P, Van den Broek AA, Hanna MG Jr (eds) In vivo immunology. Histopathology of the lymphoid system. Plenum, New York, pp 441–446

Duijvestijn AM, Schutte R, Kohler YG, Korn C, Hoefsmit EC (1983) Characterization of the population of phagocytic cells in thymic cell suspensions. A morphological and cytochemical study. Cell Tissue Res 231: 313–323

Higley HR, Rowden G (1984) Thymic interdigitating reticulum cells demonstrated by immunocytochemistry. Thymus 6: 243–253

Holtfreter HB, Cohen N (1987) In vitro behavior of thymic nurse cell-like complexes from mechanically and enzymatically dissociated tadpole thymuses. Am J Anat 179: 342–355

Hwang WS, Ho TY, Luk SC, Simon GT (1974) Ultrastructure of the rat thymus. A transmission, scanning electron microscope, and morphometric study. Lab Invest 31: 473–487

Nabarra B, Andrianarison I (1987) Ultrastructural studies of thymic reticulum. I. Epithelial component. Thymus 9: 95–121

Owen JJT, Jenkinson EJ (1984) Early events in T lymphocyte genesis in the fetal thymus. Am J Anat 170: 301–310

Raviola E, Karnovsky MJ (1972) Evidence for a blood-thymus barrier using electron-opaque tracers. J Exp Med 136: 466–498

Ritter M, Morris RJ (1980) Thy-1 antigen: selective association in lymphoid organs with the vascular basement membrane involved in lymphocyte recirculation. Immunology 39: 85–91

Sainte-Marie G (1974) Tridimensional reconstruction of the rat thymus. Anat Rec 179: 517–526

Sainte-Marie G, Peng F-S, Marcoux D (1986) The stroma of the thymus of the rat: morphology and antigen diffusion, a reconsideration. Am J Anat 177: 333–352

Scollay R, Shortman K (1984) The surface phenotype of mouse T lymphocytes. A colour-coded chart showing some of the known thymocyte subpopulations and some of their possible and likely interactions. Immunol Today 5 (6) center page

Sminia T, Van Asselt AA, Van De Ende MB, Dijkstra CD (1986) Rat thymus macrophages: an immunohistochemical study on fetal, neonatal and adult thymus. Thymus 8: 141–150

van de Wijngaert FP, Kendall MD, Schuurman HJ, Rademakers LHMP, Kater L (1984) Heterogeneity of epithelial cells in the human thymus. An ultrastructural study. Cell Tissue Res 237: 227–237

van Ewijk W (1984) Immunohistology of lymphoid and non-lymphoid cells in the thymus in the relation to T lymphocyte differation. Am J Anat 170: 311–330

van Haelst U (1967) Light and electronmicroscopical study of the normal and pathological thymus of the rat. I. The normal thymus. Z Zellforsch 77: 534–553

van Loon JJA, Secombes CJ, Egberts E, Van Muiswinkel WB (1982) Ontogeny of the immune system in fish. Role of the thymus. In: Nieuwenhuis P, Van den Broek AA, Hanna MG Jr (eds) In vivo immunology. Plenum, Oxford, pp 335–341

van Vliet E, Melis M, van Ewijk W (1984) Immunohistology of thymic nurse cells. Cell Immunol 87: 101–109

van Vliet E (1985) Stromal cells in the mouse thymus. Thesis, Erasmus University, Rotterdam

Wekerle H, Ketelson UP (1980) Thymic nurse cells – Ia-bearing epithelium involved in T-lymphocyte differentiation? Nature 283: 402–404

Williams AF, Barclay AN, Letarte-Muirhead M, Morris RJ (1977 a) Rat thy-1 antigens from thymus and brain: their tissue distribution, purification, and chemical composition. Cold Spring Harbor Symp Quant Biol 41: 51–61

Williams AF, Galfrè G, Milstein C (1977 b) Analysis of cell surfaces by xenogeneic myeloma-hybrid antibodies: differentiation antigens of rat lymphocytes. Cell 12: 663–673

Development and Aging, Thymus, Rat

C. Frieke Kuper, Rudolf B. Beems, and Victor M. H. Hollanders

Synonyms. Age-related involution; atrophy.

Introduction

The thymus consists of two poorly encapsulated lobes which arise in the embryo as separate primordia on each side of the midline in the neck region. During ontogeny, the organ migrates caudally and medially to the superior mediastinum where the two lobes become closely connected, although they do not appear to fuse. The relative weight is largest about a week after birth; the absolute weight is largest at about the age of 2 months and then gradually declines. In old rats, especially in preterminal condition, the organ can be so small that it is hardly recognizable in the mediastinal fat tissue.

The function of the thymus in the establishment of T-lymphocyte differentiation and maturation is well documented. This function is most evident before age-related size reduction starts. Other functions, especially in the adult and old thymus, are still controversial or even unknown. It is hypothesized that the thymus plays a role in non-immunological, endocrine processes such as sexual development, and as a granulopoietic and erythropoietic organ.

Overview of Development and Aging

The thymus of rodents develops from the endoderm of the ventral and a large portion of the dorsal diverticle of the third pharyngeal pouch and the ectoderm of the third pharyngeal cleft (Witschi 1962; Cordier and Haumont 1980). Based on mouse studies, it is concluded that the fourth pouch does not contribute to the development of the thymus. A small part of the dorsal diverticle of the third pouches yields the parathyroids. In nude mice which lack a lymphoid thymus, the ectoderm fails to contribute to thymic development. It is postulated that thymic cortical epithelium and at least part of the medullary epithelium are of different epithelial lineages (Cordier and Haumont 1980; Savino and Dardenne 1988).

The times at which the various stages of development are thought to happen during embryogene-

sis vary in the literature, due to strain and individual variability but probably mainly due to the imprecise fixing of the time of conception. The thymic primordia are found at about day 12 of fetal life. Around day 13, thymus and parathyroid tissues migrate caudally away from the pouches. The organs separate from each other at day 15, when the thymus moves downward into the thorax and meets its counterpart of the opposite side (Figs. 273–275). At the same time lymphocytic and connective tissue invasion can be found in the thymus. Thymic tissue in the neck becomes thin and breaks up into small fragments. These fragments may sometimes persist either embedded in the thyroid gland or as isolated thymic nests. When separation between thymus and parathyroid has been incomplete, parathyroid tissue can be found in the thorax close to the thymus. The organ is completely developed within a month after birth (see p. 249, this volume).

Generally, in healthy old rats quite a large thymus can be found. The lymphocytic component decreases with age. Although the epithelial network also decreases with age, local epithelial proliferations (cords and tubules) can be found in old animals, especially females (see p. 254, this volume). However, a relationship between these two phenomena is not yet established.

Age-related involution is probably less striking than often thought, since in most healthy old animals quite a large thymus can be found. As described below, several factors which are often encountered in old animals interfere with the aging process and disturb the interpretation of true age-related thymic changes. In addition, seasonal changes have been observed in thymic weight, although it is not known whether or not this plays a role under laboratory conditions (Kendall 1981). Age-related thymic involution is not an acute process in contrast to most induced (stress or acute) involution (see p. 293, this volume). The latter is, in most cases, reversible. It is still not clear whether aging of the thymus has to be considered as an irreversible process, or if the size of the organ is a dynamic process, mainly dependent on the establishment of peripheral T-cell populations. T cell-dependent immunity decreases with age, although it is not clear to what extent this is due to diminished thymic function.

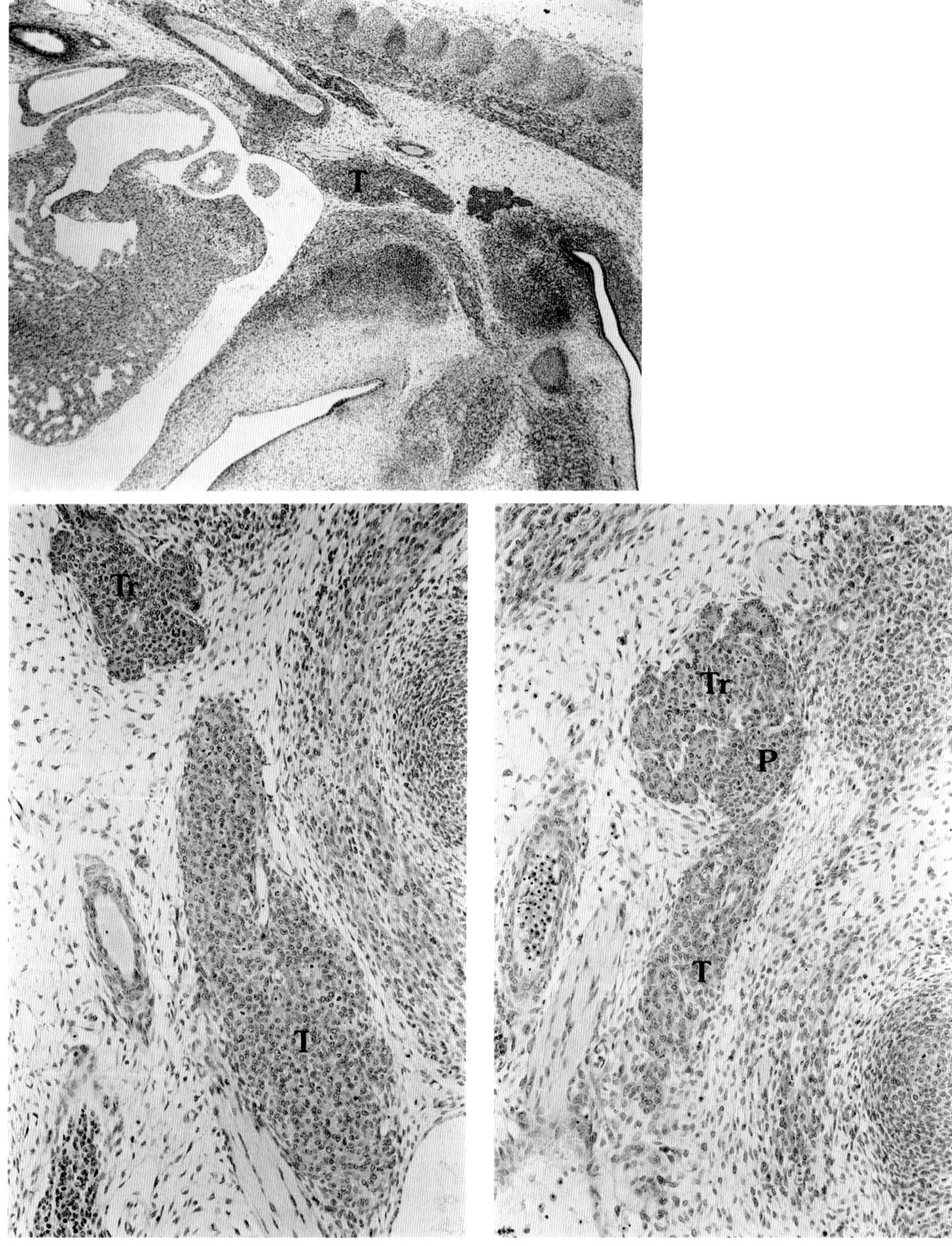

Fig. 273 *(above).* Rat embryo at day 15.5 of fetal life. Sagittal section (essentially at midline). *T,* thymus. H and E, ×33

Fig. 274 *(lower left).* Higher magnification of Fig. 273. *T,* thymus; *Tr,* thyroid. H and E, ×130

Fig. 275 *(lower right).* Rat embryo at day 15.5 of fetal life. Section about 450 μm lateral to section depicted in Figs. 273 and 274. *T,* thymus; *Tr,* thyroid; *P,* parathyroid. H and E, ×130

Factors That Influence Thymic Aging

It is generally assumed that the onset of the decline of thymic size coincides with sexual maturation. This is supported by the observations that thymic atrophy is induced by sex hormones and that thymic aging can be delayed by gonadectomy (Ross and Korenchevsky 1941). When, however, thymic aging is defined on the basis of a reduction of the cortex/medulla ratio due to a decrease in the number of cortical lymphocytes, age-related involution appears to start before sexual maturity (in Wistar rats, especially in females; Kuper et al. 1986), while the competence of the thymus for lymphocyte proliferation is maintained throughout life. The aging process, i. e., lymphocyte reduction, can be markedly accelerated by stress due to illness, deficient diet, or starvation. This can be observed in rats that are found dead or killed in extremis.

Although the age-related reduction of thymic tissue is a normal process and not a pathologic condition, it can be useful in toxicologic studies to score the degree of aging in order to investigate the influences of test compounds on the rate of aging. In chronic studies, however, illness and preterminal conditions such as stress and emaciation become more frequent and affect the morphology of the thymus. This can markedly hamper the interpretation of the results. It is therefore questionable whether in long-term toxicity studies scoring of the degree of thymic aging is appropriate.

On the other hand, it is hypothesized that the age-related decline in thymic immune function as reflected in thymic morphology in turn predisposes to the onset and/or development of disease. In a lifespan study with Wistar rats (Kuper et al. 1986), however, no consistent relationship was observed between the degree of aging of the thymus and mortality due to tumors or other causes. In the survivors, no relationship was found between thymic involution and other aging symptoms with the exception of ovarian atrophy. In some old rats a thymus was found with a relatively normal architecture but considerably larger than would be expected considering the animals' age. It is not clear whether such a so-called persisting thymus is formed by repopulation of the thymus by lymphocytes after involution or whether it has not involuted at all.

Developmental and Aging Histology

Lymphocytes

In the thymic epithelial primordium, lymphocytes can be found at about day 15 (day 14 in mice) of fetal life (Fig. 276). These lymphocytes are located in the central area near the blood capillaries, and almost all possess surface Thy-1 markers (Ritter et al. 1978; Duijvesteijn et al. 1984; Owen and Jenkinson 1984). The cells are small and round, with a relatively heterochromatic nucleus and many polyribosomes. In the subsequent days, their number increases, and they are found throughout the thymus. Between days 19 and 21 cortex and medulla can be distinguished. Lymphocyte proliferation is active in the cortex, especially in the outer zone, thereby making the distinction between cortex and me-

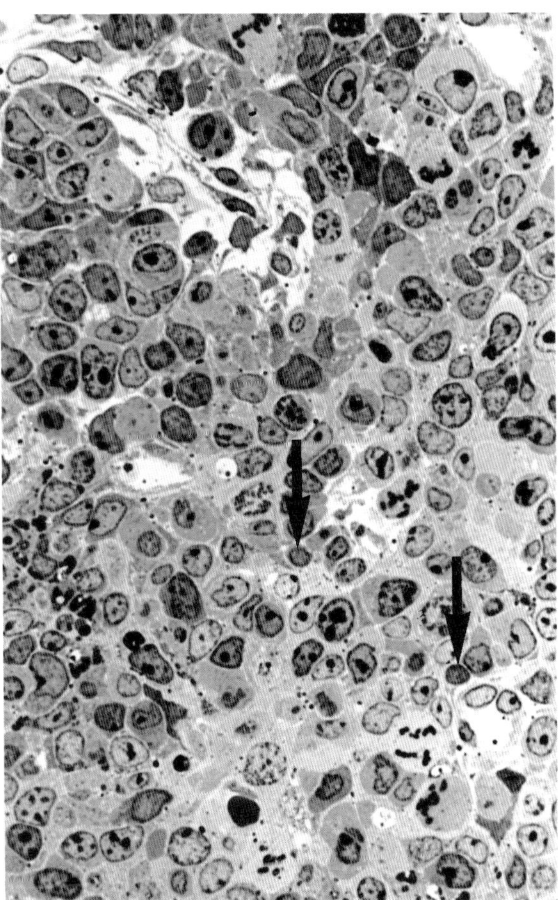

Fig. 276. Thymus, Wistar rat embryo, 15.5 day of fetal life. A few lymphocytes *(arrows)* are visible. A connective tissue strand with capillary grows from the capsule into the epithelial network. Epon-embedded, toluidine blue, × 700

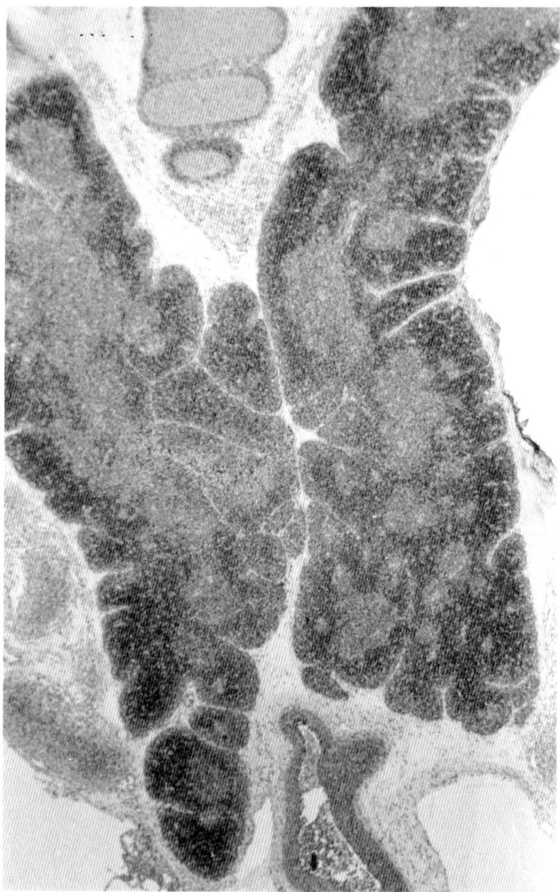

Fig. 277. Thymus with cortex-medulla differentiation. Wistar rat, 0.5 day old. H and E, ×33

Fig. 278 *(upper left).* Thymus, 23-month-old male Wistar ▶ rat. Some epithelial proliferation *(arrow).* H and E, ×33

Fig. 279 *(lower left).* Higher magnification of Fig. 278, as indicated by *arrow.* Small cyst filled with colloidal material. H and E, ×330

Fig. 280 *(upper right).* Thymus, 21-month-old female Wistar rat. Epithelial proliferation with cyst formation. H and E, ×33

Fig. 281 *(lower right).* Thymus, 17-month-old male Wistar rat. Reticulin fibers around blood vessels and crossing perivascular spaces. Some collagenous fibers are visible *(arrow).* Perfusion fixation, Gomori's stain, ×130

Macrophages and Interdigitating Cells

In addition to lymphocytes, other important bone marrow-derived cells invade the thymus during ontogeny. These include interdigitating cells, which can have an antigen-presenting function, and macrophages (Duijvesteijn et al. 1984; Owen and Jenkinson 1984). At day 17 of fetal life (day 14 in mice), some macrophages can be found in the thymus. They are irregularly shaped cells with an indented, heterochromatic, often eccentrically located nucleus and are highly phagocytic. Interdigitating cells can be found at day 19 of fetal life in the already formed medulla. They have a voluminous, pale cytoplasm and an irregular outline with cell processes interdigitating with the surrounding lymphocytes. The nucleus is indented, relatively heterochromatic, and slightly eccentric. Duijvesteijn et al. (1984) observed that the distribution pattern of these two cell populations compared well with the fully developed thymus after an obviously vascularized corticomedullary area was formed, about 1 week after birth. Interdigitating cells are Ia positive. However, it is still questionable whether the origin of Ia in the thymus is bone marrow derived or epithelial (Duijvesteijn et al. 1984; Jenkinson et al. 1980).

Epithelial Cells

The epithelial cells in the fetal thymus are interconnected with desmosomes and have numerous polyribosomes and only a few tonofilaments (Duijvesteijn et al. 1984). With age, the cells become more reticular, tonofilaments are more conspicuous, and the cytoplasm contains fewer polyribosomes. Before birth, the cortical epithelial cells differ from the medullary epithelial cells in

dulla more pronounced, and this proliferation continues for a few months after birth (Fig. 277). Not only the number but also the phenotype differs between cortical and medullary lymphocytes, although almost all are of the T-cell lineage. Cortical lymphocytes are less differentiated and mature than the medullary cells (see p. 254, this volume).

In the adult thymus, lymphocyte depletion is seen as an overall decrease of the number of thymocytes, a decrease of the cortex : medulla ratio, and an irregularity of the cortex/medulla lining. However, until an old age is reached there is often a distinct cortex and medulla visible on the basis of lymphocyte density (Fig. 276). At present, no systematic studies have been performed on age-related changes in the number and functional characteristics of thymocytes.

A few B lymphocytes can be observed in the adult and old thymus. Follicles are rare; in Wistar rats they were occasionally observed in a single rat at the age of 3 months (Kuper et al. 1986).

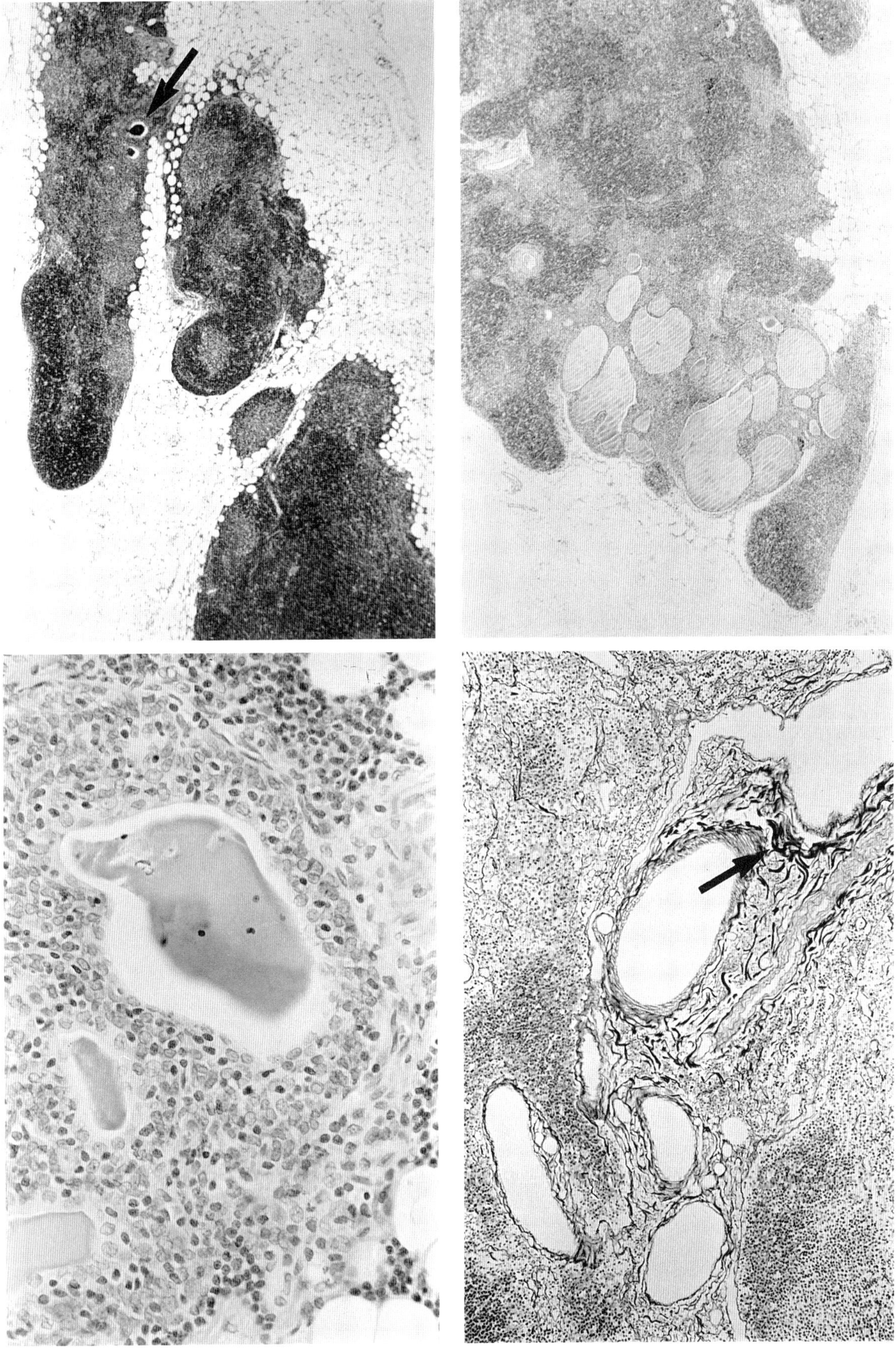

morphology and immunocytochemical identity, as in the completely developed thymus (see p. 251, this volume).

Ontogeny studies in mice revealed that epithelial cells with cytokeratin staining specific for cortical epithelial cells were detected first in fetal life (Savino and Dardenne 1988). As mentioned above, it is not clear whether early Ia-positive cells in the thymus are of epithelial (Jenkinson et al. 1980) or macrophage origin (Duijvestein et al. 1984). Age-related diminution of the epithelial reticulum is accompanied by fatty tissue development which is seen first in the septa and connective tissue capsule. Based on conventionally stained sections it appears that the cortical network diminishes the most. To our knowledge, no immunohistochemical studies on the epithelial network have been performed in old rats. In mice, the number of specific subsets of medullary epithelial cells clearly decreased with age (Savino and Dardenne 1988).

Epithelial cords can be observed at the periphery of the lobules and in the interlobular septa in almost every thymus after birth (Plagge 1946). They are more frequent and extensive in old rats, especially in females (Meihuizen and Burek 1976; Kuper et al. 1986). Small tubules occur mainly in females at about 3 months after birth. With age, these tubular structures can become fairly large and even cystic (Figs. 276–280).

The epithelial cells that form the cords and tubules are characterized by a round or irregularly shaped nucleus without prominent nucleoli and lightly stained cytoplasm. Cystic structures often contain acidophilic material that reacts positively to periodic acid-Schiff reagent. A number of the epithelial cells are ciliated and have secretory granules and a well-developed Golgi complex, indicating that the cells actively secrete a product (Cherry et al. 1967; Meihuizen and Burek 1978).

It is suggested that nonsecreted thymic hormone is stored in the granules (Meihuizen and Burek 1978; Hirokawa et al. 1982). Nabarra and Adrianarison (1987) indicated that the cord structures resemble cystic cavities found in young and adult mice.

Hassall's bodies, medullary epithelial components, are not very conspicuous in the rat thymus and appear to become even less so with aging.

Connective Tissue

In addition to the epithelial component, mesenchymal cells are part of the thymic stroma. At about day 16 of fetal life, connective tissue invades the epithelial primordia, forming a capsule and dividing the gland into lobules through septa that penetrate the parenchyma (Fig. 276). Lobulation of the organ is distinct just before birth. The septa carry along nerves and blood vessels. Reticulin fibers around the vessels increase with age, not only relatively due to involution of the organ but also because of a true increase (Fig. 281) (Christensen 1952). In 1-year-old rats, degeneration of argyrophil fibers can be observed. Collagen fibers are conspicuous in old rats.

Other Cells

Mast cells, granulocytes, and plasma cells are found normally only in minor quantities. They reside not in the thymic parenchyma but in the fibrous capsule, septae, and perivascular spaces. Changes in the number of mast cells during aging are not remarkable. Granulocytes and plasma cells increase slightly with age.

References

Cherry CP, Eisenstein R, Glucksmann A (1967) Epithelial cords and tubules of the rat thymus: effects of age, sex, castration, of sex, thyroid and other hormones on their incidence and secretory activity. Br J Exp Pathol 48: 90–106

Christensen S (1952) Studies on variations of the argyrophile network in the rat's thymus correlated with the age-groups. Acta Anat 16: 221–232

Cordier AC, Haumont SM (1980) Development of thymus, parathyroids, and ultimobranchial bodies in NMRI and Nude mice. Am J Anat 157: 227–263

Duijvestijn AM, Sminia T, Kohler YG, Janse EM, Hoefsmit ECM (1984) Ontogeny of the rat thymus micro-environment: development of the interdigitating cell and macrophage populations. Dev Comp Immunol 8: 451–460

Hirokawa K, Sato K, Makinodan T (1982) Restoration of impaired immune functions in aging animals. V. Long-term immunopotentiating effects of combined young bone marrow and newborn thymus grafts. Clin Immunol Immunopathol 22 (3): 297–304

Jenkinson EJ, Owen JJT, Aspinall R (1980) Lymphocyte differentiation and major histocompatibility complex antigen expression in the embryonic thymus. Nature 284: 177–179

Kendall MD (1981) Age and seasonal changes in the thymus. In: Kendall MD (ed) The thymus gland. Academic, New York, pp 21–37

Kuper CF, Beems RB, Hollanders VMH (1986) Spontaneous pathology of the thymus in aging Wistar (Cpb:WU) rats. Vet Pathol 23: 270-277

Meihuizen SP, Burek JD (1976) The epithelial cell component of thymic tissue in aging female BN/Bi rats. In: Ben-Shaul Y (ed) Electron microscopy, vol 2. Tal International, Israel, pp 569-570

Meihuizen SP, Burek JD (1978) The epithelial cell component of the thymuses of aged female BN/Bi rats. A light microscopic, electron microscopic and autoradiographic study. Lab Invest 39: 613-623

Nabarra B, Andrianarison I (1987) Ultrastructural studies of thymic reticulum: I. Epithelial component. Thymus 9: 95-121

Owen JJT, Jenkinson EJ (1984) Early events in T lymphocyte genesis in the fetal thymus. Am J Anat 170: 301-310

Plagge JC (1946) Some effects of prolonged massive estrogen treatment on the rat. With special reference to the thymus. Arch Pathol 42: 598-606

Ritter MA, Gordon LK, Goldschneider I (1978) Distribution of identity of Thy-1-bearing cells during ontogeny in rat hemopoietic and lymphoid tissues. J Immunol 121: 2463-2471

Ross MA, Korenchevsky V (1941) The thymus of the rat and sex hormones. J Pathol Bacteriol 52: 349-360

Savino W, Dardenne M (1988) Developmental studies on expression of monoclonal antibody-defined cytokeratins by thymic epithelial cells from normal and autoimmune mice. J Histochem Cytochem 36: 1123-1129

Witschi E (1962) Development: the rat. In: Altman PL, Dittmer DS (eds) Growth including reproduction and morphological development. Federation of American Societies for Experimental Biology, Washington DC, pp 304-314

Lymphoblastic Lymphomas, Mouse

Gerhard R. F. Krueger

Synonyms. Lymphoid neoplasm; lymphocytic leukemia; malignant lymphoma, poorly differentiated lymphocytic type (Rappaport); thymic lymphoma; T-cell lymphoma.

Gross Appearance

Most lymphoblastic lymphomas of the mouse appear to originate in the thymus, though not necessarily from thymic lymphocytes (see *Etiology* and *Pathogenesis*). The initial gross lesion is reduction in thymic size (thymic atrophy). Subsequently, one lobe enlarges by nodular lymphomatous infiltration which spreads progressively to involve the entire organ. At this time, the thymus may measure up to 1 cm in diameter, yet also unremarkable thymuses can be entirely replaced by leukemic cells (Fig. 282). The organ is pale-pink in color, has a fish flesh appearance, and is friable. Subsequently enlarged lymph nodes exhibit similar changes.

Microscopic Features

Note: The classification of these neoplasms is based entirely on cytologic/histologic criteria (Dunn 1954). Lymphoblastic lymphomas represent, however, a biologically heterogeneous group of tumors with differing etiopathogenesis and variable immunological cell types. The ultimate characterization of individual lymphoblastic lymphomas thus should include immunological cell typing (Krueger and Meyer 1982) (see p. 122, this volume).

Lymphoblastic lymphomas consist of a homogeneous population of large size lymphoid cells (9–11 μm in diameter) with a moderate amount of cytoplasm containing azurophilic, peroxidase-negative granules (Figs. 283, 284). Cells from certain, more mature lymphoblastic lymphomas may exhibit a focal paranuclear α-naphthylace-

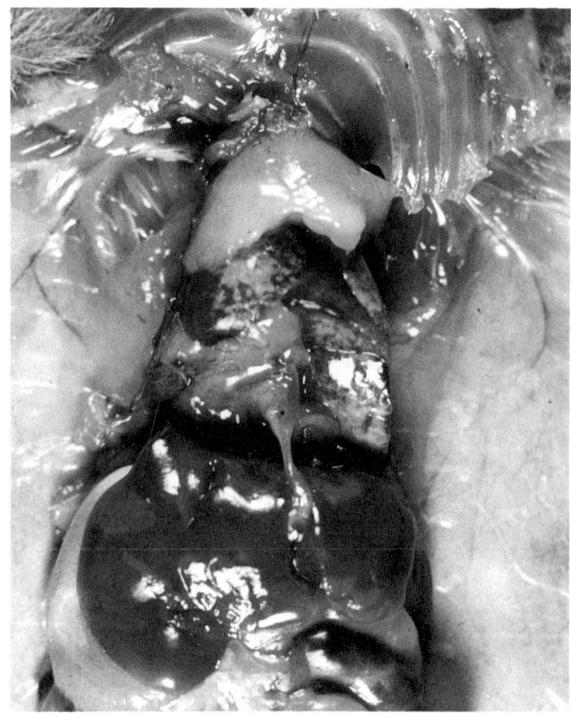

Fig. 282. M-MuLV-induced lymphoblastic lymphoma, BALB/c mouse, 20 weeks after infection. Enlarged thymus occupying the anterior part of the thoracic cavity

tate esterase reaction (ANAE) characteristic for T lymphocytes, other less mature cells a terminal deoxynucleotidyl transferase reaction (TdT). Slightly vesicular, sometimes irregular nuclei of lymphoblasts contain prominent nucleoli usually in a central location (Fig. 285). Mitoses are generally frequent, depending on the rate of cell turnover. Debris-laden macrophages may result in a "starry sky" phenomenon (Fig. 286).

Immunologic cell typing reveals T- and B-cell lymphomas at various stage of cellular differentiation, although most lymphoblastic lymphomas of the mouse are of T-cell type (Krueger and Konorza 1979; Krueger 1979; Krueger and

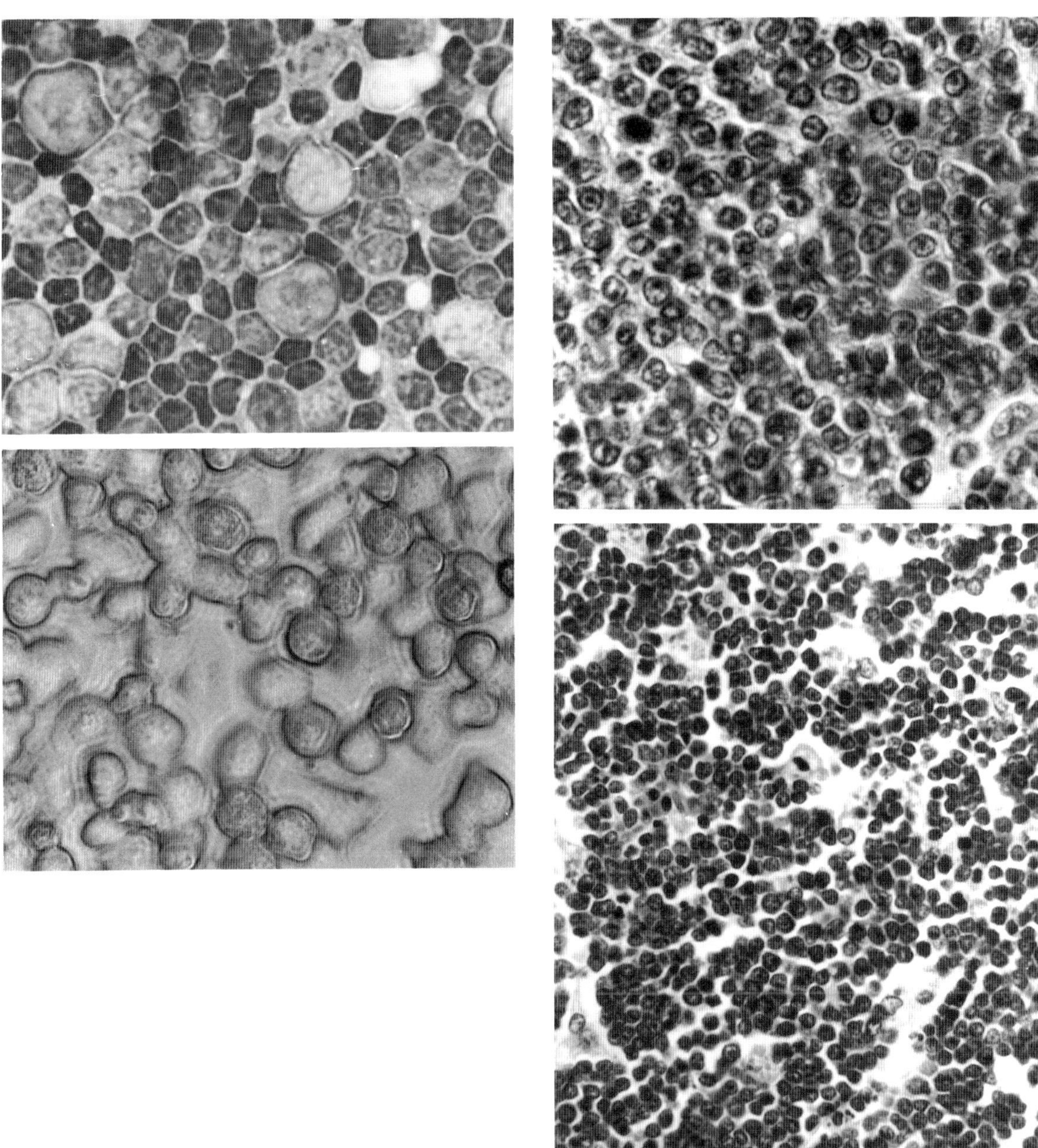

Fig. 283 *(upper left).* M-MuLV-induced lymphoblastic lymphoma, BALB/c mouse. Cytology of initial stage with large blast cells replacing thymic cortical population of small lymphocytes. Wright-Giemsa stein, × 1500

Fig. 284 *(lower left).* M-MuLV-induced lymphoblastic lymphoma, BALB/c mouse. Outgrowth of monomorphic blasts in tissue culture from thymic lymphoma. Phase contrast, × 600

Fig. 285 *(upper right).* Lymphoblastic lymphoma, lymph node, BALB/c mouse. Diffuse population of lymphoblasts with prominent nucleoli. H and E, × 470

Fig. 286 *(lower right).* Lymph node, mouse, lymphoblastic lymphoma. Scattered large macrophages producing "starry sky" pattern. H and E, × 340

Table 45. Immunotyping of mouse lymphoblastic lymphomas

Mouse	Lymphoma induction	Marker	Cell Type
BALB/cAnN	M-MuLV	Thy1, TLa, TdT	T cell
BALB/cHAN	M-MuLV	TLa, TdT	T cell prethymic
BALB/cAnN	Immunologic[a]	Thy1, TLa	T cell
BALB/c	A-MuLV	T/B marker $\varnothing$ TCRa,β germline J_{11} rearranged	T cell lineage, early stage of differentiation
C57Bl	G-MuLV	Thy1, Ly1	T cell
C57Bl	A-MuLV	like BALB/c + A-MuLV	
C57Bl	Radiation	Thy1, TdT, TLa, H2	T cell intermediate maturity
C57Bl	DMBA	Thy1, TdT, Ly1	T cell, corticomedullary
C57Bl	NBU	Thy1, Ly1,2,3	T cell, medullary
C57Br	G-MuLV	Thy1, TLa, TdT, IA	T cell, cortical activated
C57L	A-MuLV	Ly4, Fc	B cell
AKR	Spontaneous	Ly2	T cell
AKR	Spontaneous post thymectomy	TdT, Ly2,3	T cell
A	Radiation	Thy1, TLa	T cell
A	Spontaneous	Thy1, TLa, TdT	T cell
C58	Spontaneous	Thy1, TLa, TdT	T cell
B6xA	Radiation	Thy1, TLa, TdT	T cell

[a] Krueger et al. (1971).

Meyer 1982; Pattengale and Frith 1983; Frederickson et al. 1985). Table 45 summarizes the results of immunologic cell typing in various mouse lymphomas.

Ultrastructure

In semithin sections of the thymic lymphoma the majority of cells resemble immature lymphoid elements (Figs. 287–289). Such immature cells amount to 60%–70% of the total lymphoid population in the thymic cortex until about 6 weeks after birth with a rise to nearly 90% beyond the 11th week in most thymic lymphomas of young mice. There exists some variation in the course of lymphoma development, however, depending upon the kind of induction (see *Biologic Features*). Lymphoblasts contain large nuclei with quite evenly distributed chromatin. Nucleoli are always prominent. The amount of cytoplasm is usually moderate, rich in ribosomes, with few cytoplasmic organelles (Fig. 290). Reticular epithelial cells are common, with features of a more immature cell (Fig. 291). They possess a relatively large nucleus with a smooth nuclear membrane and a homogeneous distribution of chromatin. The cytoplasm contains few vacuoles, tonofibrils are scant, and short, blunt, cytoplasm processes extend between the lymphoblasts. In addition, dark stellate cells are noted, resembling degenerating reticular epithelial cells.

Quantitation of reticular epithelial cells in Moloney virus-infected mice reveals an obvious loss of this cell type preceding lymphoma development with reduction in thymopoietin production. At 12–15 weeks, degenerative changes of the reticular epithelial cells are widely manifested and lead to complete destruction of most of these cells (Heine et al. 1983; Krueger et al. 1983). Similar thymic epithelial cell changes are observed in prelymphomatous thymuses after diphenylhydantoin treatment of mice (Bedoya and Krueger 1978). In Moloney virus-induced lymphomas, C type virus particles are seen in the intercellular spaces in increasing numbers 11 weeks after virus infection, and virions are released by budding from the cytoplasmic membrane from both lymphoblasts and reticular epithelial cells (Fig. 292). In some instances, virus production is very intense, with the accumulation of numerous virions in the endoplasmic reticulum of reticular epithelial cells and in the extracellular spaces. C type particles are also noted similarly in other virus-induced lymphoblastic lymphomas as well as in chemically and immunologically induced lymphomas, although they are less numerous in the latter.

At the time of systemic development of lymphoma, atypical lymphoblastic infiltration of other tissues and organs is composed of cells as described in the thymus (except for reticular epithelial cells) associated with varying numbers of debris-laden macrophages.

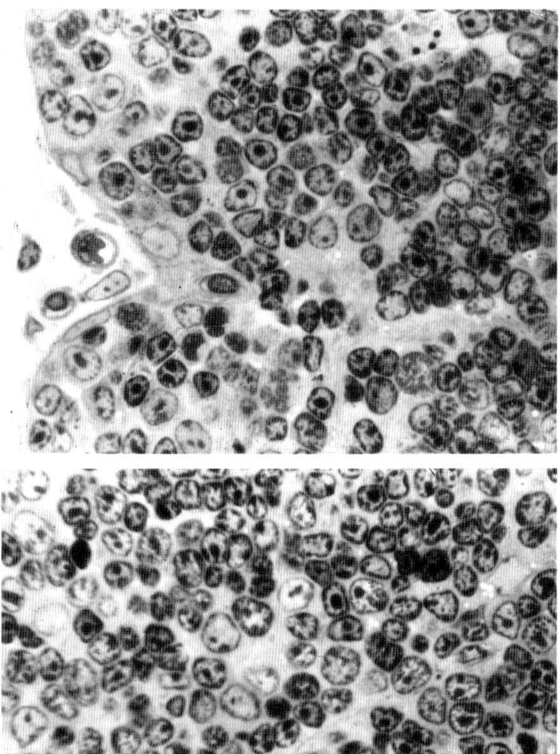

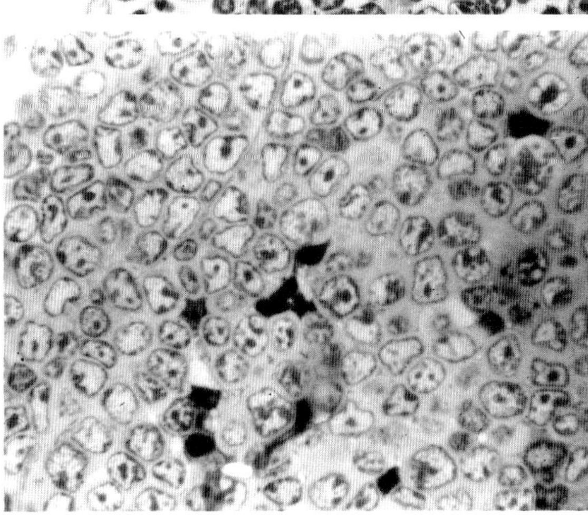

Fig. 287 *(above).* Thymus, uninfected control mouse at 11 weeks. Note mixed population of maturing small lymphoblasts/lymphocytes in cortex with subcapsular germinal layer of blasts. Toluidine blue, ×620

Fig. 288 *(middle).* Thymus, M-MuLV-infected mouse at 3 weeks after infection. Note lymphoblasts with prominent nucleoli and pale immature reticular epithelial cells. Toluidine blue, ×620

Fig. 289 *(below).* Thymus, M-MuLV-infected mouse at 11 weeks after infection. Note homogeneous population of immature lymphoblasts. Toluidine blue, ×620

Differential Diagnosis

There are no specific problems in the histologic differential diagnosis of lymphoblastic lymphomas; the uniform infiltration of involved organs by a monotonous population of typical lymphoblasts with or without the "starry sky" pattern is quite characteristic. If the Rappaport classification for human lymphomas is applied to the mouse (Krueger and Meyer 1982), in poor preparations some difficulties may arise in distinguishing lymphoblastic lymphomas convoluted cell type from poorly differentiated lymphocytic lymphomas. However, as far as we know, this has no influence on the biologic course of the disease. Poorly differentiated lymphocytic lymphomas may be somewhat more mature than lymphoblastic ones (Krueger and Meyer 1982), yet final cell typing should be accomplished by immunological methods. (It may be added that lymphoblastic lymphomas of convoluted cell type in humans are usually T-cell lymphomas; this is not so in experimental animals (Krueger and Konorza 1979).

Biologic Features

Natural History

The target organ for the development of most spontaneous and induced lymphoblastic lymphomas in the mouse is the thymus, although it is not clear whether this organ is uniformly the site of actual neoplastic transformation; chemically and virally induced lymphomas can also develop in thymectomized mice (Haran-Ghera 1980). In intact mice, lymphoma development is preceded by gross thymic atrophy which does not necessarily reflect an equally obvious quantitative loss of lymphocytes (Haas et al. 1982). During this time, "atypical" lymphoid cells (see later "preleukemic cells") can be demonstrated in the bone marrow and in the hemopoietic pulp of the spleen (prelymphomatous stage). In virus-induced lymphomas such cells frequently carry viral antigens (Krueger et al. 1978, 1980).

Subsequently, foci of lymphoblasts colonize the atrophic thymus, usually starting within one lobe (Fig. 293) and spreading from there to involve the entire thymus and the mediastinum. During the further course of the disease, distant lymphatic and nonlymphatic organs become infiltrated by lymphoblasts (Figs. 294, 295). These cells diffusely infiltrate lymphoid tissues and cause complete

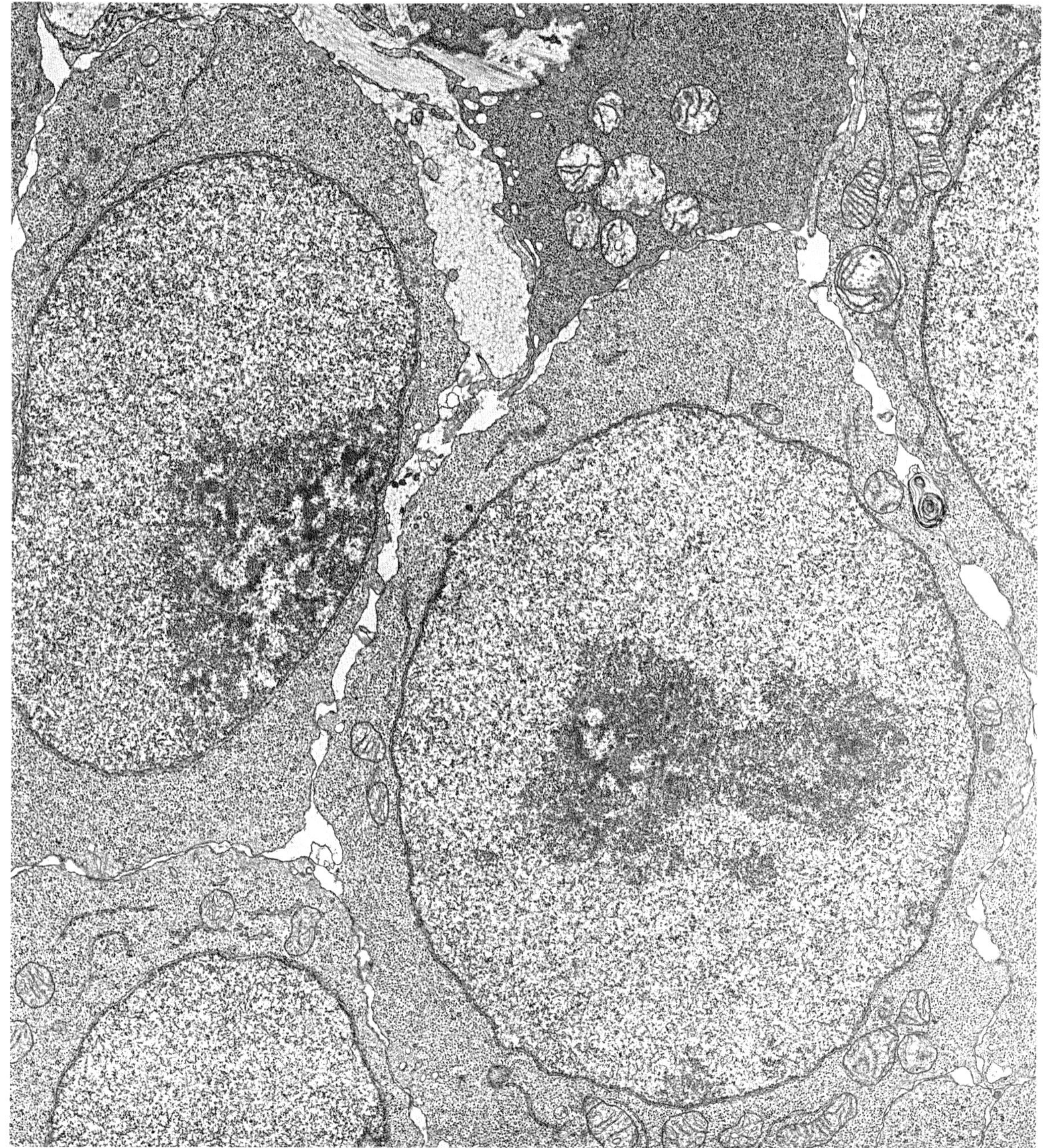

Fig. 290. Thymic lymphoma, mouse. Large immature lymphoblasts with prominent nucleoli and abundant ribosomes in cytoplasm. TEM, ×6200

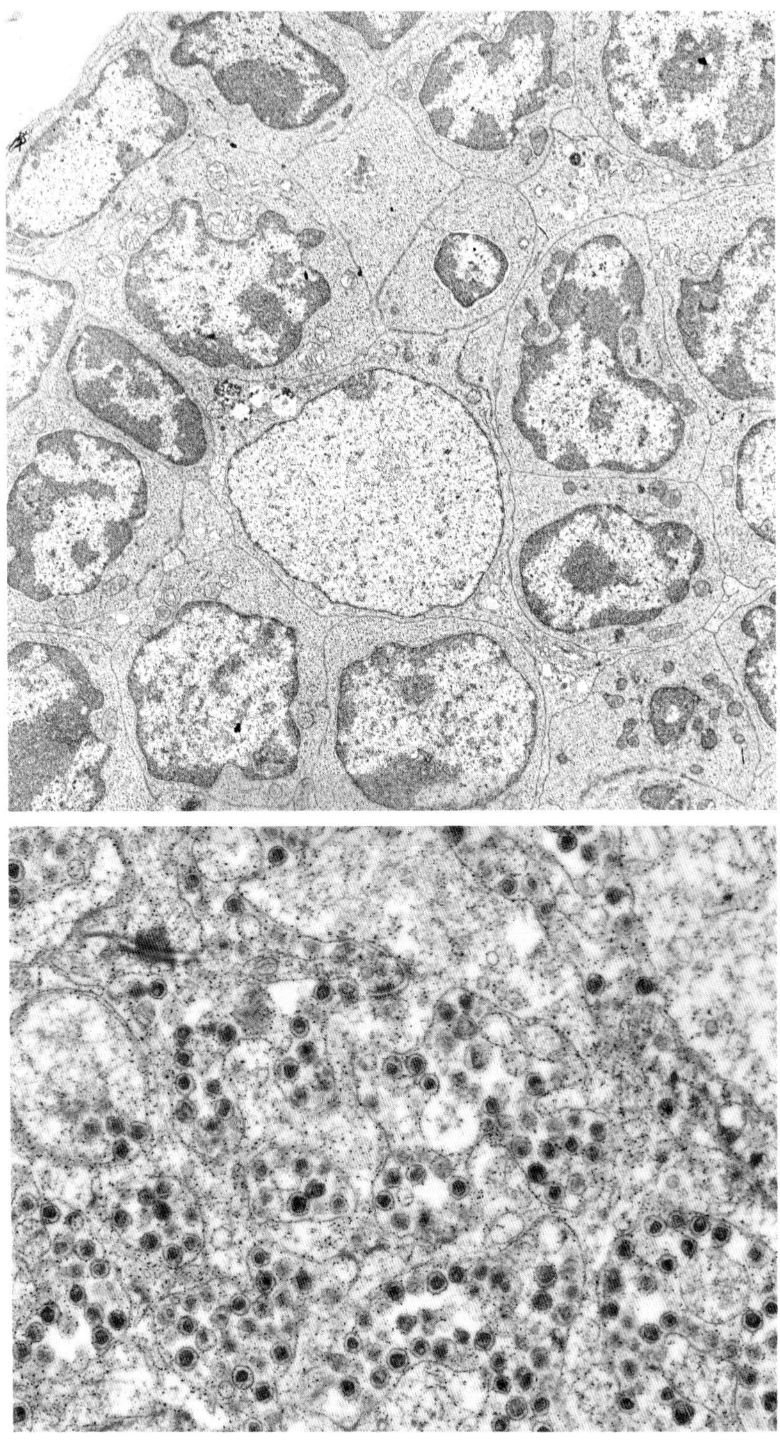

Fig. 291 *(above).* Thymus, mouse, 11 weeks after M-MuLV infection. Note immature reticular epithelial cell *(center)* with pale nucleus. TEM, ×437

Fig. 292 *(below).* Reticular epithelial cell in M-MuLV-infected mouse. Note abundant, mature, type C virions in endoplasmic spaces. Desmosomes in *upper left hand corner* characterize epithelial cell. TEM, ×21 100

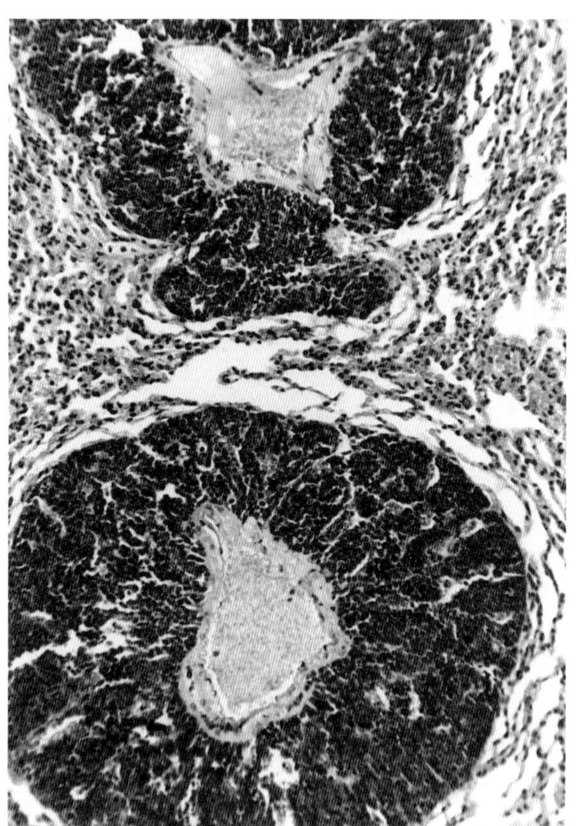

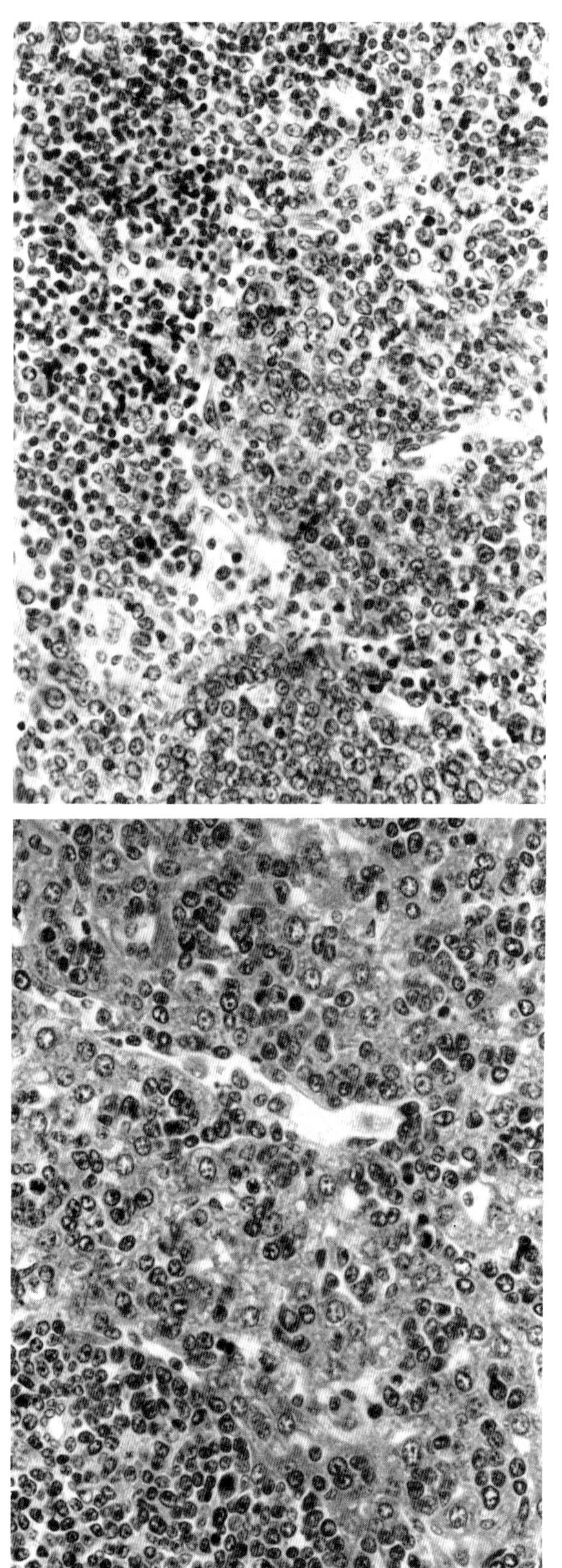

Fig. 293 *(upper left)*. Thymus, mouse, 8 weeks after M-MuLV infection. Early foci of lymphoblasts in atropic cortex indicate atypical cell proliferation. H and E, × 470

Fig. 294 *(lower left)*. Liver, mouse, 20 weeks after M-MuLV infection. Extensive nodular and sinusoidal infiltration by lymphomatous lymphoblasts. H and E, × 470

Fig. 295 *(upper right)*. Lung, mouse, 28 weeks after M-MuLV infection. Extensive nodular (perivascular and peribronchial) lymphomatous infiltration. H and E, × 120

Table 46. Incidence and latent period of some mouse lymphoblastic lymphomas

Mouse[a]	Lymphoma induction	Incidence	Latent period (L) or time of death (D)
BALB/c	M-MuLV	95%	11–12 WKS (L)
BALB/c	G-MuLV	75%	12–20 WKS (L)
BALB/c	A-MuLV	61%	4– 5 WKS (L)
BALB/c	Immunologically[b]	66%	20–24 WKS (L)
BALB/c	Spontaneous	3%	16 MOS (L)
C57Bl	A-MuLV	61%	4– 5 WKS (L)
C57Bl	NBU	95%	11 WKS (L)
C57Bl	X-ray	70%	250 D (D)
C57Bl	Phenytoin	12%	8 MOS (L)
AKR	Spontaneous	90%	12 MOS (L)
NMRI	Spontaneous	44%	18 MOS (L)
RF	Alkylating agents	16%–35%	340 D (D)
SJL	Phenytoin	25%	4– 8 MOS (L)

[a] See also the classic publication of Dunham and Stewart 1953.
[b] Krueger et al. 1971.
WKS, weeks; MOS, months; D, days.

effacement of their structure. Involvement of nonlymphoid organs is characterized by focal or diffuse lymphoblastic infiltration with secondary atrophy of parenchymal tissues rather than sarcomatous invasion and destruction. The bone marrow is regularly involved with peripheral blood lymphoblastosis; thus, in the literature lymphoblastic lymphoma and leukemia are frequently used synonymously. Cause of death appears frequently to be due to respiratory distress secondary to massive pulmonary involvement, cachexia, or failure of the central nervous system with extensive cerebral lymphoma.

The latent period of lymphoma development varies according to the type of oncogen (virus strain, carcinogen), the strain and age of the mouse, as well as the type and extent of copathogenic effects. Newborn mice are most susceptible, and following experimental induction, the tumor incidence decreases rapidly beyond 4 weeks of age (i. e., with immunologic maturity). Table 46 provides a review of incidence and latent periods of lymphoblastic lymphomas in various mice after experimental induction.

The quantitative behavior of individual lymphocyte populations during lymphoma development can be studied by immunotyping and cell sorter studies. Figures 296–299 include representative examples for such testing of thymic and lymph node lymphocytes during the development of a poorly and a well-differentiated T-cell lymphoma. Absolute cell numbers for a Moloney virus-induced BALB/c lymphoma are given in

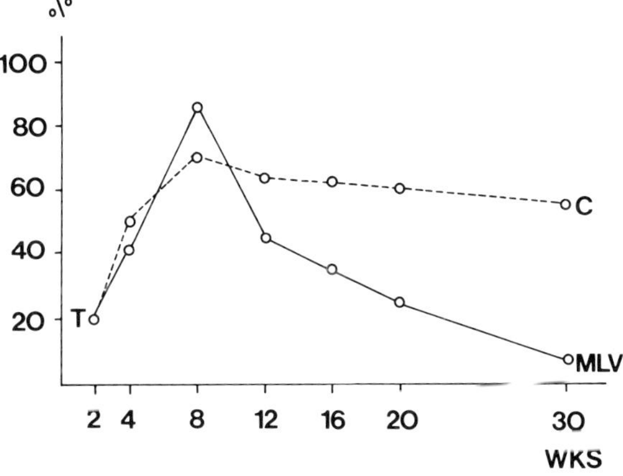

Fig. 296. Distribution of Thy+ thymic lymphocytes in thymus during M-MuLV-induced lymphomagenesis. *Solid line,* infected mice; *dotted line,* uninfected controls

Fig. 300. The data show a progressive accumulation of lymphoblasts with accompanying relative or absolute decrease in all other lymphoid populations.

Studies in cell membrane lipid fluidity indicate an increased fluidity of the cytoplasmic membrane of lymphoma cells, associated with the degree of immaturity of such cells (Krueger et al. 1987).

It may be difficult from the cell values given above to determine exactly the onset of lymphoma or, in other words, the transition from dependent (regenerative) cell proliferation to the state of autonomy. In this case, demonstration of an-

272 Gerhard R. F. Krueger

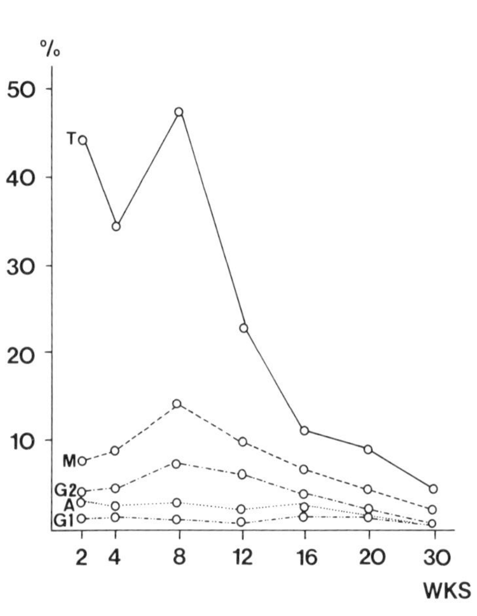

Fig. 297. Distribution of T and B lymphocytes in lymph node during M-MuLV-induced lymphomagenesis. *T,* Thy + cells; *M,* cells with IgM surface immunoglobulin; *G1, G2,* and *A,* B lymphocytes with the respective surface immunoglobulins

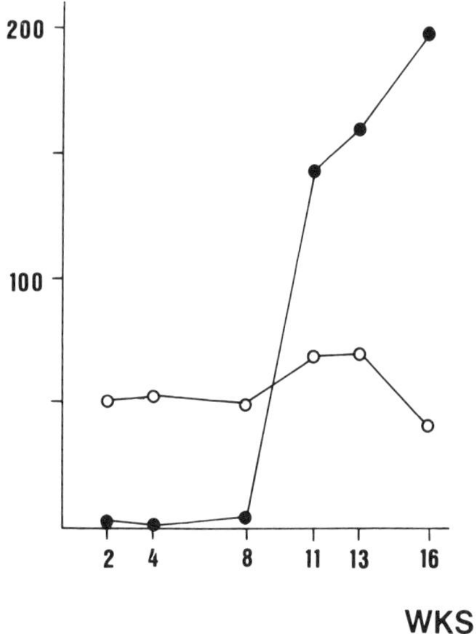

Fig. 298. Total Thy + T cells in thymus during nitrobutyl-urea-induced lymphomagenesis. *Solid circles,* treated mice (for 8 weeks); *open circles,* untreated controls

Fig. 299. Total Thy + T cells in spleen during nitrobutyl-urea-induced lymphomagenesis. *Solid circles,* treated mice; *open circles,* untreated controls

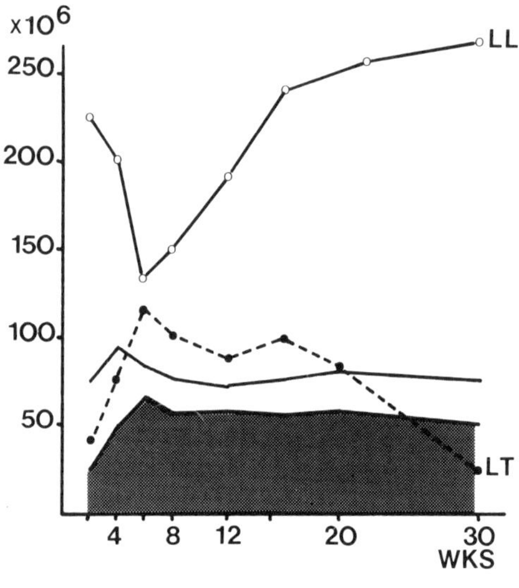

Fig. 300. Total number of lymphocytes and of Thy + T cells in thymus during M-MuLV-induced lymphomagenesis. *LL,* total lymphocytes in M-MuLV-infected mice; *LT,* total Thy + cells in M-MuLV-infected mice; *dark cross-hatched area,* total Thy + cells in uninfected controls; *light area,* total lymphocytes in uninfected controls

euploidy, chromosomal abnormalities, or expression of oncogens may be helpful, although the first two features may not be obvious in lymphoma cells. Aneuploid cells appear during the development of diphenyl-hydantoin-induced lymphoblastic lymphoma (Krueger 1970; Krueger et al. 1972).

Gross cytogenetic abnormalities such as chromosomal breakage and translocations are not equally common in experimental lymphoblastic lymphomas, especially not in virus-induced lymphomas. DNA analysis by immunoglobulin and T cell gene probing may yet reveal gene rearrangements as in human lymphomas (Pattengale et al. 1986). Such studies assist in identifying tumors as T- or B-cell lymphomas even when immunological cell typing remains inconclusive. In addition to such gene rearrangements, deregulated expression of proto-oncogenes (v-*myc*, v-*myb*, v-*mos*, v-*abl*, Ha-*ras*, etc.) can be taken to be indicative of malignant transformation (Pattengale et al. 1986; Cleveland et al. 1986).

Pathogenesis

Development of lymphoblastic lymphomas progresses through a "preleukemic stage" in which atypical cells are detected in the bone marrow, hemopoietic red pulp of the spleen, and thymus by transplantation bioassay or by the above-mentioned genetic studies without clinical manifestation of the disease. During this preleukemic stage, cell changes are observed in lymphoid tissues as shown in Figs. 296–299. Transition to malignant lymphoma is in some cases characterized by an enlarging peak of aneuploid cells in cell sorter studies. Preleukemic cells are detected in the bone marrow (prothymocytes) of AKR mice with leukemia following virus infection and radiation, for instance, as early as 10 days after infection (Haran-Ghera 1980) and in the hemopoietic red pulp of the spleen in BALB/c mice 12–14 days after infection with Moloney virus. Similar foci of atypical lymphoblasts occur in the bone marrow of chemically induced (nitrosobutylurea) T-cell lymphomas before the thymic tumor becomes overt (Hiai et al. 1973). Progression of the preleukemic stage to malignant lymphoma (a clinical definition!) is apparently dependent on specific genetic, environmental, and microenvironmental factors. Genetic control is linked to the H-2 locus of the histocompatibility complex conferring resistance or susceptibility to leukemogenesis (Lilly and Pincus 1973). Environmental factors in addition to the presence of leukemogenic viruses include coleukemogenic influences such as radiation, ultraviolet radiation, and certain chemicals. Many of these interfere with or significantly depress the state of immunological reactivity of the susceptible animal, and immune deficiency has been shown repeatedly to constitute a significant cofactor in the development of malignant lymphomas (Krueger 1972; Penn 1984).

Microenvironmental influences comprise varying effects of the cells of the thymus on cell proliferation (e. g., by mitogenic proteins of macrophages) and cell differentiation (e. g. by differentiation factors such as thymopoietins) (Krueger 1985; Krueger and Karpinski 1990). In their model, any decrease in quantity or in effectiveness of differentiation factors in favor of an absolute or relative increase in proliferation factors will support progressive (lymphomatous) lymphoproliferation. This "lymphoma-prone condition" can be brought about by quite different etiological influences.

Etiology

No unifying concept is presently available for the etiology of cancer in general or for lymphomas specifically. This problem arises in part from the fact that cancer is defined clinically, i. e., by the "social behavior" of certain "atypical" cells in a multicellular organism, while investigations in basic research primarily detect abnormalities in individual cells which taken per se may not be exclusively specific for tumor cells. Thus cancer, i. e., lymphoma in this context, appears to be a biological rather than a molecular problem (see also pathogenesis). This notion, however, should not detract from the immense accomplishments in virus tumor research, and as stated before, lymphoblastic lymphomas in the mouse to a great extent appear to be caused by viruses. The essential changes in the etiology of virus-induced lymphomas as in other viral tumors appear to be chromosomal translocation and oncogen activation (viral or cellular oncogens) leading to the synthesis of autocrine growth factors (Nowell and Croce 1986; Bishop 1986; Tronick and Aaronson 1986). Essential also for the development of malignant behavior of cells is oncogene amplification and gene dosage in a multistep mechanism (Klein 1981; Land et al. 1983; Klein 1986). Oncogene amplification uncorrected by cellular repair mechanisms seems especially important since oncogens as such are not specific for tumor cells (Duesberg 1983, 1987). Since it will exceed the task of this chapter to go into further detail, the reader may refer to the pertinent scientific literature (Phillips 1983; Notkins and Oldstone 1986).

Frequency

Lymphoblastic lymphomas occur spontaneously in certain inbred strains and may be experimentally induced by various agents. An overview is given in Table 46.

Comparison with Other Species

Lymphoblastic lymphomas of similar histology as in the mouse occur in several species, spontaneously or experimentally induced (Krueger 1977): in fish, birds, rats, *Mastomys*, cattle, pig, dogs, cats (frequent), and monkeys (frequent). In common is the growth pattern of an initial solitary nodule (thymic/mediastinal or extramediastinal) with subsequent systemic spread. A leukemic phase does not occur necessarily in all species. A large number of spontaneous lymphomas appear to be related to infection or reactivation of oncogenic viruses. The cytology of thymic lymphomas in childhood most clearly resembles that seen in other species.

Acknowledgment. Dedicated to Thelma B. Dunn, M. D., my admired and respected teacher in mouse pathology at the National Cancer Institute (1965–1972).

References

Bedoya V, Krueger GRF (1978) Ultrastructural studies on hydantoin induced lymphomas in mice. Z Krebsforsch 91: 195–204

Bishop JM (1986) Amplification of proto-oncogenes in tumorigenesis. In: Notkins AL, Oldstone MB (eds) Concepts in viral pathogenesis. Springer, Berlin Heidelberg New York, pp 71–78

Cleveland JL, Weinstein Y, Ihle JN, Askew DS, Rapp UR (1986) Transformation and insertional mutagenesis in vitro of primary hematopoietic stem cell cultures. Curr Top Microbiol Immunol 132: 44–54

Duesberg PH (1983) Retroviral transforming genes in normal cells? Nature 304: 219–226

Duesberg PH (1987) Retrovirus as carcinogens and pathogens: expectation and reality. Cancer Res 47: 1199–1220

Dunham LJ, Stewart HL (1953) A survey of transplantable and transmissible animal tumors. JNCI 13: 1299–1377

Dunn TB (1954) Normal and pathologic anatomy of the reticular tissue in laboratory mice, with a classification and discussion of neoplasms. JNCI 14: 1281–1433

Frederickson TN, Morse HC III, Yetter RA, Rowe WP, Hartley JW, Pattengale PK (1985) Multiparameter analysis of spontaneous nonthymic lymphomas occurring in NFS/N mice congenic for ecotropic murine leukemia viruses. JNCI 121: 349–360

Haas W, Deyng TH, Krueger GRF, Feaux de Lacroix W (1982) Autoradiographic and immunocytologic identification of atypical cell proliferation during Moloney virus induced lymphoma development. In: Yohn DS, Blakeslee JR (eds) Advances in comparative leukemia research 1981. Elsevier, Amsterdam, pp 241–243

Haran-Ghera N (1980) Pathogenesis of murine leukemia. In: Klein G (ed) Viral oncology. Raven, New York, pp 161–185

Heine UI, Krueger GRF, Karpinski A, Munoz E, Krueger MB (1983) Quantitative light and electron microscopic changes in thymic reticular epithelial cells during Moloney-virus-induced lymphoma development. J Cancer Res Clin Oncol 106: 102–111

Hiai H, Shisa H, Matsudaeira Y, Nishizuka Y (1973) Theta antigen in n-nitrosobutylurea leukemogenesis of the mouse. Gann 64: 197–201

Klein G (1981) The role of gene dosage and genetic transpositions in carcinogenesis. Nature 294: 313–318

Klein G (1986) Multistep scenarios in tumor development the role of oncogene activation by chromosomal translocations. In: Notkins AL, Oldstone MB (eds) Concepts in viral pathogenesis II. Springer, Berlin Heidelberg New York, pp 79–88

Krueger GRF (1970) Effect of dilantin in mice. I. Changes in the lymphoreticular tissue after acute exposure. Virchows Arch [A] 349: 297–311

Krueger GRF (1972) Chronic immunosuppression and lymphoma-genesis in man and mice. NCI Monogr 35: 183–190

Krueger GRF (1977) Comparative pathologic classification of malignant lymphomas. Z Krebsforsch 89: 253–272

Krueger GRF (1979) Morphologische und immunologische Klassifikation experimentell erzeugter maligner Lymphome. In: Krueger GRF (ed) Lymphknotentumore. Urban and Schwarzenberg, Munich, pp 55–59

Krueger GRF (1985) Klinische Immunpathologie. Kohlhammer, Stuttgart

Krueger GRF, Karpinski A (1990) Abnormal variation of the immune system as related to cancer. In: Kaiser HE (ed) Progressive stages of neoplastic growth. Kluwer, Dordrecht (in press)

Krueger GRF, Konorza G (1979) Classification of animal lymphomas: the implications of applying Rappaport's classification for human lymphomas to experimental tumors. Exp Hematol 7: 305–314

Krueger GRF, Meyer EM (1982) Classification of malignant lymphomas of the mouse using morphological, immunological, and cytochemical methods: a working proposal. J Cancer Res Clin Oncol 104: 41–52

Krueger GR, Malmgren RA, Berard CW (1971) Malignant lymphomas and plasmacytosis in mice under prolonged immunosuppression and persistent antigenic stimulation. Transplantation 11: 138–144

Krueger GRF, Harris D, Sussman E (1972) Effect of dilantin in mice. II. Lymphoreticular tissue atypia and neoplasia after chronic exposure. Z Krebsforsch 78: 290–302

Krueger GRF, Fischer KM, Flesch HG (1978) Sequential changes of T- and B-cells, virus antigen expression and primary histologic tumor diagnosis in virus-induced lymphomagenesis of mice. Z Krebsforsch 92: 41–54

Krueger GRF, Wichmann M, Huttmann G, Gregorian G, Muller C (1980) Fluidity of lymphocyte membrane during Monoley virus lymphomagenesis. In: Yohn DS, Blakeslee JR (eds) Advances in comparative leukemia research. Elsevier, Amsterdam

Krueger GRF, Karpinski A, Heine UI, Koch B (1983) Differentiation block of prethymic lymphocytes during Moloney-virus-induced lymphoma development associated with a thymic epithelial defect. J Cancer Res Clin Oncol 106: 153–157

Krueger GRF, Stolzenburg TH, Muller C (1987) Cell membrane fluidity and receptor expression in Moloney- and Friend-virus transformed cells. Fed Proc 46: 740

Land H, Parada LF, Weinberg RA (1983) Cellular oncogenes and multistep carcinogenesis. Science 222: 771–778

Lilly F, Pincus T (1973) Genetic control of murine viral leukemogenesis. Adv Cancer Res 17: 231–277

Notkins AL, Oldstone MBA (1986) Concepts in viral pathogenesis, vol II. Springer, Berlin Heidelberg New York

Nowell PC, Croce CM (1986) Oncogene activation by chromosome translocation. In: Notkins AL, Oldstone MD (eds) Concepts in viral pathogenesis II. Springer, Berlin Heidelberg New York, pp 89–97

Pattengale PK, Frith CH (1983) Immunomorphologic classification of spontaneous lymphoid cell neoplasms occurring in female BALB/c mice. JNCI 70: 169–179

Pattengale P, Leder A, Kuo A, Stewart T, Leder P (1986) Lymphohematopoietic and other malignant neoplasms occurring spontaneously in transgenic mice carrying and expressing MTV/myc fusion genes. In: Melchers F, Potter M (eds) Mechanisms in B-cell neoplasia. Springer, Berlin Heidelberg New York, pp 9–16 (Current topics in microbiology and immunology, vol 132)

Penn I (1984) Allograft transplant cancer registry. In: Purtilo DT (ed) Immune deficiency and cancer. Plenum, New York, pp 281–308

Phillips LA (1983) Viruses associated with human cancer. Dekker, New York

Tronick SR, Aaronson SA (1986) Oncogenes, Growth Factors, and Receptors. In: Notkins AL, Oldstone MBA (eds) Concepts in viral pathogenesis II. Springer, Berlin Heidelberg New York, pp 98–109

Thymoma, Lymphocytic, Rat

Mutsushi Matsuyama

Synonyms. Benign thymoma; epithelial thymoma.

Gross Appearance

Large thymomas form a lobular mass occupying a large part of the thoracic cavity in old rats of susceptible strains, compressing the heart and lungs, and measuring 2–4 cm in diameter. In medium-sized thymomas, enlarged right and left lobes are usually demarcated by an anterior midline cleft. They are yellowish-white in color and soft in consistency. The surface is smooth, being surrounded by a distinct tissue capsule and clearly separated from the surrounding tissues. Small thymoma nodules may not be visible with the naked eye in younger rats of the susceptible strains because of their constitutively large thymuses, but they may be discernible in the involuted thymuses of Fl hybrid rats between the susceptible and resistant strains (Matsuyama et al. 1988).

Microscopic Features

Thymomas of the lymphocytic type are essentially composed of darkly stained, cortexlike tissues, which are richly infiltrated with small lymphocytes (Fig. 301). A few medium- and large-sized lymphocytes, sometimes with mitotic figures, pale epithelial cells, and macrophages, are intermingled, with a "starry sky" pattern. The epithelial cells, which are thought to be neoplastic in nature (Matsuyama and Amo 1977), are scattered throughout the thymoma and are polygonal in shape and larger than those in the adjacent involuted thymic tissues (Fig. 302). No medulla is discernible, but a few lightly stained areas, similar to the "foci of medullary differentiation" described in human thymoma (Rosai and Levine 1976), are found (Fig. 301). The foci consist of large epithelial cells, small lymphocytes, macrophages, and interdigitating reticulum cells.

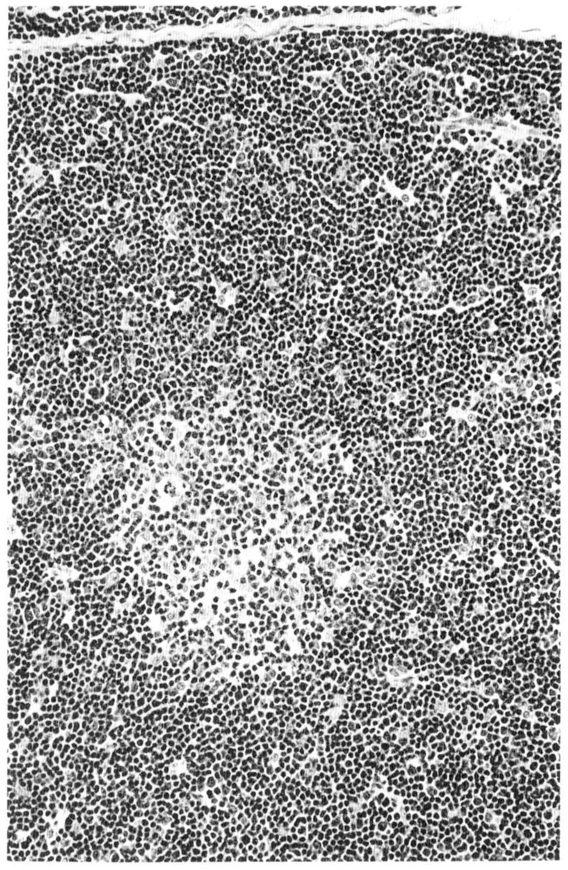

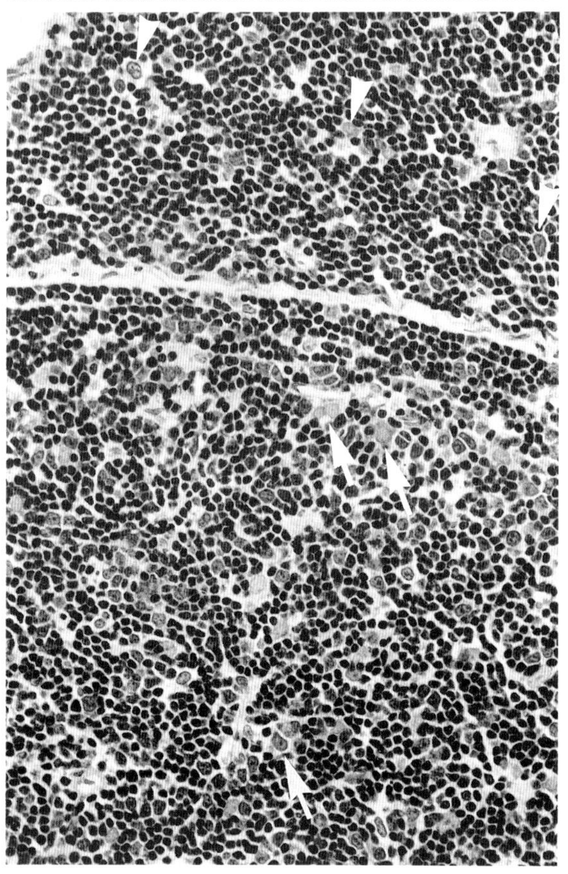

◀ **Fig. 301** *(above).* Thymoma, lymphocytic type, rat. It is composed predominantly of small lymphocytes and a few epithelial cells. A focus of "medullary differentiation" is also seen. H and E, ×35

Fig. 302 *(below).* Thymoma, lymphocytic type, rat. Thymoma nodule *(lower two-thirds).* Involuted thymic lobule *(upper third).* Epithelial cells in the nodule *(arrows)* are larger than those in the involuted thymic lobule *(arrowheads).* H and E, ×270

All thymomas contain thymic epithelium, but in many, lymphoid cells predominate (lymphocytic thymoma), and in a few others, the epithelium predominates (epithelial type) (see p. 280, this volume).

Ultrastructure

Epithelial cells of thymomas extend extremely attenuated cytoplasmic processes, forming a network that contains a large number of lymphocytes (Fig. 303) and sometimes rests on the basal laminae. Many of the epithelial cells have well-developed rough-surfaced endoplastic reticulum and bundles of tonofilaments localized around the nuclei and attached to the desmosomes (Matsuyama et al. 1975; Hinsull and Bellamy 1977; Murray et al. 1985). Rarely, membrane-bound bodies, which are characteristic of thymic epithelial cells in rodents, can be found. Three-dimensional examinations of the thymomas by SEM reveal a complicated network consisting of planklike cytoplasmic processes of epithelial cells embracing lymphocytes (Fig. 304).

Differential Diagnosis

Thymoma of the lymphocytic type can easily be differentiated from malignant lymphoma of the thymus. Lymphocytes are small and have no cellular atypism in thymoma, whereas lymphoma cells are large, with severe atypism. Staining with keratin-specific antisera, preferentially in alcohol-fixed specimens, is useful for detecting epithelial cells in the thymomas.

Biologic Features

The incidence of the spontaneous development of thymoma is high in some susceptible inbred strains (Dunning and Curtis 1946; Pollard and

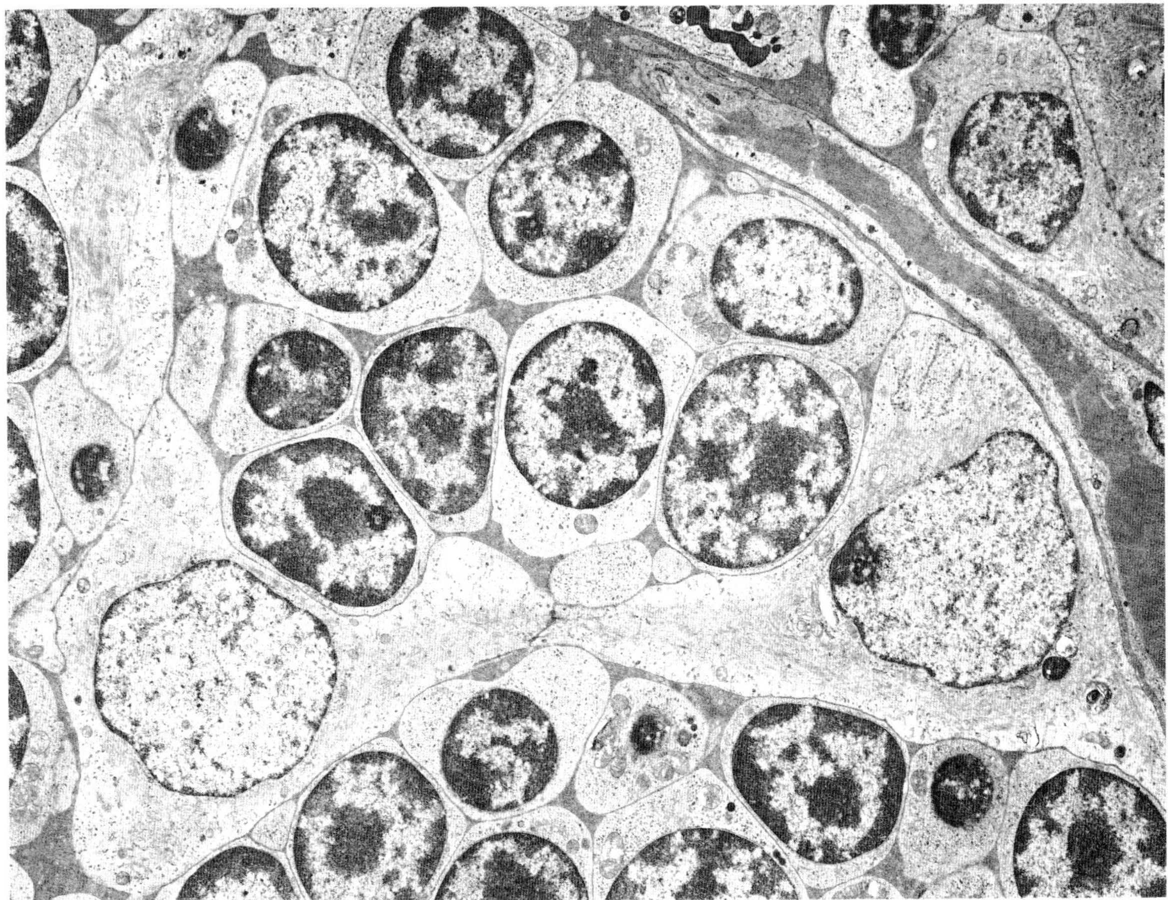

Fig. 303. Thymoma, lymphocytic type, rat. Epithelial cells form a network with elongated cytoplasmic processes which surround numerous lymphocytes. Tonofilaments, desmosomes, and membrane-bound bodies are characteristic in the epithelial cells. TEM, × 4100

Kajima 1970; Yamada et al. 1973; Hinsull and Bellamy 1977; Katayama and Kitamura 1983; Murray et al. 1985; Matsuyama et al. 1988) but extremely low in resistant strains (Table 47). In rats of susceptible strains, these tumors occur as multiple, small, round nodules in the substance of the thymuses that undergo less pronounced physiological involution (Matsuyama et al. 1988). Such small nodules develop into medium- and large-sized thymomas of the lymphocytic type and then into those of the mixed epithelial/lymphocytic and epithelial types in a few long-lived rats. The development of the thymoma is regulated by genetic factors, susceptible and resistant genes (Matsuyama et al. 1986), and suppressed in the heterozygote rats by introduction of the rat nude gene, *rnu* (Matsuyama et al. 1987). No method is known to induce thymoma experimentally in rats of the resistant strains. However, weak carcinogens, such as urethane, may accelerate tumor progression from the lymphocytic type

to the epithelial type in rats of susceptible strains (Matsuyama et al. 1972).

Comparison with Other Species

In humans thymoma is one of the most common neoplasms in the mediastinum (Rosai and Levine 1976; Marchevsky and Kaneko 1984). The tumors are, microscopically, subdivided into 4 types, predominantly lymphocytic, mixed, epithelial, and spindle cell (Bernatz et al. 1961). They have recently been subdivided into 3 types: cortical, mixed, and medullary, by their stainability to various monoclonal antibodies against cortical and medullary epithelial cells (Müller-Hermelink et al. 1986). The spindle cell thymoma is often associated with pure red cell anemia or hypogammaglobulinemia, and lymphocytic and mixed type thymomas, containing polygonal epithelial cells, are often related to myasthenia gra-

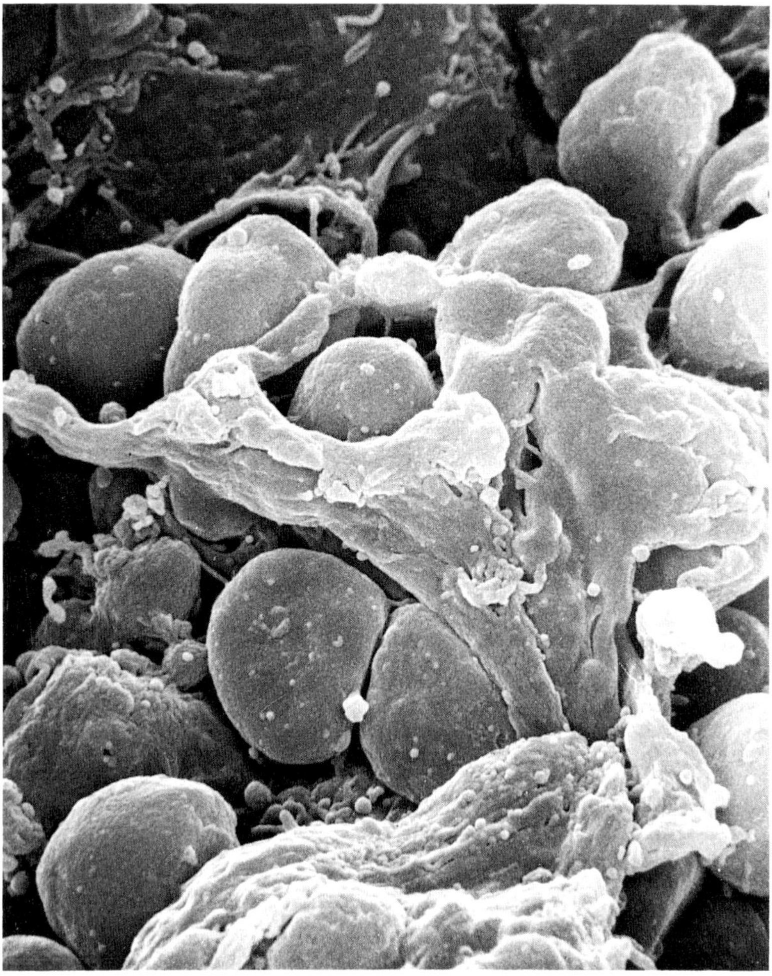

Fig. 304. Thymoma, lymphocytic type, rat. Cytoplasmic processes of epithelial cells enfold lymphocytes and extend small, but thick processes. SEM, × 8700

vis (Rosai and Levine 1976; Marchevsky and Kaneko 1984).

Thymomas are exceedingly rare in cattle, horses, sheep, goats, swine, dogs, cats, rabbits, duck, and mice. However, a high percentage of mice inoculated with polyomavirus develops epithelial type thymoma (Dawe et al. 1959). *Praomys (Mastomys) natalensis* also develop lymphocytic type thymoma at a moderate rate (Stewart and Snell 1968). These spontaneous thymomas in animals, including rats, are predominantly of the lymphocytic type, with a few of the mixed and epithelial types, which might correspond to the cortical type. Spindle cell type thymoma, which might correspond to the human medullary type, is not frequently described in animals. Microscopic and ultrastructural features of these lymphocytic type thymomas are not significantly different in rat, *Mastomys,* and humans. Myositis, myocardi-

tis, and sialodacryoadenitis develop in *Mastomys* with thymic abnormalities (Stewart and Snell 1968), and muscle atrophy and nephropathy are associated in rats of a strain highly susceptible to thymoma (Kato and Watanabe 1982; Kato et al. 1983; Nakamura et al. 1986; Matsuyama et al. 1987).

References

Bernatz PE, Harrison EG, Clagett OT (1961) Thymoma: a clinicopathologic study. J Thorac Cardiovasc Surg 42: 424–444

Crain RC (1958) Spontaneous tumors in the Rochester strain of the Wistar rat. Am J Pathol 34: 311–335

Dawe CJ, Law LW, Dunn TB (1959) Studies of parotid-tumor agent in cultures of leukemic tissues of mice. JNCI 23: 717–797

Dunning WF, Curtis MR (1946) The respective roles of longevity and genetic specificity in the occurrence of

Table 47. Incidences of thymoma in susceptible and resistant strains of rats

Strain	Sex	Observation period	Thymoma per 100 rats	References
Copenhagen	Female	over 12 months	15	Dunning and Curtis 1946
	Male		9	
Buffalo	Female	over 12 months	39	Yamada et al. 1973
	Male		54	
BUF/Mna	Female	over 50 weeks	100	Matsuyama et al. 1988
	Male		100	
Wistar	Not specified	over 24 months	50 or 9[a]	Pollard and Kajima 1970
WAB	Not specified	over 24 months	23	Hinsull and Bellamy 1977
SD/Os	Female	12 months	80	Katayama and Kitamura 1983
	Male		56	
W/Nhg	Female	over 21 months	97	Murray et al. 1985
	Male		22	
Fischer	Female	over 58 weeks	0	Jacobs and Huseby 1967
	Male		0	
Rochester	Female	over 18 months	0	Crain 1958
	Male		0	
Sprague-Dawley	Female	7-32 months	0	Thompson et al. 1961
	Male		0	
ACl/N	Female	over 30 weeks	3	Maekawa and Odashima 1975
	Male		0	
Donryu	Female	over 47 weeks	1	Maekawa et al. 1986
	Male		1	
F-344/DuCrj	Female	over 12 months	0	Maekawa et al. 1983 a
	Male		1	
Wistar/Slc	Female	over 43 weeks	0	Maekawa et al. 1983 b
	Male		1	

[a] May depend on the difference of the diets or generations of matings.

spontaneous tumors in the hybrids between two inbred lines of rats. Cancer Res 6: 61-81

Hinsull SM, Bellamy D (1977) Spontaneous thymoma in an inbred strain of rat. JNCI 58: 1609-1614

Jacobs BB, Huseby RA (1967) Neoplasms occurring in aged Fischer rats, with special reference to testicular, uterine, and thyroid tumors. JNCI 39: 303-309

Katayama S, Kitamura H (1983) Spontaneous thymoma in rats. I. Age and sex related incidence. Proceedings of the Japanese Cancer Association 42nd annual meeting, p 61

Kato F, Watanabe M (1982) Motor dysfunction in thymoma rats: comparison between fast and slow muscles. J Pharmacobiodyn 5: 1005-1011

Kato F, Watanabe M, Matsuyama M (1983) Nephrotic syndrome in spontaneous thymoma rats, Buffalo/Mna. Biomed Res 4: 105-109

Maekawa A, Odashima S (1975) Spontaneous tumors in ACI/N rats. JNCI 55. 1437-1445

Maekawa A, Kurokawa Y, Takahashi M, Kokubo T, Ogiu T, Onodera H, Tanigawa H, Ohno Y, Furukawa F, Hayashi Y (1983 a) Spontaneous tumors in F-344/DuCrj rats. Gann 74: 365-372

Maekawa A, Onodera H, Tanigawa H, Furuta K, Koda ma Y, Horiuchi S, Hayashi Y (1983 b) Neoplastic and non-neoplastic lesions in aging Slc: Wistar rats. J Toxicol Sci 8: 279-290

Maekawa A, Onodera H, Tanigawa H, Furuta K, Matsuoka C, Kanno J, Ogiu T, Hayashi Y (1986) Spontaneous neoplastic and nonneoplastic lesions in aging Donryu rats. Jpn J Cancer Res (Gann) 77: 882-890

Marchevsky AM, Kaneko M (1984) Surgical pathology of the mediastinum. Raven, New York, pp 58-116

Matsuyama M, Amo H (1977) Host origin of lymphoid cells in thymomas developed from subcutaneous thymus grafts in Buffalo rats. Gann 68: 293-300

Matsuyama M, Suzuki H, Ito M, Yamada S, Nagayo T (1972) Strain difference in carcinogenesis by urethan administration to suckling rats. Gann 63: 209-215

Matsuyama M, Suzuki H, Yamada S, Ito M, Nagayo T (1975) Ultrastructure of spontaneous and urethan-induced thymomas in Buffalo rats. Cancer Res 35: 2771-2779

Matsuyama M, Yamada C, Hiai H (1986) A single dominant susceptible gene determines spontaneous development of thymoma in BUF/Mna rat. Jpn J Cancer Res (Gann) 77: 1066-1068

Matsuyama M, Yamada C, Kojima A (1987) Possible single dosage effects of the nude gene: suppression of spontaneous development of thymoma and nephropathy in BUF/Mna-rnu/+rats. Jpn J Cancer Res (Gann) 78: 40-44

Matsuyama M, Matsuyama T, Ogiu T, Kojima A (1988) Nodular development of spontaneous epithelial thymoma in (ACI/NMs X BUF/Mna)Fl rats. Jpn J Cancer Res (Gann) 79: 1031-1038

Müller-Hermelink HK, Marino M, Palestro G (1986) Pathology of thymic epithelial tumors. In: Muller-Hermelink HK (ed) The human thymus: histophysiology and pathology. Springer, Berlin Heidelberg New York, pp 207-268

Murray AB, Schäffer E, Nüssel M, Luz A (1985) Incidence, morphology, and ultrastructure of spontaneous thymoma – the most common neoplasm in W/Nhg rats. JNCI 75: 369-379

Nakamura T, Oite T, Shimizu F, Matsuyama M, Kazama T, Koda Y, Arakawa M (1986) Sclerotic lesions in the glomeruli of Buffalo/Mna rats. Nephron 43: 50-55

Pollard M, Kajima M (1970) Lesions in aged germfree Wistar rats. Am J Pathol 61: 25-36

Rosai J, Levine GD (1976) Tumors of the thymus. In: Firminger HI (ed) Atlas of tumor pathology. 2nd series, Fasc. 13, Armed Forces Institute of Pathology, Washington DC, pp 34-161

Stewart HL, Snell KC (1968) Thymomas and thymic hyperplasia in *praomys (Mastomys) natalensis*. Concomitant myositis, myocarditis, and sialodacryoadenitis. JNCI 40: 1135-1159

Thompson SW, Huseby RA, Fox MA, Davis CL, Hunt RD (1961) Spontaneous tumors in the Sprague-Dawley rat. JNCI 27: 1037-1057

Yamada S, Masuko K, Ito M, Nagayo T (1973) Spontaneous thymoma in Buffalo rats. Gann 64: 287-292

Thymoma, Epithelial, Rat

C. Frieke Kuper and Rudolf B. Beems

Synonyms. Epithelioma; lymphoepithelioma; mixed tumor, thymic carcinoma; epithelial thymoma.

Gross Appearance

Thymomas are usually found in the anterior thorax as encapsulated, smoothly surfaced or coarsely lobulated tumors, consisting of firm, gray-white to pink-white tissue which does not adhere to adjacent tissue. Their diameter can be up to 3 cm. Smaller tumors are generally found incidentally. They are seen as distinct nodules or as local thickening in the thymus, which disturb the symmetrical appearance of the organ. Larger tumors are more likely to cause clinical signs and be a possible cause of death due to compression of intrathoracic organs. Rarely, gross infiltration of the tumor into the surrounding tissues is seen. Careful collection and examination of residual normal thymus tissue is often helpful in differential diagnosis.

Microscopic Features

Thymomas are defined as tumors of the thymus with involvement of the thymic epithelial cells. They are generally well circumscribed, partly en-

Fig. 305 *(upper left).* Thymoma with medullary differentiation, 20-month-old female Wistar rat. H and E, × 160 ▶

Fig. 306 *(lower left).* Thymoma, 24-month-old female Wistar rat. Focus of pale epithelial cells in the lymphocyte-rich areas with medullary differentiation. H and E, × 640

Fig. 307 *(upper right).* Thymoma, 28-month-old male Wistar rat. Predominantly lymphocytic. H and E, × 640

Fig. 308 *(lower right).* Thymoma, 26-month-old female Wistar rat. Predominantly epithelial. H and E, × 400

capsulated by a fibrous capsule, and noninvasive. The tumors represent a local process as evidenced by occasional remnants of atrophic thymus in close association with the capsule. They usually consist of a mixture of proliferating epithelial cells, which are considered to be the neoplastic cells, and small dark lymphocytes, which usually are without distinct neoplastic features. Thymomas can be divided in two types, tumors with and without medullary differentiation. The former probably represents a well-differentiated variety of thymoma. Medullary differentiation is characterized by small, pale-staining areas throughout the tumor in which lymphocytes are much less abundant and which occasionally contain Hassall's bodies, giving the tumor an organoid appearance (Fig. 305). Associated with the

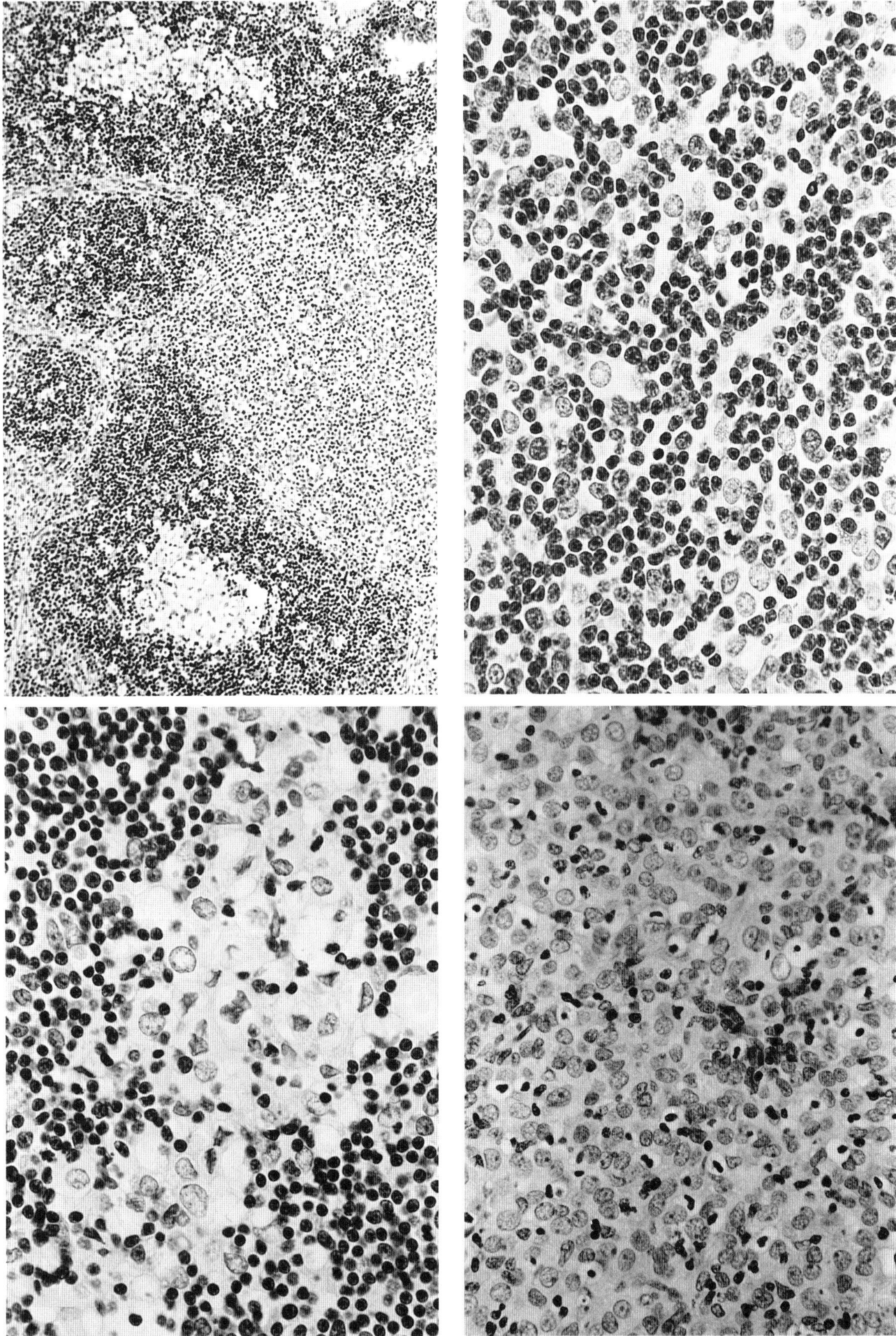

medullary areas are fibrous trabeculae which subdivide the tumor into lobules. Within these trabeculae epithelial cells occasionally form cords, tubules, and cysts, similar to those observed in age-associated thymic involution. A characteristic feature is the presence of foci of large, pale, epithelial cells, generally dispersed in the lymphocyte-rich or cortical areas of the tumor (Fig. 306).

Thymomas without medullary differentiation consist of a mixture of small dark lymphocytes and of epithelial cells of various shapes but predominantly with vesicular nuclei and clear cytoplasm (Figs. 307, 308). Occasionally, small groups or nodules of epithelial cells are observed which may compress the adjacent lymphocytes.

The epithelial involvement in thymomas varies considerably; sometimes the tumor is exclusively composed of epithelial cells. The type of cells ranges from spindle-shaped to pale ovoid cells with large nuclei or cells undergoing squamous differentiation (Figs. 309, 310).

Immunocytochemistry reveals that the neoplastic epithelial cells contain low molecular weight cytokeratins (Fig. 311).

The epithelial cytology can vary considerably in different parts of the same tumor, but atypia is rare. In the lymphocyte-rich areas normal mitotic figures may be frequent. These areas frequently have a "starry sky" appearance due to scattered macrophages containing phagocytized material. Large perivascular spaces occupied by plasma and lymphocytes, frequently present in human thymomas, have incidentally been observed in the rat (Fig. 312).

Small aggregates of lymphocytes are occasionally present in or outside the fibrous capsule but are not considered indicative of the neoplastic involvement of lymphocytes.

Ultrastructures

The ultrastructural features of the epithelial cells in thymoma (rat: Matsuyama et al. 1975; Murray et al. 1985; Kuper et al. 1986; human: Levine and Bearman 1980) are reminiscent of those of the epithelial cells in the normal thymus (Nabarra and Andrianarison 1987). The nuclei of the cells often have no distinct nucleolus and only a marginal concentration of chromatin, giving the nucleus a more lucent aspect than that of the surrounding lymphocytes (Fig. 313). Most cells are also larger than lymphocytes and have extended processes. Subcapsular and perivascular epithel-

Fig. 309 *(upper left).* Invasive tumor, thought to originate ▶ from the thymus, 24-month-old male Wistar rat. The tumor grows in sheets and cords and has undergone squamous differentiation. H and E, × 400

Fig. 310 *(lower left).* Thymoma, 21-month-old female Wistar rat. Squamous differentiation. H and E, × 400

Fig. 311 *(upper right).* Cytokeratin staining of epithelial cells in thymoma shown in Fig. 307. Carnoy fixation, paraffin embedding, polyclonal wide spectrum cytokeratin-specific serum, light counterstain with H, × 400

Fig. 312 *(lower right).* Thymoma, spindle cell type, 28-month-old female Wistar rat. Perivascular space. H and E, × 400

ial cells have a clear, often thickened basement membrane. The presence of desmosomes and bundles of tonofilaments is critical for the establishment of the epithelial nature of the cells (Fig. 314). They are observed in varying numbers and sometimes have a quite bizarre appearance. Thymomas rich in epithelial cells appear to have a higher number of tonofilaments and more prominent desmosomes than thymomas with a less prominent epithelial cell component (Matsuyama et al. 1975; Murray et al. 1985).

Lymphocytes in thymomas do not generally have abnormal features. However, so-called transformed lymphocytes with euchromatin-rich nuclei, prominent nucleoli, electron-lucent mitochondria, and abundant polyribosomes have been described. Multilayered membraneous formations derived from rough endoplasmic reticulum in dividing lymphocytes are possibly indicative of increased activity of these cells in thymoma (Levine and Bearman 1980; Murray et al. 1985).

Differential Diagnosis

The differential diagnosis of thymomas is usually not difficult despite many variations in morphology: The presence of considerable numbers of normal lymphocytes, medullary differentiation, and the epithelial nature of the neoplastic cell are indicative. Nevertheless, it may be difficult to distinguish some thymomas from other mediastinal tumors. Lymphocyte-rich thymomas can be mistaken for (thymic) lymphomas if medullary differentiation is absent. Careful search for the neoplastic epithelial cell component is then warranted, if necessary, aided by ultrastructural or immunohistochemical studies. Also, lymphomas

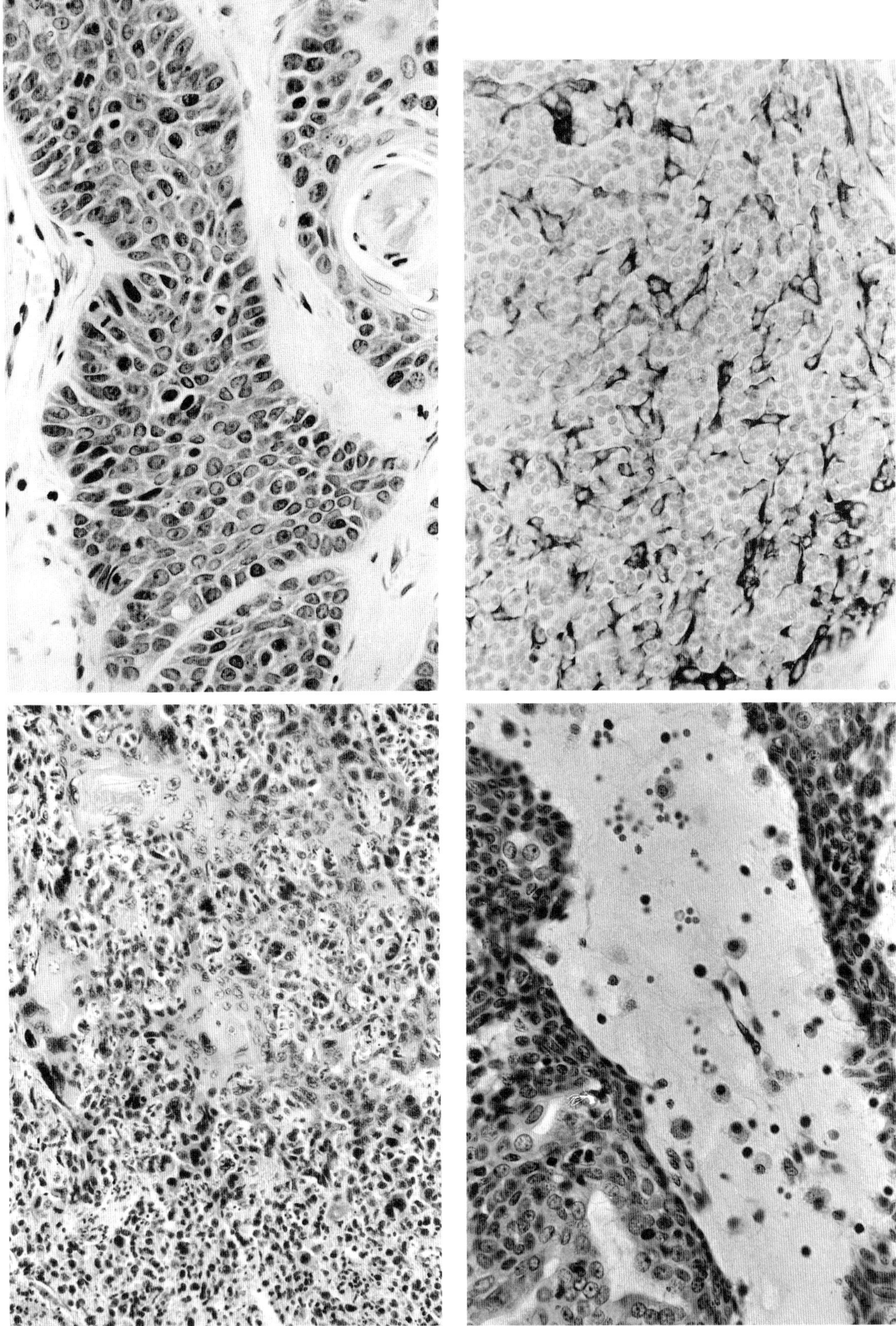

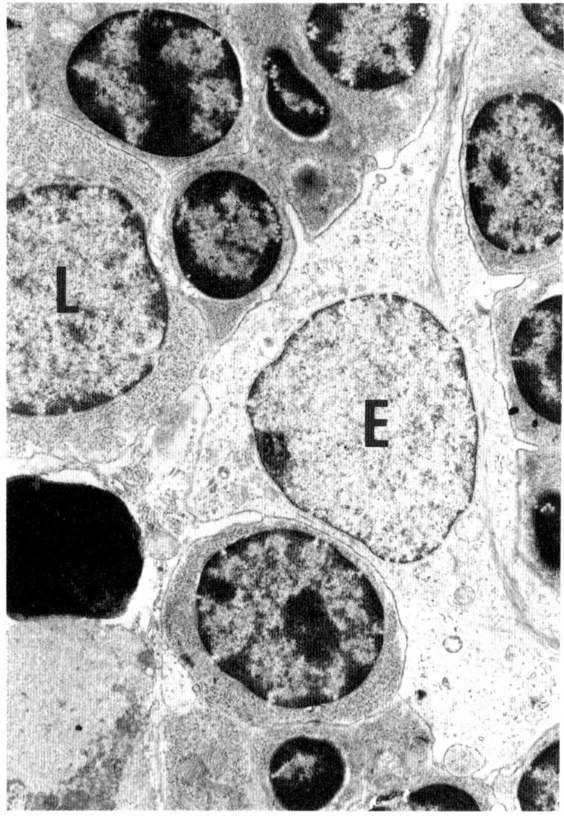

◄ **Fig. 313** *(above)*. Thymoma, 27-month-old female Wistar rat. *E,* nucleus of gray epithelial cell; *L,* nucleus of lymphoblast with polyribosome-rich cytoplasm. TEM, ×5700

Fig. 314 *(below)*. Thymoma, rat. Same tumor as Fig. 313. Cytoplasm of epithelial cell with tonofilaments and desmosomes. TEM, ×5700

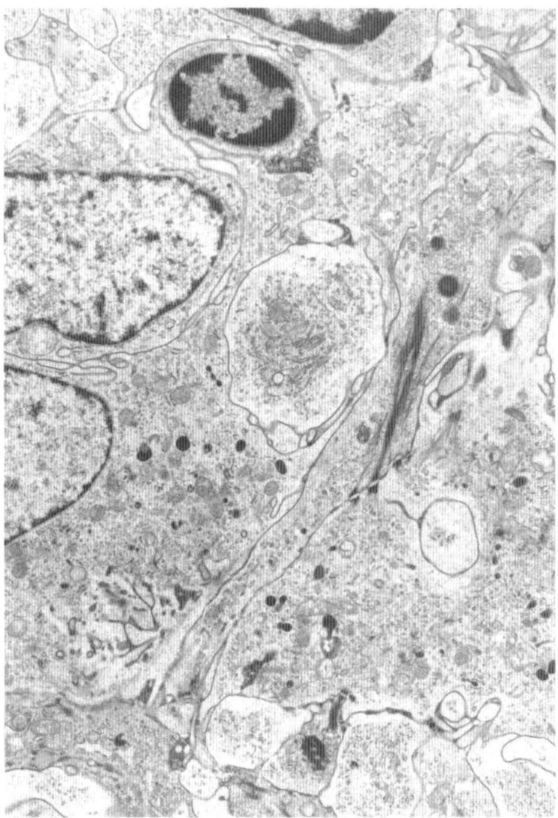

often involve peripheral lymphoid organs in contrast to thymomas which are usually restricted to the thymus. In humans, thymic carcinoid presents a problem in the differential diagnosis of thymoma. The presence of dense-core granules in the cells (electron microscopy) is indicative for carcinoid. Thymic carcinoid is rare in rats. Naylor et al. (1988) describe a neuron specific-enolase positive carcinoid in Sprague-Dawley rats. Electron microscopy or immunohistochemistry may also be needed to distinguish spindle cell-type epithelial thymomas from infiltrating mesenchymal tumors. Finally, it will not always be possible to establish the exact origin of carcinomas that involve several thoracic organs including the thymus.

Occasionally, old rats have a persisting or hyperplastic thymus, seen as a gland with a relatively normal architecture, but considerably larger than would be expected in adult or aged animals. In contrast to thymoma, which represents a localized process, persistent thymus involves the whole organ; the normal cortical and medullary architecture is preserved.

Biologic Features

Most thymomas are benign tumors. Thymic tumors which invade adjacent tissues are very rare in the rat, and metastases appear to be extremely unusual (Abott and Cherry 1982). Most thymomas grow slowly and expansively and only become manifest in old age in most rat strains. However, among female W/Hng rats and male BUF/Mna rats, the onset of thymomas occurs at a relatively early age. In some of the literature it is not always clear whether thymomas are epithelial tumors or thymic lymphomas. It can, however, be concluded that the incidence of thymomas in most rat strains is lower than 5% except for a few strains with a high incidence such as the above-mentioned female W/Hng and male BUF/Mna rats (Altmann and Goodman 1979; Murray et al. 1985; Kuper et al. 1986). The occurrence of strains and sublines with low and high incidence is suggestive of a genetically determined susceptibility to thymoma in rats. In BUF/Mna rats, a gene has been identified that is though to regulate the development of thymoma in this strain (Matsuyama et al. 1986). In most strains, thymomas occur more frequently in females than in males, and thus sex hormones perhaps play a role in the pathogenesis. Further evidence is provided by the observation that early castration or ovariectomy increases the incidence of thymomas in an inbred subline of WAB rats (Hinsull and Bellamy 1977). Epithelial cell hyperplasia as observed in old rats (see p. 257, this volume) also occurs more frequently in females than in males. It is unclear whether the hyperplasia has any significance in the pathogenesis of thymoma.

Thymomas in rats are generally well differentiated, as evidenced by the presence of lymphocytes in mitotic phases and the frequent occurrence of medullary differentiation. Lymphocytes in mitotic phases indicate that the epithelial cells retain the property of producing humoral factors that stimulate lymphopoiesis (Matsuyama et al. 1975). Thymomas are not associated with lymphocytosis or lymphoid hyperplasia in other lymphoid tissues, indicating that the lymphocytes do not migrate to the peripheral lymphoid organs (Hinsull and Bellamy 1977; Kuper 1986).

Advanced thymomas often cause dyspnea and other symptoms due to compression of thoracic organs. In BUF/Mna rats, thymoma is associated with increased muscle fatigability (Kato and Watanabe 1982) and nephrotic syndrome (Kato et al. 1983), which are possible autoimmune disorders. Interestingly, although the tumor in W/Nhg rats is symptomless, immunosuppressive agents reduced the incidence of thymomas in male rats, suggesting an association of the tumor with immune disorders (Murray et al. 1985).

The majority of induced thymic tumors in rodents are lymphomas (see p. 275, this volume), and most of these studies have been done with mice. We are aware of only one study in which the neoplastic response of thymic epithelial cells was modulated. In that study the subcutaneous injection of urethan in suckling Buffalo rats caused a shift from the mainly lymphocytic type to the mainly epithelial type of thymoma. However, the overall incidence of thymoma was not increased (Matsuyama et al. 1972).

Comparison with Other Species

In humans, thymic tumors are among the most common neoplasms of the mediastinum (Rosai and Levine 1976; Otto 1984). The term thymic carcinoma is often used for malignant thymoma, based either on biological behaviour or on cytological characteristics. Human thymomas may undergo medullary differentiation, while distinct perivascular spaces are more common than in rats. There is no clear evidence for a sex difference in occurrence as in rats. About half of the human thymomas produce no clinical signs. The other half are associated with signs caused by compression of thoracic organs and/or with systemic diseases that are thought to have an autoimmune basis, as in myasthenia gravis.

In most laboratory and domestic animals, thymomas are uncommon (laboratory animals: Squire et al. 1978; hamster: Ghadially and Illman 1965; Deerberg et al. 1987; mouse: Barness et al. 1968; dog: Robinson 1974; Aronsohn 1985). An exception is *Praomys (Mastomys) natalensis,* which has an incidence of thymoma varying between 8% and 40% (Kurokawa et al. 1968; Stewart and Snell 1968; Solleveld 1981).

Acknowledgement. We thank Dr. M. C. Bosland, Institute of Environmental Medicine, New York University Medical Center, New York, for critically reading the manuscript.

References

Altmann NH, Goodman DG (1979) Neoplastic diseases. In: Baker HJ, Lindsey JR, Weisbroth SH (eds) The laboratory rat, vol I. Academic, New York, pp 353–355

Abbott DP, Cherry CP (1982) Malignant mixed thymic tumor with metastases in a rat. Vet Pathol 19: 721 723

Aronsohn M (1985) Canine thymoma. Vet Clin North Am [Small Anim Pract] 15: 755–767

Barnes RD, Tuffrey MA, Berry CL (1968) Auto-immune disease in (NZB × CFW) Fl mice. J Pathol 95: 391–403

Deerberg F, Fuchs I, Rapp KG, Sickel E, Kaspareit J (1987) Spontaneous mortality and incidence of spontaneous tumours in Han: CHIN hamsters. Z Versuchstierkd 29: 120–143

Ghadially FN, Illman O (1965) Naturally occurring thymomas in the European hamster. J Pathol 90: 465–469

Hinsull SM, Bellamy D (1977) Spontaneous thymoma in an inbred strain of rat. JNCI 58: 1609–1614

Kato F, Watanabe M (1982) Motor dysfunction in thymoma rats: comparison between fast and slow muscles. J Pharm Dyn 5: 1005–1011

Kato F, Watanabe M, Matsuyama M (1983) Nephrotic syndrome in spontaneous thymoma rats, Buffalo/Mna. Biomed Res 4: 105–110

Kuper CF, Beems RB, Hollanders VMH (1986) Spontaneous pathology of the thymus in aging Wistar (Cpb:WU) rats. Vet Pathol 23: 270–277

Kurokawa Y, Fujii K, Suzuki M, Sato H (1968) Spontaneous tumors of the thymus in mastomys (Rattus natalensis). Gann 59: 145–150

Levine D, Bearman RM (1980) The pathological thymus. In: Johannesen JV (ed) Electron microscopy in human medicine, vol 5. Cardiovascular system, lymphoreticular and hemopoietic system. McGraw-Hill, New York, pp 228–254

Matsuyama M, Suzuki H, Ito M, Yamada S, Nagayo T (1972) Strain difference in carcinogenesis by urethan administration to suckling rats. Gann 63: 209–215

Matsuyama M, Suzuki H, Yamada S, Ito M, Nagayo T (1975) Ultrastructure of spontaneous and urethan-induced thymomas in Buffalo rats. Cancer Res 35: 2771–2779

Matsuyama M, Yamada C, Hiai (1986) A single dominant susceptible gene determines spontaneous development of thymoma in BUF/Mna rat. Gann 77: 1066–1068

Murray AB, Schäffer E, Nüssel M, Luz A (1985) Incidence, morphology, and ultrastructure of spontaneous thymoma – the most common neoplasm in W/Nhg rats. JNCI 75: 369–379

Nabarra B, Andrianarison I (1987) Ultrastructural studies of thymic reticulum. I. Epithelial component. Thymus 9: 95–121

Naylor DC, Krinke GJ, Ruefenacht HJ (1988) Primary tumours of the thymus in the rat. J Comp Pathol 99: 187–203

Otto HF (1984) Epitheliale thymustumoren (Thymome). In: Doerr W, Seifert G (eds) Pathologie des thymus. Spezielle pathologische anatomie, vol 17. Springer, Berlin Heidelberg New York, pp 127–197

Robinson M (1974) Malignant thymoma with metastases in a dog. Vet Pathol 11: 172–180

Rosai J, Levine GD (1976) Tumors of the thymus. In: Firminger HI (ed) Atlas of tumor pathology. 2nd series, Fasc 13. Armed Forces Institute of Pathology, Washington DC, pp 34–161

Solleveld HA (1981) Praomys (Mastomys) natalensis in aging research. With emphasis on autoimmune phenomena. Thesis, Leiden

Squire RA, Goodman DG, Valerio MG, Fredrickson T, Strandberg JD, Levitt MH, Lingeman CH, Harshbarger JC, Dawe CJ (1978) Tumors. In: Benirschke K, Garner FM, Jones TC (eds) Pathology of laboratory animals, vol II. Springer, Berlin Heidelberg New York, pp 1051–1262

Stewart HL, Snell KC (1968) Thymomas and thymic hyperplasia in Praomys (Mastomys) natalensis. Concomitant myositis, myocarditis and sialodacryoadenitis. JNCI 40: 1135–1159

T-Cell Lymphoma, Thymic Origin, Rat

Toshiaki Ogiu

Synonyms. Thymic lymphoma; thymic leukemia; malignant lymphoma of the thymus; thymic lymphosarcoma.

Gross Appearance

T-cell lymphomas of thymic origin are yellowish or pearly white tumors in the cranial mediastinum. The surface of the tumor is not always smooth and sometimes contains a few small or large nodules. At an advanced stage, tumor cells invade surrounding tissues, involving the mediastinal lymph nodes, epicardium, adipose tissue around the trachea and aorta, pleura adjacent to the sternum, and sometimes intercostal muscles. Bloody or milky fluid containing many tumor cells may be demonstrated in the epicardial cavity in the early stages and may later involve the pleural cavity. Enlarged lymph nodes are frequently seen in mediastinal, portal, mesenteric, cervical, and axillary locations. Inguinal and retroperitoneal lymph nodes and Peyer's patches are occasionally involved. Edema around the salivary glands, sometimes extending to the cranial half of the body, and dilatation of the subcutaneous veins of the abdominal wall are seen when large tumors occupy the mediastinum. The spleen and liver are slightly or moderately enlarged in many cases, but the kidney, adrenal glands, and other organs are rarely involved until the final stages.

Microscopic Features

Most of the tumors are composed of monotonous sheets of lymphoid cells and a few macrophages which give the appearance, at low magnification, of a prominent "starry sky" pattern. Neoplastic lymphocytes are variable in maturation and size and often are in mitosis. Rat T-cell

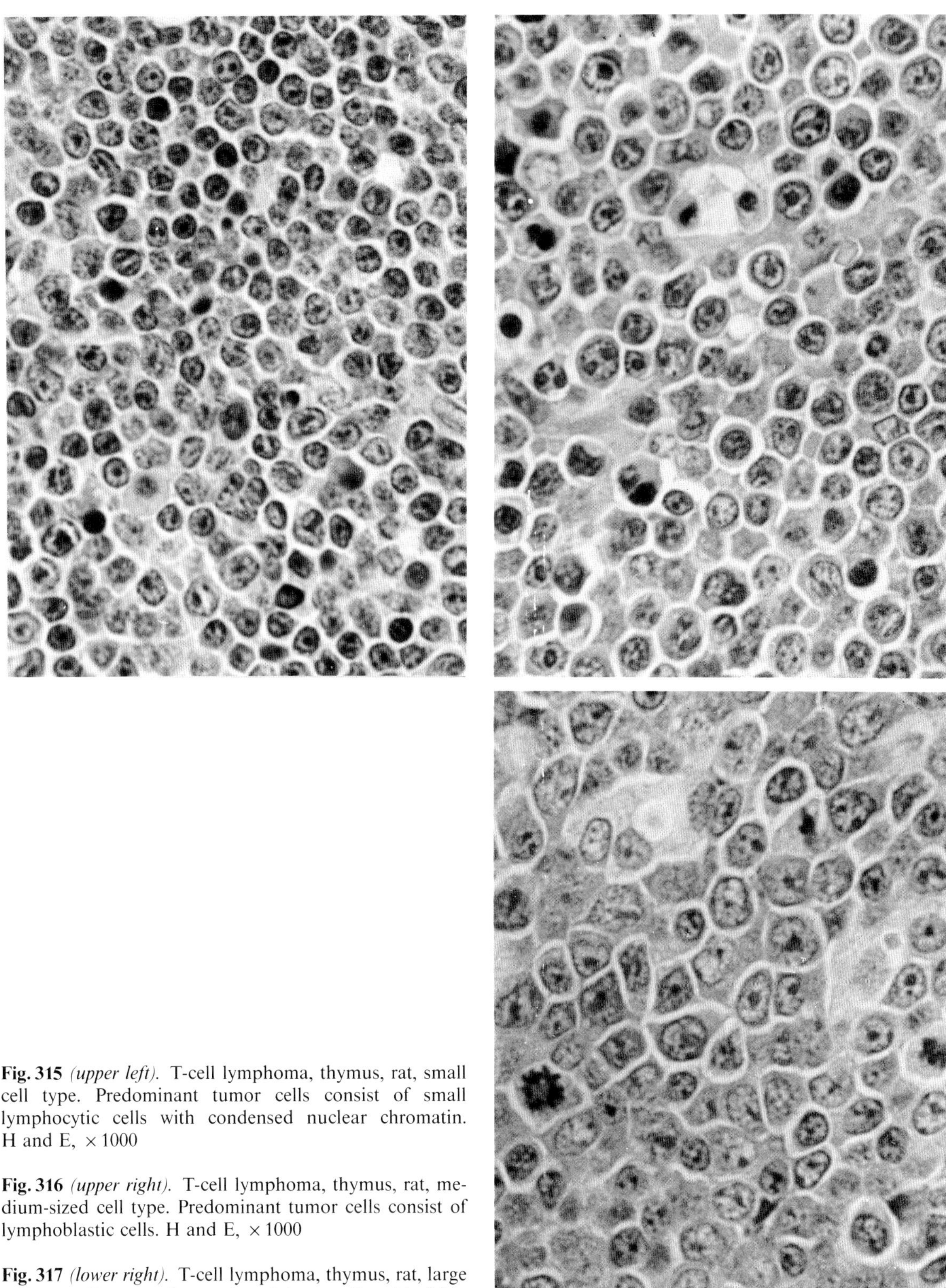

Fig. 315 *(upper left).* T-cell lymphoma, thymus, rat, small cell type. Predominant tumor cells consist of small lymphocytic cells with condensed nuclear chromatin. H and E, × 1000

Fig. 316 *(upper right).* T-cell lymphoma, thymus, rat, medium-sized cell type. Predominant tumor cells consist of lymphoblastic cells. H and E, × 1000

Fig. 317 *(lower right).* T-cell lymphoma, thymus, rat, large cell type. Tumor cells consist of large cells with fairly abundant cytoplasm and vesicular nuclei. H and E, × 1000

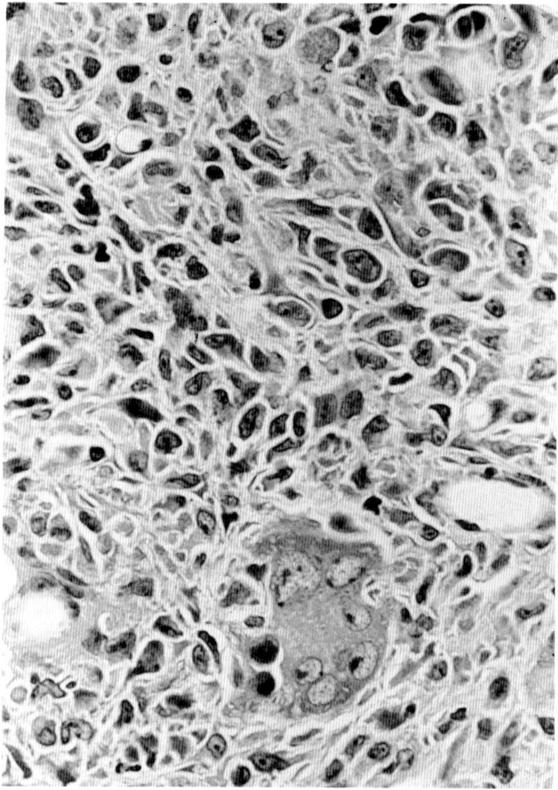

Fig. 318 *(above).* T-cell lymphoma, thymus, rat, pleomorphic type. This tumor consists of two major types of cells, histiocytic large cells and lymphoid small cells. H and E, ×550

Fig. 319 *(below).* Higher magnification of tumor in Fig. 318. Many lymphoid cells with various sizes and morphologies are observed between the histiocytic cells. H and E, ×1000

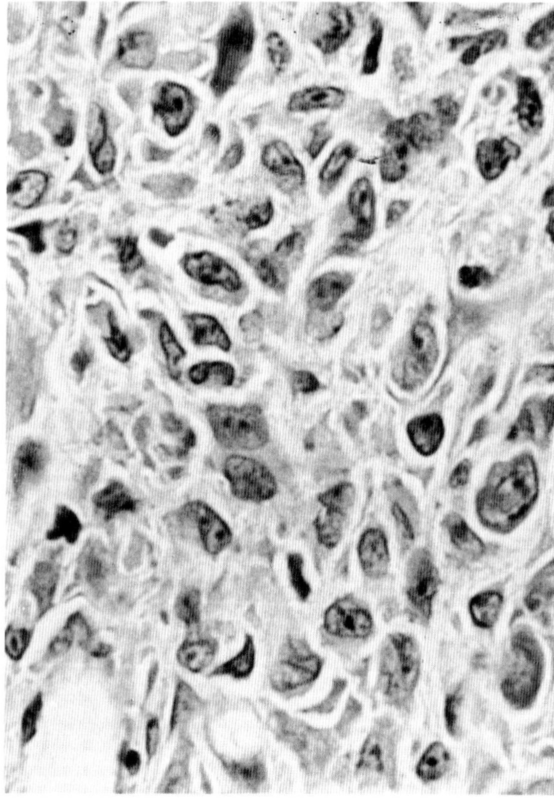

lymphomas may be classified into a few subtypes in conformity to the classifications of human malignant lymphomas (Suchi et al. 1979; The Non-Hodgkin's Lymphoma Pathologic Classification Project 1982): small cell type, medium-sized cell or lymphoblastic type, and large cell type according to size of the dominant tumor cells. Tumor cells of small cell type closely resemble small lymphocytes with scanty and well-circumscribed, compact cytoplasm and deeply stained, round nuclei (Fig. 315). The medium-sized cell type is made up of lymphoblastic cells with round or oval nuclei and scant, fairly well-circumscribed cytoplasm (Fig. 316). The cells of the large cell type are larger than the lymphoblastic type and consist of fairly abundant and well-circumscribed cytoplasm with vesicular and round or oval nuclei (Fig. 317). The nucleoli are usually conspicuous in the center of the nucleus.

Morphologic characteristics of another specific pleomorphic type were reported by Suzuki et al. (1984). Tumors of this type consist of two types of cells: large histiocytic cells and atypical lymphoid cells (Figs. 318, 319).

Cells of the former are pleomorphic in size and shape, often with a whorled arrangement. Their cytoplasm is abundant but pale, and the nuclei are irregularly shaped. Lymphoid cells are found among the histiocytic cells and are sometimes in mitosis. The size of the cells is varied, and they have twisted nuclei and slightly eosinophilic cytoplasm. A few macrophages, multinucleated giant cells, granulocytes, and plasma cells are also scattered among the admixture of histiocytic and lymphoid cells. Most of the chemically induced lymphomas are of the medium-sized cell type. (See also histiocytic tumors, p. 54, this volume.)

Ultrastructure

Tumor cells of small cell, medium-sized, or large cell types resemble normal lymphoid cells and are round or oval with round or sometimes in-

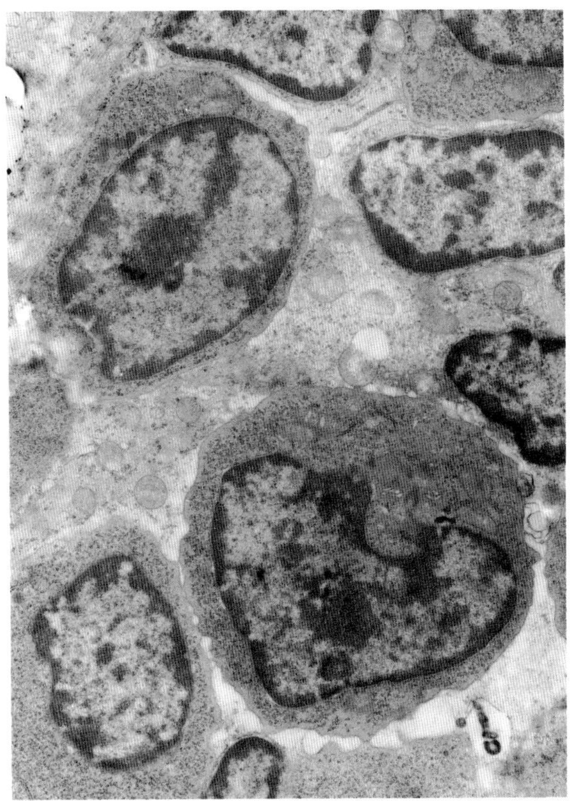

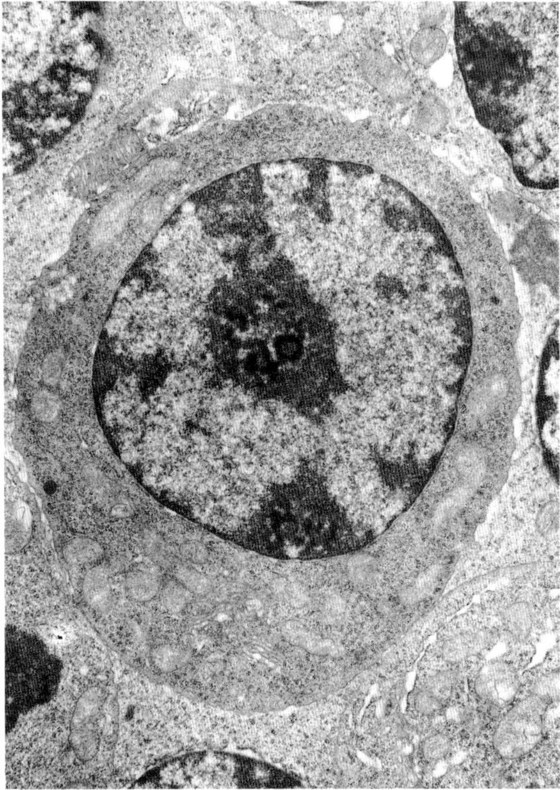

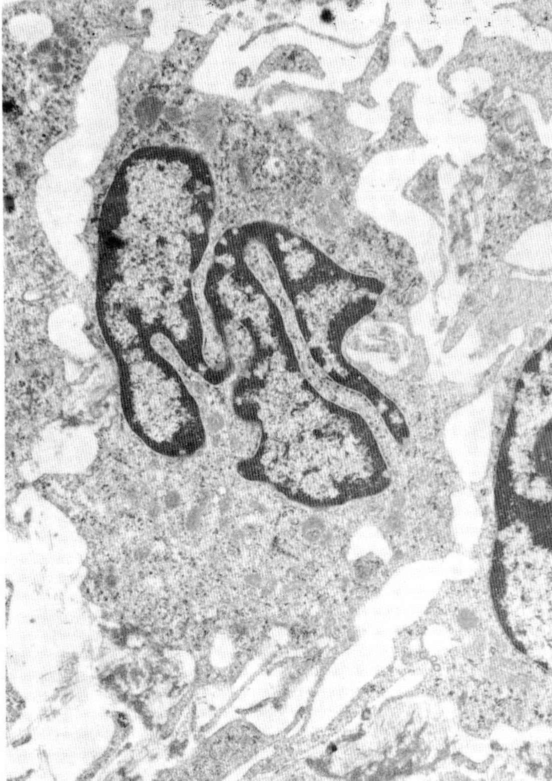

Fig. 320 *(upper left).* T-cell lymphoma, thymus, rat, medium-sized cell type. Scanty cytoplasm with a few cytoplasmic organelles are seen. Uranyl acetate and lead, TEM, × 8200. (Courtesy of Suzuki et al. 1984)

Fig. 321 *(upper right).* T-cell lymphoma, thymus, rat, large cell type. Note large nucleus with several nucleolar organizing regions and abundant polyribosomes. Uranyl acetate and lead, TEM, × 8200. (Courtesy of Suzuki et al. 1984)

Fig. 322 *(lower right).* T-cell lymphoma, thymus, rat, pleomorphic cell type. Severely infolded nuclei and elongated cytoplasmic processes are characteristic. Deparaffinized. Uranyl acetate and lead, TEM, × 8500. (Courtesy of Suzuki et al. 1984) dented nuclei (Figs. 320, 321). Chromatin is condensed to the nuclear membrane; the cytoplasm is scant and well circumscribed in smaller tumor cells and fairly abundant in larger cells. Moderate to numerous numbers of free ribosomes and polyribosomes are observed, depending on cell maturation. Golgi apparatus are poorly to moderately well developed. Clustered or isolated dense bodies are sometimes observed in smaller cells while they are rare or few in larger cells.

Pleomorphic type tumors consist mainly of histiocytic and lymphoid cells. The histiocytic cells are identified as interdigitating reticular cells. Variable-sized lymphoid cells have moderately abundant cytoplasm with thin processes. The cytoplasm contains many polyribosomes and rare clustered dense bodies. The nucleus, which is severely indented or infolded, has one or two moderately developed spherical nucleoli and a rim of condensed chromatin along the nuclear membrane (Fig. 322; see p. 249, this volume).

Differential Diagnosis

Although the term "thymoma" has been used synonymously for malignant lymphoma of the thymus in experimental and domestic animals in many reports, the term "thymoma" is restricted to the thymic neoplasm arising from thymic epithelial cells in our classification in accordance with the concepts of Rosai and Levine (1976) concerning human thymic tumors.

T-cell lymphomas of thymic origin should be distinguished from thymomas and nonthymic lymphomas. One of the distinguishing features of T-cell lymphomas is their gross appearance. Thymomas are found as a diffuse enlargement of the thymus without involving the surrounding tissues (Yamada et al. 1973). Thymic T-cell lymphomas appear as a large mass which involves the surrounding tissues. The presence of metastasis in lymphatic tissues and of leukemic cells in the peripheral blood is also helpful for diagnosis. Microscopically, thymic lymphoma generally consists of homogeneous tumor cells with a few or frequent "starry sky" patterns, while the lymphocyte-predominant type of thymoma consists of epithelial reticular cells and small lymphocytes with a medullary differentiation pattern. Metastasis of tumor cells into lymph nodes is not observed in thymomas. (See lymphocytic thymoma, p. 275, this volume.)

The absence of macroscopic and microscopic involvement of the thymus with tumor cells is an important finding in the diagnosis of nonthymic lymphoma. Immunohistologic diagnosis with T-cell-specific antibody and immunoglobulin-specific antisera is useful to distinguish a tumor of T-cell origin from one originating from B cells (Imamura et al. 1981; Imamura and Okada 1982; Moriuchi et al. 1981).

Biologic Features

Spontaneous thymic T-cell lymphomas rarely develop in rats (Swaen and Van Heerde 1973). Two possible targets of thymic lymphomagenic agents are suggested: pre-T cells (precursor of thymic lymphocytes existing in the bone marrow) and intrathymic lymphocytes. Recently, it was reported that rat thymic T-cell lymphoma originated from intrathymic lymphocytes after chemical lymphomagenesis, although their subset is still unknown (Ogiu and Fukami 1987).

Sequential changes of the thymus in rat thymic lymphoma development were examined in N-methyl-N-nitrosourea (MNU)-induced thymic lymphomas in Sprague-Dawley rats (Koestner et al. 1977) and in N-propyl-N-nitrosourea (PNU)-induced thymic lymphomas in F344 rats (Ogiu et al. 1985). A few days after carcinogen treatment, the thymus becomes atrophic, with a decrease in cortical thymocytes, and the corticomedullary border becomes unclear. Recovery follows with normal-appearing thymocytes. Among regenerating tissues, foci of growth of relatively large lymphoblastic cells are observed in the deep cortex of the thymus. Development of lymphoma is seen in one lobe at first; subsequently, tumor cells infiltrate and grow in other lobes; and finally, the lymphoma becomes leukemic, and tumor cells metastasize into many other tissues such as the lymph nodes, splenic white pulp, intestinal Peyer's patches, bone marrow, and liver.

Experimental Induction. A few methods have been reported for the successful induction of thymic T-cell lymphomas in rats. They have been induced in 7%–50% of Sprague-Dawley rats given a magnesium-deficient diet for more than 8 weeks (Bois et al. 1969), in 100% of Sprague-Dawley rats continuously fed 0.05% 4(5)-(3,3-dimethyl-l-triazeno)imidazole-5(4)-carboxamide in the diet (Skibba et al. 1970, in almost all Sprague-Dawley rats given intragastric administration of MNU (Koestner et al. 1977), in 45% of F344 rats given intraperitoneal administration of

MNU (Imaida et al. 1984), and in almost all F344 rats given continuously a 0.04% solution of PNU as drinking water (Sakura et al. 1984). It was demonstrated, however, that the incidences of PNU-induced thymic lymphomas are different among some strains of rats (Shisa and Hiai 1985). Thymic lymphomas were also induced in rats following inoculation with the murine leukemia viruses including Gross, Friend, or Rauscher viruses (Gross et al. 1961; Kunii and Furth 1964; Dawson et al. 1966; Kobayashi et al. 1969; Swaen 1966).

Comparison with Other Species

In humans, the incidence of malignant lymphoma is about 10% of total mediastinal tumors (Wychulis et al. 1971). The majority of them are considered to originate in the lymph nodes present in this location, and T-cell lymphoma of thymic origin is rare (Rosai and Levine 1976). In the mouse, thymic T-cell lymphomas are one of the most common neoplasms. They occur spontaneously, the frequency dependent on the mouse strain (Furth et al. 1933; Law and Miller 1950), and can be induced by viruses, radiation (Kaplan 1967), and chemicals, including urethan (ethylcarbamate) (Tannenbaum and Maltoni 1962), dimethylbenz[*a*]anthracene (Rappaport and Baroni 1962) and *N*-alkylnitrosoureas (Terracini and Testa 1970; Yokoro et al. 1970). The spontaneous development of thymic T-cell lymphomas and the detection of leukemogenic viruses have been reported in the cat (Jarrett 1971) and cow (Devare et al. 1976). Lymphoid tumors were also induced in chickens by viruses; Marek's disease virus (MDV), a herpesvirus, causes tumors of T- and B-cell origin (Hudson and Payne 1973), but avian leukemia virus (ALV), a retrovirus, causes lymphoid leukosis of B-cell origin (Cooper et al. 1968). Although the spontaneous occurrence of lymphomas was reported in rabbits, guinea pigs, and hamsters, T-cell lymphomas of thymic origin were rare.

References

Bois P, Sandborn EB, Messier PE (1969) Study of thymic lymphosarcoma developing in magnesium-deficient rats. Cancer Res 29: 763–775
Cooper MD, Payne LN, Dent PB, Burmester BR, Good RA (1968) Pathogenesis of avian lymphoid leukosis. JNCI 41: 373–389
Dawson PJ, Rose WM, Fieldsteel AH (1966) Lymphatic leukaemia in rats and mice inoculated with Friend virus. Br J Cancer 20: 114–121
Devare SG, Stephenson JR, Sarma PS, Aaronson SA, Chander S (1976) Bovine lymphosarcoma: development of radioimmunologic technique for detection of the etiologic agent. Science 194: 1428–1430
Furth J, Sibold HR, Rathbone RR (1933) Experimental studies on lymphomatosis of mice. Am J Cancer 19: 21–604
Gross L, Dreyfuss Y, Moore LA (1961) Induction of leukemia in rats with mouse leukemia (passage A) virus. Proc Soc Exp Biol Med 106: 890–893
Hudson L, Payne LN (1973) An analysis of the T and B cells of Marek's disease lymphomas of the chicken. Nature New Biol 241: 52–53
Imaida K, Fukushima S, Shirai T, Masui T, Ogiso T, Ito N (1984) Promoting activities of butylated hydroxyanisole, butylated hydroxytoluene and sodium L-ascorbate on forestomach and urinary bladder carcinogenesis initiated with methylnitrosourea in F344 male rats. Gann 75: 769–775
Imamura N, Okada K (1982) Immunological analysis of *N*-nitrosourea-induced rat leukemia and experimental trials for therapy of human leukemia. Acta Hematol Jpn 45: 1307–1313
Imamura N, Saito O, Dohy H, Ogiu T (1981) T-Cell leukemia induced by l-propyl-l-nitrosourea in Fischer rats. Experientia 37: 1339–1340
Jarrett WFM (1971) Feline leukemia. Int Rev Exp Pathol 10: 243–263
Kaplan HS (1967) On the natural history of the murine leukemias. Presidental address. Cancer Res 27: 1325–1340
Kobayashi H, Hosokawa M, Takeichi N, Sendo F, Kodama T (1969) Transplantable Friend virus-induced tumors in rats. Cancer Res 29: 1385–1392
Koestner AW, Ruecker FA, Koestner A (1977) Morphology and pathogenesis of tumors of the thymus and stomach in Sprague-Dawley rats following intragastric administration of methyl nitrosourea (MNU). Int J Cancer 20: 418–426
Kunii A, Furth J (1964) Inhibition of lymphoma induction in virus-infected rats by thymectomy. An affinity of the lymphoma virus for myeloid cells. Cancer Res 24: 493–497
Law LW, Miller JH (1950) Observations on the effect of thymectomy on spontaneous leukemias in mice of the high-leukemic strains, RIL and C58. JNCI 11: 253–262
Moriuchi T, Kasai M, Yamaguchi N, Kobashi N (1981) Characterization and classification of rat leukemias and lymphomas by membrane markers. Cancer Res 41: 1938–1949
Ogiu T, Fukami H (1987) Existence of *N*-nitroso-*N*-propylurea target cells in the thymus of F344 rats in thymic lymphomagenesis. JNCI 79: 179–183
Ogiu T, Sakura Y, Maekawa A (1985) Sequential observations of thymic lymphoma development in 10-week-old F344 rats by *N*-propyl-*N*-nitrosourea. Acta Pathol Jpn 35: 1191–1200
Rappaport H, Baroni C (1962) A study of the pathogenesis of malignant lymphoma induced in the Swiss mouse by 7,12-dimethylbenz[*a*]anthracene injected at birth. Cancer Res 22: 1067–1074

Rosai J, Levine GD (1976) Malignant lymphoma. In: Atlas of tumor pathology, 2nd Series, Fascicle 13, Tumors of the thymus. AFIP, Washington DC, pp 191–205

Sakura Y, Ogiu T, Imamura N, Furuta K, Matsuoka C, Odashima S (1984) Development of thymic lymphomas by oral administration of N-nitroso-N-propylurea and establishment of transplantable lines of thymic lymphoma in F344 rats. JNCI 73: 757–762

Shisa H, Hiai H (1985) Genetically determined susceptibility of Fischer 344 to propylnitrosourea-induced thymic lymphomas. Cancer Res 45: 1483–1487

Skibba JL, Ertürk E, Bryan GT (1970) Induction of thymic lymphosarcoma and mammary adenocarcinomas in rats by oral administration of the antitumor agent, 4(5)-(3,3-dimethyl-l-triazeno)imidazole-5(4)-carboxamide. Cancer 26: 1000–1005

Suchi T, Tajima K, Nanba K, Wakasa H, Mikata A, Kikuchi M, Mori S, Watanabe S, Mohri N, Shamoto M, Harigaya K, Itagaki T, Matsuda M, Kirino Y, Takagi K, Fukunaga S (1979) Some problems on the histopathological diagnosis of non-Hodgkin's malignant lymphoma – a proposal of a new type. Acta Pathol Jpn 29: 755–776

Suzuki Y, Matsuyama M, Ogiu T (1984) Morphologic characteristics of thymic lymphomas induced by N-nitroso-N-propylurea in F344 rats. JNCI 72: 367–373

Swaen GJV (1966) Development of thymic neoplasms in rats inoculated with a murine leukemia virus (Rauscher). JNCI 36: 1027–1048

Swaen GJV, Van Heerde P (1973) Tumours of the haematopoietic system. In: Turusov VS (ed) Pathology of tumours in laboratory animals, vol I. Tumours of the rat. IARC Sci Publ 5 (1): 185–214

Tannenbaum A, Maltoni C (1962) Neoplastic response of various tissues to the administration of the urethan. Cancer Res 22: 1105–1112

Terracini B, Testa MC (1970) Carcinogenicity of a single administration of N-nitrosomethylurea: a comparison between newborn and 5-week-old mice and rats. Br J Cancer 24: 588–598

The Non-Hodgkin's Lymphoma Pathologic Classification Project (1982) National Cancer Institute sponsored study of classifications of non-Hodgkin's lymphomas: summary and description of a working formulation for clinical usage. Cancer 49: 2112–2135

Wychulis AR, Payne WS, Clagett OT, Woolner LB (1971) Surgical treatment of mediastinal tumors: a 40 year experience. J Thorac Cardiovasc Surg 62: 379–392

Yamada S, Masuko K, Ito M, Nagayo T (1973) Spontaneous thymoma in Buffalo rats. Gann 64: 287–291

Yokoro K, Imamura N, Takizawa S, Nishihara H, Nishihara E (1970) Leukemogenic and mammary tumorigenic effects of N-nitrosobutylurea in mice and rats. Gann 61: 287–289

Atrophy of Thymus Induced by Cytostatic Chemicals, Rat

Kiyoshi Imai

Gross Appearance

The weight of an affected thymus decreases, because of atrophy. The color of the thymus is normal, but occasionally has increased opacity. Sometimes hemorrhagic foci are noted, especially in the medulla. In advanced cases, the thymus cannot be distinguished from the surrounding adipose tissue.

Microscopic Features

In the cortex a decrease in the number of thymic lymphocytes is noted, and abundant pyknotic thymic lymphocytes are present (Fig. 323). Therefore, the reticular and epithelial cells are prominent, frequently swollen, and contain cell debris of necrotic thymic lymphocytes (Fig. 324). As described above, these changes are sometimes associated with small hemorrhagic foci. In the medulla, the thymic lymphocytes are slightly increased in number, and the corticomedullary junction is not sharply demarcated at low magnification. In advanced cases, cortical thymic lymphocytes are completely destroyed, and the cortex is not evident (Fig. 325).

Ultrastructure

The ultrastructural features of this lesion in rats have not been described.

Differential Diagnosis

The thymus is an organ most sensitive to the effects of aging. Therefore, it is very important to differentiate chemical-induced thymic atrophy from the effect of aging. The thymus undergoes atrophy with aging, and its weight is gradually reduced (Fig. 326). Atrophy is more remarkable

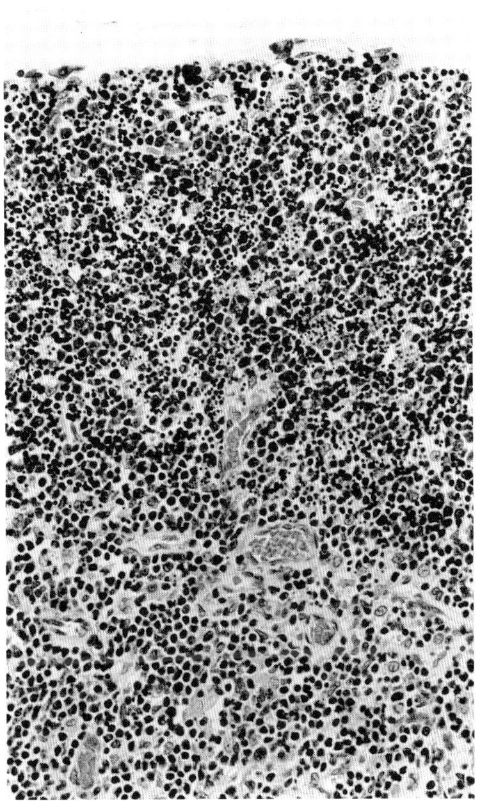

Fig. 323. Thymic necrosis and atrophy, rat treated with cyclophosphamide. Cortical lymphocytes are decreased, and the corticomedullary junction is not distinct. H and E, × 300

in the cortex than in the medulla. Histologically, it may be evident that the number of cortical lymphocytes reduces with age, and the thickness of the cortex is diminished, but necrotic or degenerative changes of cortical lymphocytes are not observed. In advanced cases of thymic atrophy related to aging, marked infiltration of adipose tissue is also noted in the cortex.

An apparent proliferation of thymic epithelial cells is often seen in aging rats (older than 2 years) (Meihuizen and Burek 1978). The epi-

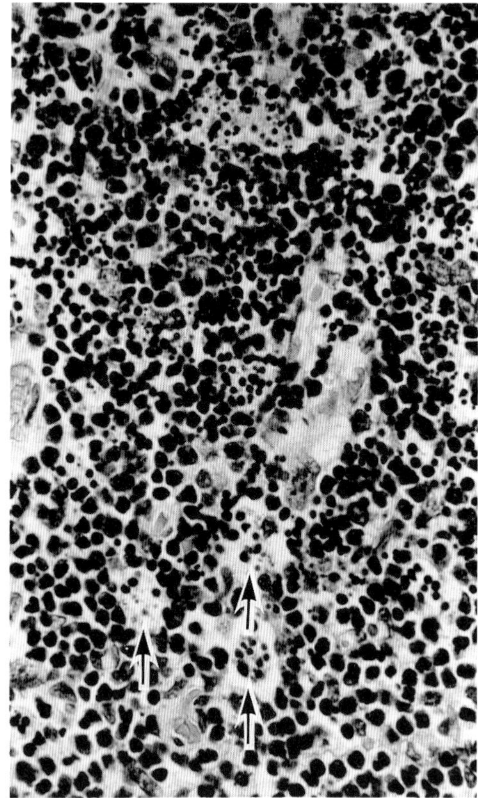

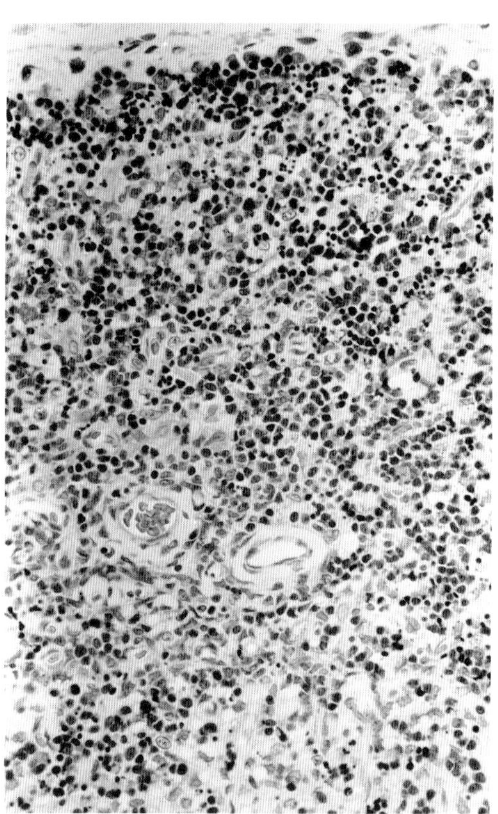

Fig. 324. Higher magnification of Fig. 323. Many necrotic lymphocytes are present in the reticuloepithelial cells as cell debris *(arrows).* H and E, × 600

Fig. 325. Atrophy of thymus, rat treated with cyclophosphamide. Cortex is not identified because of marked decrease of cortical lymphocytes. H and E, × 300

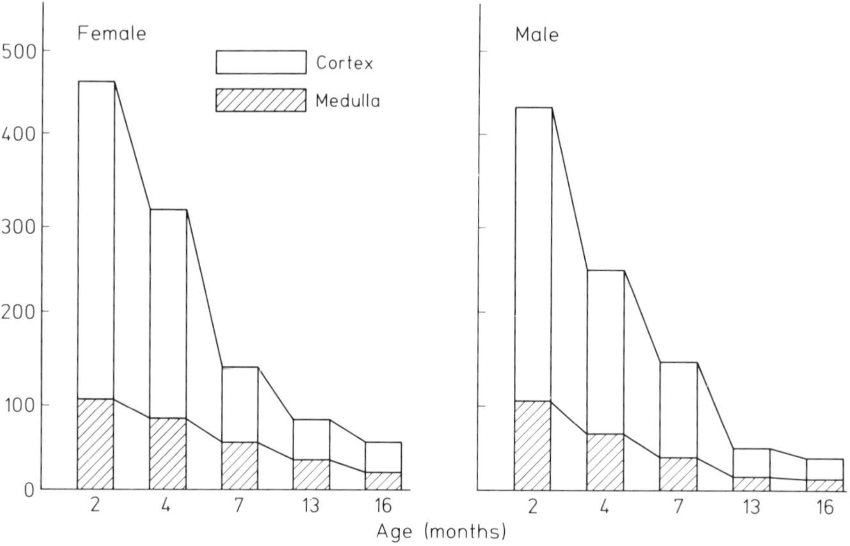

Fig. 326. Changes in thymic weight with aging. The weight of each component was calculated as follows: cortex, total weight (mg) × cortical area/total area; medulla, total weight (mg) × medullary area/total area

thelial elements form tubular structures which occasionally contain pink homogenous products.

In general, nonspecific stress can also induce thymic atrophy through the elevation of blood corticoid levels. It is very difficult, however, to differentiate histologically between chemical-induced and stress-associated thymic atrophy.

Biologic Features

Many cytostatic chemicals such as busulfan, cyclophosphamide, and corticosteroids have an inhibitory effect on DNA or protein synthesis. They also have a strong affinity for hemopoietic cells, causing necroses and suppression of immunologic responses. Subsequently, these cytostatic chemicals cause atrophy of all lymphoid tissues including the thymus. Occasionally, secondary infections occur, and the animals can develop multiple abscesses in the brain, eye, liver, kidney, or lung (Tonelli 1966).

Some chemicals which do not have cytostatic effects such as polybrominated biphenyl (Gupta et al. 1983), 3,3',4,4'-tetra-chloroazobenzene (Olson et al. 1984), fluoroxene (Dersham et al. 1983), 2,3,7,8-tetrachlorodibenzo-p-dioxin (van Logten et al. 1980), trialkyltin (Snoeij et al. 1985), or methoxyacetic acid (Miller et al. 1982) also induce atrophy of the thymus, but the mechanism of action is not clear.

Comparison with Other Species

Due to the characteristic structure of the thymus, these changes may be found frequently in various species of laboratory animals as well as in human beings.

References

Dersham G, McMartin D, Dunber D, Kaminsky L (1983) Trifluorinated ether anesthetic lethality in rats: the role of bacterial infection. Toxicol Appl Pharmacol 71: 93–100

Gupta BN, McConnell EE, Goldstein JA, Harris MW, Moore JA (1983) Effects of a polybrominated biphenyl mixture in the rat and mouse. I. Six-month exposure. Toxicol Appl Pharmacol 68: 1–18

Meihuizen SP, Burek JD (1978) The epithelial cell component of the thymuses of aged female BN/Bi rats. A light microscopic electron microscopic and autoradiographic study. Lab Invest 39: 613–622

Miller RR, Carreon RE, Young JT, McKenna JM (1982) Toxicity of methoxyacetic acid in rats. Fundam Appl Toxicol 2: 158–160

Olson LJ, Hsai MT, Kreamer BL, Hinsdill RD (1984) Immunosuppression in weanling and adult Sprague-Dawley rats induced by acute exposure to 3,3',4,4'-tetrachloroazobenzene. Toxicology 32: 287–296

Snoeij NJ, van Iersel AAJ, Penninks AH, Seinen W (1985) Toxicology of triorganotin compounds: comparative in vivo studies with a series of trialkyltin compounds and triphenyltin chloride in male rats. Toxicol Appl Pharmacol 81: 274–286

Tonelli G (1966) Acute toxicity of corticosteroids in the rat. Toxicol Appl Pharmacol 8: 250–258

van Logten MJ, Gupta BN, McConnell EE, Moore JA (1980) Role of the endocrine system in the action of 2,3,7,8-tetrachlorodibenzo-p-dioxin (TCDD) on the thymus. Toxicology 15: 135–144

Other Hemopoietic Tissues

Bronchus-Associated Lymphoid Tissue, Rat, Normal Structure

Taede Sminia, Gerda van der Brugge-Gamelkoorn, and Marja B. van der Ende

Gross Appearance

Large numbers of lymphoid cells that belong functionally to the immune system occur dispersed in the lamina propria and the epithelial lining of the respiratory tract. At certain sites the lymphoid cells are organized into smaller and larger lymphoid aggregates. These permanent aggregates of lymphatic nodules, called previously bronchus-associated lymphoid units (BALU; Sminia et al. 1989), are now described under the name bronchus-associated lymphoid tissue (BALT; Bienenstock et al. 1973a). With respect to its structure and function BALT is comparable with gut-associated lymphoid tissue (GALT), and together they constitute the common mucosal immune system (Bienenstock et al. 1973b). BALT can be detected in the respiratory tract under the dissecting microscope; when the bronchus is cut open, the affected bronchus epithelium has a whiter appearance due to the underlying lymphoid tissue. After fixation in situ white mucosal patches can be seen throughout the bronchial tree. These patches, which represent BALUs, are randomly distributed along the bronchial tract but consistently present around bifurcations. According to Plesch (1982) there are 30–50 BALUs per adult rat. A BALU always lies directly beneath the bronchus epithelium and is situated between an artery and a bronchus, and a nerve or group of neurons often accompanies it (for schematic drawing see Fig. 327).

Microscopic Features

The epithelium covering a BALU is different with respect to its cell composition and (nonepithelial) infiltrating cells from the rest of the bronchial epithelium. The main difference is the relative absence of mucous cells and the lower number of ciliated cells (Fig. 328). Moreover, numerous lymphocytes, macrophages, and granulocytes are often present in between the epithelial cells. Intratracheal administration of antigen induces a decrease in the number of ciliated cells in BALU epithelium in favor of the number of nonciliated cells (Van der Brugge-Gamelkoorn et al. 1986); moreover, Ia expression (MHC class II molecules) by the epithelial cells occurs. In addi-

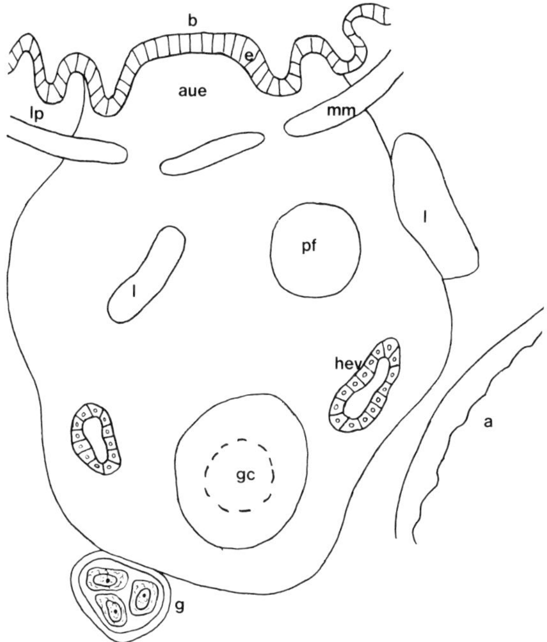

Fig. 327. Schematic drawing of a bronchus-associated lymphoid unit, rat. *a*, artery; *aue*, area under the epithelium; *b*, bronchus; *e*, epithelium; *g*, ganglion; *gc, germinal center; hev*, high endothelial venule; *l*, lymph vessel; *lp*, lamina propria; *mm*, muscularis mucosae; *pf*, primary follicle

tion, the number of mobile nonepithelial cells that infiltrate the BALU epithelium increases remarkably upon stimulation, and among them are numerous lymphocytes (Racz et al. 1977; Van der Brugge-Gamelkoorn et al. 1986).

Just beneath the epithelium in the lamina propria and submucosa lies the lymphoid tissue. A BALU is not separated from its surroundings by a capsule of connective tissue. Therefore, BALUs are not considered true lymphoid organs but represent local aggregations of lymphoid and nonlymphoid cells within the connective tissue compartment of the respiratory tract.

During the development of a BALU lymphocytes break through the smooth-muscle layer (tunica muscularis mucosae) of the bronchus, thus forming the area under the epithelium (Gregson et al. 1979; Plesch et al. 1983) (Fig. 329). The T and B lymphocytes in this area are intermingled. Underneath the tunica muscularis mucosae, lymphocytes are situated in T- and B-cell areas. Most

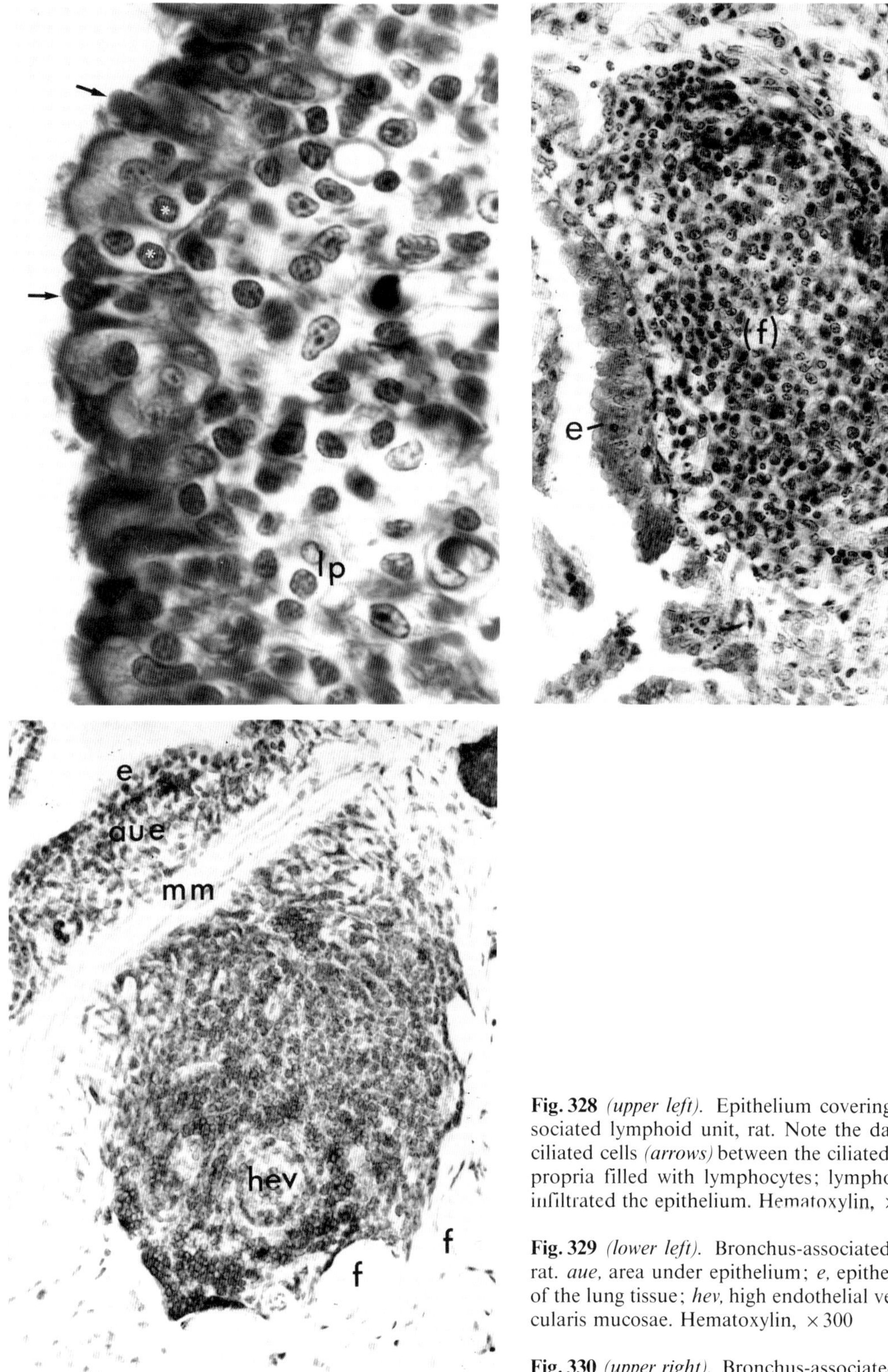

Fig. 328 *(upper left).* Epithelium covering a bronchus-associated lymphoid unit, rat. Note the dark-stained, non-ciliated cells *(arrows)* between the ciliated cells. *lp*, lamina propria filled with lymphocytes; lymphocytes have also infiltrated the epithelium. Hematoxylin, × 1200

Fig. 329 *(lower left).* Bronchus-associated lymphoid unit, rat. *aue*, area under epithelium; *e*, epithelium; *f*, fat cells of the lung tissue; *hev*, high endothelial venule; *mm*, muscularis mucosae. Hematoxylin, × 300

Fig. 330 *(upper right).* Bronchus-associated lymphoid unit with B-cell follicle *(f)* in the center and T cells around it, rat. *e*, epithelium; *lt*, lung tissue. Hematoxylin, × 300

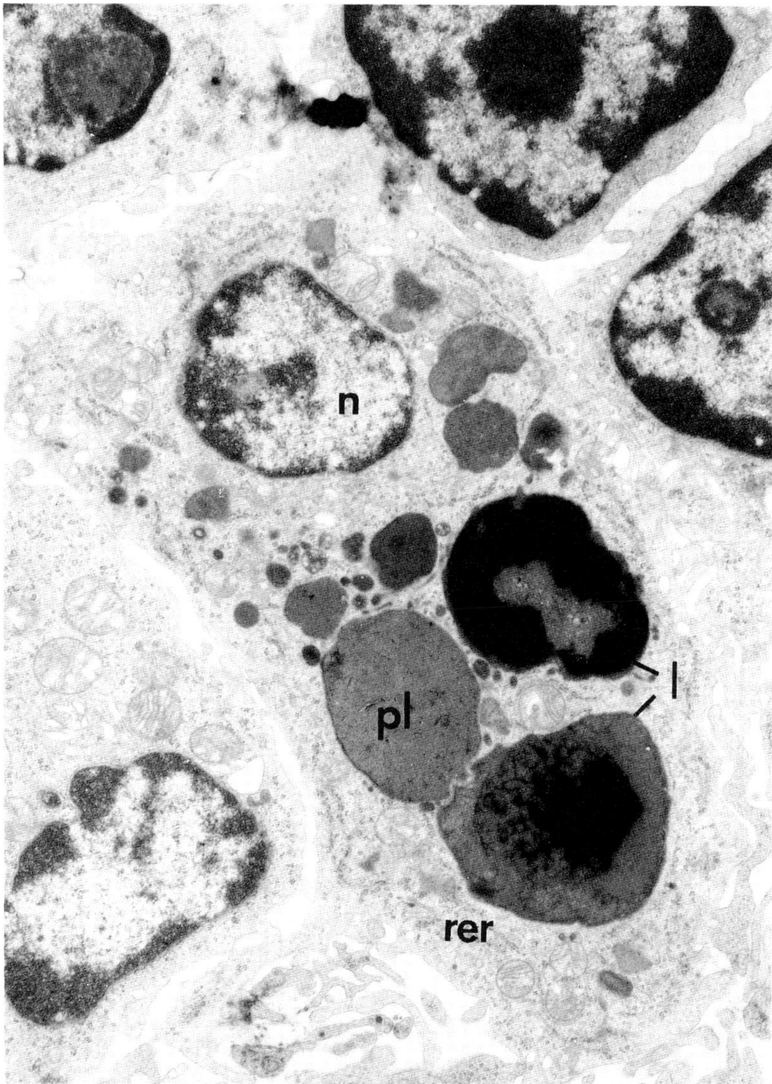

Fig. 331. Tingible body macrophage, rat. *l*, lysosomes filled with digested lymphocytes; *n*, nucleus; *pl*, primary lysosomes; *rer*, rough endoplasmic reticulum. TEM, × 4000

B cells seem globular, thus forming a B-cell follicle. Among them, the IgM- and IgG-bearing cells were evenly distributed in BALUs in approximately equal numbers, whereas IgA-positive cells were remarkably fewer in number. The majority of the T cells are concentrated around these follicles, in inter- or parafollicular areas (Fig. 330). In the various parts of the BALT, T- and B-cell areas do not occupy the same location with regard to the position of the bronchus and the artery. For example, at some points the B-cell areas are located close to the bronchus; in others, the opposite is the case (Plesch 1982; Van der Brugge Gamelkoorn and Sminia 1985). This is striking, considering the fixed position T- and B-cell areas always have in other lymphoid organs in relation to the site from which antigens are transported.

Several types of nonlymphoid cells are present in BALUs: fibroblasts, reticulum cells, macrophages, IDC, and follicular dendritic cells. The morphology of these fibroblasts and reticulum cells is similar to that in other lymphoid organs (Siminia et al. 1989). The only difference between BALUs, lymph nodes, and the spleen appears to be that BALUs have a relatively high proportion of collagen and reticular fibrils. The macrophage population of BALUs is heterogeneous. In addition to (classic) scavenger macrophages that occur throughout a BALU, tingible body macrophages and interdigitating cells are present. Tingible body macrophages, which are

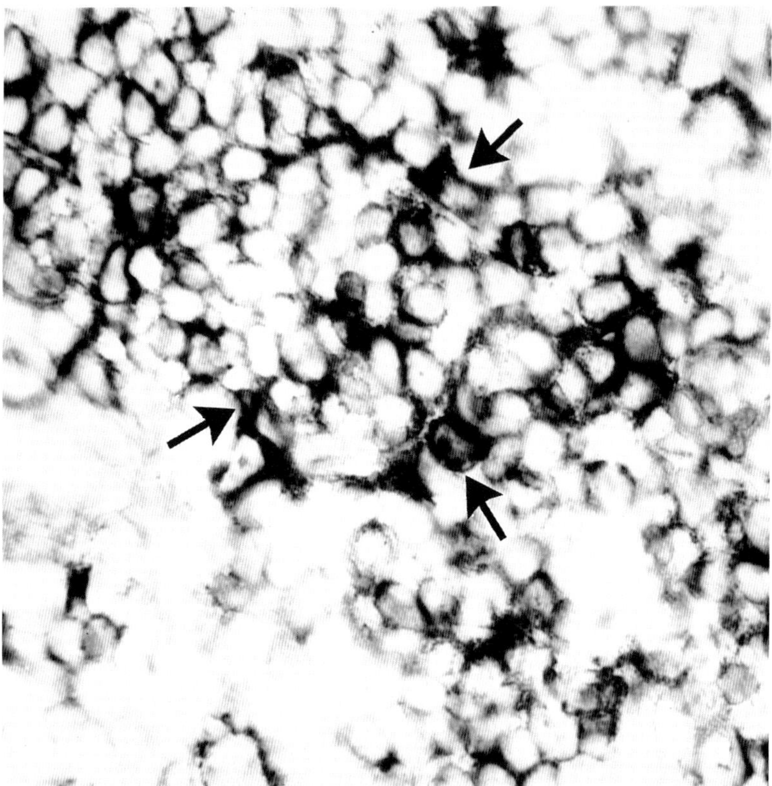

Fig. 332. Rat, part of the T-cell area of a bronchus-associated lymphoid unit with branched interdigitating cells *(arrows)* which are strongly Ia-positive. Stained with Ia-specific antibodies, × 800

almost confined to the B-cell areas, are thought to play a part in the removal and digestion of derailed B lymphocytes within B-cell follicles (Fig. 331). Interdigitating cells are the antigen-presenting cells characteristic of T-cell areas (Veerman and Van Ewijk 1975); they are often in intimate contacts with T cells and are strongly Ia-positive (Fig. 332) (Van der Brugge-Gamelkoorn et al. 1985a; Simecka et al. 1986). The nonlymphoid cell type characteristic of B-cell follicles is the follicular dendritic cell. These cells retain immune complexes on the cell surface and probably originate from reticulum cells (Dijkstra et al. 1984). They are OX-2-positive (Barclay 1981) but poorly developed in unstimulated BALUs. After antigenic stimulation they exhibit their typical morphological feature of long dendritic cell processes between the B cells. BALUs lack defined afferent lymphatics: Efferent lymph vessels arise in and around the BALUs and drain into peripheral sinuslike vessels through which the lymph flows to the draining paratracheal and hilar lymph nodes. BALUs contain arteriolar capillaries and venules, among them high-endothelial venules (Fig. 333). Studies on the T/B-cell speci-

ficity of these specialized blood vessels through which lymphocytes migrate from the blood to the lymphoid tissue have shown that T and B lymphocytes adhere in about equal numbers to high endothelial venules in BALUs (Van der Brugge-Gamelkoorn and Kraal 1985). This specificity of high endothelial venules of BALU reflects the actual in situ distribution of the two cell populations in this organ; a BALU is comprised of about 45% T and about 55% B lymphocytes.

Ultrastructure

BALU epithelium is characterized by the presence of nonciliated, microvilli-bearing cells, which are intermingled with the ciliated cells, the common cell type of bronchus epithelium (Fig. 334). The microvilli-bearing cells contain numerous free ribosomes, short cisterns of rough endoplasmic reticulum, a few mitochondria, and an inconspicuous Golgi apparatus. Based on the degree of electron density and on the presence or absence of cytoplasmic granules, two subtypes of microvilli-bearing cells can be distinguished (Van

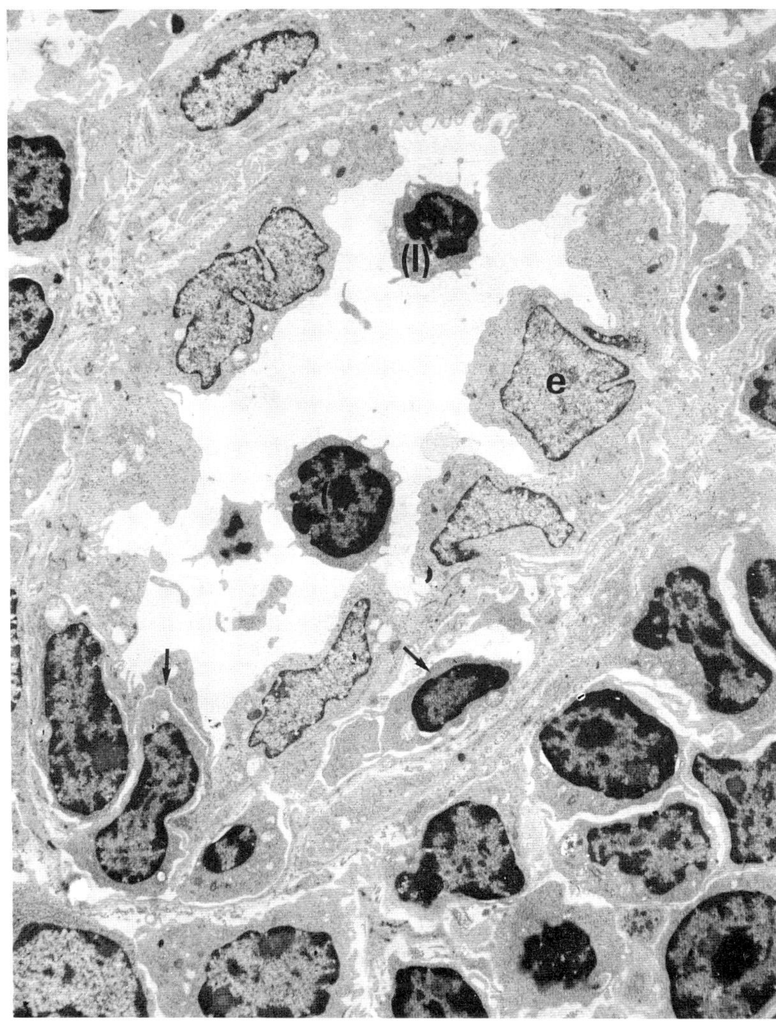

Fig. 333. High endothelial venule with lymphocytes *(l)* in the lumen, in the wall between the endothelial cells *(e; arrows)*, and in the surrounding connective tissue. TEM, × 3000

der Brugge-Gamelkoorn et al. 1986). Those with cytoplasmic granules have some resemblance to the serous cells described in the airway epithelium and are believed to be the site of production of the secretory component involved in the epithelial transfer of secretory IgA (Van der Brugge-Gamelkoorn et al. 1986). In those without cytoplasmic granules, invaginations of the apical cell membrane and cytoplasmic vacuoles are often present, suggesting active endocytosis. Using tracers such as horseradish peroxidase and latex particles, it could be shown that these microvilli-bearing cells are involved in the uptake and transport of soluble and particulate antigens from the bronchus lumen to the BALUs (Gregson et al. 1982; Van der Brugge-Gamelkoorn et al. 1985b). Functionally, they are presumably comparable to the M cells in the epithelium covering Peyer's patches in the gut (Owen and Jones 1974) as they are involved in antigen uptake and because they are in intimate contact with the infiltrated cells, in particular, macrophages and dendritic cells. However, in contrast to the antigen-sampling BALU epithelial cells, M cells form a kind of umbrella above a cluster of infiltrated lymphocytes and macrophages.

Interdigitating cells in BALUs of unstimulated (control) animals have an immature appearance; they have only a few short cell processes, and the vesicular complex is not conspicuous (Fig. 335) (Van der Brugge-Gamelkoorn et al. 1985a). Mature IDCs having the ultrastructural characteristics of spleen and lymph node IDCs (Veerman and Van Ewijk 1975) can be found after antigenic stimulation. At the ultrastructural level these cells are characterized by an electron-lucent cyto-

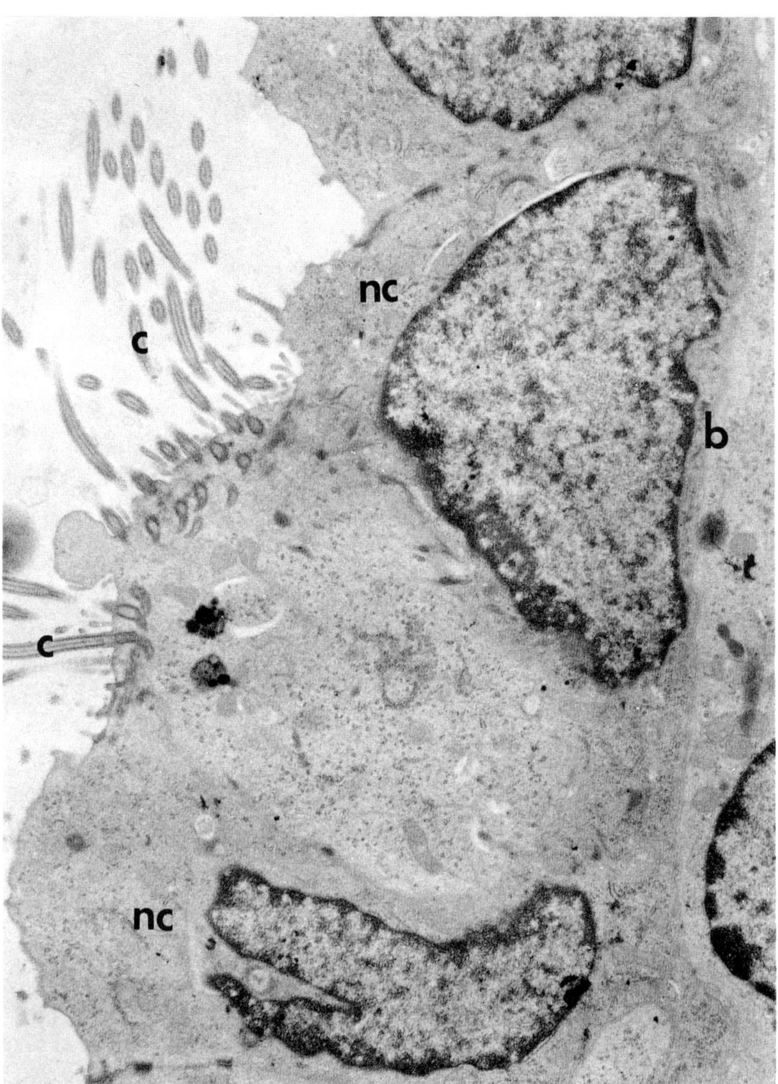

Fig. 334. Epithelium covering a bronchus-associated lymphoid unit with three nonciliated cells *(nc)* and a ciliated cell between them, rat. *c,* cilia; *b,* basal lamina. TEM, × 8000

plasm and by blunt cell processes that interdigitate with fingerlike extensions of adjacent lymphocytes. Well-developed Golgi bodies are located around the cytocenter, together with small lymsosomes. Furthermore, numerous vesicles forming a vesicular complex, small mitochondria; and a varying number of cisterns of the rough endoplasmic reticulum occur. FDCs in BALUs are less conspicuous than in other lymphoid organs. Although they share the ultrastructural characteristics of their counterparts in the spleen and lymph nodes, BALU follicular dendritic cells have shorter and less irregular cytoplasmic processes between the surrounding B lymphocytes (Van der Brugge-Gamelkoorn et al.

1985a). Moreover, they have another phenotype. Monoclonal antibodies which specifically recognize nonlymphoid cells, in particular follicular dendritic cells in the B-cell follicles of the spleen and lymph nodes, do not react with BALU follicular dendritic cells (Jeurissen and Dijkstra 1986). It may be that these phenotypic differences between BALU and non-mucosal follicular dendritic cells are related to their function in the induction of IgA responses during the Ig switch, which is assumed to take place in germinal centers (Kraal et al. 1982).

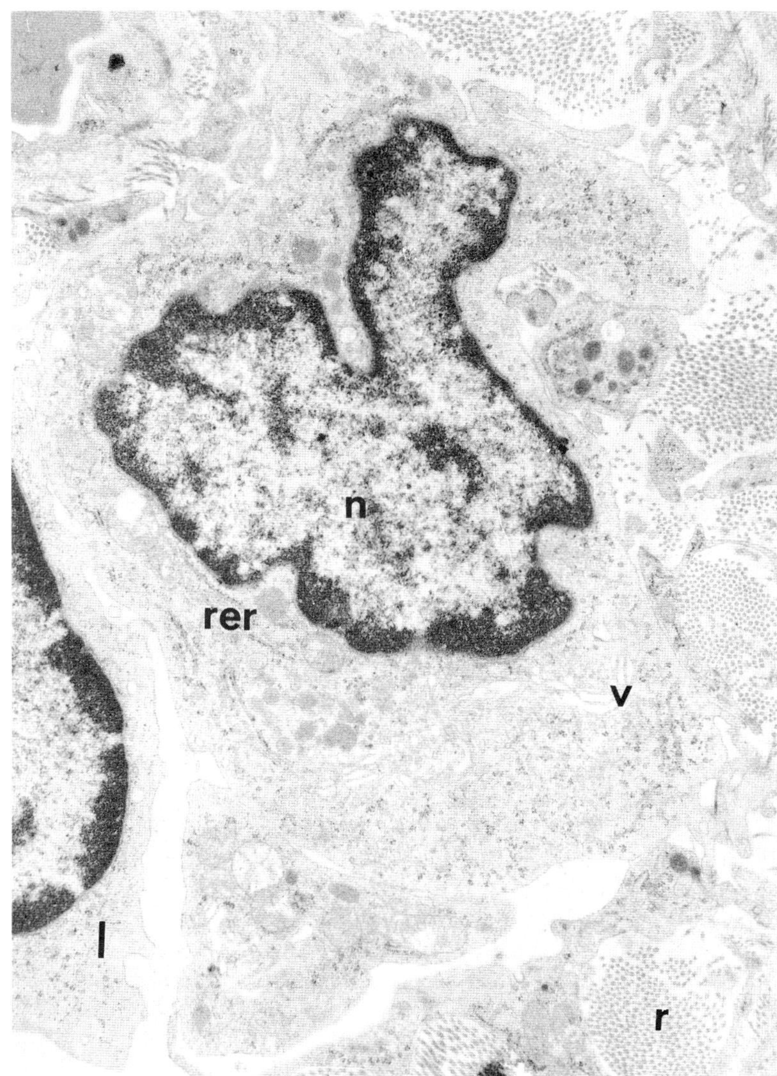

Fig. 335. Interdigitating cell surrounded by a lymphocyte *(l)* and reticular fibrils *(r)*, rat. *n*, nucleus; *rer*, rough endoplasmic reticulum; *v*, vesicular complex. TEM, × 4000

Biologic Features

BALUs are strategically located along the bronchial tract, in particular around bifurcations. They are involved in the uptake and transport of intratracheally administered antigens. As mentioned, antigens can reach a BALU directly via the BALU epithelium or indirectly, bound to alveolar macrophages that migrate from the lung alveoli to the BALUs. BALUs are also involved in cellular and humoral immune responses, which can remain local or become part of the common mucosal immune system (Bienenstock et al. 1973a) or even part of the systemic immune system. There is much debate about the precise role of BALT in local and systemic immune re-

sponses. Its function in the humoral immune response has been investigated by antigen administration in aerosols and in drops given intratracheally. After a single or repeated administration of antigen, specific antibody-forming cells occur in the paratracheal lymph node – the draining lymph node of BALT – and in the lung parenchyma, but not in BALT itself (Van der Brugge-Gamelkoorn 1986). Based on these observations and results of migration studies on alveolar macrophages, it has been suggested that antigen-laden alveolar macrophages migrate to the lung draining lymph nodes to induce an immune response. After proliferation and differentiation, the lymphoid cells migrate as blast cells to the lung parenchyma to secrete their antibodies locally. Although plasma cells have not been found in BALUs, morphologic changes do occur upon antigen stimulation. The most prominent changes are: enlargement of the BALUs, high infiltration of the epithelium by lmyphocytes and macrophages, dilated high endothelial venules, and the formation of secondary follicles with germinal centers, and the occurrence of prominent FDCs. A very interesting observation is the occurrence of immune complexes in the germinal centers. Based on these data, it can be suggested that BALT is not primarily involved in local antibody formation, but most likely it is the main site of generation of memory cells. It may well be that the FDCs in BALUs play by the presentation of immune complexes a main role in the formation of IgA memory cells, in addition ot other environmental elements, among which are IgA-specific T cells.

Comparison with Other Species

BALT has been observed in the lungs of a number of mammalian species (rabbit, rat, mouse, and guinea pig) including humans and is also present in the lungs of chickens (Bienenstock et al. 1973a). BALT is not confined to mammals and birds but also occurs in reptiles (turtle; unpublished own observations), which suggests that it is widespread in vertebrates. It must be stressed that there are clear interspecies differences relative to the development and organization of BALT (Bienenstock et al. 1973a; Van der Brugge-Gamelkoorn et al. 1986; Breel et al. 1988). For example, the morphology of guinea pig BALT is widely different from that of rat BALT. In guinea pig BALT the alternating T- and B-cell areas are more constant in their localization. In 1875 Klein described a slight difference in number and cell density between the lymphoid follicles in the rabbit lung and those in the guinea pig lung. In the lung of the Syrian golden hamster, no BALT has been found (Bienenstock et al. 1973a), and in various strains of mice (C57Bl/6, BALB/c, and [C3D2]F1) BALT is present but not well developed (Breel et al. 1988). In the chicken, BALT is localized in fingerlike mucosal projections protruding into the bronchial lumen, and the trachea of this animal contains more lymphoid tissue than the rabbit (Bienenstock et al. 1973a). So in conclusion we can say that BALT may or may not be present in the lungs, and, when present, there is a large variation in structure and development in various species. The functional significance of the observed structural differences is unknown. As mentioned already, the extensiveness of BALT within a certain species appears to be highly dependent on the antigen load of the individual. In humans it has been shown that BALT can undergo considerable proliferation following infections of the respiratory tract (Meuwissen et al. 1982; Herbert et al. 1985).

References

Barcley AN (1981) Different reticular elements in rat lymphoid tissue identified by localization of Ia, Thy-1 and MRC 0 × 2 antigens. Immunology 44: 727–736

Bienenstock J, Johnston N, Perey DYE (1973a) Bronchial lymphoid tissue. I. Morphologic characteristics. Lab Invest 28: 686–692

Bienenstock J, Johnston N, Perey DYE (1973b) Bronchial lymphoid tissue. II. Functional characteristics. Lab Invest 28: 693–698

Breel M, Van de Ende M, Sminia T, Kraal G (1988) Subpopulations of lymphoid and non-lymphoid cells in bronchus associated lymphoid tissue (BALT) of the mouse. Immunology 63: 657–662

Dijkstra CD, Kamperdijk EWA, Dopp EA (1984) The ontogenetic development of the follicular dendritic cell. An ultrastructural study by means of intravenously injected horseradish peroxidase (HRP)-anti-HRP complexes as a marker. Cell Tissue Res 236: 203–207

Gregson RL, Davey JJ, Prentice DE (1979) Postnatal development of bronchus-associated lymphoid tissue (BALT) in the rat, *Rattus norvegicus*. Lab Anim 13: 231–238

Gregson RL, Edmondson NA, Plesch BEC (1982) Preferential uptake of soluble antigen by respiratory tract epithelium overlying bronchus-associated lymphoid tissue in the rat. In: Nieuwenhuis P, Van den Broek AA, Hanna MG (eds) In vivo immunology. Plenum, New York, pp 499–505

Herbert A, Walters MT, Cawley MID, Godfrey RC (1985) Lymphocytic interstitial pneumonia identified as lymphoma of mucosa associated lymphoid tissue. J Pathol 146: 129–134

Jeurissen SHM, Dykstra CD (1986) Characteristics and functional aspects of non-lymphoid cells in rat germinal centers recognized by two monoclonal antibodies ED$_5$ and ED$_6$ Eur J Immunol 6: 562–568

Kraal G, Weissman IL, Butcher EC (1982) Germinal centre B cells: antigen specificity and changes in heavy chain class expression. Nature 298: 377–379

Meuwissen HJ, Hussain M (1982) Bronchus-associated lymphoid tissue in human lung: correlation of hyperplasia with chronic pulmonary disease. Clin Immunol Immunopathol 23: 548–552

Owen JL, Jones AL (1974) Epithelial cell specialization within human Peyer's patches: an ultrastructural study of intestinal lymphoid follicles. Gastroenterology 66: 189–203

Plesch BEC (1982) Histology and immunohistochemistry of bronchus-associated lymphoid (BALT) in the rat. In: Nieuwenhuis P, van de Broek AA, Hanna MG (eds) In vivo immunology. Plenum, New York, pp 491–497

Plesch BC, Gamelkoorn GJ, Van de Ende MB (1983) Development of bronchus-associated lymphoid tissue (BALT) in the rat, with special reference to T- and B-cells. Dev Comp Immunol 7: 179–188

Racz RP, Tenner Racz K, Myrvik QN, Painter LK (1977) Functional architecture of bronchial associated lymphoid tissue and lymphoepithelium in pulmonary cell-mediated reactions in the rabbit. J Reticuloendothel Soc 22: 59–83

Simecka JW, Davis JK, Cassel SH (1986) Distribution of Ia antigens and T-lymphocyte subpopulations in rat lungs. Immunology 57: 93–98

Sminia T, van der Brugge-Gamelkoorn GJ, Jeurissen SHM (1989) Structure and function of bronchus-associated lymphoid tissue (BALT). CRC Crit Rev Immunol 9: 119–150

Van der Brugge-Gamelkoorn GJ (1986) Structure and function of bronchus-associated lymphoid tissue (BALT) in the rat. Thesis, Free University, Amsterdam

Van der Brugge-Gamelkoorn GJ, Kraal G (1985) The specificity of the high endothelial venule in bronchus-associated lymphoid tissue (BALT). J Immunol 134: 3746–3750

Van der Brugge-Gamelkoorn GJ, Sminia T (1985) T cells and T cell subsets in rat bronchus associated lymphoid tissue (BALT) in situ and in suspension. In: Klaus GGB (ed) Microenvironments in the lymphoid system. Plenum, New York, pp 323–329

Van der Brugge-Gamelkoorn GJ, Van de Ende MB, Sminia T (1985a) Non-lymphoid cells of bronchus-associated lymphoid tissue of the rat in situ and in suspension, with special reference to interdigitating and follicular dendritic cells. Cell Tissue Res 239: 177–182

Van der Brugge-Gamelkoorn GJ, Van de Ende MB, Sminia T (1985b) Uptake of antigens and inert particles by bronchus-associated lymphoid tissue (BALT) epithelium in the rat. Cell Biol Int Rep 9: 524

Van der Brugge-Gamelkoorn GJ, Van de Ende MB, Sminia T (1986) Changes occurring in the epithelium covering bronchus-associated lymphoid tissue (BALT) after intratracheal challenge with horseradish peroxidase. Cell Tissue Res 245: 439–444

Veerman AJP, Van Ewijk W (1975) White pulp compartments in the spleen of rats and mice. Cell Tissue Res 156: 417–441

Gut-Associated Lymphoid Tissue, Rodent, Normal Structure and Function

Taede Sminia and S. H. M. Jeurissen

Gross Appearance

The gut-associated lymphoid tissue (GALT) is part of the mucosa-associated lymphoid tissue (MALT) that is comprised of lymphoid tissues and organs located directly beneath the mucosal epithelium (Bienenstock et al. 1973; McDermott et al. 1979; Börsch 1984). Single B and T lymphocytes are present in the lamina propria and within the gut epithelium. Aggregates of lymphocytes occur as solitary follicles in the lamina propria and when stimulated by antigen are large enough to extend down into the submucosa. Collections of unencapsulated lymphoid follicles develop during the first 3 weeks after birth independent of antigenic stimulation (Mayrhofer et al. 1983; Wilders et al. 1983a). These are mainly present in the walls of the small intestine, particularly the ileum, and are called Peyer's patches. Other permanent aggregates of lymphoid follicles which belong to the GALT are colonic lymphoid patches (Bland and Britton 1984), tonsiles, and the appendix. This paper will primarily deal with Peyer's patches, as in rodents these structures are well developed and have been studied

extensively. It must be stressed, however, that the basic structure and function of Peyer's patches, tonsils, and the appendix are comparable. Peyer's patches lack defined afferent lymphatics; gut antigens reach the lymphoid tissue via the mucosal epithelium (Bockman and Cooper 1973; Owen 1977). Specific mucosal immunity is characterized by the local production of polymeric IgA by plasma cells in the lamina propria; this IgA is then taken up by a receptor on the surfaces of gut epithelial cells and transported into the gut lumen (Brandtzaeg 1984; Mestecky 1987).

Microscopic Features

Peyer's patches consist of a number of relatively large B-cell follicles separated by small interfollicular T-cell areas. Each follicle consists of a germinal center surrounded by a corona. Between a follicle and the overlying gut epithelium, a (subepithelial) dome area is present (Fig. 336). Each of these compartments has in a framework of reticular cells its own characteristic lymphoid and

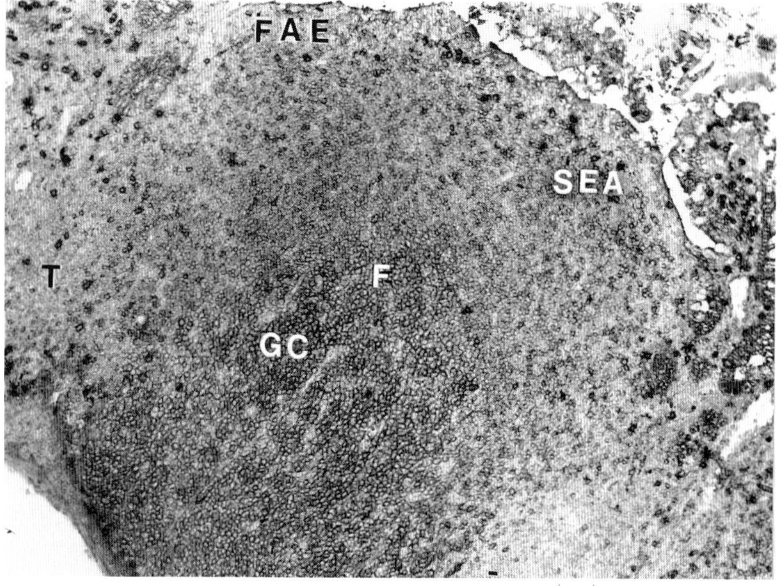

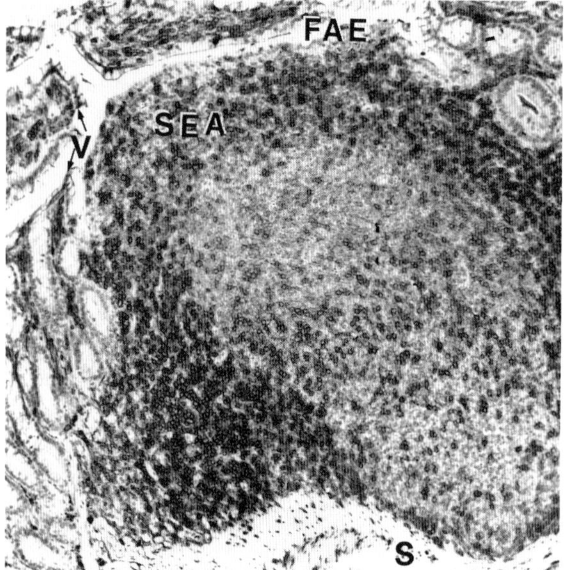

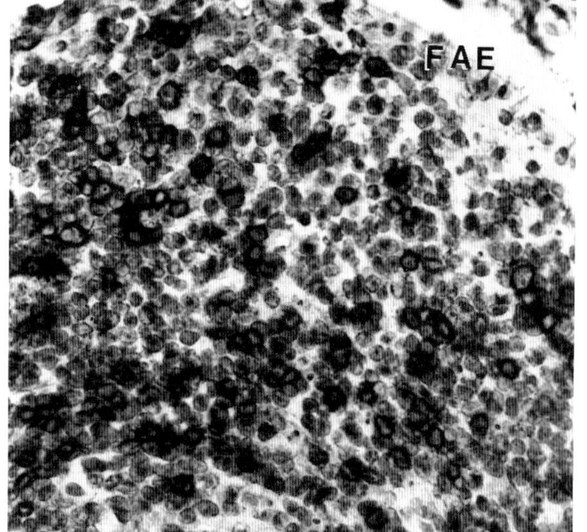

Fig. 336 *(above).* Peyer's patch, rat. Surface IgA-positive cells are predominantly present in the B-cell follicle *(F);* cells having cytoplasmic IgA *(black dots)* are mainly present in the subepithelial area *(SEA)* and the villi. *FAE,* follicle-associated epithelium; *GC,* germinal center, *T,* T-cell area. Cryostat section. Stained with IgA-specific antibodies, × 300

Fig. 337 *(lower left).* Peyer's patch, rat. T-helper cells *(black cells)* in the T-cell area, the subepithelial area *(S),*

and also in the follicle. *FAE,* follicle-associated epithelium; *S,* serosa; *V,* villi. Stained for T-helper cells, × 200

Fig. 338 *(lower right).* Peyer's patch, rat. Higher magnification of subepithelial area in Fig. 337. T-helper cells *(black cells)* are both present in follicle-associated epithelium *(FAE; arrows)* and subepithelial area. Stained for T-helper cells, × 600

nonlymphoid cell population (Sminia and Plesch 1982; Sminia et al. 1983). Silver staining for the detection of reticular fibers illustrates that the T-cell area is comprised of a dense meshwork of fibers and that the follicle is almost devoid of reticular fibers.

The germinal center is made up of a dark and a light area. The dark area, located at the serosal side of the follicle, contains many lymphoblasts with basophilic cytoplasm and mitotic figures. In the light area numerous large lymphocytes and only a few plasma cells are present. Most of the

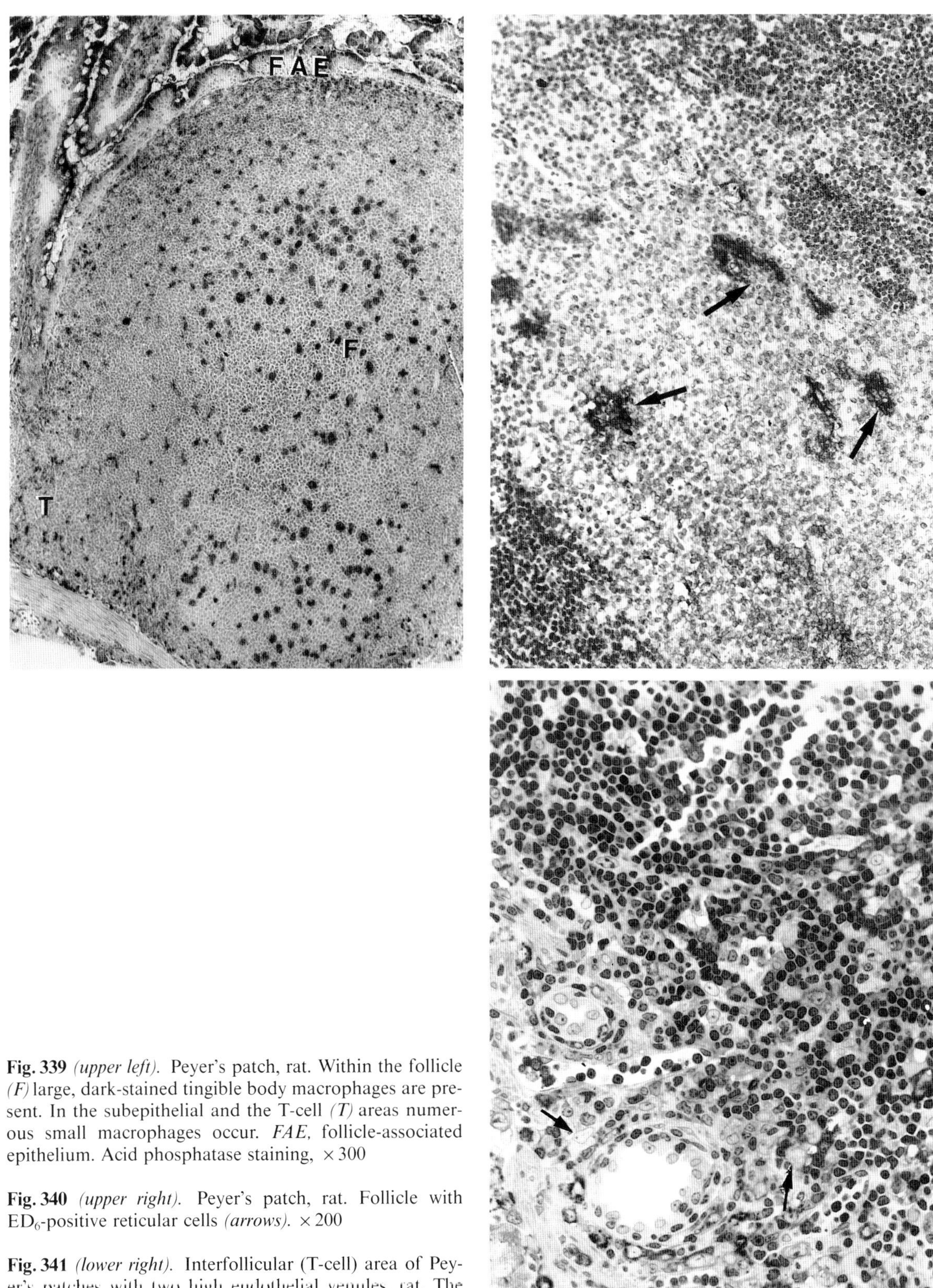

Fig. 339 *(upper left).* Peyer's patch, rat. Within the follicle *(F)* large, dark-stained tingible body macrophages are present. In the subepithelial and the T-cell *(T)* areas numerous small macrophages occur. *FAE,* follicle-associated epithelium. Acid phosphatase staining, × 300

Fig. 340 *(upper right).* Peyer's patch, rat. Follicle with ED$_6$-positive reticular cells *(arrows).* × 200

Fig. 341 *(lower right).* Interfollicular (T-cell) area of Peyer's patches with two high endothelial venules, rat. The light cells *(arrows)* are interdigitating cells. Semithin plastic section, × 400 lymphoid cells in the germinal center are B cells, although T-helper cells are also present (Figs. 337, 338). Most B cells (more than 70%) bear surface IgA (Butcher et al. 1982).

In addition to lymphoid cells, several populations of nonlymphoid cells are present in the germinal centers, such as tingible body macrophages and follicular dendritic cells. Tingible body macrophages are large macrophages with a high content of lysosomal enzymes which are dispersed in the germinal center (Fig. 339). They contain lymphocytes in various stages of digestion and are thought to play a role in the removal of lymphocytes that should not leave the Peyer's patches. Although these cells morphologically resemble their splenic and lymph node counterparts, our recent observations (unpublished) suggest that they have another enzyme content and different lectin-binding capacities.

Follicular dendritic cells are mainly confined to the light area. These cells have long cytoplasmic processes and bind immune complexes on their surface. They probably originate from reticular cells (Dijkstra et al. 1984). Recently, Jeurissen and Dijkstra (1986) have shown in the rat that the monoclonal antibody ED_5 reacts with follicular dendritic cells in the spleen and lymph nodes but not in the Peyer's patches, indicating that the phonotype of these cells in the Peyer's patches differs from that in the spleen and lymph nodes. Moreover, these authors report the presence of another type of reticular cell in the germinal centers, the so-called ED_6-positive cell (Fig. 340). This finding points to heterogeneity among reticular cells within the B-cell follicles.

The corona (mantle, cap) is a ring of densely packed small lymphocytes which surrounds about half of the germinal center but is thickest toward the epithelium among which both B and T cells are present.

The dome, situated between the follicle and the epithelium, covers the Peyer's patch. In this area B and T lymphocytes, plasma cells, scavenger macrophages, and dendritic cells are present.

The interfollicular area, which forms only a small part of a Peyer's patch between the follicles, contains predominantly T lymphocytes (Sminia and Plesch 1982). About twice as many T-helper cells as T-suppressor cells are present and intermingled at random (Jeurissen et al. 1985; see Figs. 337, 338). The most conspicuous nonlymphoid cell in the T-cell areas is the interdigitating cell. They have a dendritic appearance; their cytoplasmic processes are in intimate contact with the surrounding T cells. The strong Ia-positivity (MHC class II antigens) of these cells suggests that they are involved in antigen-presentation to the T cells. The interfollicular area is further characterized by high endothelial venules (postcapillary venules) (Fig. 341). These specialized blood vessels are the major sites by which lymphocytes leave the blood circulation (Butcher et al. 1980) and enter the Peyer's patches. After entry, the lymphocytes localize in their respective T- and B-cell areas.

The follicle-associated epithelium covering the Peyer's patches forms the barrier between the gut lumen and the lymphoid tissue. Unlike the villous epithelium, this epithelium has reduced numbers of goblet cells and is heavily infiltrated with lymphocytes and nonlymphoid cells among which are "veiled" cells (Wilders et al. 1983b). With respect to the infiltrated lymphocytes, Rell et al. (1987) have shown that lymphocytes are non-randomly distributed in the follicle-associated epithelium and often occur in groups. The lymphocytes in the villus epithelium, in contrast to the follicle-associated epithelium, are scattered randomly. Observations on the phenotype of intra- und subepithelial lymphocytes in the Peyer's patches have shown that they are predominantly T-helper cells (Figs. 337, 338). The majority of the intraepithelial lymphocytes of the villi belong to the T-suppressor/cytotoxic phenotype (Lyscom and Brueton 1982). The most characteristic feature of the follicle-associated epithelium is the presence of a special type of epithelial cell, the microfold cell (Owen and Jones 1974; Bye et al. 1984). This M cell differs from enterocytes by having typical ultrastructural features (see Ultrastructure). Under the light microscope these cells are difficult to find. M cells have been shown to play an important part in antigen transport from the gut lumen toward the lymphoid tissue (Owen 1977).

Peyer's patches do not have a separate blood supply: Their microcirculation is part of the general circulation of the gut. Apart from high endothelial venules, a meshwork of capillaries is present in the dome area: The number of capillaries in the B-cell follicle is low (Fig. 342). Using retrograde injection of pontamic blue, Anderson and coworkers (1982) demonstrated that the lymphatics of the villi, situated on the top of a Peyer's patch, drain into the underlying interfollicular areas, whereas the B-cell follicles are completely devoid of lymph vessels (Fig. 343).

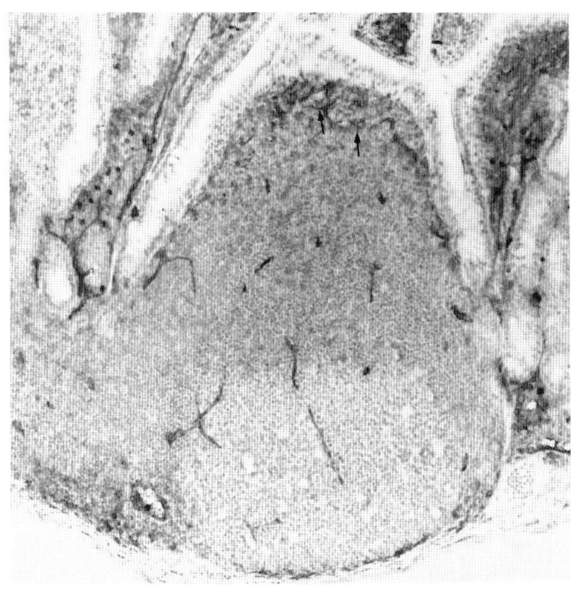

◄ **Fig. 342** *(above).* Peyer's patches, mouse, surrounded by villi (stained with the monoclonal antibody MECA-20, a general marker for endothelium in mice). A network of capillaries is present in the dome (subepithelial) area *(arrows)* and in the villi. Only a few capillaries are present in the follicle. × 300

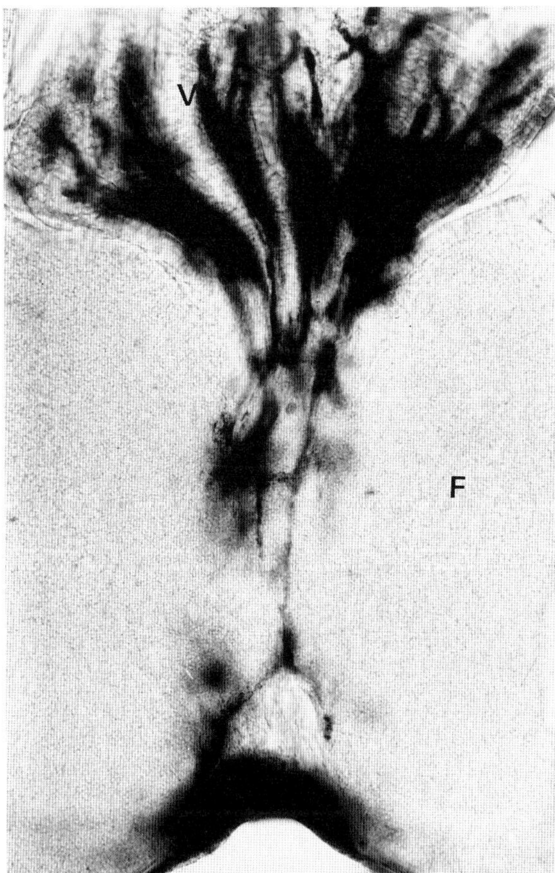

Fig. 343 *(below).* Peyer's patches, mouse. Two follicles *(F)* separated by interfollicular area, above which villi *(V)* are present. Retrograde injection of pontamic blue into the subserosal lymphatics fill the lymph vessels in the villi and the interfollicular area. × 300

Ultrastructure

Studies with the electron microscope have revealed detailed information about the M cells in the follicle-associated epithelium and the non lymphoid cells (interdigitating and follicular dendritic cells) in the Peyer's patches. In ultrathin sections, and M cell is seen as a rim of apical cytoplasm that bridges the space between the adjacent enterocytes (Fig. 344).

The cell bears irregularly shaped microvilli (microfolds), and morphological signs of endocytosis (invaginations of the apical cell membrane, coated vescicles) can always be seen. M cells form a kind of umbrella above the infiltrated lymphocytes and nonlymphoid cells (macrophages and dendritic cells). Tracer studies with horseradish peroxidase and ferritin have shown that the M cells endocytose and transport antigens from the gut lumen, without digestion, towards the infiltrated cells and the underlying lymphoid tissue (Owen 1977; Bye et al. 1984). The porous structure of the basement membrane of the follicle-associated epithelium also facilitates bidirectional migration of antigens, lymphoid and nonlymphoid cells from the epithelium to the Peyer's patches (McClugage et al. 1986).

The antigen-presenting interdigitating cells in the T-cell areas of the Peyer's patches resemble morphologically those in other lymphoid organs (Sminia et al. 1982).

Follicular dendritic cells have a typical morphologic feature: long slender cell processes that run among the lymphocytes present in the germinal center of the follicle (Sminia et al. 1982). The population of reticular cells to which follicular dendritic cells belong is heterogeneous with respect to morphology and probably also to function (Jeurissen and Dijkstra 1986).

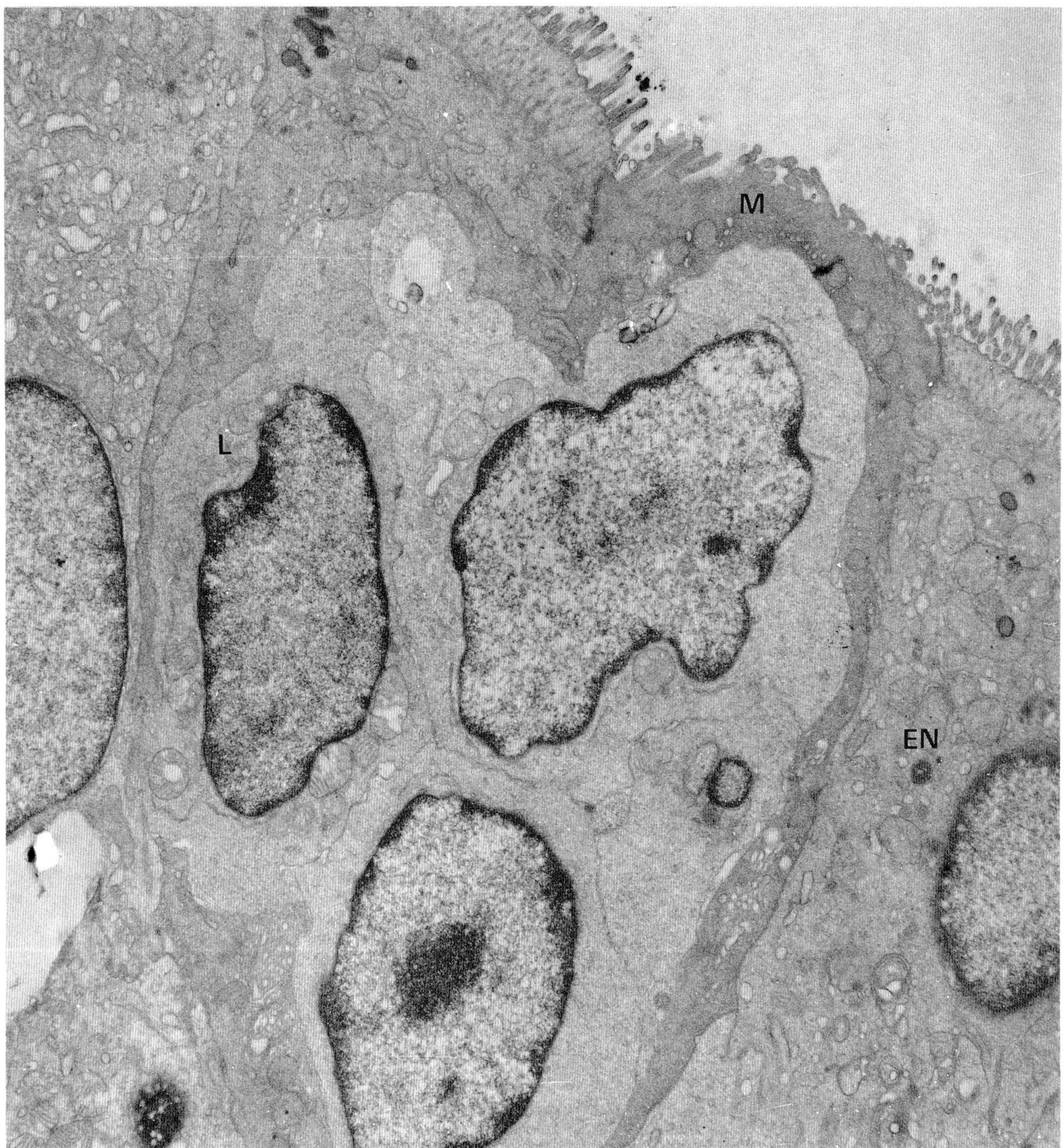

Fig. 344. Peyer's patch, mouse. M cell *(M)* in follicle-associated epithelium. *EN,* enterocyte; *L,* lymphocytes that have infiltrated the epithelium. TEM, ×7500

Biologic Features

The interaction of antigens with the gut-associated immune system has been studied extensively. The immune response varies between a state of tolerance, extensive cellular or humoral reactivity, and hypersensitivity, depending on the kind of antigen, the dose, and the frequency of administration (e. g., Mowat 1987). Peyer's patches are thought to play a crucial role in the regulation of these immune response and are involved in the generation of antigen-specific suppressor cells (Kagnoff 1978; Elson et al. 1986). Subsequent migration of T-suppressor cells (Fig. 345) derived from the Peyer's patches to the mesenteric lymph nodes and the spleen is thought to be responsible for systemic suppression (tolerance) in combination with a local humoral immune response (Mattingly and Waksman 1978; Jeurissen et al. 1984).

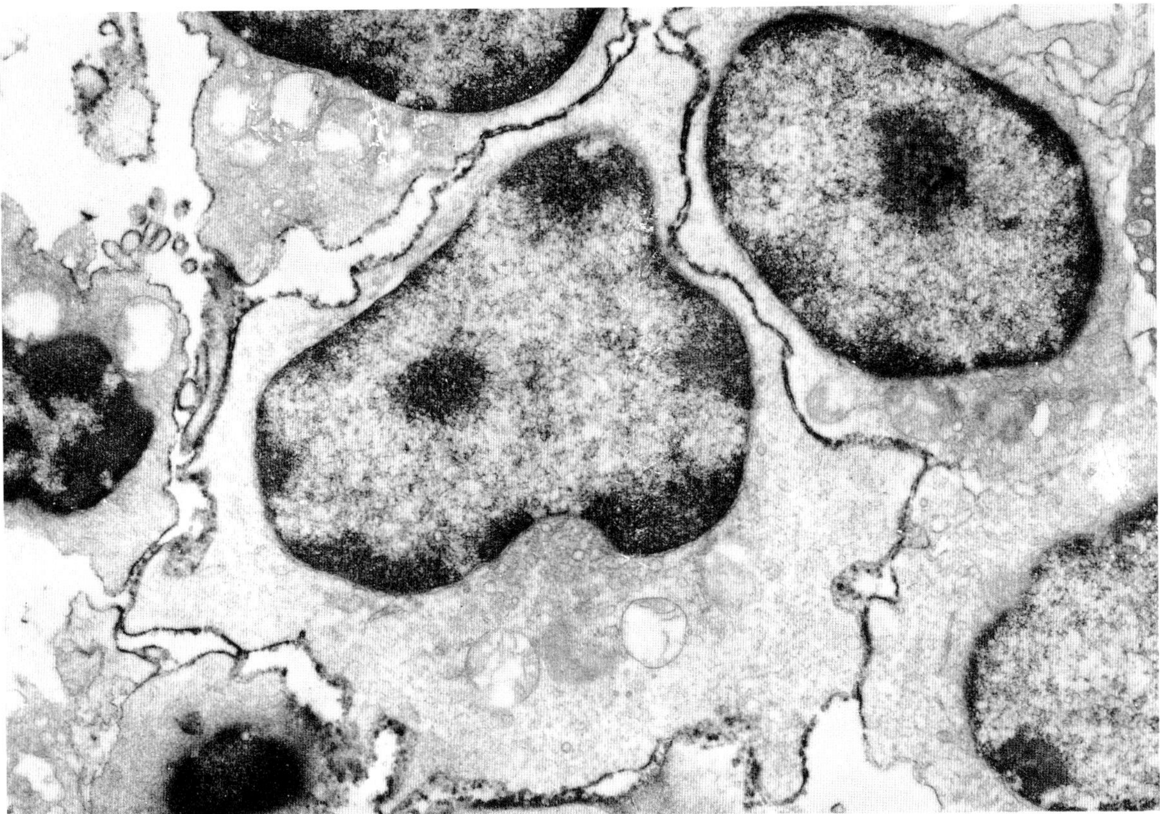

Fig. 345. Peyer's patch, mouse. T-suppressor cell in the T-cell area. Note the reaction product on the cell membrane. Stained with the monoclonal OX-8, TEM, ×8000

The humoral immune response to intestinal antigens is characterized by the production of predominantly IgA immunoglobulins synthesized in plasma cells present in the lamina propria of the gut (Mestecky 1987). Precursor cells of these IgA-producing plasma cells are shown to be derived from the Peyer's patches (Craig and Cebra 1971). The induction of IgA-committed B lymphocytes is thought to be regulated by IgA-specific T-helper cells in the Peyer's patches (Elson et al. 1986), in combination with antigen-specific immune complexes which have been shown to localize in germinal centers of the Peyer's patches (Jeurissen et al. 1987b). Migration studies in which IgA lymphoblasts and plasma cells obtained from mesenteric lymph nodes and Peyer's patches were intravenously injected have shown that these cells preferentially localize in mucosa-associated lymphoid tissue (Roux et al. 1981). These data imply that antigen-reactive cells will tend to return to the sites at which they are likely to meet the appropriate antigens. High endothelial venules play an important role in this regulated migration of lymphocytes (Kraal et al. 1987).

High endothelial venules in the Peyer's patches appear to have a marked preference for B lymphocytes. For every T cell, four to six B cells were found to bind onto or migrate through the high endothelial venules in the Peyer's patches (Stevens et al. 1982). This preferential immigration of B lymphocytes into the Peyer's patches is reflected by the in situ distribution of lymphocytes, of which 80% is B cells. T cells of the helper phenotype localize 1.5 times as well in the Peyer's patches than T-suppressor/cytotoxic cells (Kraal et al. 1983). This relative preference of T-helper cells also parallels their in situ distribution in the Peyer's patches.

Comparison with Other Species

GALT is common among mammals, although the amount of lymphoid tissue and the internal organization may differ. In ruminants (calves and sheep) Peyer's patches are present both in the ileum and jejunum (Reynolds and Morris 1983; Landsverk 1987). The jejunal Peyer's patches resemble those of rodents, but the ileal Peyer's patches of ruminants are unique with respect to size and development, and lymphopoiesis takes place in them in the absence of antigenic stimulation (Reynolds 1987). Less information is available on GALT in other classes of vertebrates. In aves (chickens, fowl, and turkey) (Burns and Maxwell 1986; Jeurissen et al. 1988) Peyer's patches occur and are similar in many respects to those found in mammals. Although in reptiles (Solas and Zapata 1980), amphibians (Ardavin 1982a,b), and fishes (Davina et al. 1980) accumulation of lymphoid cells are present in the gut, these structures are regarded as infiltrates rather than true structured lymphoid aggregates such as Peyer's patches. These data suggest that in contrast to mammals and birds, cold-blooded vertebrates do not have Peyer's patches.

References

Anderson AO, Anderson ND, White JD (1982) Lymphatics in the intestines of mice. In: Hay JB (ed) Animal models of immunological processes. Academic, New York, pp 25–32

Ardavin CF, Zapata A, Villena A, Solas MT (1982a) Gut-associated lymphoid tissue (GALT) in the amphibian urodele *Pleurodeles waltlii*. J Morphol 173: 35–41

Ardavin CF, Zapata A, Garrido E, Villena A (1982b) Ultrastructure of gut-associated lymphoid tissue (GALT) in the amphibian urodele *Pleurodeles waltlii*. Cell Tissue Res 224: 663–671

Bienenstock J, Johnston N, Perey DYE (1973) Bronchial lymphoid tissue. I. Morphologic characteristics. Lab Invest 28: 686–692

Bland PW, Britton DC (1984) Morphological study of antigen-sampling structures in the rat large intestine. Infect Immun 43: 693–699

Bockman DE, Cooper MD (1973) Pinocytosis by epithelium associated with lymphoid follicles in the bursa of Fabricius, appendix, and Peyer's patches. An electron microscopic study. Am J Anat 136: 455–477

Börsch G (1984) Der Gastrointestinaltrakt als Immunorgan: das darmassoziierte Immunsystem. Klin Wochenschr 62: 699–709

Brandtzaeg P (1984) Immune functions of human nasal mucosa and tonsils in health and disease. In: Bienenstock J (ed) Immunology of the lung and upper respiratory tract. McGraw-Hill, New York, pp 28–95

Burns RB, Maxwell MH (1986) Ultrastructure of Peyer's patches in the domestic fowl and turkey. J Anat 147: 235–243

Butcher EC, Scollay RG, Weissman IL (1980) Organ specificity of lymphocyte migration: mediation by highly selective lymphocyte interaction with organ-specific determinants on high endothelial venules. Eur J Immunol 10: 556–561

Butcher EC, Reichert RA, Coffman RL, Nottenburg C, Weissman IL (1982) Surface phenotype and migratory capability of Peyer's patch germinal center cells. Adv Exp Med Biol 149: 765–772

Bye WA, Allan CH, Trier JS (1984) Structure, distribution, and origin of M-cells in Peyer's patches of mouse ileum. Gastroenterology 86: 789–801

Craig SW, Cebra JJ (1971) Peyer's patches: an enriched source of precursors for IgA-producing immunocytes in the rabbit. J Exp Med 134: 188–200

Davina JHM, Parmentier HK, Rombout JHWM, Timmermans LPM, Van Muiswinkel WB (1980) Lymphoid and non-lymphoid cells in the intestine of cyprinid fish. In: Horton JD (ed) Development and differentiation of the vertebrate lymphocytes. Elsevier, Amsterdam, pp 129–140 (Developments in Immunology, vol 8)

Dijkstra CD, Kamperdijk EWA, Dopp EA (1984) The ontogenetic development of the follicular dendritic cell. An ultrastructural study by means of intravenously injected horseradish peroxidase (HRP)-anti-HRP complexes as a marker. Cell Tissue Res 236: 203–206

Elson CO, Kagnoff MF, Fiocchi C, Befus AD, Targan S (1986) Intestinal immunity and inflammation: recent progress. Gastroenterology 91: 746–768

Jeurissen SHM, Dijkstra CD (1986) Characteristics and functional aspects of non-lymphoid cells in rat germinal centers, recognized by two monoclonal antibodies ED5 and ED6. Eur J Immunol 16: 562–568

Jeurissen SHM, Sminia T, Kraal G (1984) Selective emigration of suppressor T cells from Peyer's patches. Cell Immunol 85: 264–269

Jeurissen SHM, Schmidt ED, Sminia T, Kraal G (1985) Effects of a single oral dose of dinitrochlorobenzene on T lymphocyte distribution and migration in the gut. Int Arch Allergy Appl Immunol 77: 384–389

Jeurissen SHM, Duijvestijn AM, Sonntag Y, Kraal G (1987a) Lymphocyte migration into the lamina propria of the gut is mediated by specialized HEV-like blood vessels. Immunology 62: 273–277

Jeurissen SHM, Kraal G, Sminia T (1987b) The role of Peyer's patches in intestinal humoral immune responses is limited to memory formation. Adv Exp Med Biol 216A: 257–266

Jeurissen SHM, Janse EM, Koch G, de Boer GF (1988) The monoclonal antibody CVI-CHN6-68.1 recognizes cells of the monocytemacrophage lineage in chickens. Dev Comp Immunol 12: 855–864

Kagnoff MF (1978) Effects of antigen-feeding on intestinal and systemic immune responses. II. Suppression of delayed-type hypersensitivity responses. J Immunol 120: 1509–1513

Kraal G, Weissman IL, Butcher EC (1983) Differences in "in vivo" distribution and homing of T cell subsets to mucosal vs non-mucosal lymphoid organs. J Immunol 130: 1097–1102

Kraal G, Duijvestijn AM, Hendriks HH (1987) The endothelium of the high endothelial venule: a specialized endothelium with unique properties. Exp Cell Biol 55: 1–10

Landsverk T (1987) The follicle-associated epithelium of the ileal Peyer's patch in ruminants is distinguished by its shedding of 50 nm particles. Immunol Cell Biol 65: 251–261

Lyscom N, Brueton MJ (1982) Intraepithelial, lamina propria and Peyer's patch lymphocytes of the rat small intestine: isolation and characterization in terms of immunoglobulin markers and receptors for monoclonal antibodies. Immunology 45: 775–783

Mattingly JA, Waksman BH (1978) Immunologic suppression after oral administration of antigen. I. Specific suppressor cells formed in rat Peyer's patches after oral administration of sheep erythrocytes and their systemic migration. J Immunol 121: 1878–1883

Mayrhofer G, Pugh CW, Barclay AN (1983) The distribution, ontogeny and origin in the rat of Ia-positive cells with dendritic morphology and of Ia antigen in epithelia, with special reference to the interstine. Eur J Immunol 13: 112–122

McClugage SG, Low FN, Zimmy ML (1986) Porosity of the basement membrane overlying Peyer's patches in rats and monkeys. Gastroenterology 91: 1128–1133

McDermott MR, Bienenstock J (1979) Evidence for a common mucosal immune system. I. Migration of B immunoblasts into intestinal, respiratory, and genital tissues. J Immunol 122: 1892–1898

Mestecky J (1987) The common mucosal immune system and current strategies for induction of immune responses in external secretions. J Clin Immunol 7: 265–276

Mowat AMmcL (1987) The regulation of immune response to dietary protein antigens. Immunol Today 8: 93–98

Owen RL (1977) Sequential uptake of horseradish peroxidase by lymphoid follicle epithelium of Peyer's patches in normal unobstructed mouse intestine: an ultrastructural study. Gastroenterology 72: 440–451

Owen RL, Jones AL (1974) Epithelial cell specialization within human Peyer's patches: an ultrastructural study of intestinal lymphoid follicles. Gastroenterology 66: 189–203

Rell KW, Lamprech J, Sicinski P, Bem W, Rowinski J (1987) Frequency of occurrence and distribution of the intra-epithelial lymphoid cells in the follicle-associated epithelium in phenotypically normal and athymic nude mice. J Anat 152: 121–131

Reyolds JD, Morris B (1983) The evolution and involution of Peyer's patches in foetal and postnatal sheep. Eur J Immunol 13: 627–635

Reynolds JD (1987) Mitotic rate maturation in the Peyer's patches of fetal sheep and in the bursa of Fabricius of the chick embryo. Eur J Immunol 17: 503–507

Roux ME, McWilliams M, Phillips-Quagliata JM, Lamm ME (1981) Differentiation pathway of Peyer's patch precursors of IgA plasma cells in the secretory immune system. Cell Immunol 61: 141–153

Sminia T, Plesch BEC (1982) An immunohistochemical study of cells with surface and cytoplasmic immunoglobulins in situ in Peyer's patches and lamina propria of rat small intestine. Virchows Arch (B) 40: 181–189

Sminia T, Janse EM, Wilders MM (1982) Antigen-trapping cells in Peyer's patches of the rat. Scand J Immunol 16: 481–485

Sminia T, Wilders MM, Janse EM, Hoefsmit ECM (1983) Characterization of non-lymphoid cells in Peyer's patches of the rat. Immunobiology 164: 136–143

Solas MT, Zapata A (1980) Gut-associated lymphoid tissue (GALT) in reptiles: intraepithelial cells. Dev Comp Immunol 4: 87–97

Stevens SK, Weissman IL, Butcher EC (1982) Differences in the migration of B and T lymphocytes: organ-selective localization in vivo and the role of lymphocyte-endothelial cell recognition. J Immunol 128: 844–851

Wilders MM, Sminia T, Plesch BEC, Drexhage HA, Weltevreden EF, Meuwissen SGM (1983a) Large mononuclear Ia-positive veiled cells in Peyer's patches. II. Localization in rat Peyer's patches. Immunology 48: 461–471

Wilders MM, Sminia T, Janse EM (1983b) Ontogeny of non-lymphoid and lymphoid cells in the rat gut with special reference to large mononuclear Ia-positive dendritic cells. Immunology 50: 303–314

Intraepithelial Leukocytes, Murine

Angela C. Hanglow, Peter B. Ernst, and John Bienenstock

Synonyms. Intraepithelial lymphocytes; IEL.

Gross Appearance

These cells are not seen with the unaided eye.

Microscopic Features

Intraepithelial leukocytes were first described in 1864 as a heterogenous population of mononuclear cells located between the epithelial cells of both the small and large intestine (Eberth 1864, cited by Heidenheim 1888). These cells comprise approximately 10%–15% of all cells within the normal intestinal epithelium. They are located above the basal lamina between, but never within, the epithelial cells (Fig. 346). Most intraepithelial leukocytes are found at the base of the epithelial cells but do not form junctional contacts with them (Collan 1972; Marsh 1975). They are usually found as single cells, but they have also been observed in groups of between 5 and 10 cells. They do not migrate up the villus with the epithelial cells, suggesting that they are not all effete cells in the process of being shed in-

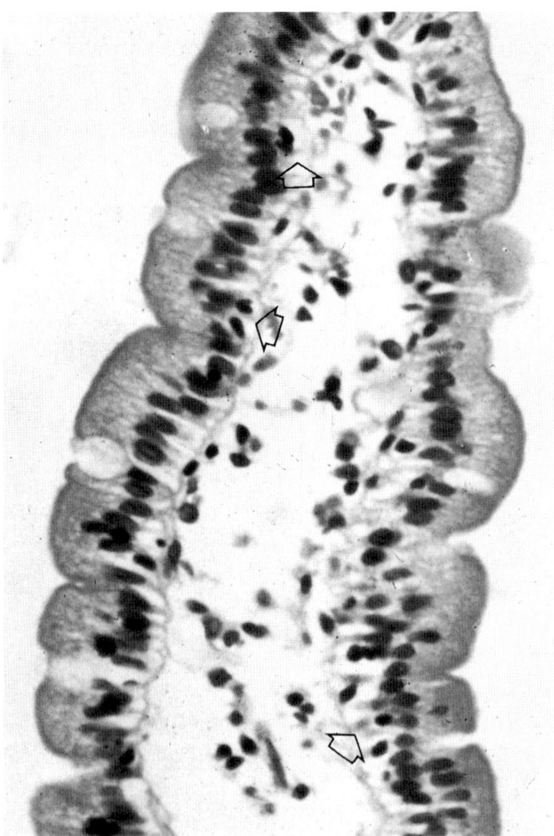

Fig. 346. Villus, small intestine, normal mouse. Note the presence of nucleated cells located between the intestinal epithelial cells, the intraepithelial leukocyte population *(arrowheads)*. H and E, ×250

Fig. 347 *(lower)*. Suspension of normal mouse intraepi-▶ thelial leukocytes. Note morphologic heterogeneity. Approximately ×750. (Reproduced from Ernst et al. 1985, *European Journal of Immunology,* with permission)

Fig. 348 *(below)*. Granulated intraepithelial leukocyte isolated from normal mouse small intestine. It contains three membrane-bound electron-dense granules located close to the Golgi apparatus. TEM, ×6000

to the intestinal lumen but rather that they perform an important biologic role.

Close examination of isolated intraepithelial leukocytes shows why intraepithelial lymphocyte is an inadequate term to describe all the nonepithelial cells within the gut epithelium; intraepithelial leukocyte is more appropriate to describe this extremely heterogenous population of cells, only some of which definitely belong to the lymphocyte lineage. In both mouse and rat, approximately 97% of intraepithelial leukocytes are mononuclear cells, including nongranular and granular leukocytes (Collan 1972). In nude rats, it has been demonstrated that the majority of the intraepithelial leukocytes are OX-8-positive, a marker for large granular lymphocytes (Ward et al. 1983).

The intraepithelial leukocyte population does not contain either B or plasma cells; they are confined to the lamina propria (Carmen et al. 1986). In both rats (Collan 1972) and mice (Petit et al. 1985) the lamina propria contains considerably

more neutrophils, eosinophils, macrophages, and mast cells than are found within the epithelium.

Only a small percentage of these cells are seen in mitosis. For example, in normal rat ileum 2%–3% of them are undergoing DNA synthesis at any one time (Fichtelius 1968). Generally, those cells in mitosis are found within the intestinal crypts. Degenerated leukocytes are present within the villus epithelium, and although it has been suggested that such cells are excreted into the gut lumen, most intraepithelial leukocytes undoubtedly have an active role to play within the intestinal environment.

Ultrastructure

Murine intraepithelial leukocytes are approximately 5–9 cm in diameter and contain sparse cytoplasmic organelles including mitochondria, ribosomes (both isolated and polyribosomes), endoplasma reticulum (rough: smooth = 2:1), and a small Golgi complex (Fig. 347). Nucleoli are often present in these cells. Up to 60% have between 2 and 5 large membrane-bound intracytoplasmic granules (Fig. 348). These granules correspond to the azurophilic-staining granules in Giemsa and Wright preparations and are reported to be lysosomal in nature (Collan 1972). Such characteristics suggest that intraepithelial leukocytes resemble the large granular lymphocytes which are found in many tissues including blood, spleen, liver, and lung and appear to correspond to natural killer cells (Timonen et al. 1981).

Biologic Features

Isolation and Quantification of Intraepithelial Leukocytes

Various techniques have been employed to isolate these cells from different species. Essentially these methodologies involve freeing the intestinal

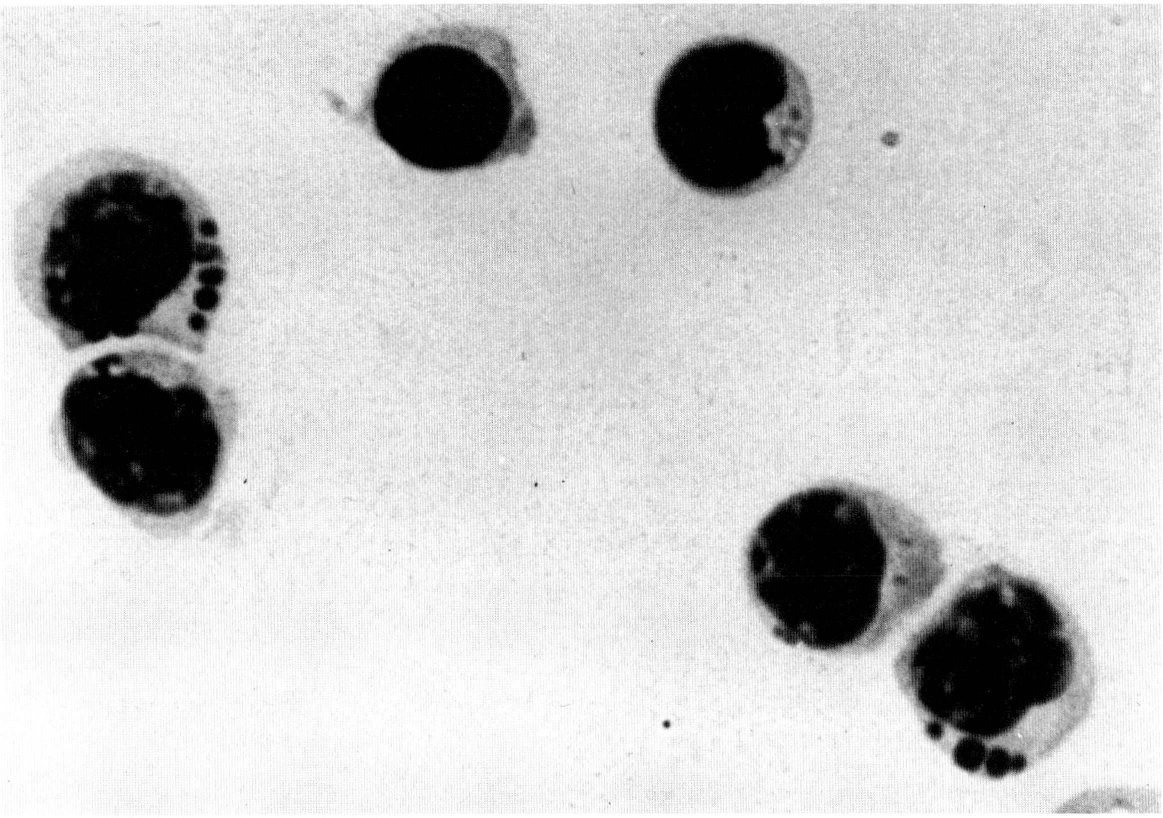

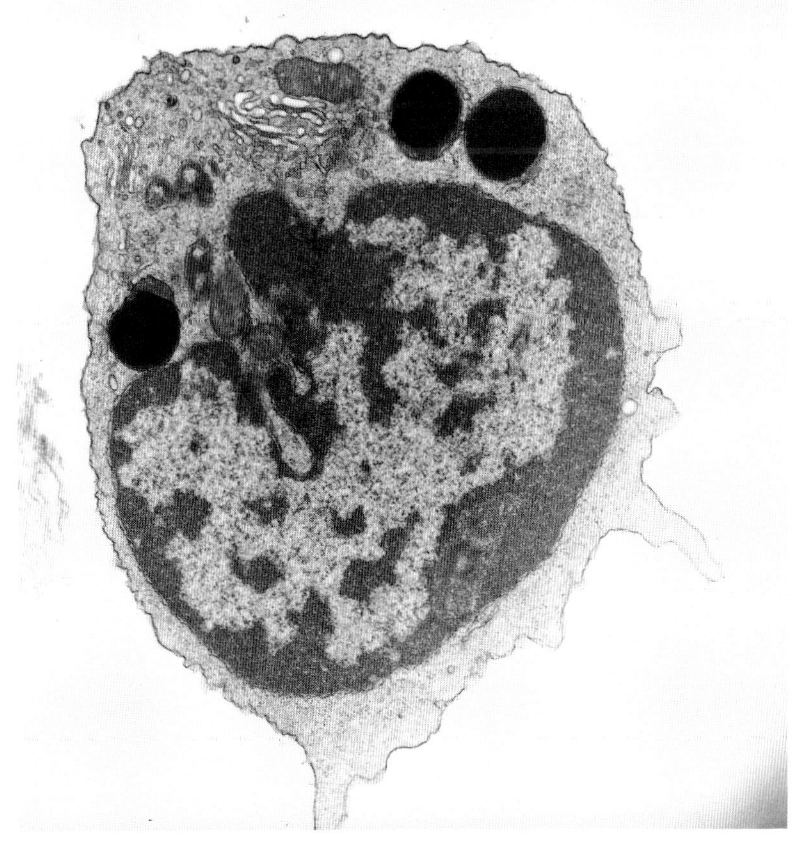

epithelium containing the leukocyte population from the underlying basement membrane, leaving the lamina propria intact. In mice this has been successfully achieved using a calcium-free isolation solution, but mechanical techniques have been the preferred means to dislodge the epithelium in rats. The leukocytes are subsequently separated from contaminating epithelial cells by a series of filtrations through nylon or cotton wool, followed by centrifigation over a discontinuous Percoll density gradient (Mayrohofer and Whately 1983).

Accurate in situ quantification of intraepithelial leukocytes has proved to be very difficult. These cells can be enumerated in relation to either the number of epithelial cells within a villus/crypt unit or the length of the underlying mucosa muscularis (Dobbins 1986). However, whatever method is employed, these assessments are founded on arbitrary criteria.

Surface Phenotype

Intraepithelial leukocytes have been isolated from the small intestine of mice and rats by the methods outlined above. Following isolation, these cells have been characterized using monoclonal antibodies directed against cell surface molecules which differentiate between distinct cell subsets.

In mice the following cell surface markers have been used to characterize these cells: Thy 1 (T cell), Ly 1 or L3T4 (helper T cell), Ly 2 (cytotoxic/suppressor cell), and asialo-GM 1 (mixed population containing cytotoxic cells with natural killer activity). Approximately 30% of these cells in the mouse bear the phenotype Thy 1^+, Ly 2^+, indicating a cytotoxic/suppressor T cell. In contrast, approximately 5% of Thy 1^+ intraepithelial leukocytes from normal mice bear the specific T helper cell marker, L3T4. It is the Thy 1^+ populations that are absent in athymic mice, indicating that they have a thymic-dependent origin. A major proportion of intraepithelial leukocytes (50%) bear an unusual phenotype: Thy 1^-, Ly 1^-, Ly 2^+ (Petit et al. 1985). Taken together, these observations may suggest that a major population of such cells in mice is not thymus-dependent because 50% are Thy 1^- even though they express the T cell-associated antigen Ly 2. Only 10% of these cells in mice are asialo-GM 1^+, suggesting that they belong to a population of cells with natural killer cytotoxic activity.

In the rat 92% of intraepithelial leukocytes express the leukocyte-common antigen (OX-1) and the class I major histocompatibility antigen detected by OX-18 (Mayrhofer and Pitts 1986). Very few cells in the normal rat gut are OX-19^+, antibody specific for rat T cells, although 80% are detected by the less specific T-cell marker W3/13 (van der Heijden 1986). Approximately 80% of these cells in rats have a cytotoxic/suppressor marker (OX-8^+), whereas only 3% have the helper marker (W3/25^+) (Fig. 349). Taken together, these results confirm those of the mouse and support the hypothesis that over 50% of these cells from rats are not T cells or may be very unusual T cells whose significance has yet to be determined.

Origin and Differentiation of Intraepithelial Leukocytes

Very few of these leukocytes are present in normal mice at birth (fewer than 2 per 100 epithelial cells), but they increase in number during the first few weeks of life (to 14–16 per 100 epithelial cells) (Ferguson and Parrott 1972). They are present in reduced numbers in antigen-deprived mice (Ferguson and Parrott 1972). These observations suggest that environmental antigens are responsible for the increase in numbers of such cells in the neonate.

Studies in rats and mice have indicated that both granulated and nongranulated cells in the gut epithelium do not originate there (Guy-Grand et al. 1978) but are derived from cells within the primary mucosal lymphoid tissue which migrate to the epithelium. At this site they divide, giving rise to smaller, long-lived intraepithelial leukocytes (Ferguson 1977). There is some controversy over whether all such cells have a thymus-dependent origin, i. e., whether they are T cells. In vivo experiments in the rat suggest that both granulated and nongranulated cells differentiate from the bone marrow without passing through the thymus and are, therefore, not T cell in origin (Mayrhofer and Pitts 1986). Although a few groups of researchers propose that the majority of the cells in the rat and mouse are T cells (Guy-Grand et al. 1978), most evidence supports the view that over 50% of them are thymus-independent. In addition to the evidence from the phenotypic analyses described above, these cells are present in spontaneously athymic mice (Klein et al. 1986) and rats (Ward et al. 1983), supporting a thymus-independent origin for the majority of these cells.

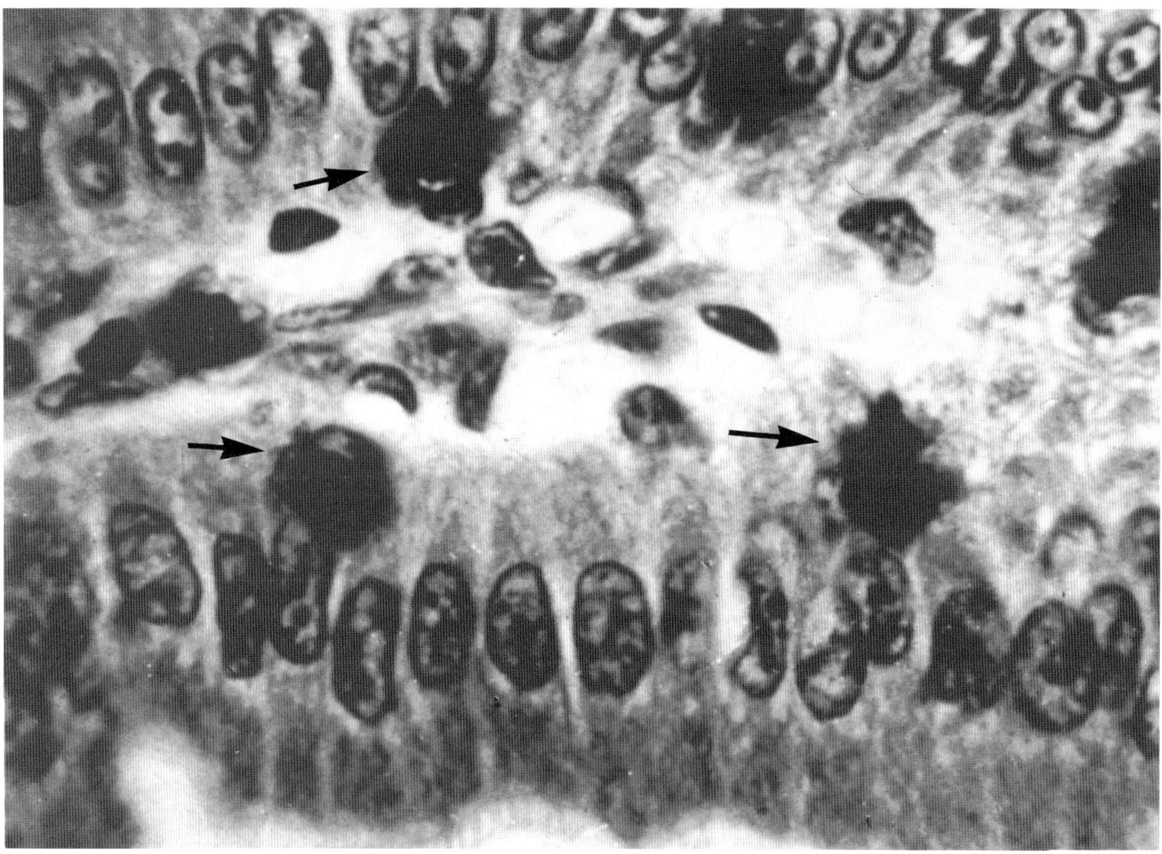

Fig. 349. Immunohistochemical staining of OX-8$^+$ cells *(arrows)* within the small intestine of nude (athymic) rat. × 1300. (Reproduced from Ward et al. 1983 and American Association of Immunologists)

Recent work by Goodman and Lefrancois (1988) has shown that many Thy1$^-$ mouse intraepithelial leukocytes of the suppressor/cytotoxic phenotype express $\gamma\,\delta$ T-cell receptors but not $\alpha\,\beta$ T-cell receptors. The authors suggest that these cells may represent "a phenotypically diverse and anatomically restricted population of T lymphocytes" which may not be thymus-dependent.

Functions of Intraepithelial Leukocytes

The biological role played by these cells in vivo remains to be determined. However, because they are located in intimate association with luminal antigens, it is often speculated that they provide an important line of defense in the prevention of enteric infection.

The majority of studies have shown that these cells of murine origin have a low spontaneous replication rate in vivo (Marsh 1975). Furthermore, they are less responsive to stimulation by mitogens in vitro than are cells isolated from the spleen (Dillon and MacDonald 1984; Mowat et al. 1986). However, it is possible that the isolation procedures used to obtain these cells may affect their function, and behavior in vitro may not be an accurate reflection of function in vivo (Bland et al. 1979).

There is good evidence that among intraepithelial leukocytes are both specific and nonspecific (i. e., natural killer) cytotoxic cells (Tagliabue et al. 1982). Furthermore, these leukocytes from antigenically naive mice can kill virally infected target cells (Carman et al. 1986), again suggesting that they have a role to play in protecting against enteric infection. Evidence is also available to suggest that these cells contain precursors for cytotoxic T cells (Ernst et al. 1985).

Interactions may occur between the intestinal epithelium and intraepithelial leukocytes. For example, in the rat, these leukocytes have been shown to secrete a factor (probably gamma interferon) which inhibits the growth of intestinal epithelial cells and induces their expression of class II major histocompatibility antigens (Ia)

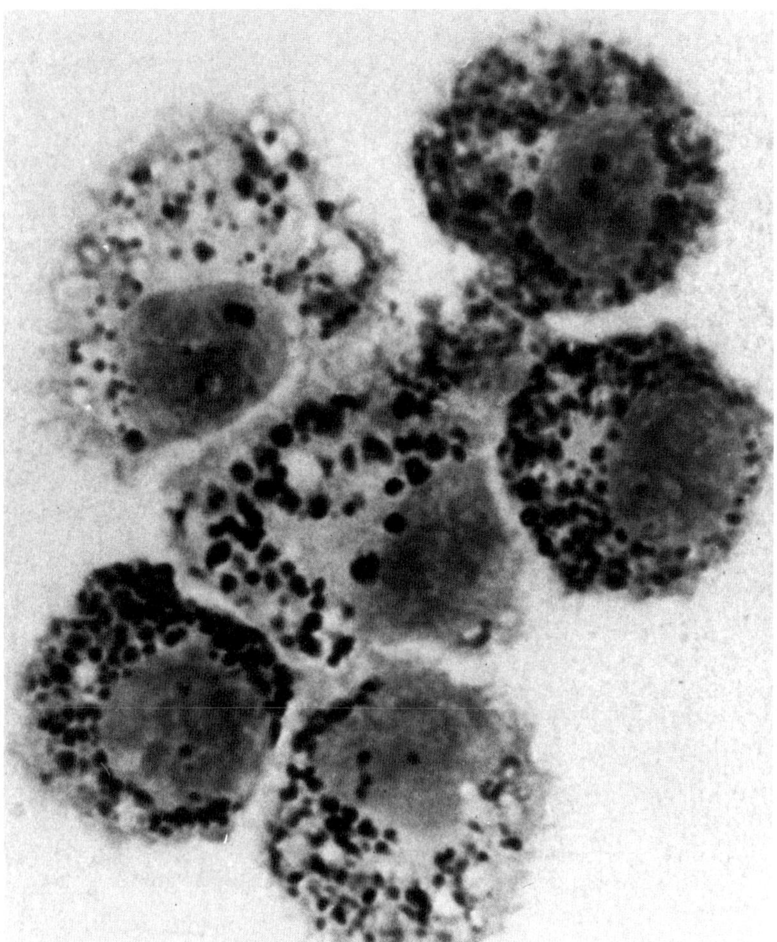

Fig. 350. Mouse, intraepithelial leukocyte cultured in IL-3-containing supernatants. These cells are larger than freshly isolated cells and contain many small granules typical of mast cells. Giemsa stain, ×750. (Reproduced from Ernst et al. 1985, European Journal of Immunology, with permission)

(Cerf-Bensussan et al. 1984). This suggests that intestinal epithelial cells may in turn present antigen to the intraepithelial leukocytes. If further experimental evidence continues to support this view, it will be a major contribution toward the understanding of how immune responses are initiated and/or suppressed within the environment of the gut.

Disease States

Intraepithelial leukocytes can increase in number during the enteric inflammation occurring in a "graft versus host reaction" or parasitic infection, for example, by *Nippostrongylus brasiliensis*. It has been proposed that under these conditions intraepithelial leukocytes are responsible for the changes in the mucosal architecture (Mowat and Ferguson 1982). For example, they may release lymphokines, inducing the increased crypt cell proliferation observed in these diseases. In addition, the mast cell population increase dramatically in these inflammatory states, and it is possible that such cells originate from precursors within the intraepithelial leukocyte population (Schrader et al. 1983) (Fig. 350). Mast cell mediators may be responsible for at least some of the pathological changes seen in the gut during inflammation. However, intraepithelial leukocytes are not mast cells nor are they derived from mast cells. The granules in intraepithelial leukocytes do not contain histamine and do not possess the high affinity receptors for IgE characteristic of mast cells (Petit et al. 1985).

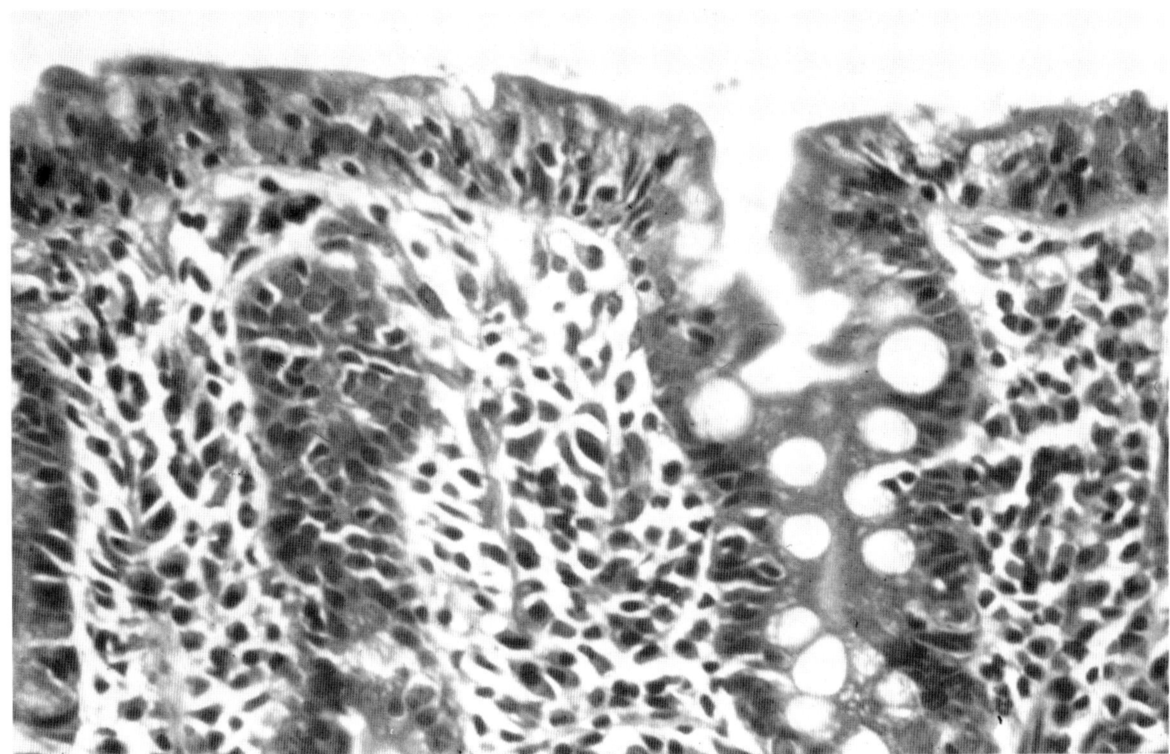

Fig. 351. Human bowel from a patient with celiac disease (gluten-sensitive enteropathy). Note the flattened mucosa and numerous intraepithelial leukocytes. H and E, × 200

Comparison with Other Species

Intraepithelial leukocytes have been described in a number of other species, including humans (Selby et al. 1984; Cerf-Bensussan et al. 1983) and rabbits (Rudzik and Bienenstock 1974). As many as 60% of rabbit or human intraepithelial leukocytes are granulated cells. In human subjects these leukocytes do not contain B cells and only very few macrophages, mast cells, or polymorphonuclear cells. In the human small intestine 80%–90% of intraepithelial leukocytes express T-cell markers (Leu-1$^+$, T3$^+$), 70%–80% of them being of the suppressor/cytotoxic phenotype (T8$^+$, Leu-2a$^+$). Only 10% express the helper phenotype (T4$^+$, Leu-3a$^+$) (Cerf-Bensussan et al. 1983; Janossy et al. 1980). This is in marked contrast to results in rats and mice for which available evidence indicates that a significant majority of intraepithelial leukocytes do not bear specific T-cell markers.

Several studies performed on intraepithelial leukocytes isolated from human colon suggest that these leukocytes can kill autologous colonic epithelial cells (Targan et al. 1983). Consequently, they may have a role to play in the pathogenesis of inflammatory bowel disease, although this is a controversial issue. Furthermore, in the inflamed bowel these leukocytes often have numerous elongated cytoplasmic projections in intimate contact with adjacent epithelial cell membranes (Dobbins 1986). It has been proposed that the increased numbers of intraepithelial leukocytes observed in the gut of individuals with celiac disease (gluten-sensitive enteropathy) are responsible for the flattening of the intestinal villi associated with this condition (Fig. 351). In contrast, the leukocytes do not increased in number in patients with Crohn's disease or ulcerative colitis (Selby et al. 1984), and there is no obvious change in the proportion of suppressor/cytotoxic and helper cells in these inflammatory conditions. Therefore, their exact role in the pathogenesis of inflammatory bowel disease is not yet fully understood.

References

Bland PW, Richens ER, Britton DC, Lloyd JV (1979) Isolation and purification of human large bowel mucosal lymphoid cells: effect of separation technique on functional characteristics. Gut 20: 1037–1046

Carman PS, Ernst PB, Rosenthal KL, Clark DA, Befus AD, Bienenstock J (1986) Intraepithelial leukocytes contain a unique subpopulation of NK-like cytotoxic cells active in the defense of gut epithelium to enteric murine coronavirus. J Immunol 136: 1548–1553

Cerf-Bensussan N, Schneeberger EE, Bhan AK (1983) Immunohistologic and immunoelectron microscopic characterization of the mucosal lymphocytes of human small intestine by the use of monoclonal antibodies. J Immunol 130: 2615–2622

Cerf-Bensussan N, Quaroni A, Kurnick JT, Bhan AK (1984) Intraepithelial lymphocytes modulate Ia expression by intestinal epithelial cells. J Immunol 132: 2244–2252

Collan Y (1972) Characteristics of nonepithelial cells in the epithelium of normal rat ileum, a light and electron microscopical study. Scand J Gastroenterol (Suppl 7) 17: 1–66

Dillon SB, MacDonald TT (1984) Functional properties of lymphocytes isolated from murine small intestinal epithelium. Immunology 52: 501–509

Dobbins WO (1986) Human intestinal intraepithelial lymphocytes. Gut 27: 972–985

Ernst PB, Petit A, Befus AD, Clark D, Rosenthal KL, Ishizaka T, Bienenstock J (1985) Murine intestinal intraepithelial lymphocytes. II. Comparison of freshly isolated and cultured intraepithelial lymphocytes. Eur J Immunol 15: 216–221

Ferguson A (1977) Intraepithelial lymphocytes of the small intestine. Gut 18: 921–937

Ferguson A, Parrott DMV (1972) The effect of antigen deprivation on thymus-dependent and thymus independent lymphocytes in the small intestine of the mouse. Clin Exp Immunol 12: 477–488

Fichtelius KE (1968) The gut epithelium – a first level lymphoid organ? Exp Cell Res 49: 87–104

Goodman T, Lefrançois L (1988) Expression of the $\gamma\delta$ T-cell receptor on intestinal CD8$^+$ intraepithelial lymphocytes. Nature 333: 855–858

Guy-Grand D, Griscelli C, Vassalli P (1978) The mouse gut T lymphocyte, a novel type of T cell. Nature, origin and traffic in normal and graft-versus-host conditions. J Exp Med 148: 1661–1677

Heidenhein R (1888) Pfluegers Arch 43 [Suppl]: 23

Janossy G, Tidman N, Selby WS, Thomas JA, Granger S, Kung PC, Goldstein G (1980) Human T lymphocytes of inducer and suppressor type occupy different microenvironments. Nature 288: 81–84

Klein JR (1986) Ontogeny of the Thy 1$^-$, Ly-2$^+$ murine intestinal intra-epithelial lymphocyte. Characterization of a unique population of thymus-independent cytotoxic effector cells in the intestinal mucosa. J Exp Med 164: 309–314

Marsh MN (1975) Studies of intestinal lymphoid tissue. I. Electron microscopic evidence of 'blast transformation' in epithelial lymphocytes of mouse small intestinal mucosa. II. Aspects of proliferation and migration of epithelial lymphocytes in the small intestine of mice. Gut 16: 665–682

Mayrhofer G, Pitts R (1986) A comparison of some properties of mast cells and other granulated cells. In: Befus AD et al. (eds) Mast cell differentiation and heterogeneity. Raven, New York, pp 141–157

Mayrhofer G, Whately RJ (1983) Granular intraepithelial lymphocytes of the rat small intestine. 1. Isolation, presence in T-lymphocyte deficient rats and bone marrow origin. Int Arch Allergy Appl Immunol 71: 317–327

Mowat AM, Ferguson A (1982) Intraepithelial lymphocyte count and crypt hyperplasia measure the mucosal component of the graft-versus-host reaction in mouse small intestine. Gastroenterology 83: 417–423

Mowat AM, MacKenzie S, Baca ME, Felstein MV, Parrott DMV (1986) Functional characteristics of intraepithelial lymphocytes from mouse small intestine. II. In vivo and in vitro responses of intraepithelial lymphoytes to mitogenic and allogeneic stimuli. Immunology 58: 627–634

Petit A, Ernst PB, Befus AD, Clark DA, Rosenthal KL, Ishazaki T, Bienenstock J (1985) Murine intestinal intraepithelial lymphocytes. I. Relationship of a novel Thyl-1, Lyt-1$^-$, Ly-2$^+$, granulated subpopulation to natural killer cells and mast cells. Eur J Immunol 15: 211–215

Rudzik O, Bienenstock J (1974) Isolation and characteristics of gut mucosal lymphocytes. Lab Invest 30: 260–266

Schrader JW, Scollay R, Battye F (1983) Intramucosal lymphocytes of the gut: Ly-2 and Thy-1 phenotype of the granulated cells and evidence for the presence of both T cells and mast cell precursors. J Immunol 130: 558–564

Selby WS, Janossy G, Bofill M, Jewell DP (1984) Intestinal lymphocyte subpopulations in inflammatory bowel disease: an analysis by immunohistological and cell isolation techniques. Gut 25: 32–40

Tagliabue A, Befus AD, Clark DA, Bienenstock J (1982) Characteristics of natural killer cells in the murine intestinal epithelium and lamina propria. J Exp Med 155: 1785–1796

Targan S, Britvan L, Kendal R, Vimadalal S, Soll A (1983) Isolation of spontaneous and interferon inducible natural killer like cells from human colonic mucosa: lysis of lymphoid and autologous epithelial target cells. Clin Exp Immunol 54: 14–22

Timonen T, Ortaldo JR, Herberman RB (1981) Characteristics of human large granular lymphocytes and relationship to natural killer and K cells. J Exp Med 153: 569–582

van der Heijden FL (1986) Mucosal lymphocytes in the rat small intestine: phenotypical characterization *in situ*. Immunology 59: 397–399

Ward JM, Argilan F, Reynolds CW (1983) Immunoperoxidase localization of large granular lymphocytes in normal tissues and lesions of athymic nude rats. J Immunol 131: 132–139

Subject Index*
